Geriatrics: A Clinical Approach

Geriatrics: A Clinical Approach

Edited by Roger Simpson

hayle
medical

New York

Hayle Medical,
750 Third Avenue, 9th Floor,
New York, NY 10017, USA

Visit us on the World Wide Web at:
www.haylemedical.com

ISBN: 978-1-63241-452-6

The publisher's policy is to use permanent paper from mills that operate a sustainable forestry policy. Furthermore, the publisher ensures that the text paper and cover boards used have met acceptable environmental accreditation standards.

Trademark Notice: Registered trademark of products or corporate names are used only for explanation and identification without intent to infringe.

Printed in the United States of America.

Cataloging-in-Publication Data

   Geriatrics : a clinical approach / edited by Roger Simpson.
      p. cm.
   Includes bibliographical references and index.
   ISBN 978-1-63241-452-6
   1. Geriatrics. 2. Older people--Health and hygiene. 3. Older people--Diseases. I. Simpson, Roger.
RC952 .G47 2017
618.97--dc23

Table of Contents

Preface

Geriatrics is a speciality that focuses on health care for elderly people. It strives on promoting health care of the elderly by preventing and treating diseases and disabilities. The topics covered in this extensive book deal with the core aspects of this specialty. This book discusses the sub-fields of geriatrics like cardiogeriatics, geriatric pharmacotherapy, etc. amongst others. It also elucidates the various techniques and strategies that are meant for the well-being of the elderly people. This book is a valuable source of information for students, researchers and doctors working in this field. The extensive content of this book provides the readers with a thorough understanding of the subject.

This book has been the outcome of endless efforts put in by authors and researchers on various issues and topics within the field. The book is a comprehensive collection of significant researches that are addressed in a variety of chapters. It will surely enhance the knowledge of the field among readers across the globe.

It gives us an immense pleasure to thank our researchers and authors for their efforts to submit their piece of writing before the deadlines. Finally in the end, I would like to thank my family and colleagues who have been a great source of inspiration and support.

Editor

Reduced Functional Reserve in Patients with Age-Related White Matter Changes: A Preliminary fMRI Study of Working Memory

Martin Griebe[1]*[9], **Michael Amann**[2,3][9], **Jochen G. Hirsch**[4], **Lutz Achtnichts**[2], **Michael G. Hennerici**[1], **Achim Gass**[1], **Kristina Szabo**[1]

1 Department of Neurology, MR Research Neurology, UniversitätsMedizin Mannheim, University of Heidelberg, Mannheim, Germany, 2 Department of Neurology, University Hospital Basel, Basel, Switzerland, 3 Division of Diagnostic and Interventional Neuroradiology, Department of Radiology, Basel, Switzerland, 4 Fraunhofer MEVIS, Institute for Medical Image Computing, Bremen, Germany

Abstract

Subcortical age-related white matter changes (ARWMC) are a frequent finding in healthy elderly people suggested to cause secondary tissue changes and possibly affecting cognitive processes. We aimed to determine the influence of the extent of ARWMC load on attention and working memory processes in healthy elderly individuals. Fourteen healthy elderly subjects (MMSE >26; age 55–80 years) performed three fMRI tasks with increasing difficulty assessing alertness, attention (0-back), and working memory (2-back). We compared activation patterns in those with only minimal ARWMC (Fazekas 0–1) to those with moderate to severe ARWMC (Fazekas 2–3). During the fMRI experiments, the study population showed activation in brain areas typically involved in attention and working memory with a recruitment of cortical areas with increasing task difficulty. Subjects with higher lesion load showed a higher activation at all task levels with only sparse increase of signal with increasing complexity. In the lower lesion load group, rising task difficulty lead to a significant and widely distributed increase of activation. Although the number of patients included in the study is small, these findings suggest that even clinically silent ARWMC may affect cognitive processing and lead to compensatory activation during cognitive tasks. This can be interpreted as a reduction of functional reserve and may pose a risk for cognitive decline in these patients.

Editor: Jie Tian, Institute of Automation, Chinese Academy of Sciences, China

Funding: The study was supported by the Deutsche Forschungsgemeinschaft (DFG), Sonderforschungsbereich (SFB) 636. URL: http://www.sfb636.de. The funders had no role in study design, data collection and analysis, decision to publish, or preparation of the manuscript.

Competing Interests: The authors have declared that no competing interests exist.

* Email: griebe@neuro.ma.uni-heidelberg.de

[9] These authors contributed equally to this work.

Introduction

As cerebral white matter lesions are highly prevalent in healthy elderly individuals – having been reported in 27%–92% of this population [1,2] – these findings have also been termed age-related white matter changes (ARWMC). Their extent seemingly corresponds to a continuum from normal functioning to clinically overt neurological syndromes in subcortical vascular encephalopathy (SVE) with apraxia of locomotion, gait disturbance, working memory deficits and executive dysfunction [3]. Using diffusion tensor imaging (DTI) and planimetry of the corpus callosum we have recently demonstrated a loss of tissue integrity and atrophy of the corpus callosum secondary to spatially remote – and per se clinically silent – lesions in the peri- and paraventricular white matter in ARWMC in healthy elderly individuals [4]. In a study of cognitive correlates of subclinical structural brain disease in elderly healthy control subjects, even modest volumes of ARWMC were found to be functionally associated with a decline in cognitive performance [5]; in particular, ARWMC have been suggested to be an important cause of age-related attentional and executive dysfunction in the elderly [6]. The functional processes underlying the transition to SVE, with affection of cognitive skills - especially attention, working memory, and cognitive processing speed are poorly understood. Substantial fMRI research into the pathophysiology of aging has focused on task related brain activity changes in the elderly [7,8]. An intriguing finding is the recruitment of larger brain areas interpreted as compensation – either with or without clinical correlation [9,10].

The aim of our study was to determine the influence of ARWMC load on attention and working memory task performance with increasing complexity in healthy elderly individuals. We used a three task paradigm with increasing task difficulty (alertness<attention<working memory) and compared subjects with no or mild ARWMC to those with moderate to severe ARWMC. We hypothesized that increasing difficulty of presented tasks might be compensated in patients with progressive ARWMC by extended recruitment of normally silent brain areas.

Methods

Ethics Statement

The local ethics committee (Medical Ethics Committee 2, Medical Faculty Mannheim, University of Heidelberg) approved this study. All participants gave written informed consent before study entry.

Study design/Inclusion and exclusion criteria

We included healthy elderly subjects aged >55 years with no or only minimal disability in their instrumental activities of daily living (IADL). Exclusion criteria were a history of stroke or other neurological or psychiatric diseases, head and neck surgery, hearing loss, impaired vision or physical disabilities, left-handedness and contraindications to perform MRI. Furthermore duplex ultrasound examinations of the carotid arteries and the arteries of the circle of Willis were performed to exclude arterial stenosis. Twenty-five subjects participated in the study. The participants were split according to the extent of ARWMC in two groups with a low and a high lesion load (see data analysis). The data sets of nine subjects had to be discarded due to excessive motion during the fMRI experiment (see data analysis). Two further subjects in the low lesion load group were excluded to adjust both groups with respect to sample size and age, resulting in groups with seven participants each. For subject characteristics see *Table 1*.

Stimuli

Before the experiment itself, participants were instructed and practised the tasks. Three cognitive tasks were presented blockwise during fMRI. 1.) We used an alertness task to assess basic attentional function. During this task, the digit "2" was presented visually for 1 s in pseudo-randomized intervals between 1.2 s and 2.8 s. During a 36 s period 18 stimuli were presented to which subjects were asked to respond as fast as possible by pressing the button on a response device in the right hand. 2.) To assess attention we used a 0-back task. In this task, random numbers from 1–9 were presented. Subjects had to respond by pressing the button, when the number "2" was displayed. In one task block, 18 numbers appeared in intervals of 2 s (1 s on, 1 s off). 3.) Finally, a 2-back working memory task was used, during which the numbers were presented in the same way as in the 0-back task. A response was requested if a currently shown number was identical to the second last one.

Data acquisition

During the fMRI measurement, the stimulus was presented as a movie with the use of the "Integrated Functional Imaging System" (IFIS, Invivo, Orlando, USA) via an LCD screen attached to the MRI head coil. Subjects with visual impairment were provided with MR-compatible corrective lenses. Performance of subjects was monitored visually and via the IFIS response units. The MR scan was performed on a 1.5 T whole body scanner (Magnetom Sonata, Siemens Medical, Erlangen, Germany). A three-dimensional T1-weighted whole brain data set was acquired (MPRAGE; TR/TE/flip angle = 1.900 ms/3.9 ms/15°) with an isotropic resolution of $1 \times 1 \times 1$ mm^3 for anatomical reference. A FLAIR data set was acquired to identify individual lesion load (TR/TE/TI/turbo factor = 9000 ms/108 ms/2400 ms/25; voxel size $1 \times 1 \times 4$ mm^3). For the three BOLD fMRI scans, a T2*w EPI sequence was used (TR/TE/flip angle = 2000 ms/55 ms/90°) with an in-plane resolution of 4×4 mm^2. Per volume, 20 slices (4 mm thick, 2 mm gap) parallel to the inferior borders of the corpus callosum were scanned in interleaved order. For each fMRI experiment an identical blocked design was used which consisted of five baseline blocks of 18 volumes (black screen with fixation cross, 1 s on, 1 s off) and four task blocks of 18 volumes. Each fMRI scan started with two dummy scans which were discarded automatically by the scanner to minimize non-equilibrium T1 effects, resulting in a total measurement time of 5 min 28 s. Anatomical data sets and all three fMRI runs were scanned in one session.

Data analysis

Structural and functional MRI data were analysed by independent investigators. The degree of ARWMC severity on MRI was rated using a modified version of the visual scale of Fazekas [11], ranging from 0 to 3, that scores deep and subcortical white matter lesions in three categories of mild (1), moderate (2), and severe (3) ARWMC. The study participants were classified into 2 groups: subjects with no or mild ARWMC (0–1) and those with moderate to severe ARWMC (2–3).

The fMRI data sets were pre-processed using AFNI [12]. After slice timing correction, a rigid body six-parameter motion correction was performed for each of the fMRI runs. Spatial smoothing with a Gaussian filter (FWHM = 8 mm) was applied to the data, and global intensity normalization was carried out. The T1-weighted anatomical data sets were then realigned to the EPI volumes. Statistical maps were created for each subject and for each task by performing a multiple linear regression (MLR) analysis. The ideal function was modelled as a boxcar function convolved with the hemodynamic response function. In the MLR, the whole brain signal time course and motion parameters were treated as regressors of no interest. The resulting signal per cent change maps (activation versus baseline) were transformed to

Table 1. Subject characteristics.

	Low lesion load	High lesion load	P value
Number of subjects (N)	7	7	
Age, years (median, range)	66 (55-72)	68 (56-79)	0.427
Sex, male (N)	3	5	0.127
MMSE (median, range)	30 (28-30)	30 (28-30)	0.701
Education, high degree (N)	3	2	0.403
IADL (median, range)	8 (7-8)	8 (8-8)	0.655
Hypertension (N)	3	6	**0.022 ***
Diabetes mellitus (N)	2	3	0.403
Hyperlipidemia (N)	2	3	0.403
Smoking (N)	0	0	1.000

Talairach space [13] using the transformation parameters of the respective anatomical data set. For the second level analysis, only those subjects were included with less than 2 mm absolute motion in all three fMRI experiments. Thus, the signal change maps of seven subjects in the low lesion load group and of seven subjects in the high lesion load group underwent a three-factor analysis of variance (ANOVA). Group and task were treated as fixed factors and the subjects as the random factor (AxBxC(A)-ANOVA). The following statistical maps were created as we have described in a previous study [14]: first, a main effect map for each task pooled over all subjects; second, a contrast map between both groups for each task; and third, the different task conditions contrasted separately for each group. The resulting t-maps were converted to Gaussian Z-scores and thresholded at $Z > 3.3$ and at a corrected cluster significance level of $p < 0.01$. Based on the group/task contrast map, the average per cent signal change of specific brain areas was evaluated for both groups separately. Regions of interest (ROI) were located in areas that showed either a significant task effect for the low lesion load group alone or for both groups [14]. Separately for both groups, the mean regional per cent signal change for each task was calculated and t-tests were performed.

Results

For patient characteristics see *Table 1*. ARWMC grades were distributed as follows: Fazekas 0 in 1, Fazekas 1 in 6, Fazekas 2 in 3 and Fazekas 3 in 4 subjects, respectively. Data analysis of the study population (n = 14) showed recruitment of cortical areas parallel to increasing task difficulty (see *Figure 1* and *Table 2*). During all three tasks, the anterior insula (AI) bilaterally, as well as medial frontal and precentral areas were significantly activated. In the n-back tasks, additionally recruitment of bilateral posterior parietal areas was found.

During all three tasks, the high lesion load group showed slightly higher activation compared to the low lesion group. In the alertness task, higher activation was found in the left anterior insula/inferior frontal cortex, in 0-back, differences were found in right middle temporal areas, and in 2-back in the right posterior insula/superior temporal gyrus (*Figure 2* and *Table 3*).

There were significantly different characteristics of both groups with regard to the increase of activation parallel to task difficulty. In the low lesion load group, a significant and widely distributed change of activation in both 2-back versus 0-back, and 2-back versus alertness was observed (*Figure 3* and *Table 4*), including signal increase in medial frontal, bilateral parietal and dorsolateral frontal areas and decrease in the posterior insula and in cingulate and hippocampal areas. In contrast, in the high lesion load group only sparse increase of signal was found in medial frontal parts for 2-back versus 0-back and in bilateral middle frontal areas for 2-back versus alertness (*Figure 4* and *Table 5*).

The ROI analysis of the signal change maps further characterized these effects (*Figure 5*). In the middle frontal cortex bilaterally, the supplemental motor area, and the right parietal cortex, the low lesion load group showed higher signal increase for the 2-back task compared to both the 0-back and the alertness task. In this group we also found a significant signal decrease between the 2-back and the 0-back task in the anterior and posterior cingulate gyrus and in the right hippocampal gyrus. Subjects in the high lesion load group showed higher activation even in the less demanding tasks in the right middle frontal cortex, in the supplemental motor area, and in the right parietal cortex. Accordingly, they demonstrated a decreased signal for the alertness and 0-back task in both anterior and posterior cingulated gyrus. Hence, the regional signal contrasts between the different tasks remained non-significant in this group of subjects.

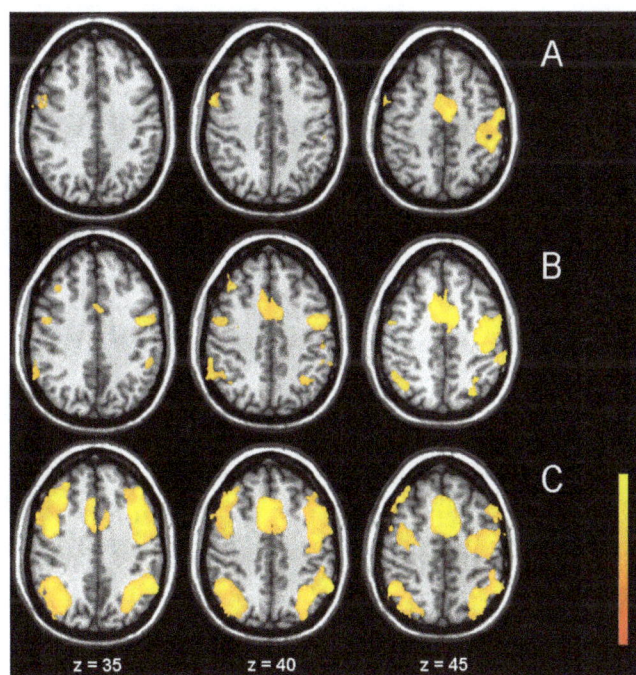

Figure 1. fMRI main effects. Group activation map over all subjects for the three different tasks alertness (A), 0-back (B), and 2-back (C) (Z>3.3, corrected p<0.01). Statistical maps are superimposed onto the MNI structural template. All MR Images shown here are in radiological order (image left is anatomical right).

Table 2. Areas of activated regions in the three different tasks (pooled over all subjects).

	Talairach-Tournoux Coordinates (mm)			max. Z-scores	p-values (corrected)
	x	y	z		
Alertness – Main effect					
Left medial frontal/left SMA	−5	−8	51	5.44	<0.01
Left precentral/postcentral	−46	−17	48	4.29	<0.01
Left superior temporal	−49	−41	28	4.01	<0.01
Right anterior insula	45	12	0	5.18	<0.01
Left anterior insula	−45	1	−2	4.06	<0.01
Right inferior/middle temporal	56	−63	−3	4.45	<0.01
Right cerebellum	19	−50	−22	4.09	<0.01
Left cerebellum	−33	−55	−26	4.73	<0.01
0-back – Main effect					
Left superior parietal	−32	−59	59	3.43	<0.01
Medial frontal/SMA	1	−8	58	5.00	<0.01
Right inferior/superior parietal	38	−62	46	3.18	<0.01
Left precentral	−33	−20	45	4.52	<0.01
Right middle/superior temporal	51	−41	9	5.26	<0.01
Right anterior insula	38	15	8	4.53	<0.01
Left anterior insula	−33	16	7	4.36	<0.01
Left cerebellum	−36	−51	−27	3.43	<0.01
Right precentral gyrus	38	−16	59	3.59	<0.01
2-back – Main effect					
Right middle/superior frontal/right precentral	28	−4	53	5.04	<0.01
Left middle/superior frontal/left precentral	−46	−10	49	4.2	<0.01
Medial frontal/anterior cingulate	−8	5	47	5.58	<0.01
Right inferior/superior parietal/right angular	45	−49	40	4.21	<0.01
Left inferior/superior parietal/left angular	−37	−57	38	4.43	<0.01
Left inferior frontal	−41	0	23	5.27	<0.01
Right inferior frontal	45	3	21	5.11	<0.01
Left anterior insula	−44	11	8	6.24	<0.01
Right anterior insula	35	17	7	5.82	<0.01
Right inferior temporal	49	−53	−15	3.55	<0.01
Left cerebellum	−33	−49	−32	5.05	<0.01
Right cerebellum	24	−59	−36	3.84	<0.01

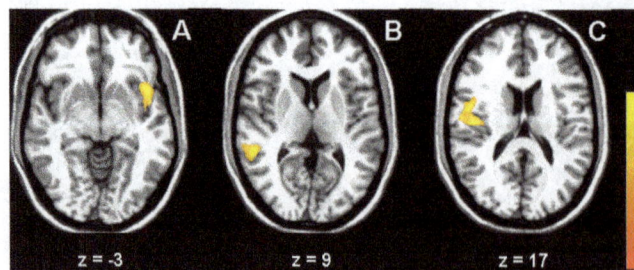

Figure 2. Effect of ARWMC lesion load. Difference in activation between the high lesion load group and the low lesion load group for the tasks alertness (A), 0-back (B) and 2-back (C) (Z>3.3, corrected p<0.01).

Table 3. Task main effect: differences between the low lesion load group and the high lesion load group.

	Talairach-Tournoux Coordinates (mm)			max. Z-scores	p-values (corrected)
	x	y	z		
Alertness – Contrast high-low lesion load					
Left insula/left inferior frontal	−42	13	−3	4.22	<0.01
0-back – Contrast high-low lesion load					
Right superior/middle temporal	51	−40	9	4.51	<0.05
2-back – Contrast high-low lesion load					
Right posterior insula/right superior temporal	45	−16	17	4.27	<0.01

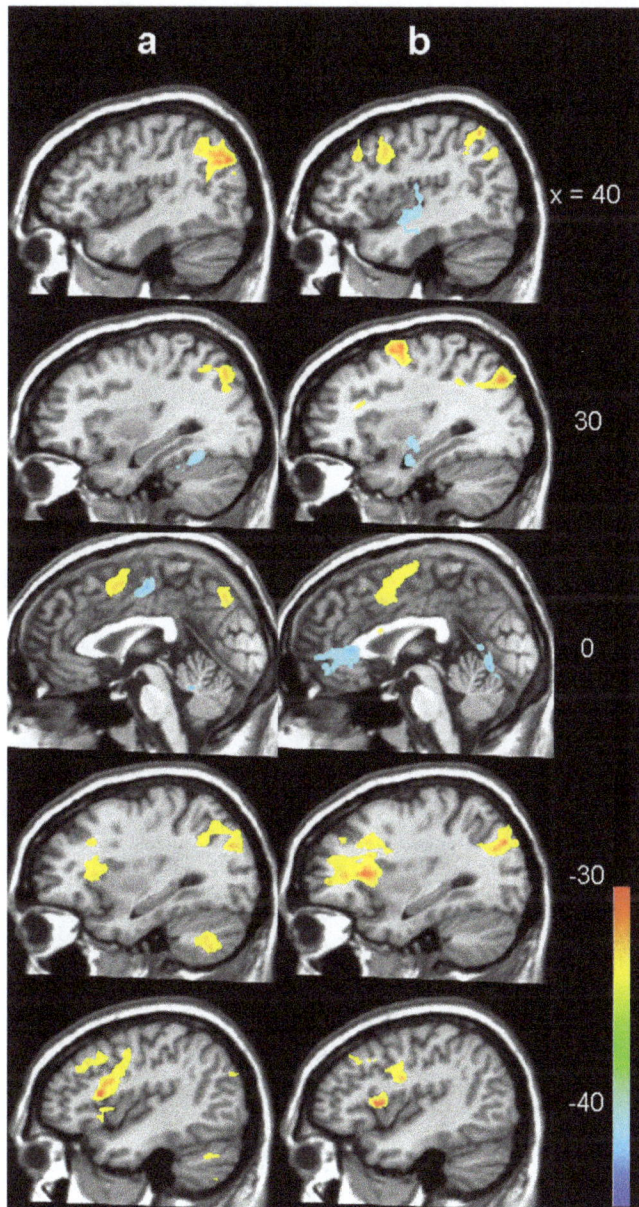

Figure 3. Increasing task difficulty in low lesion load. Activation change for the low lesion load group between 2-back and alertness (a) and between 2-back and 0-back (b). Blue to green means decreased activation for 2-back, yellow to red means increased activation (Z>3.3, corrected p< 0.01).

Table 4. Changes between task classes in the low lesion load group.

	Talairach-Tournoux Coordinates (mm)			max. Z-scores	p-values (corrected)
	x	y	z		
Contrast 2-back – alertness					
Left medial frontal/left (pre-) SMA	−4	5	47	4.47	<0.01
Left precentral/left middle frontal	−41	25	35	4.23	<0.01
Right angular/right precuneus/right middle temporal	39	−72	31	4.42	<0.01
Left superior occipital/left angular/left precuneus/left middle temporal	−32	−75	27	3.88	<0.01
Left anterior insula/left inferior frontal	−41	16	14	5.35	<0.01
Left cerebellum	−42	−63	−27	3.63	<0.01
Contrast alertness – 2back					
Paracentral lobule/left medial frontal/left cingulate	14	−12	50	4.77	<0.01
Right insula/right postcentral	44	−15	11	4.77	<0.01
Right cerebellum	26	−47	−22	4.52	<0.01
Contrast 2-back – 0-back					
Cingulate/medial frontal	−5	2	48	4.29	<0.01
Right inferior parietal	43	−50	42	2.89	<0.01
Right middle frontal/right inferior frontal	42	9	38	3.81	<0.01
Right precuneus/right inferior parietal	29	−72	36	4.13	<0.01
Left precentral/left middle frontal	−32	18	34	3.12	<0.01
Left precuneus/left cuneus	−27	−76	30	4.77	<0.01
Left precentral/left inferior frontal	−37	−5	25	4.70	<0.01
Left precentral/left insula/left inferior frontal	−42	11	8	5.08	<0.01
Contrast 0-back – 2back					
Left posterior cingulate/left lingual	−9	−55	1	3.96	<0.01
Left anterior cingulate	−5	39	−3	3.93	<0.01
Left posterior insula	−39	−16	1	4.16	<0.05
Right insula	41	−6	−6	4.34	<0.05
Right hippocampus/right parahippocampal	20	−14	−10	2.86	<0.05
Left hippocampus/left parahippocampal	−32	−13	−12	3.83	<0.05
Contrast 0-back – alertness					
–	–	–	–	–	
Contrast alertness – 0-back					
–	–	–	–	–	

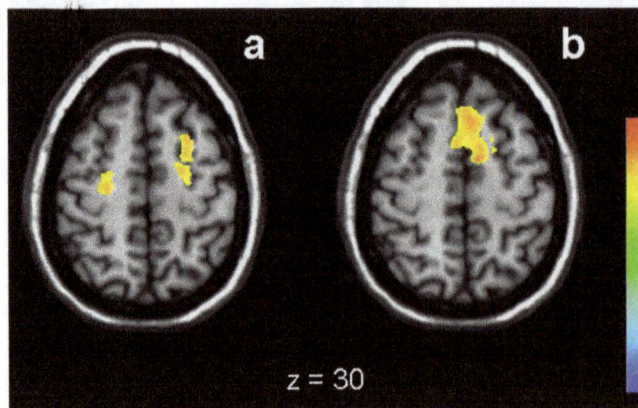

Figure 4. Increasing task difficulty in high lesion load. Activation change for the high lesion load group between 2-back and alertness (a) and between 2-back and 0-back (b). Yellow to red: increased activation (Z>3.3, corrected p<0.01).

Table 5. Changes between task classes in the high lesion load group.

	Talairach-Tournoux Coordinates (mm)			max. Z-scores	p-values (corrected)
	x	**y**	**z**		
Contrast 2-back – alertness					
Left middle frontal	−15	−7	57	4.21	<0.05
Right middle frontal	19	−20	56	3.96	<0.05
Contrast alertness – 2back					
–	–	–	–	–	
Contrast 2-back – 0-back					
Left medial frontal	−8	−3	48	4	<0.01
Contrast 0-back – 2back					
–	–	–	–	–	
Contrast 0-back – alertness					
–	–	–	–	–	
Contrast alertness – 0-back					
–	–	–	–	–	

Discussion

While numerous studies have attributed a decrease in grey matter volume to cognitive decline and especially to working memory dysfunction, far less have addressed the effect of ARWMC on functional brain changes during working memory tasks. In this study we attempted to identify subclinical changes in brain activation in cognitive processing in individuals with different stages of asymptomatic ARWMC. We used a stimulation paradigm that provided very stable activation patterns. Although we had to discard nine datasets due to large motion artefacts in our cohort of elderly individuals, the paradigm itself was simple to perform and provided increasing degrees of complexity while using the same stimulation set-up ensuring robustness and the opportunity to relate the findings of each part of the experiment to the other.

Task specific activation patterns showed only subtle differences between the subjects with low or high ARWMC lesion load. In all three tasks, activation was found in the motor network including the contralateral primary motor cortex and the supplemental motor area, as expected for the motor response. Additionally, activation was found in the AI bilaterally in all three tasks. The AI is considered to integrate the sensory signals associated with voluntary movements [15]. A recent study also suggested that the bilateral AI may exert executive control by selectively biasing processing in favour of task-relevant information in an fMRI study investigating the neural correlates of perceptual load induced attentional selection [16]. Roski et al. analysed age-dependent differences and observed both selective increases and decreases in resting-state functional connectivity with age in regions associated with both attention and sensorimotor systems (rostral supplementary motor area and bilateral anterior insula) [17]. In both short-term memory tasks, a typical pattern of activation was found including bilateral dorsolateral prefrontal (BA9/46), inferior frontal (BA6/44) and parietal (BA7/40) areas. This pattern became more prominent with higher memory load. This result parallels findings in other studies using N-back paradigms [14,18–20]. The inferior parietal cortex (BA40) is considered a locus of the storage component of working memory, whereas the inferior frontal cortex is involved in the rehearsal process [21,22].

We found distinct changes of brain activity with increasing difficulty of the tasks. Subjects with a low lesion load showed a variety of activation differences between the three tasks, namely a signal increase parallel to task difficulty, but also recruitment of additional cortical areas and signal decrease in other areas such as the cingulum, the right insula, and the hippocampus. In contrast, only sparse task-dependent activation changes could be observed in the group with high lesion load. It might seem contradictory that we found distinct task-dependent activity changes for both groups, but almost no inter-group task effect differences. In several regions including the anterior cingulum, the right middle frontal gyrus, and supplemental motor areas, the activation level in the high lesion load group was already higher during the simplest task (alertness) than in subjects with low lesion load. In other regions such as the middle frontal areas in both hemispheres and right hippocampus, the maximal BOLD amplitude for the 2-back task was lower in the high lesion load group. Due to the lower BOLD signal range, the inter-task differences in subjects with high lesion load remained non-significant. Additionally, higher inter-individual variances were observed in the high lesion load group, particularly in bilateral parietal and cingulate areas, which also led to a reduced statistical significance. The higher inter-individual variances could also be an indication of different functional compensatory mechanisms with respect to the variable impairments of a higher lesion load.

All these findings may be interpreted as normal adaptation processes to task complexity in low ARWMC lesion load, while it could be postulated that those subjects with a high lesions load may already have compensatory activation at the level of the simplest task. In a very recent fMRI study of motor performance examining a cohort quite similar to ours, Linortner et al. observed an increased recruitment of supplemental motor areas in individuals with advanced ARWMC in a simple motor paradigm of ankle movement representing an element of gait. In line with our interpretations, they conclude that the alterations match the clinical phenomenology of SVE and speculate that a disruption of frontosubcortical networks might be its pathoanatomical correlate [23]. Nordahl and co-workers used ARWMC as a marker for white matter degeneration to demonstrate that increases in both global and regional dorsal prefrontal cortex ARWMC volume

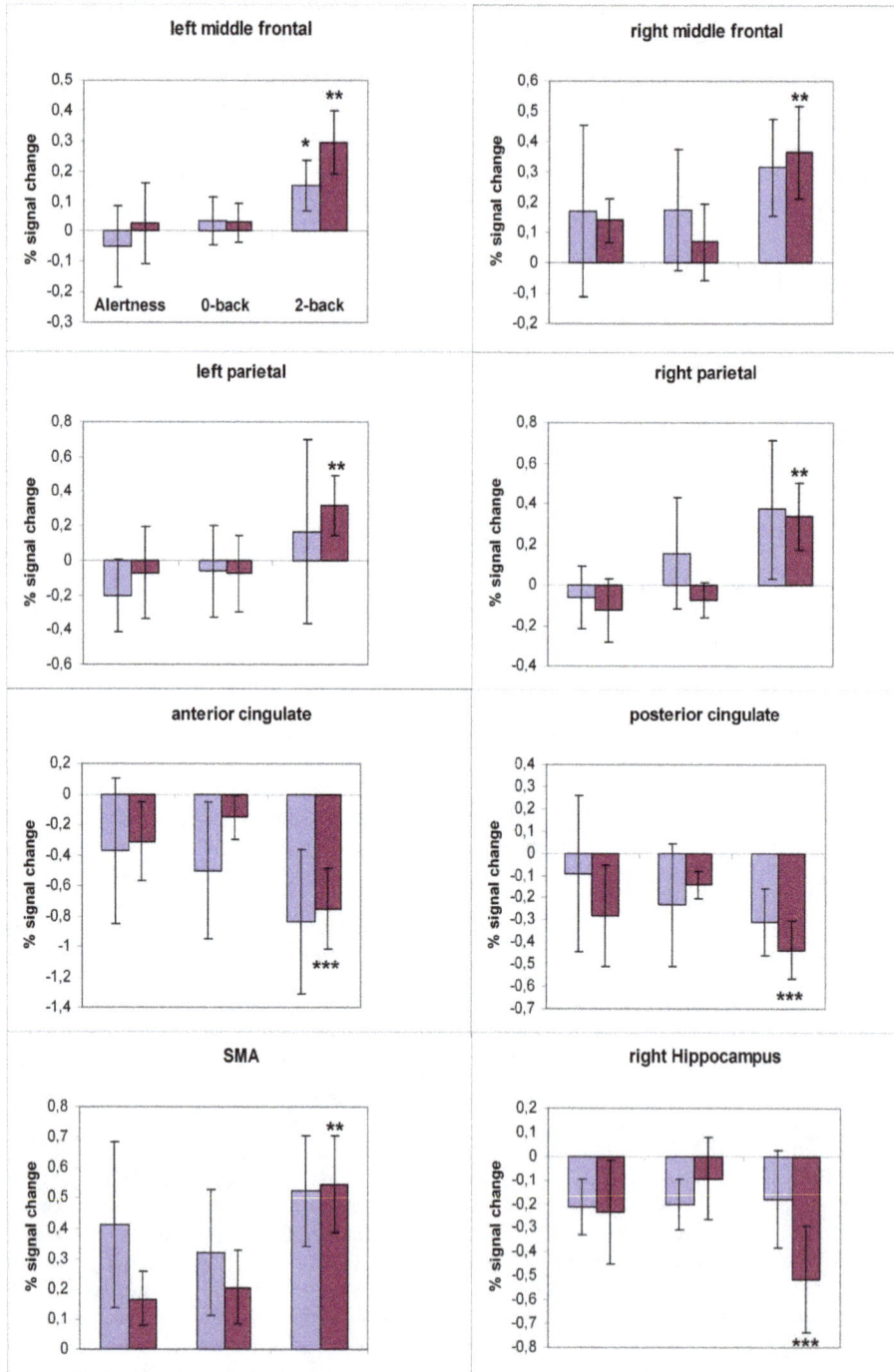

Figure 5. Quantification of task-dependent signal response. Regional mean percent signal change for different cortex areas defined by significant clusters in the task effect maps. The low lesion load group is shown in red bars, the high lesion load group in blue bars. The standard error is indicated by error bars. * significantly different to the alertness task (p<0.01); ** significantly different to the 0-back task (p<0.01); *** significantly different to both the alertness and 0-back tasks (p<0.01).

were associated with decreases in prefrontal cortex activity and decreased activity in the posterior parietal and anterior cingulate cortex during working memory performance [24]. Charlton et al. performed MRI and cognitive testing in 84 middle-aged and elderly adults at baseline and after two years and showed a correlation of diffusion tensor imaging (DTI) in white matter histograms with a change in working memory function [25]. A more recent study found significant increases in fMRI activation in the left dorsal and ventral lateral prefrontal cortices with increased working memory load and also with increased age that correlated with DTI derived fractional anisotropy (FA) in frontal brain regions [26]. A study addressing a similar hypothesis as ours, reported a reduction in the up-regulation of prefrontal and parietal regions in response to increasing working memory task demand along with a reduction in the down-regulation of default mode network regions with increasing cognitive load in the elderly compared to a younger group [27]. However the study did not report ARWMC. More pronounced brain activation might be interpreted as potential additional recruitment or reduction of inhibitory activity. Both have been interpreted as compensatory mechanisms preserving neurological function in the presence of structural tissue damage. An fMRI study examining the correlates of age-related reduction in working memory capacity, found that at higher working memory loads with worse performance older subjects had relatively reduced activity in prefrontal regions implicating a decline in performance past a threshold of physiological compensation [28].

Theoretically, different degrees of microangiopathy could lead to different BOLD responses. In functional magnetic resonance imaging (fMRI), neuronal activity is detected indirectly via the blood oxygenation level dependent (BOLD) effect [29]. Neuronal events induce an increase in local blood flow, but can also alter the BOLD signal by influencing several other factors like cerebral blood volume and cerebral blood oxygen consumption. This neurovascular coupling could be altered by microvascular disease thus affecting the BOLD signal. The anatomical scans prior to our fMRI experiments showed that none of the subjects had asymptomatic incidental pathology (e.g. lacunar stroke, cortical lesions). To exclude subtle influences of microangiopathy to the fMRI results, we focussed on group-by-task interactions and not on main effects in BOLD response between both groups [30]. Additionally, the ROI analysis demonstrated that the maximum amplitude of signal change was similar in both groups, which may indicate a comparable response range to stimulation. This would

argue against differences induced by vascular pathology and microangiopathy. However, our study has two main limitations: first, the small sample size for an fMRI cohort study [31]. To preserve a high standard of our data we had to exclude a number of subjects due to intolerable movement artefacts. It has to be taken into account that our study cohort consisted of healthy but aged individuals. In contrast to young volunteers in many cognitive fMRI studies, our participants had no previous experience with being examined in an MR scanner or even with using computers as necessary for the cognitive tasks. Second, the performance data could not be used as regressors because a technical transmission error lead to incomplete data recording. However, the paradigms were designed and reviewed to be feasible for our cohort. All subjects were able to solve the paradigms in the training runs, and during the fMRI experiments their responses were continuously monitored.

The results of this study indicate that clinically silent ARWMC may affect cognitive processing and lead to compensatory activity in cognitive tasks. This can be interpreted as a reduction of functional reserve and may pose a risk for cognitive decline in these patients. However, these hypotheses need further substantiation in a consecutive study with larger patient numbers.

Author Contributions

Conceived and designed the experiments: MG AG KS. Performed the experiments: MG LA. Analyzed the data: MG MA JGH LA. Contributed reagents/materials/analysis tools: MA JGH AG. Wrote the paper: MG MA MGH KS.

References

1. Breteler MM, van Swieten JC, Bots ML, Grobbee DE, Claus JJ, et al. (1994) Cerebral white matter lesions, vascular risk factors, and cognitive function in a population-based study: the Rotterdam Study. Neurology 44: 1246–1252.
2. de Leeuw FE, de Groot JC, Achten E, Oudkerk M, Ramos LM, et al. (2001) Prevalence of cerebral white matter lesions in elderly people: a population based magnetic resonance imaging study. The Rotterdam Scan Study. Journal of neurology, neurosurgery, and psychiatry 70: 9–14.
3. Guttmann CR, Benson R, Warfield SK, Wei X, Anderson MC, et al. (2000) White matter abnormalities in mobility-impaired older persons. Neurology 54: 1277–1283.
4. Griebe M, Forster A, Wessa M, Rossmanith C, Bazner H, et al. (2011) Loss of callosal fibre integrity in healthy elderly with age-related white matter changes. Journal of neurology 258: 1451–1459.
5. Cook IA, Leuchter AF, Morgan ML, Conlee EW, David S, et al. (2002) Cognitive and physiologic correlates of subclinical structural brain disease in elderly healthy control subjects. Archives of neurology 59: 1612–1620.
6. O'Brien JT, Wiseman R, Burton EJ, Barber B, Wesnes K, et al. (2002) Cognitive associations of subcortical white matter lesions in older people. Ann N Y Acad Sci 977: 436–444.
7. Eyler LT, Sherzai A, Kaup AR, Jeste DV (2011) A review of functional brain imaging correlates of successful cognitive aging. Biological psychiatry 70: 115–122.
8. Spreng RN, Wojtowicz M, Grady CL (2010) Reliable differences in brain activity between young and old adults: a quantitative meta-analysis across multiple cognitive domains. Neuroscience and biobehavioral reviews 34: 1178–1194.
9. Kalpouzos G, Persson J, Nyberg L (2012) Local brain atrophy accounts for functional activity differences in normal aging. Neurobiology of aging 33: 623 e621–623 e613.
10. McIntosh AR, Sekuler AB, Penpeci C, Rajah MN, Grady CL, et al. (1999) Recruitment of unique neural systems to support visual memory in normal aging. Current biology : CB 9: 1275–1278.
11. Wahlund LO, Barkhof F, Fazekas F, Bronge L, Augustin M, et al. (2001) A new rating scale for age-related white matter changes applicable to MRI and CT. Stroke; a journal of cerebral circulation 32: 1318–1322.
12. Cox RW (1996) AFNI: software for analysis and visualization of functional magnetic resonance neuroimages. Computers and biomedical research, an international journal 29: 162–173.
13. Talairach J, Tournoux P (1988) Co-planar stereotaxic atlas of the human brain : 3-dimensional proportional system : an approach to cerebral imaging. Stuttgart; New York: Georg Thieme. 122 p. p.
14. Amann M, Dossegger LS, Penner IK, Hirsch JG, Raselli C, et al. (2011) Altered functional adaptation to attention and working memory tasks with increasing complexity in relapsing-remitting multiple sclerosis patients. Human brain mapping 32: 1704–1719.
15. Farrer C, Frith CD (2002) Experiencing oneself vs another person as being the cause of an action: the neural correlates of the experience of agency. NeuroImage 15: 596–603.
16. Wei P, Szameitat AJ, Muller HJ, Schubert T, Zhou X (2013) The neural correlates of perceptual load induced attentional selection: an fMRI study. Neuroscience 250: 372–380.
17. Roski C, Caspers S, Langner R, Laird AR, Fox PT, et al. (2013) Adult age-dependent differences in resting-state connectivity within and between visual-attention and sensorimotor networks. Front Aging Neurosci 5: 67.
18. Braver TS, Cohen JD, Nystrom LE, Jonides J, Smith EE, et al. (1997) A parametric study of prefrontal cortex involvement in human working memory. NeuroImage 5: 49–62.
19. Cader S, Cifelli A, Abu-Omar Y, Palace J, Matthews PM (2006) Reduced brain functional reserve and altered functional connectivity in patients with multiple sclerosis. Brain : a journal of neurology 129: 527–537.
20. Cohen JD, Perlstein WM, Braver TS, Nystrom LE, Noll DC, et al. (1997) Temporal dynamics of brain activation during a working memory task. Nature 386: 604–608.
21. Baddeley A (2003) Working memory: looking back and looking forward. Nature reviews Neuroscience 4: 829–839.
22. Smith EE, Jonides J (1997) Working memory: a view from neuroimaging. Cognitive psychology 33: 5–42.
23. Linortner P, Fazekas F, Schmidt R, Ropele S, Pendl B, et al. (2012) White matter hyperintensities alter functional organization of the motor system. Neurobiol Aging 33: 197 e191–199.
24. Nordahl CW, Ranganath C, Yonelinas AP, Decarli C, Fletcher E, et al. (2006) White matter changes compromise prefrontal cortex function in healthy elderly individuals. J Cogn Neurosci 18: 418–429.
25. Charlton RA, Landau S, Schiavone F, Barrick TR, Clark CA, et al. (2008) A structural equation modeling investigation of age-related variance in executive function and DTI measured white matter damage. Neurobiol Aging 29: 1547–1555.
26. Schulze ET, Geary EK, Susmaras TM, Paliga JT, Maki PM, et al. (2011) Anatomical correlates of age-related working memory declines. J Aging Res 2011: 606871.

27. Prakash RS, Heo S, Voss MW, Patterson B, Kramer AF (2012) Age-related differences in cortical recruitment and suppression: implications for cognitive performance. Behav Brain Res 230: 192–200.

28. Mattay VS, Fera F, Tessitore A, Hariri AR, Berman KF, et al. (2006) Neurophysiological correlates of age-related changes in working memory capacity. Neurosci Lett 392: 32–37.

29. Kim SG, Ogawa S (2012) Biophysical and physiological origins of blood oxygenation level-dependent fMRI signals. Journal of Cerebral Blood Flow and Metabolism 32: 1188–1206.

30. D'Esposito M, Deouell LY, Gazzaley A (2003) Alterations in the BOLD fMRI signal with ageing and disease: a challenge for neuroimaging. Nature reviews Neuroscience 4: 863–872.

31. Thirion B, Pinel P, Meriaux S, Roche A, Dehaene S, et al. (2007) Analysis of a large fMRI cohort: Statistical and methodological issues for group analyses. Neuroimage 35: 105–120.

2

A Circulating MicroRNA Profile Is Associated with Late-Stage Neovascular Age-Related Macular Degeneration

Felix Grassmann[1], Peter G. A. Schoenberger[1], Caroline Brandl[1,2], Tina Schick[3], Daniele Hasler[4], Gunter Meister[4], Monika Fleckenstein[5], Moritz Lindner[5], Horst Helbig[2], Sascha Fauser[3], Bernhard H. F. Weber[1]*

1 Institute of Human Genetics, University of Regensburg, Regensburg, Germany, 2 Department of Ophthalmology, University Hospital Regensburg, Regensburg, Germany, 3 Department of Ophthalmology, University Hospital of Cologne, Cologne, Germany, 4 Biochemistry Center Regensburg (BZR), Laboratory for RNA Biology, University of Regensburg, Regensburg, Germany, 5 Department of Ophthalmology, University of Bonn, Bonn, Germany

Abstract

Age-related macular degeneration (AMD) is the leading cause of severe vision impairment in Western populations over 55 years. A growing number of gene variants have been identified which are strongly associated with an altered risk to develop AMD. Nevertheless, gene-based biomarkers which could be dysregulated at defined stages of AMD may point toward key processes in disease mechanism and thus may support efforts to design novel treatment regimens for this blinding disorder. Circulating microRNAs (cmiRNAs) which are carried by nanosized exosomes or microvesicles in blood plasma or serum, have been recognized as valuable indicators for various age-related diseases. We therefore aimed to elucidate the role of cmiRNAs in AMD by genome-wide miRNA expression profiling and replication analyses in 147 controls and 129 neovascular AMD patients. We identified three microRNAs differentially secreted in neovascular (NV) AMD (hsa-mir-301-3p, $p_{corrected} = 5.6*10^{-5}$, hsa-mir-361-5p, $p_{corrected} = 8.0*10^{-4}$ and hsa-mir-424-5p, $p_{corrected} = 9.6*10^{-3}$). A combined profile of the three miRNAs revealed an area under the curve (AUC) value of 0.727 and was highly associated with NV AMD ($p = 1.2*10^{-8}$). To evaluate subtype-specificity, an additional 59 AMD cases with pure unilateral or bilateral geographic atrophy (GA) were analyzed for microRNAs hsa-mir-301-3p, hsa-mir-361-5p, and hsa-mir-424-5p. While we found no significant differences between GA AMD and controls neither individually nor for a combined microRNAs profile, hsa-mir-424-5p levels remained significantly higher in GA AMD when compared to NV ($p_{corrected} < 0.005$). Pathway enrichment analysis on genes predicted to be regulated by microRNAs hsa-mir-301-3p, hsa-mir-361-5p, and hsa-mir-424-5p, suggests canonical TGFβ, mTOR and related pathways to be involved in NV AMD. In addition, knockdown of hsa-mir-361-5p resulted in increased neovascularization in an *in vitro* angiogenesis assay.

Editor: Torben L. Sørensen, Copenhagen University Hospital Roskilde and the University of Copenhagen, Denmark

Funding: This study was supported in part by grants from the Deutsche Forschungsgemeinschaft (WE 1259/19-1 to BHFW, FL 658/4-1 to MF), Novartis Pharma (grant #3625340) and the Alcon Research Institute (to BHFW). The funders had no role in study design, data collection and analysis, decision to publish, or preparation of the manuscript.

Competing Interests: ML and MF received research support from Genentech and Heidelberg Engineering. FG, PGS, CB, TS, DH, GM, HH, SF, and BHW have declared that no competing interests exist.

* Email: bweb@klinik.uni-regensburg.de

Introduction

Age-related macular degeneration (AMD) is a highly prevalent cause of severe vision impairment among people aged 55 years and older [1]. It is a degenerative disorder of the central retina involving predominantly the rod photoreceptors, the retinal pigment epithelium (RPE), Bruchs membrane and the underlying choriocapillaris [2]. The disease aetiology is complex and is influenced by a combination of multiple genetic susceptibility factors and environmental components.

An early sign of AMD is the appearance of drusen, yellowish extracellular deposits of protein and lipid material within and beneath the RPE. Advanced AMD manifests essentially as two distinct late-stage lesions – geographic atrophy (GA) and neovascular (NV) AMD. GA occurs in up to 50% of cases and is clinically defined as a discrete area of RPE atrophy with visible choroidal vessels in the absence of neovascularization in the same eye [2–5]. It may or may not involve the fovea. NV AMD describes the development of new blood vessels beneath and within the retina and is characterized by serous or hemorrhagic detachment of either the RPE or the sensory retina, the presence of subretinal fibrous tissue and eventually widespread RPE atrophy. Progression to visual loss can be rapid in NV AMD [1].

The precise aetiology of AMD is still not fully understood, although risk factors such as age, smoking, and genetic components are known to strongly contribute to disease development [2]. In Western societies, AMD reveals an age-dependent prevalence of almost 1 in 5 people aged 85 and above [3–5]. Across a number of epidemiological studies, smoking has consistently been associated with increased risk of developing advanced AMD with an estimated odds ratio of approximately 2 [6]. The exact mechanism, however, by which smoking affects the retina is unknown.

Twin studies and familial aggregation studies suggested a significant genetic contribution of up to 70% in disease risk [7]. Subsequently, several genes have been implicated in AMD pathology by candidate gene studies as well as genome wide association studies. Genetic variants in complement factor H (CFH) and ARMS2/HtrA Serine Protease 1 (HTRA1) were found to be strongly associated with odds ratios over 2.5 per risk allele. In addition, multiple medium to low effect size gene variants were discovered in a large number of loci across the genome. A recent meta-analysis of genome wide association studies found a total of 19 independently associated loci by comparing over 17,000 cases and 60,000 controls [8].

The combined effect of the major risk variants on AMD was estimated by modelling risk scores [9]. The multiple logistic regression model was found to have an area under the curve (AUC) of about 82%, which is suitable for classifying individuals in high and low risk groups. Accordingly, roughly 50% of AMD cases and 50% of healthy controls can now reliably be predicted. However, a large proportion of AMD cases do not have the expected genetic risk profile despite their given disease status. Consequently, other components, genetic or environmental, may influence disease development. This makes it crucial to identify these components possibly by defining disease biomarkers correlating with the underlying genetic or environmental factors and eventually reflecting a defined disease stage.

Recently, circulating microRNAs (cmiRNAs) were found in blood plasma or blood serum where they are carried by nanosized exosomes or microvesicles [10,11]. Origin and effects of these cmiRNAs are unclear although some studies suggested functional involvement in cell-to-cell signalling [12]. In general, cmiRNAs are potential biomarkers which can be used for diagnostics and prognostics of human diseases [13]. Additionally, synthetic microRNAs in artificial exsosomes could be applicable for therapeutic approaches by modulating cmiRNA levels.

In this study, we aimed to elucidate the role of cmiRNAs in AMD and performed a genome-wide expression profiling in patients affected by late stage neovascular manifestation. Such analyses provide a promising approach to define biomarkers for AMD which could be helpful to identify as of yet unknown gene targets involved in defined aspects of AMD pathology. Such biomarkers could also serve as the long sought-after variable needed to monitor treatment effects in future clinical trials for AMD.

Results

Study design

We applied a three stage design to identify significantly associated cmiRNAs. First, RNASeq was performed to screen for miRNA candidates in 9 cases and 9 controls from the Regensburg study. The cmiRNAs with a nominal significance of p>0.1 were then validated in an unrelated set of 45 NV cases and 68 controls from the Regensburg study (**Table 1**). Finally, candidate cmiRNAs with a nominal significant association (p< 0.05, adjusted or unadjusted for glaucoma) and an odds ratio above 2 or below 0.5 were then replicated in a population based study (Cologne study, **Table 1**) consisting of 75 NV cases and 70 controls. In total, the combined study included 129 patients with NV AMD and 147 AMD-free controls (**Table 1**). Additionally, 59 AMD patients with pure GA were assessed for candidate cmiRNAs to test for specificity of the findings in NV AMD.

Identification of cmiRNAs in NV AMD (discovery study)

To search for candidate cmiRNAs, we first performed next-generation sequencing of cmiRNAs extracted from plasma of 9 AMD NV cases and 9 matched controls. Overall, in the 18 samples we identified 203 different cmiRNA species. Of these, 10 cmiRNAs were significantly associated with late-stage NV AMD ($p_{uncorrected} < 0.1$) (**Table 2**).

Circulating miRNAs associated with NV AMD (replication study)

To replicate the initial findings, qRT-PCR was performed for the significant 10 cmiRNAs in 113 samples consisting of 45 NV AMD cases and 68 controls. Three cmiRNAs were identified (hsa-mir-301-3p, hsa-mir-361-5p, and hsa-mir-451a-5p) which showed (1) an association signal in the same direction as in the discovery study, (2) an odds ratio over 2 or under 0.5 and (3) an uncorrected (one-sided) p-value below 0.1. These three cmiRNAs showed reduced levels in the serum of CNV cases compared to AMD free controls. The association was robust also when adjusting for covariates such as age, gender, smoking (measured in packyears), genetic risk score (GRS) or levels of the housekeeping cmiRNA hsa-mir-451a-5p (**Table 3**). Of note, two cmiRNAs (hsa-mir-301-3p and hsa-mir-361-5p) were strongly confounded by glaucoma disease status and showed stronger association signals when adjusting for glaucoma.

Circulating miRNAs hsa-mir-301-3p, hsa-mir-361-5p, and hsa-mir-424-5p were then analyzed by qRT-PCR in an additional replication study (Cologne study) consisting of 75 NV cases and 70 controls. In concordance with the Regensburg study, we also found reduced levels of those three cmiRNAs in NV cases compared to controls in the Cologne study. The results of the two replications were pooled and jointly analyzed (**Figure 1, Table S1**). We found raw (one-sided) p-values of 2.78×10^{-7}, 4.09×10^{-6}, and 4.75×10^{-5} for hsa-mir-301-3p, hsa-mir-361-5p, and hsa-mir-424-5p, respectively. The p-values were adjusted by a conservative Bonferroni correction, assuming 203 statistical tests based on the number of microRNAs detected in the serum of cases and controls. After correction, the p-values for hsa-mir-301-3p, hsa-mir-361-5p, and hsa-mir-424-5p were 5.63×10^{-5}, 8.03×10^{-4}, and 9.64×10^{-3}, respectively. A cmiRNA profile including hsa-mir-301-3p, hsa-mir-361-5p, and hsa-mir-424-5p was significantly associated with AMD in the combined study (129 NV AMD versus 147 controls, $p = 1.17 \times 10^{-8}$) as well as in the Cologne study alone (75 NV cases and 70 controls, $p = 2.43 \times 10^{-5}$).

Testing of cmiRNAs specificity in NV and GA AMD

The expression of hsa-mir-301-3p, hsa-mir-361-5p, and hsa-mir-424-5p was analyzed by qRT-PCR in the serum of 59 GA AMD patients from the Cologne and Bonn study and compared to all controls (**Figure 1, Table S1**). There was no statistically significant association of cmiRNA levels with GA compared to controls ($p_{corrected} > 0.05$). We also found no significant association of the cmiRNA profile including hsa-mir-301-3p, hsa-mir-361-5p, and hsa-mir-424-5p with GA AMD versus controls (p = 0.084).

Circulating miRNA hsa-mir-424-5p showed significantly higher levels in GA compared to NV ($p_{corrected} < 0.005$), while hsa-mir-301-3p and hsa-mir-361-5p were not significant ($p_{corrected} > 0.05$).

Pathway analysis

Pathway enrichment analysis was performed for 3,516 genes predicted by microT-CDS to be regulated by either hsa-mir-301-3p, hsa-mir-361-5p, or hsa-mir-424-5p. A total of 410 genes was predicted to be regulated by at least two of the three cmiRNAs and

Table 1. Summary characteristics of the study.

	Regensburg	Bonn	Cologne
Study type	**Case/Control**	**Case/Control**	**Population based**
Number of individuals	131	18	186
Controls	77	0	70
Cases	54	18	116
Geographic atrophy	0	18	41
Neovascular AMD	54	0	75
Mean age cases (S.D.) [years]	75.15 (6.75)	74.60 (8.70)	80.22 (9.24)
Mean age controls (S.D.) [years]	73.26 (8.00)	-	78.44 (8.76)
Female cases [%]	59.3	61.1	56.9
Female controls [%]	54.5	-	55.7
Glaucoma in cases [%]	11.1	5.5	NA
Glaucoma in controls [%]	83.1	-	NA

35 genes were regulated by the three cmiRNAs jointly (**Figure S1**). Evaluation with miRSystem implicated the canonical TGF-β and mTOR pathways as well as related pathways such as WNT signaling, focal adhesion, neutrophin signaling and insulin metabolism as the top regulated pathways. This is in agreement with the results of mirPATH v2.0, which implicated mTOR (KEGG ID: hsa04150, $p<10^{-13}$) and TGF-β pathways (KEGG ID: hsa04350, $p<10^{-14}$) as top regulated pathways (**Table 4**).

Functional characterization of candidate miRNAs in human endothelial cells

MicroRNA hsa-mir-361-5p was shown earlier to influence the expression level of VEGFA [14] and thus should also influence angiogenesis. In order to test this hypothesis *in vitro*, we designed antisense oligoribonucleotides against hsa-mir-361-5p but also against hsa-mir-301a-3p and hsa-mir-424-5p and performed tube formation assays with human umbilical vein endothelial cells (HUVEC). We show that a knockdown of hsa-mir-361-5p significantly alters tube formation *in vitro* ($p_{corrected}<0.05$, **Figure 2, Figure S2 and S3**). Knockdown of hsa-mir-301a-3p and hsa-mir-424-5p also showed elevated average tube lengths, however, this was not statistically significant after adjustment for multiple testing ($p_{corrected}>0.05$).

Classification

The raw AUC value for the cmiRNA profile was 0.727 for NV AMD and controls from the Regensburg study and 0.802 when restricting the analysis to NV AMD and controls from the Cologne study. Additionally, we used the weights obtained from the Regensburg study of each cmiRNA in the profile to predict the outcome (case or no case) in the Cologne study and found an AUC value of 0.722. To estimate non-parametric confidence intervals, we performed a 2,000 fold bootstrap analysis in the pooled study. The bootstrapped AUC value for the profile was 0.730 (95% CI: 0.544–0.877) indicating a good classification accuracy.

Discussion

To our knowledge, this is the first study to evaluate the relative abundance of cmiRNAs in the serum of late stage AMD patients. We identified three cmiRNAs (hsa-mir-301a-3p, hsa-mir-361-5p, and hsa-mir-424-5p) which were significantly altered in NV AMD patients compared to AMD-free controls. Even when conditioned on covariates such as age, gender, smoking or genetic risk scores computed from known AMD-associated variants, the three cmiRNAs showed little alteration in their association strength, indicating a true association with late stage NV AMD. In contrast,

Table 2. Association of circulating microRNAs with AMD in the Regensburg discovery study (9 NV cases and 9 controls).

microRNA	uncorrected p-value	mean cases (95% CI)	mean controls (95% CI)
hsa-miR-142-5p	0.012	1.21 (1.14–1.28)	1.00 (0.93–1.07)
hsa-miR-192-5p	0.010	1.29 (1.20–1.38)	1.00 (0.91–1.09)
hsa-miR-194-5p	0.028	1.28 (1.19–1.38)	1.00 (0.89–1.11)
hsa-miR-26a-5p	0.082	0.90 (0.83–0.96)	1.00 (0.94–1.06)
hsa-miR-301a-3p	0.084	0.83 (0.72–0.93)	1.00 (0.90–1.10)
hsa-miR-335-5p	0.094	1.34 (1.17–1.50)	1.00 (0.84–1.16)
hsa-miR-361-5p	0.056	0.74 (0.56–0.91)	1.00 (0.85–1.15)
hsa-miR-424-5p	0.028	0.52 (0.30–0.73)	1.00 (0.84–1.16)
hsa-miR-4732-5p	0.086	1.24 (1.12–1.36)	1.00 (0.88–1.12)
hsa-miR-505-5p	0.048	1.29 (1.13–1.44)	1.00 (0.85–1.15)

Table 3. Sensitivity analysis in the Regensburg study by multiple logistic regression models.

covariate	hsa-miR-301a-3p	hsa-miR-361-5p	hsa-miR-424-5p
none	0.31 (0.10–0.86)*	0.50 (0.19–1.27)	0.28 (0.12–0.59)*
age [years]	0.33 (0.13–0.92)*	0.49 (0.19–1.26)	0.27 (0.12–0.59)*
packyears [years]	0.31 (0.10–0.86)*	0.50 (0.19–1.27)	0.27 (0.12–0.59)*
gender	0.29 (0.09–0.82)*	0.48 (0.18–1.23)	0.28 (0.12–0.59)*
genetic risk score	0.38 (0.10–1.33)	0.53 (0.13–2.12)	0.21 (0.07–0.56)*
glaucoma	0.15 (0.04–0.54)*[1]	0.23 (0.06–0.78)*[1]	0.24 (0.08–0.65)*
hsa-mir-451a-5p	0.38 (0.12–1.08)	0.68 (0.24–1.85)	0.35 (0.14–0.78)*

[1]strong increase in association signal by adjusting for glaucoma as a covariate.
*statistically significant association (p<0.05).

there was no association of cmiRNAs hsa-mir-301a-3p, hsa-mir-361-5p, or hsa-mir-424-5p with GA AMD, suggesting subtype-specific cmiRNA profiles for late stage AMD. A global screening strategy similar to the one applied in this study may be suited to eventually characterize a GA AMD specific cmiRNA profile.

Our initial discovery study comprised 9 NV AMD cases and 9 matched controls and identified several cmiRNA candidates with altered expression levels although none reached statistical significance after adjustment for multiple testing (n = 203 equivalent to the discovery of 203 cmiRNAs). A recent study compared cmiRNA levels in long-surviving versus short-surviving patients with lung cancer and found fold changes of significantly altered cmiRNAs between 1.60 and 7.15 [15] and Cohen's effect sizes between 0.92 and 1.54 which are considered to be large [16]. Given the number of samples in our discovery study, we calculated the power to detect comparable effect sizes after adjustment for

multiple testing between 4.2% and 33.2%. This would imply a power to identify between 4 and 33 cmiRNAs out of 100 in our discovery study at the assumed effect size or higher. To compensate for lower effect sizes, we increased our sample size to 276 individuals (129 NV cases and 147 AMD-free controls) in the replication and retested individually the top 10 cmiRNAs hits from discovery. This uncovered a statistically significant association of NV AMD with cmiRNAs hsa-mir-301a-3p, hsa-mir-361-5p, and hsa-mir-424-5p.

Bioinformatical pathway analysis for genes suggested to be regulated by the NV AMD associated cmiRNAs were performed with two independent programs including the miRSystem and mirPATH v2.0. Both revealed concurring results and implicated the TGF-β and mTOR pathways in neovascular AMD pathology. Interestingly, this is in agreement with a recently published GWAS which also implicated the TGF-β and the mTOR pathways in late

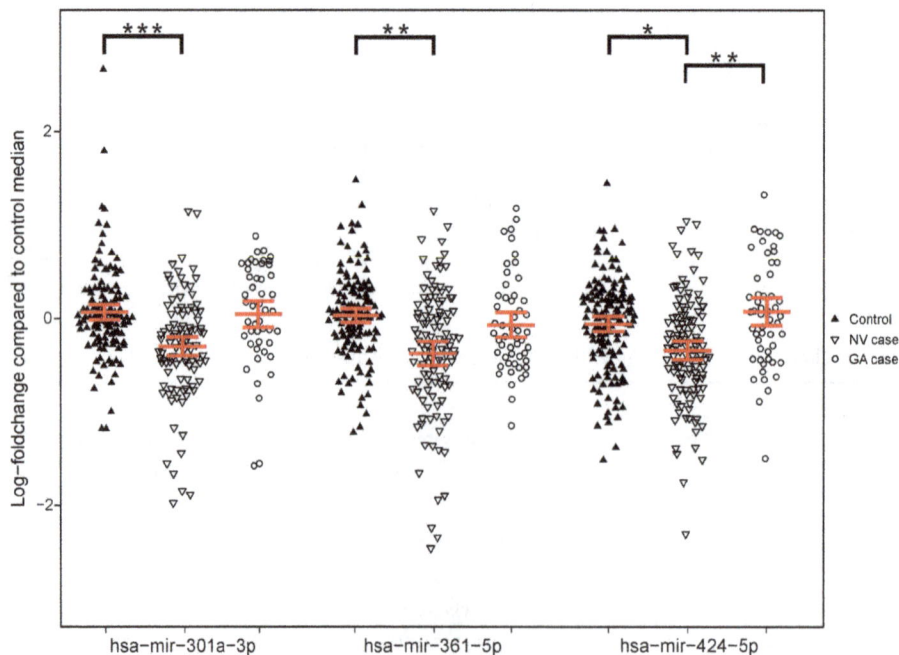

Figure 1. Expression analysis of three cmiRNAs (hsa-mir-301a-3p, hsa-mir-361-5p and hsa-mir-424-5p) in 129 NV AMD cases, 59 GA AMD cases and 147 healthy controls. Expression values for all samples were normalized by the median expression value in controls. Broad horizontal bars represent the mean value in each group (NV cases, GA cases or controls) for each cmiRNA. Smaller horizontal bars represent the 95% confidence intervals for each mean (see Table S1). Significant differences between means are indicated by asterix. * = $p_{corrected}$<0.05; ** = $p_{corrected}$<0.005; *** = $p_{corrected}$<0.0005.

Table 4. Pathway enrichment analysis performed with miRSystem and mirPATH2.

Canonical pathway (ID[2])	genes observed/genes in pathway		genetic association reported[1]
	miRSystem	mirPATH2	
TGF-β signaling (hsa04350)	25/84	35/80	TGFBR1 [8]
mTOR signaling (hsa04150)	16/52	33/60	VEGFA [17]
Neutrophin signaling (hsa04722)	38/127	-	-
WNT signaling (hsa04310)	48/150	-	
Focal adhesion (hsa04510)	43/199	-	VEGFA [17]
Insulin signaling (hsa04910)	35/137	-	
Melanogenesis (hsa04916)	28/101	-	

[1]genetic associations were reported in or near genes in this pathway by genome wide association studies.
[2]KEGG pathway ID (http://www.genome.jp/kegg/).

stage AMD by identifying risk associated genetic variants near or within the genes encoding the transforming growth factor, beta receptor 1 (*TGFBR1*) and the vascular endothelial growth factor A (*VEGFA*) [8,17]. The TGF-β as well as the mTOR pathway are involved in cellular responses to stress and injury and also regulate angiogenesis. Consequently, we performed *in vitro* tube formation assays and reduced the levels of hsa-mir-424-5p, hsa-mir-301a-3p, and hsa-mir-361-5p by antisense oligoribonucleotides to evaluate the impact of decreased miRNA levels on angiogenesis. Knock-down efficiency reduced microRNA levels in the test system on average by about two-fold. Antisense treatment of hsa-mir-361-5p lead to a significant increase in tube formation and, thus, angiogenesis in vitro. Results for hsa-mir-424-5p and hsa-mir-301a-3p revealed a similar direction of effect but were not statistically significant due to correction for multiple testing. Together, the data are promising and support our bioinformatical analyses.

Additionally, pathways closely related to the mTOR pathway were implicated by our analysis including WNT signaling, focal adhesion, neutrophin signaling and the insulin pathway. These pathways are involved in (neural) cell survival and therefore are reasonable candidate pathways for the pathogenesis of AMD. However, so far no genetic association with late stage AMD was observed for any genes associated with these signaling pathways. In this context, it should be noted that until now only few studies evaluated a genetic association for progression and severity of AMD [18,19]. These studies mainly focused on strong (and known) signals associated with increased risk for AMD and therefore may have missed possible existing associations. The present study has now identified cmiRNAs hsa-mir-301a-3p, hsa-mir-361-5p, and hsa-mir-424-5p as new biomarkers for late stage neovascular AMD. Furthermore, our data show that these biomarkers are not associated with GA AMD implying that different biomarkers and thus different biological pathways are

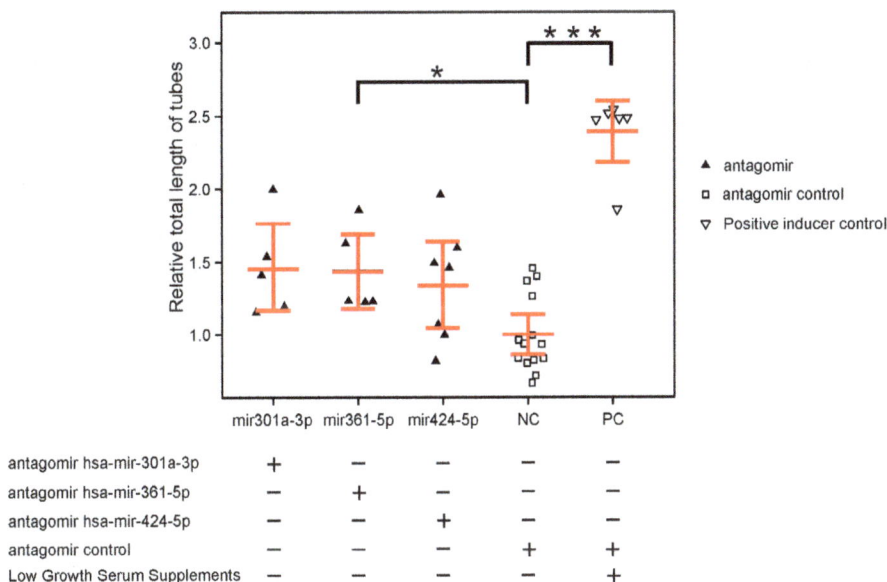

Figure 2. *In vitro* **tube formation assays in human endothelial cells.** HUVEC cells were transfected with antagomirs for hsa-mir-301a-3p, hsa-mir-361-5p or hsa-mir-424-5p or with control antagomirs (see **Figure S2**) and seeded on Geltrex/Matrigel. Cumulative tube length was quantified with Angiogenesis Analyzer implemented in ImageJ. Each measurement point indicates one independent transfection. Low Serum Growth Supplements (Life) were used as a positive inducer control. Representative images are shown in **Figure S3**. Significant differences between means are indicated by asterix. * = p_corrected<0.05; *** = p_corrected<0.0005.

likely involved in subtype-specific manifestations of late stage AMD. If confirmed, this could have major implications for designing treatment regiments for AMD.

A recent study investigated a treatment option for patients with stroke by increasing a disease-related reduction in plasma levels of hsa-mir-424-5p [20]. In an inducible mouse model of acute stroke which also revealed a down-regulation of hsa-mir-424-5p in plasma as well as in brain, lentiviral overexpression of hsa-mir-424-5p in the murine brain prior to induction of ischemic stroke significantly lowered the infarct volume as well as the brain edema levels [20]. A similar approach could be envisioned for treating AMD lesions. The identification of cmiRNAs that are dysregulated in NV AMD patients, now offers a number of novel starting points for therapeutic regimens. For example, such targets could be the genes that are regulated by the cmiRNAs or, alternatively, could directly address the dysregulated cmiRNAs itself. Specifically, the latter approach would initially entail prescreening of patients for altered cmiRNAs levels. Reduced expression of a diagnostic cmiRNA (as pre-microRNA or mature microRNA) could be supplemented by lentiviral transduction, nano-particle aided transfection or by delivery of the dysregulated cmiRNA via synthetic microRNAs in artificial exsosomes. Therapies to modify up- or down-regulated genes are also conceivable. This could be done by using small molecules to influence gene activity [21], protein activity and stability [22] or by targeting proteins or interacting proteins with specific antibodies [23].

In summary, this study has identified three cmiRNAs with a significantly altered expression profile in the serum of NV AMD patients when compared to AMD-free control individuals. This finding opens up a number of new avenues in understanding disease mechanisms and designing targeted treatment options. Another important aspect of our finding pertains to monitoring treatment effects in clinical trial settings. Although proof of concept is still waranted, measuring drug responses as a means of measuring changes in the cmiRNA profil from blood samples of AMD patients may proof a direct and little invasive approach in the future.

Materials and Methods

Ethics statement

This study followed the tenets of the declaration of Helsinki and was approved by the Ethics Review Board at the University of Regensburg, Germany (ID: 12-101-0241), University of Bonn, Germany and University of Cologne, Germany. Informed written consent was obtained from each proband after explanation of the nature and possible consequences of the study.

Recruitment of AMD cases and control individuals

The case-control sample included 54 individuals with seemingly non-familial NV AMD and 77 age- and gender-matched AMD-free controls from the Regensburg study, 116 cases and 70 controls from the Cologne study, and 18 GA AMD cases from the Bonn Eye Clinic (**Table 1**). Inclusion and exclusion criteria have been described elsewhere [8,24–26].

Genotyping of samples

Genotyping was carried out as described elsewhere [9]. Briefly, genomic DNA was extracted from peripheral blood leukocytes. Ten single nucleotide polymorphisms (SNPs, **Table S2**) were genotyped either by direct sequencing, restriction enzyme digestion of PCR products (RFLP) or TaqMan SNP Genotyping (Applied Biosystems, Foster City, USA).

Isolation of cmiRNAs from stabilized blood samples and serum

To reduce degradation of microRNAs and other RNA species [27], for the Regensburg and Bonn samples peripheral venous blood was drawn in PAXgene Blood RNA tubes (PreAnalytiX GmbH, Hombrechtikon, CH) and immediately stored at −80°C. To isolate RNA, tubes were thawed at room temperature on a rocker and centrifuged for 5 minutes at 1500 rcf at 4°C. The RNA isolation was carried out with the mirVANA microRNA isolation kit (Ambion, Austin, TX, USA) as described elsewhere [28]. Briefly, 300 µl of the supernatant were mixed with 600 µl of binding/lysis buffer. Then, 90µl of microRNA homogenate additive was added, thoroughly mixed for 30s and incubated on ice for 10 minutes. An equal amount of acid/phenol/chloroform (Ambion) was then added to each aliquot and vortexed for 1 minute at maximum setting. The solution was spun for 10 minutes at 10,000 g at room temperature. The resulting aqueous (upper) phase was mixed with 1.25 volumes of 100% ACS grade ethanol and passed through a mirVANA column in sequential 700 µl steps. The columns were then washed according to the manufactures protocol and the RNA was eluted with 50 µl nuclease-free water (preheated to 95°C).

For the Cologne samples, RNA isolation from blood serum was carried out with the miRNeasy Serum/Plasma kit (Qiagen) according to the manufacturer's recommendations. Typically, we used 200 ul of serum and eluted the RNA in 24 ul of nuclease-free water.

Sequencing of cmiRNAs and data analysis (discovery study)

cDNA libraries were constructed using the Ion Total RNA-Seq v2 kit (Life Technologies) according to the manufacturers recommendations for 9 NV AMD cases and 9 control samples. The resulting cDNA libraries were purified by AMPure beads (Beckman Coulter), and their concentrations and sizes distribution were determined on an Agilent BioAnalyzer DNA high-sensitivity Chip (Agilent Technologies). Emulsion PCR and enrichment of cDNA conjugated particles were performed with an Ion OneTouch 200 Template Kit v2 DL (Life Technologies) according to the manufacturer's instructions. The final particles were loaded on an Ion 316 chip and sequenced on a Personal Genome Machine with 200 bp read length (Life Technologies).

The data obtained were analyzed with the mirDEEP2 package [29]. Briefly, all reads were mapped to the human genome. Reads that failed to align were excluded. Remaining reads were then mapped to the pre-microRNA and microRNA sequences obtained from mirbase.org (Release 19, August 2012) and quantified. Reads per microRNA were normalized to the overall number of reads and normalized to 100,000 reads. The data were transformed with the natural logarithm to obtain a normal distribution of expression values. In order to account for batch effects in the data, we employed an empirical Bayesian batch effect correction algorithm known as ComBat [30]. For each microRNA, mean values of cases were compared to mean values of controls via t-test. Nominal significant associations with a (two-sided) p-value<0.1 were considered for replication.

Quantitative (q)RT-PCR and data analysis (replication study)

Circulating miRNA was extracted from blood as described above and reverse transcription followed by qRT-PCR was performed according to Hurteau et al. [31]. Briefly, 10 µl of purified cmiRNA solution were modified by *E. coli* Poly (A)

Polymerase I (E-PAP) by the addition of a polyA tail (Ambion, Austin, TX, USA). Reverse transcription was performed with Superscript III reverse transcriptase (Invitrogen Carlsbad, CA) and a Universal RT oligonucleotide primer, which contains a polyT stretch of DNA that binds to the newly synthesized polyA tail (**Table S3**). The RT solution was diluted 1:50, of which 4:μl were used per qRT-PCR reaction. Each qRT-PCR master mix was prepared according to the protocol of the Power SYBR Green Master Mix (Applied Biosystems, Foster, CA, USA) and run on an ABI Viia-7 (Applied Biosystems, Paisley, UK). Each microRNA was assayed in triplicates. Primers that performed poorly (<50% qRT-PCR efficiency) were excluded from further analysis. We further excluded measurements with a standard deviation greater than 0.4 Ct values in the triplicates. In order to normalize the Ct-values according to the amount of isolated RNA and reverse transcription efficiency, we used hsa-mir-451-5p as a housekeeping cmiRNA. This microRNA showed the least variance between cases and controls and within each group in our discovery study and was therefore regarded suitable as a housekeeper. The normalized Ct values of each individual were then normalized versus the median of the Ct values of the controls. We considered associated cmiRNAs with an odds ratio greater than 2 or lower than 0.5 for further replication.

The standard student's t-tests was applied to evaluate a statistically significant association as implemented in R [32]. In the final dataset, we adjusted the observed raw p-values ($p_{uncorrected}$) by a conservative Bonferroni correction ($p_{corrected}$). Adjusted p-values below 0.05 were considered significant. Sensitivity analysis was carried out by fitting logistic regression models adjusted for possible confounding variables.

Target prediction for cmiRNAs

We used miRSystem [33] and DIANA mirPATH v2.0 [34] to identify canonical pathways involved in AMD pathogenesis based on differentially regulated microRNAs. We used the default settings in miRSystem to identify target genes and to find canonical KEGG pathways. With mirPATH v2.0, targets predicted by microT-CDS were selected with a threshold of 0.7. The intersection of pathways which showed an involvement of all investigated microRNAs (p-value threshold: 0.005, with Conservative Stats) was considered. We excluded KEGG pathways with more than 200 genes to increase specificity and to exclude pathways considered to be too general. Furthermore, we excluded validated cmiRNA targets as well as cancer pathways such as prostate cancer (hsa05215) or glioma (hsa05214), as the majority of the cmiRNA work has been in the field of oncology and thus cancer pathways are expected by design to be among the top findings.

Classification of cases and controls

Area under the curve (AUC) measurements were carried out with the function lroc from the package "epicalc" [35]. We used a bootstrap (n = 2000) approach to calculate robust mean and confidence interval estimates for the AUC measurements by randomly selecting half of the cases and half of the controls (with replacement) and calculating the risk model with this sub-sample (training data). A randomly selected sample of half of the cases and half of the controls (with replacement) was then used to calculated the AUC (test data).

In vitro angiogenesis assay

Pooled human umbilical vein endothelial cells (HUVECs) were purchased from Life Technologies and cultured in Medium 200PRF with Low Serum Growth Supplement and Gentamicin/

Amphotericin Solution (Life Technologies). Transfection of HUVECs was carried out as described in Bonauer et al. 2009 [36]. Briefly, cells were subcultured to passage 3 and grown until 70% confluent. 2′O-methyl antisense oligoribonucleotides against hsa-mir-424-5p (5′-UUCAAAACAUGAAUUGCUGCUG-3′), hsa-mir-301a-3p (5′-GCUUUGACAAUACUAUUGCACUG-3′) or hsa-mir-361-5p (5′-ACAGGCCGGGACAAGUG-CAAUA-3′) or GFP (5′-AAGGCAAGCUGACCCUGAAGUU-3′) were synthesized by VBC Biotech and 50 nM were transfected with GeneTrans II (MoBiTec) according to the manufacturer's protocol. After 24 h the medium was changed to full growth medium with supplements and antibiotics. 48 h after transfection, 3.5×10^4 HUVECs of each transfection were sown onto one well of a 24 well plate coated with 150 μl Geltrex (Life Technologies). As a positive inducer control, cells were cultured in full growth medium with supplements. Total tube length was quantified after 24 hours by measuring the cumulative tube length in four random fields (area in each field: 2.25 mm^2) using the Angiogenesis Analyzer in ImageJ [37]. In total, we performed between 5 and 14 independent transfections for each knockdown or control experiment. In order to assess the transfection efficiency, miRNAs were isolated with the mirVANA microRNA isolation kit (Ambion, Austin, TX, USA) according to the manufacturer's protocol. cDNA synthesis and qRT-PCR was carried out as described above.

Supporting Information

Figure S1 Venn diagram of target genes predicted by microT-CDS. Target genes were predicted with microT-CDS with a microT threshold of 0.7. In total, 3,516 target genes were predicted.

Figure S2 Knockdown of candidate miRNAs in human endothelial cells. Mean relative reduction in miRNA levels compared to control antagomir (mock). Whiskers represent the standard error of the mean.

Figure S3 Representative images of *in vitro* tube formation assays in human endothelial cells. The measured cumulative tube length in each image was close to the mean cumulative tube length measured in all images of the respective treatment.

Acknowledgments

We are grateful to the patients and control subjects for their participation in this study. We also want to thank Kerstin Meier for her excellent technical support.

Author Contributions

Conceived and designed the experiments: FG GM BHW. Performed the experiments: FG PGS. Analyzed the data: FG PGS. Contributed reagents/ materials/analysis tools: PGS CB TS DH MF ML HH SF. Contributed to the writing of the manuscript: FG BHW. Recruited and phenotyped patients and control individuals: PGS CB TS MF ML HH SF.

References

1. Swaroop A, Branham KE, Chen W, Abecasis G (2007) Genetic susceptibility to age-related macular degeneration: a paradigm for dissecting complex disease traits. Hum Mol Genet 16 Spec No: R174–82.

2. Fritsche LG, Fariss RN, Stambolian D, Abecasis GR, Curcio CA, et al. (2014) Age-Related Macular Degeneration: Genetics and Biology Coming Together. Annu Rev Genomics Hum Genet.

3. Jonasson F, Arnarsson A, Eiríksdottir G, Harris TB, Launer LJ, et al. (2011) Prevalence of age-related macular degeneration in old persons: Age, Gene/ environment Susceptibility Reykjavik Study. Ophthalmology 118: 825–830.

4. Friedman DS, O'Colmain BJ, Muñoz B, Tomany SC, McCarty C, et al. (2004) Prevalence of age-related macular degeneration in the United States. Arch Ophthalmol 122: 564–572.

5. VanNewkirk MR, Nanjan MB, Wang JJ, Mitchell P, Taylor HR, et al. (2000) The prevalence of age-related maculopathy: the visual impairment project. Ophthalmology 107: 1593–1600.

6. Tomany SC, Wang JJ, Van Leeuwen R, Klein R, Mitchell P, et al. (2004) Risk factors for incident age-related macular degeneration: pooled findings from 3 continents. Ophthalmology 111: 1280–1287.

7. Seddon JM, Cote J, Page WF, Aggen SH, Neale MC (2005) The US twin study of age-related macular degeneration: relative roles of genetic and environmental influences. Arch Ophthalmol 123: 321–327.

8. Fritsche LG, Chen W, Schu M, Yaspan BL, Yu Y, et al. (2013) Seven new loci associated with age-related macular degeneration. Nat Genet 45: 433–9, 439e1–2.

9. Grassmann F, Fritsche LG, Keilhauer CN, Heid IM, Weber BHF (2012) Modelling the genetic risk in age-related macular degeneration. PLoS One 7: e37979.

10. Gallo A, Tandon M, Alevizos I, Illei GG (2012) The majority of microRNAs detectable in serum and saliva is concentrated in exosomes. PLoS One 7: e30679.

11. Turchinovich A, Weiz L, Burwinkel B (2012) Extracellular miRNAs: the mystery of their origin and function. Trends Biochem Sci 37: 460–465.

12. Zhang Y, Liu D, Chen X, Li J, Li L, et al. (2010) Secreted monocytic miR-150 enhances targeted endothelial cell migration. Mol Cell 39: 133–144.

13. Lässer C (2012) Exosomal RNA as biomarkers and the therapeutic potential of exosome vectors. Expert Opin Biol Ther 12 Suppl 1: S189–97.

14. Kanitz A, Imig J, Dziunycz PJ, Primorac A, Galgano A, et al. (2012) The expression levels of microRNA-361-5p and its target VEGFA are inversely correlated in human cutaneous squamous cell carcinoma. PLoS One 7: e49568.

15. Hu Z, Chen X, Zhao Y, Tian T, Jin G, et al. (2010) Serum microRNA signatures identified in a genome-wide serum microRNA expression profiling predict survival of non-small-cell lung cancer. J Clin Oncol 28: 1721–1726.

16. Cohen J (1988) Statistical power analysis for the behavioral sciences. 2nd ed. Hillsdale, NJ: Lawrence Erlbaum Associates.

17. Yu Y, Bhangale TR, Fagerness J, Ripke S, Thorleifsson G, et al. (2011) Common variants near FRK/COL10A1 and VEGFA are associated with advanced age-related macular degeneration. Hum Mol Genet 20: 3699–3709.

18. Leveziel N, Puche N, Richard F, Somner JEA, Zerbib J, et al. (2010) Genotypic influences on severity of exudative age-related macular degeneration. Invest Ophthalmol Vis Sci 51: 2620–2625.

19. Klein ML, Ferris FL, Francis PJ, Lindblad AS, Chew EY, et al. (2010) Progression of geographic atrophy and genotype in age-related macular degeneration. Ophthalmology 117: 1554–9, 1559.e1.

20. Zhao H, Wang J, Gao L, Wang R, Liu X, et al. (2013) MiRNA-424 Protects Against Permanent Focal Cerebral Ischemia Injury in Mice Involving Suppressing Microglia Activation. Stroke 44: 1706–1713.

21. Koh JT, Zheng J (2007) The new biomimetic chemistry: artificial transcription factors. ACS Chem Biol 2: 599–601.

22. Hagan EL, Banaszynski LA, Chen L, Maynard-Smith LA, Wandless TJ (2009) Regulating protein stability in mammalian cells using small molecules. Cold Spring Harb Protoc 2009: pdb.prot5172.

23. Scott AW, Bressler SB (2013) Long-term follow-up of vascular endothelial growth factor inhibitor therapy for neovascular age-related macular degeneration. Curr Opin Ophthalmol 24: 190–196.

24. Ferris FL, Davis MD, Clemons TE, Lee L-Y, Chew EY, et al. (2005) A simplified severity scale for age-related macular degeneration: AREDS Report No. 18. Arch Ophthalmol 123: 1570–1574.

25. Ristau T, Paun C, Ersoy L, Hahn M, Lechanteur Y, et al. (2014) Impact of the Common Genetic Associations of Age-Related Macular Degeneration upon Systemic Complement Component C3d Levels. PLoS One 9: e93459.

26. Dreyhaupt J, Mansmann U, Pritsch M, Dolar-Szczasny J, Bindewald A, et al. (2005) Modelling the natural history of geographic atrophy in patients with age-related macular degeneration. Ophthalmic Epidemiol 12: 353–362.

27. Köberle V, Pleli T, Schmithals C, Alonso EA, Haupenthal J, et al. (2013) Differential Stability of Cell-Free Circulating microRNAs: Implications for Their Utilization as Biomarkers. 8: 1–11.

28. Kosaka N, Izumi H, Sekine K, Ochiya T (2010) microRNA as a new immune-regulatory agent in breast milk. Silence 1: 7.

29. Friedlaender MR, Chen W, Adamidi C, Maaskola J, Einspanier R, et al. (2008) Discovering microRNAs from deep sequencing data using miRDeep. Nat Biotechnol 26: 407–415.

30. Johnson WE, Li C, Rabinovic A (2007) Adjusting batch effects in microarray expression data using empirical Bayes methods. Biostatistics 8: 118–127.

31. Hurteau GJ, Spivack SD, Brock GJ (2006) Potential mRNA degradation targets of hsa-miR-200c, identified using informatics and qRT-PCR. Cell Cycle 5: 1951–1956.

32. R Core Team (2013). R: A language and environment for statistical computing. R Foundation for Statistical Computing, Vienna, Austria. Available at http://www.R-project.org/.

33. Lu T-P, Lee C-Y, Tsai M-H, Chiu Y-C, Hsiao CK, et al. (2012) miRSystem: an integrated system for characterizing enriched functions and pathways of microRNA targets. PLoS One 7: e42390.

34. Vlachos IS, Kostoulas N, Vergoulis T, Georgakilas G, Reczko M, et al. (2012) DIANA miRPath v.2.0: investigating the combinatorial effect of microRNAs in pathways. Nucleic Acids Res 40: W498–504.

35. Virasakdi Chongsuvivatwong (2012). epicalc: Epidemiological calculator. R package version 2.15.1.0. Available at http://CRAN.R-project.org/package=epicalc.

36. Bonauer A, Carmona G, Iwasaki M, Mione M, Koyanagi M, et al. (2009) MicroRNA-92a controls angiogenesis and functional recovery of ischemic tissues in mice. Science 324: 1710–1713.

37. Carpentier G, Martinelli M, Courty J, Cascone I (2012) Angiogenesis Analyzer for ImageJ. 4th ImageJ User and Developer Conference proceedings, 198–201, Mondorf-les-Bains, Luxembourg, ISBN 2-919941-18-6.

3

Comparison of Estimated Glomerular Filtration Rate by the Chronic Kidney Disease Epidemiology Collaboration (CKD-EPI) Equations with and without Cystatin C for Predicting Clinical Outcomes in Elderly Women

Wai H. Lim[1,2*¶], Joshua R. Lewis[1,3¶], Germaine Wong[4,5¶], Robin M. Turner[6], Ee M. Lim[2,7], Peter L. Thompson[8], Richard L. Prince[1,3]

1 University of Western Australia School of Medicine and Pharmacology, Sir Charles Gairdner Hospital Unit, Perth, Australia, 2 Department of Renal Medicine, Sir Charles Gairdner Hospital, Perth, Australia, 3 Department of Endocrinology and Diabetes, Sir Charles Gairdner Hospital, Perth, Australia, 4 Centre for Kidney Research, Children's Hospital at Westmead, Sydney, Australia, 5 School of Public Health, Sydney Medical School, The University of Sydney, Sydney, Australia, 6 School of Public Health, The University of New South Wales, Sydney, Australia, 7 PathWest, Sir Charles Gairdner Hospital, Perth, Australia, 8 Department of Cardiovascular Medicine, Sir Charles Gairdner Hospital, Perth, Australia

Abstract

Background: Reduced estimated glomerular filtration rate (eGFR) using the cystatin-C derived equations might be a better predictor of cardiovascular disease (CVD) mortality compared with the creatinine-derived equations, but this association remains unclear in elderly individuals.

Aim: The aims of this study were to compare the predictive values of the Chronic Kidney Disease Epidemiology Collaboration (CKD-EPI)-creatinine, CKD-EPI-cystatin C and CKD-EPI-creatinine-cystatin C eGFR equations for all-cause mortality and CVD events (hospitalizations±mortality).

Methods: Prospective cohort study of 1165 elderly women aged>70 years. Associations between eGFR and outcomes were examined using Cox regression analysis. Test accuracy of eGFR equations for predicting outcomes was examined using Receiver Operating Characteristic (ROC) analysis and net reclassification improvement (NRI).

Results: Risk of all-cause mortality for every incremental reduction in eGFR determined using CKD-EPI-creatinine, CKD-EPI-cystatin C and the CKD-EPI-creatinine-cystatic C equations was similar. Areas under the ROC curves of CKD-EPI-creatinine, CKD-EPI-cystatin C and CKD-EPI-creatinine-cystatin C equations for all-cause mortality were 0.604 (95%CI 0.561–0.647), 0.606 (95%CI 0.563–0.649; p = 0.963) and 0.606 (95%CI 0.563–0.649; p = 0.894) respectively. For all-cause mortality, there was no improvement in the reclassification of eGFR categories using the CKD-EPI-cystatin C (NRI -4.1%; p = 0.401) and CKD-EPI-creatinine-cystatin C (NRI -1.2%; p = 0.748) compared with CKD-EPI-creatinine equation. Similar findings were observed for CVD events.

Conclusion: eGFR derived from CKD-EPI cystatin C and CKD-EPI creatinine-cystatin C equations did not improve the accuracy or predictive ability for clinical events compared to CKD-EPI-creatinine equation in this cohort of elderly women.

Editor: Antonio Carlos Seguro, University of São Paulo School of Medicine, Brazil

Funding: Dr. Lewis was supported by Raine Medical Research Foundation Priming Grant and Dr. Turner was supported by National Health and Medical Research Council (NHMRC) program grant #633003 to the Screening & Test Evaluation Program. The authors had full access to all of the data in the study and take responsibility for the integrity of the data and the accuracy of the data analysis. The study was supported by Kidney Health Australia, Healthway Health Promotion Foundation of Western Australia and by project grants 254627, 303169 and 572604 from the National Health and Medical Research Council of Australia. The funders had no role in study design, data collection and analysis, decision to publish, or preparation of the manuscript.

Competing Interests: The authors have declared that no competing interests exist.

* Email: wai.lim@health.wa.gov.au

¶ These authors contributed equally to this work.

¶ These authors are co-first authors on this work.

Introduction

Chronic kidney disease (CKD) is a major public health burden worldwide. Patients with CKD, especially those on dialysis, suffer from reduced life expectancy and quality of life [1]. CKD is a multi-system disease with established evidence demonstrating reduced kidney function increases the risk of cardiovascular disease (CVD) mortality [2–5], infections and cancer [6]. Previous meta-analyses reported the risk of associated disease such as CVD mortality commences with an estimated glomerular filtration rate (eGFR) of less than 60 ml/min/1.73 m^2 and increases exponentially as one approaches end-stage renal disease (ESRD) requiring dialysis. However, epidemiological studies have also shown that eGFR between 60–74.9 mL/min/1.73 m^2 is associated with a higher risk of CVD-related death compared to eGFR of ≥75 mL/min/1.73 m^2 in patients following myocardial infarction suggesting that the risk of adverse clinical events is not confined to those with eGFR of less than 60 mL/min/1.73 m^2 [7]. Although it is generally accepted that early identification of CKD may slow the progression to advanced stage kidney disease and provides a window of opportunity to prevent associated illness such as CVD and cancer [8], the threshold of reduced kidney function that prompts early intervention remains undefined suggesting that determining precise GFR in individuals may not be absolutely critical.

Chronic Kidney Disease Epidemiology Collaboration (CKD-EPI) equation [3] has been shown to be a more reliable marker of measured GFR and is superior in predicting the risk of adverse clinical outcomes such as mortality and stroke compared to Modification of Diet in Renal Disease (MDRD) [9] or the Cockcroft-Gault equations [10]. Although these equations are widely used in the community, previous studies have shown that serum creatinine-based equations may underestimate actual kidney function, especially in elderly individuals. As serum creatinine is affected by multiple factors including muscle mass and age, [11], alternative filtration markers such as cystatin C have been evaluated for GFR estimation.

Several newly-derived eGFR equations such as the CKD-EPI cystatin C and CKD-EPI creatinine-cystatin C equations have shown improvement in the precision and accuracy of determining GFR compared to CKD-EPI creatinine equation, but uncertainties remain as to the clinical significance and cost-effectiveness of using cystatin C-derived eGFR estimations over creatinine-derived eGFR estimations in the general population, particularly in elderly individuals. A recent meta-analysis of sixteen population cohorts reported both CKD-EPI cystatin C and combined CKD-EPI creatinine-cystatin C equations improved the accuracy in predicting all-cause and CVD mortality compared to CKD-EPI creatinine equation, but the majority of the included population cohorts were younger individuals of mixed gender with dissimilar proportion of muscle mass [12]. There have been no prior studies examining the clinical utility of these newly derived cystatin C equations in predicting adverse clinical outcomes exclusively in the older female population. The aims of this study were to determine the association of reduced kidney function as measured by CKD-EPI creatinine, CKD-EPI cystatin C and CKD-EPI creatinine-cystatin C equations and all-cause mortality and CVD events and also to assess the accuracy of these newly derived cystatin C-based eGFR equations in the prediction of clinical events in a cohort of elderly women mainly without prevalent CKD and with two-thirds of women with eGFR above 60 mL/min/1.73 m^2.

Subjects and Methods

Study Population

One thousand five hundred women were recruited in 1998 to a five-year prospective, randomized, controlled trial of oral calcium supplements (1.2 g of elemental calcium daily or matching placebo) to prevent osteoporotic fractures, the Calcium Intake Fracture Outcome study (CAIFOS; Australian Clinical Trials Registry Registration Number: ACTRN012607000055404) [13]. Details of recruitment are published elsewhere [13]. Our population-based study is representative of the general elderly population in Western Australia. Participants were women aged over 70 years who were selected using the electoral roll and contacted by mail. Registration on this electoral roll is a standard and compulsory requirement of citizenship in Australia. Of the 5,586 women who responded to a letter inviting participation, 1510 eligible women were randomly selected. Participants had similar disease burden and pharmaceutical consumption to the whole population of this age but they were more likely to be from higher socio-economic groups [13]. The University of Western Australia Human Ethics Committee had approved the study and written informed consents were obtained from all participants. The present study is to evaluate the utility of creatinine and/or cystatin-derived eGFR equations in a cohort of elderly women recruited in 1998 in predicting 10-year clinical outcomes up to 2008.

Baseline medical history including the presence of diabetes, hypertension, smoking history (current/former smokers or non-smokers) and medications were obtained from all participants. Blood pressure was measured on the right arm with a mercury column manometer using an adult cuff after the participants have been seated in an upright position and had rested for 5 minutes. An average of three blood pressure readings was recorded.

Fasting blood samples were collected at baseline (i.e. at time of randomisation in 1998) with sera stored in −70°C freezer until analysis. Creatinine and cystatin C measurements were performed using stored sera after 2008 and results were available in 1165 women (77%). Serum creatinine was analysed using an isotope dilution mass spectrometry (IDMS) traceable Jaffe kinetic assay for creatinine on a Hitachi 917 analyser (Roche Diagnostics GmbH, Mannheim Germany). Serum cystatin C was measured on the Siemens Dade Behring Nephelometer, traceable to the International Federation of Clinical Chemistry Working Group for Standardization of Serum cystatin C and the Institute for Reference Materials and Measurements certified reference materials. eGFR was estimated by three equations derived by *Inker et al* and these are presented in Table S1 – CKD-EPI creatinine equation, CKD-EPI cystatin C equation and CKD-EPI creatinine-cystatin C equation [14].

Assessment of clinical outcomes

Participants' general practitioners verified their medical histories and medications where possible, and were coded using the International Classification of Primary Care–Plus (ICPC-Plus) method [15]. Prevalent CVD was determined from hospital discharge data between 1980 and 1998 and were defined using diagnosis codes from the International Classification of Diseases, Injuries and Causes of Death Clinical Modification (ICD-9-CM, 309-459) [16]. Prevalent renal disease was collected between 1980 and 1998 using International Classification of Diseases, Injuries and Causes of Death Clinical Modification (ICD-9-CM) 17. These codes included glomerular diseases (ICD-9-CM codes 580–583); renal tubulo-interstitial diseases (ICD-9-CM codes 593.3–593.5, 593.7); renal failure (ICD-9-CM codes 584–586); and hypertensive renal disease (ICD-9-CM code 403). The search for renal disease hospitalizations included any diagnosis code.

The primary outcomes of the study were all-cause mortality and CVD hospitalizations and/or mortality retrieved from the Western Australian Data Linkage System (WADLS) for each of the study participants from 1998 until 10 years following their initial study visit. CVD hospitalizations and mortality were defined using primary diagnosis codes from ICD-9-CM, 390-459 [16] and the International Statistical Classification of Diseases and Related Health Problems, 10th Revision, Australian Modification (ICD-10-AM), I00-I99 [17]. All diagnosis text fields from the death certificate were used to ascertain the cause(s) of deaths where these data were not yet available from the WADLS.

Statistical Analysis

Baseline characteristics were expressed as mean and standard deviation (SD) for continuous variables or as number and proportion for categorical variables. Association between eGFR and all-cause mortality and CVD hospitalization and/or mortality was examined using Cox proportional hazard regression model and results were expressed as hazard ratio (HR) with 95% confidence interval (CI) for every incremental reduction in eGFR to allow comparison between equations. The covariates included in the Cox regression models were age, smoking history, body mass index (BMI), diabetes, antihypertensive medications, systolic blood pressure, treatment code, prevalent renal and CVD.

To assess performance of the different equations for estimating eGFR, we assessed the discrimination of the three different models using the Area Under Curve (AUC). Discrimination refers to how well the model distinguishes individuals with and without the outcomes of interests. To assess discrimination, we calculated the area under the receiver operating characteristic (ROC) curve (AUC). An area of 1 implies perfect discrimination, whereas an area of 0.5 represents random discrimination. The sidak option provides adjusted p-values comparing the ROC areas between

eGFR equations, assuming a "gold standard" being the CKD-EPI creatinine equation. For net reclassification improvement (NRI), participants were classified into three eGFR categories for all-cause and CVD hospitalization and/or mortality (≥75, 60–74.9 and <60 mL/min/1.73 m^2), and then reclassified into new eGFR categories with CKD-EPI cystatin C equation and CKD-EPI creatinine-cystatin C equation as compared with CKD-EPI creatinine equation. P-values of less than 0.05 in two tailed testing were considered statistically significant. The data was analysed using SPSS (version 15; SPSS Inc, Chicago, IL) and STATA (version 11 StataCorp LP, College Station, TX).

Results

Baseline characteristics

The baseline characteristics of study cohort as of 1998 are shown in table 1. The mean $\pm$ SD age of the participants was 75 ± 2.7 years. Among them, 42.7% had hypertension, 6.7% had diabetes and 36.5% were former/current smokers at the inception of the study. Using hospital discharge records, 23.4% of participants were deemed to have prevalent CVD (defined as having prior hospitalizations for CVD) and 1.5% prevalent renal disease (defined as having prior hospitalizations of any renal disease) between 1980 to study randomization. The mean $\pm$ SD eGFRs calculated by CKD-EPI creatinine equation, CKD-EPI cystatin C equation and CKD-EPI creatinine-cystatin C equation were 66.6 ± 13.3, 65.3 ± 14.8 and 65.7 ± 13.0 mL/min/1.73 m^2 respectively.

Association between eGFR, cardiovascular events and all-cause mortality

There was at least over 30% increase in CVD events between participants with eGFR of <60 mL/min/1.73 m^2 compared to those with eGFR of ≥75 mL/min/1.73 m^2 as measured by the CKD-EPI creatinine, CKD-EPI cystatin C and the CKD-EPI

Table 1. Baseline characteristics of the cohort.

Baseline Characteristics	All participants (n = 1,165)
Age, mean ± SD, years	75.2±2.7
Body mass index, mean ± SD, kg/m²	27.2±4.7
Systolic blood pressure, mean ± SD, mmHg	138.0±17.9
Diastolic blood pressure, mean ± SD, mmHg	73.1±11.0
Anti-hypertensive medications, No. (%)	497 (42.7)
Smoked ever, No. (%)	427 (36.5)
Diabetes, No. (%)	78 (6.7)
Cardiovascular disease at baseline (I00-I99), No. (%)	273 (23.4)
Renal disease at baseline, No. (%)	17 (1.5)
Calcium supplements, No. (%)	614 (52.7)
Biochemistry	
Creatinine, mean ± SD, mg/dL	0.9±0.2
Cystatin C, mean ± SD, mg/L	1.1±0.2
Estimated glomerular filtration rate by the CKD-EPI equations	
CKD-EPI creatinine-derived eGFR, mean ± SD, mL/min/1.73 m²	66.6±13.3
CKD-EPI Cystatin C-derived eGFR, mean ± SD, mL/min/1.73 m²	65.3±14.8
CKD-EPI Creatinine-cystatin C-derived eGFR, mean ± SD, mL/min/1.73 m²	65.7±13.0

Results are mean ± SD or number and (%). CVD cardiovascular disease, eGFR estimated glomerular filtration rate, CKD-EPI Chronic Kidney Disease EPIdemiology.

Table 2. Hazard ratios for clinical outcomes stratified by categories of eGFR in ml/min/1.73 m^2.

Characteristics (n = 1,165)	Hazard Ratio (95% CI)	P value
All-cause mortality (n = 231)		
CKD-EPI creatinine equation		0.318
≥75 ml/min/1.73 m^2	Referent	
60–74.9 ml/min/1.73 m^2	0.89 (0.63–1.26)	
<60 ml/min/1.73 m^2	1.14 (0.81–1.60)	
CKD-EPI cystatin C equation		0.208
≥75 ml/min/1.73 m^2	Referent	
60–74.9 ml/min/1.73 m^2	0.76 (0.53–1.07)	
<60 ml/min/1.73 m^2	0.96 (0.68–1.35)	
CKD-EPI creatinine-cystatin C equation		0.278
≥75 ml/min/1.73 m^2	Referent	
60–74.9 ml/min/1.73 m^2	0.80 (0.56–1.14)	
<60 ml/min/1.73 m^2	1.01 (0.71–1.45)	
Cardiovascular disease hospitalization/mortality (n = 469)		
CKD-EPI creatinine equation		0.028
≥75 ml/min/1.73 m^2	Referent	
60–74.9 ml/min/1.73 m^2	1.08 (0.84–1.39)	
<60 ml/min/1.73 m^2	1.36 (1.06–1.76)	
CKD-EPI cystatin C equation		0.031
≥75 ml/min/1.73 m^2	Referent	
60–74.9 ml/min/1.73 m^2	1.06 (0.81–1.37)	
<60 ml/min/1.73 m^2	1.35 (1.04–1.75)	
CKD-EPI creatinine-cystatin C equation		0.021
≥75 ml/min/1.73 m^2	Referent	
60–74.9 ml/min/1.73 m^2	1.21 (0.92–1.57)	
<60 ml/min/1.73 m^2	1.46 (1.11–1.91)	

Results are age and multivariable-adjusted hazard ratio (mean 95% CI) by eGFR categories by the three equations. eGFR - estimated glomerular filtration rate, CKD-EPI - Chronic Kidney Disease EPIdemiology equation. Multivariable adjustment includes age, body mass index, previous cardiovascular disease, previous renal disease, systolic blood pressure, antihypertensive medications, diabetes, smoking history and treatment.

creatinine-cystatic C equations (Table 2). However, there was no association between eGFR reduction and all-cause mortality for the three eGFR equations (Table 2). For CKD-EPI creatinine equation, the proportion of participants with prevalent renal disease in those with eGFR of <60, 60–75 and >75/mL/min/1.73 m^2 were 0.9%, 0.6% and 1.9% respectively (χ^2 3.01, p = 0.222), which was similar for CKD-EPI cystatin C and CKD-EPI creatinine-cystatin C equations.

Model discrimination

For prediction of all-cause mortality, the AUCs varied between 0.604 (95%CI 0.561, 0.647), 0.606 (95%CI 0.563, 0.649; Sidak p-value 0.963) and 0.606 (95%CI 0.563, 0.649; Sidak p-value 0.894) respectively using the CKD-EPI creatinine, CKD-EPI cystatin C and CKD-EPI creatinine-cystatin C equations adjusted for age, BMI, hypertension, diabetes, systolic blood pressure, prevalent renal disease and CVD, smoking history and treatment group (Figure 1). The correlation between the predicted probabilities of the adjusted model for all cause mortality using CKD-EPI creatinine equation compared with CKD-EPI creatinine-cystatin C equation is shown in Figure 2.

For the prediction of CVD hospitalization and/or mortality, the AUCs varied between 0.660 (95%CI 0.622, 0.712), 0.659 (95%CI 0.621, 0.710; Sidak p-value 0.974) and 0.660 (95%CI 0.622, 0.712; Sidak p-value 0.996) respectively using the CKD-EPI creatinine, CKD-EPI cystatin C and CKD-EPI creatinine-cystatin C equations adjusted for age, BMI, hypertension, diabetes, systolic blood pressure, prevalent renal disease and CVD, smoking history and treatment group (Figure 3). The correlation between the predicted probabilities of the adjusted model for CVD hospitalization and/or mortality using CKD-EPI creatinine equation compared with CKD-EPI creatinine-cystatin C equation is shown in Figure 4.

Net reclassification improvement

The reclassification of eGFR categories in predicting all-cause mortality and CVD hospitalization and/or mortality between CKD-EPI cystatin C and CKD-EPI creatinine-cystatin C equations compared with CKD-EPI creatinine equation is shown in Tables 3 and 4. For all-cause mortality, there was no significant improvement in net reclassification of eGFR categories with CKD-EPI cystatin C equation (NRI -4.1%, p = 0.401) or CKD-EPI creatinine-cystatin C equation (NRI -1.2%, p = 0.748) compared with CKD-EPI creatinine equation. For CVD hospitalization and/or mortality, there was no significant improvement in net reclassification of eGFR categories for CVD hospitalization

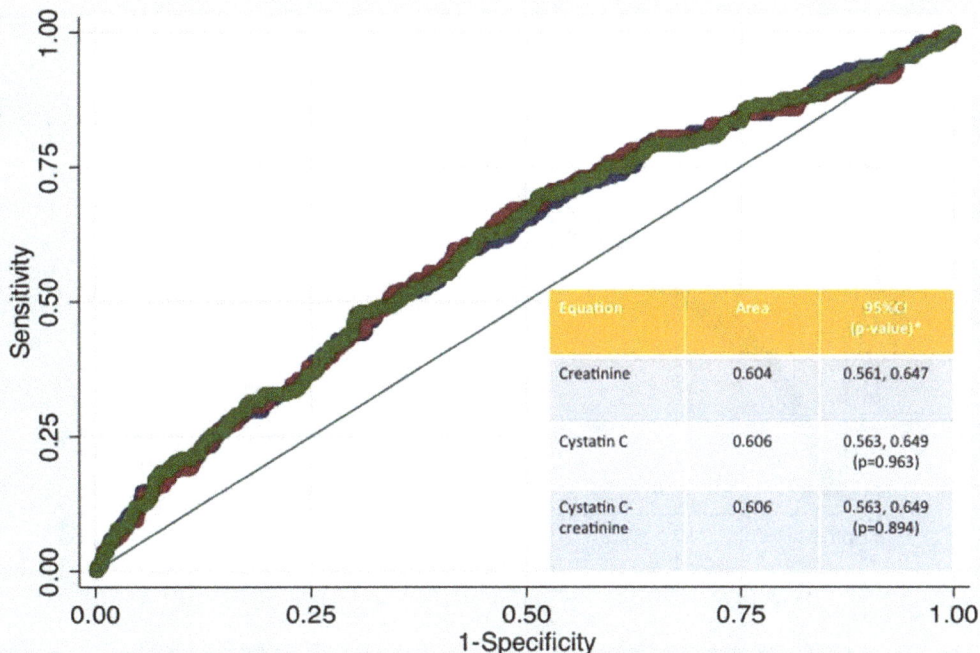

Equation	Area	95%CI (p-value)*
Creatinine	0.604	0.561, 0.647
Cystatin C	0.606	0.563, 0.649 (p=0.963)
Cystatin C-creatinine	0.606	0.563, 0.649 (p=0.894)

ROC adjusted for BMI, hypertension, diabetes, prevalent renal disease and CVD, smoker, treatment group
Sidak p-value compared to creatinine eGFR

Figure 1. Receiver Operating Characteristic curves of CKD-EPI creatinine, CKD-EPI cystatin C and CKD-EPI creatinine-cystatin C eGFR equations for all-cause mortality. Fully adjusted models include body mass index, previous cardiovascular disease, previous renal disease, anti-hypertensive medications, diabetes, smoking history and treatment code.

and/or mortality with CKD-EPI cystatin C equation (NRI 2.0%, p = 0. 614) and creatinine-cystatin C equation (NRI 3.0%, p = 0.351) compared with CKD-EPI creatinine equation.

Discussion

In elderly individuals, the accurate evaluation of eGFR for CKD staging is critical to determine correct drug dosing and risk

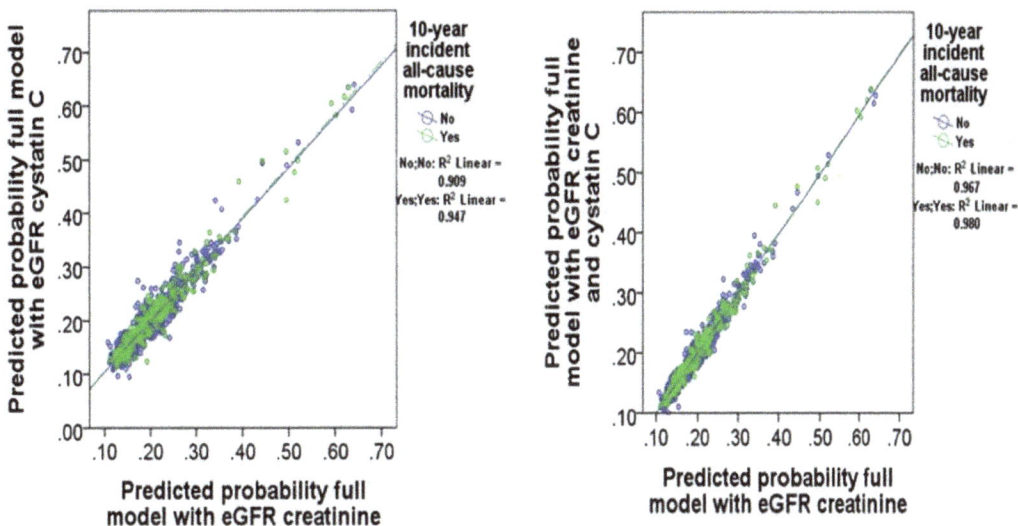

Figure 2. Receiver Operating Characteristic curves of CKD-EPI creatinine, CKD-EPI cystatin C and CKD-EPI creatinine-cystatin C eGFR equations for cardiovascular disease hospitalization and/or mortality. Fully adjusted models include body mass index, previous cardiovascular disease, previous renal disease, anti-hypertensive medications, diabetes, smoking history and treatment code.

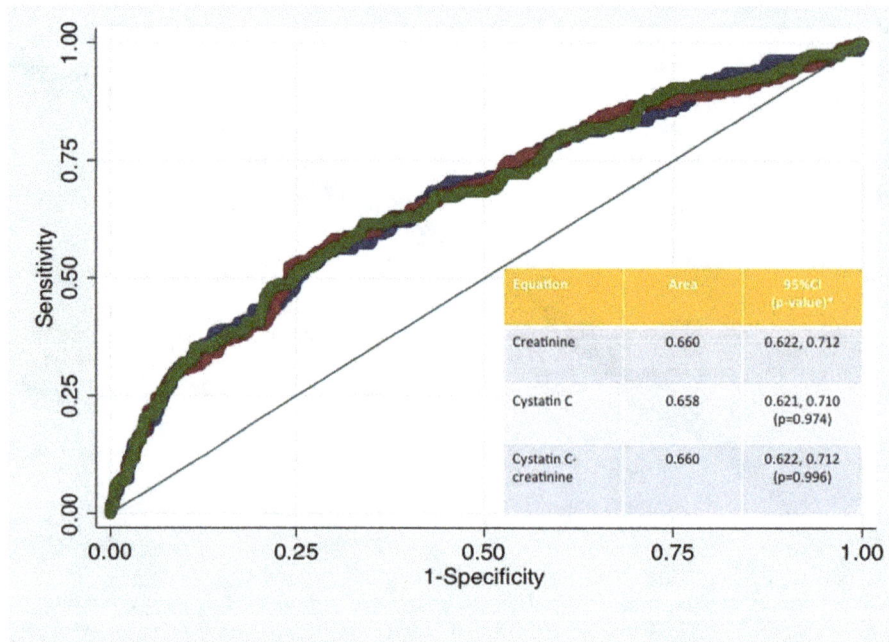

Equation	Area	95%CI (p-value)*
Creatinine	0.660	0.622, 0.712
Cystatin C	0.658	0.621, 0.710 (p=0.974)
Cystatin C-creatinine	0.660	0.622, 0.712 (p=0.996)

ROC adjusted for BMI, hypertension, diabetes, prevalent renal disease and CVD, smoker, treatment group
Sidak p-value compared to creatinine eGFR

Figure 3. Correlation of the predicted probabilities for cardiovascular disease hospitalization and/or mortality of CKD-EPI creatinine and CKD-EPI creatinine-cystatin C equations. Fully adjusted models include body mass index, previous cardiovascular disease, previous renal disease, anti-hypertensive medications, diabetes, smoking history and treatment code.

stratification for major clinical events including CVD and all-cause mortality. Our study findings suggest that the association between reduced GFR and clinical outcomes is similar for eGFR equations with and without cystatin C. In addition, the combined CKD-EPI creatinine-cystatin C eGFR or CKD-EPI cystatin C prediction equations were not superior in predicting or reclassifying CVD hospitalization and/or mortality or all-cause mortality over the CKD-EPI creatinine eGFR equation in a cohort of elderly women.

Cystatin C appears to be a superior GFR marker compared to creatinine [18,19]. Cystatin C is a low molecular weight protein (13 kDa) that is produced at a constant rate by all cells in the body, is freely filtered by the glomeruli and is completely reabsorbed and catabolised by the proximal tubules. Unlike creatinine, cystatin C is less likely to be influenced by muscle mass or diet and therefore may be a more reliable marker of GFR, particularly in older individuals, females and those with reduced muscle mass [20]. In

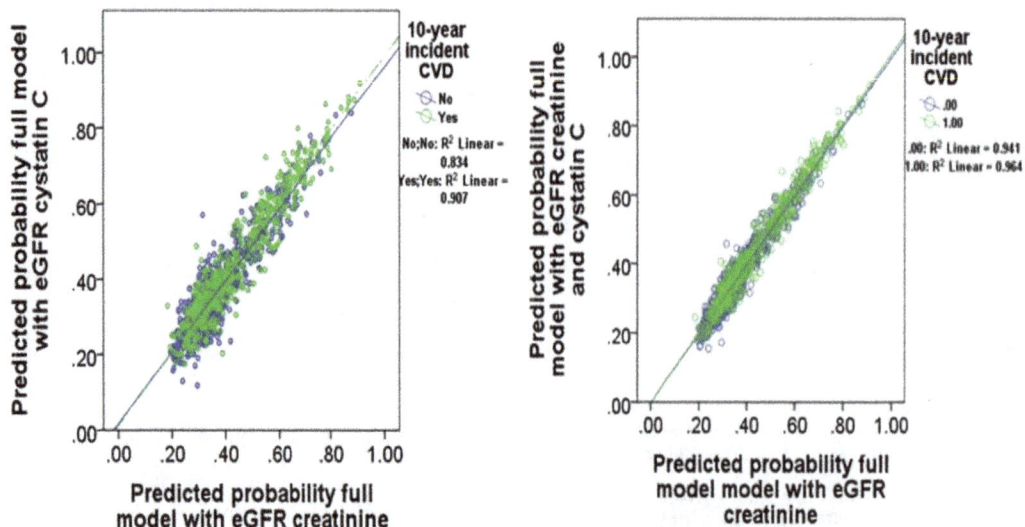

Figure 4. Correlation of the predicted probabilities for all-cause mortality of CKD-EPI creatinine and CKD-EPI creatinine-cystatin C equations. Fully adjusted models include body mass index, previous cardiovascular disease, previous renal disease, anti-hypertensive medications, diabetes, smoking history and treatment code.

Table 3. Net reclassification improvement of eGFR categories for all-cause mortality and cardiovascular disease hospitalization and/or mortality using CKD-EPI cystatin C equation compared with CKD-EPI creatinine equation.

All-cause mortality (Net reclassification improvement -4.1%, p = 0.401)						
	eGFR with CKD-EPI cystatin C equation					
eGFR with CKD-EPI creatinine equation	≥75	60–74.9	<60	Reclassified higher eGFR	Reclassified lower eGFR	Correctly reclassified
	Participants who died (n = 231)					
≥75	32	19	9	48 (20.8%)	50 (21.6%)	2 (0.8%)
60–74.9	22	37	22			
<60	6	20	64			
	Participants who did not die (n = 934)					
≥75	124	105	38	195 (20.9%)	241 (25.8%)	46 (4.9%)
60–74.9	95	191	98			
<60	20	80	183			
Cardiovascular disease hospitalization and/or mortality (Net reclassification improvement 2.0%, p = 0.614)						
	eGFR with CKD-EPI cystatin C equation					
eGFR with CKD-EPI creatinine equation	≥75	60–74.9	<60	Reclassified higher eGFR	Reclassified lower eGFR	Correctly reclassified
	Participants with an event (n = 469)					
≥75	50	42	18	91 (19.4%)	116 (24.7%)	25 (5.3%)
60–74.9	37	83	56			
<60	9	45	129			
	Participants without an event (n = 696)					
≥75	106	82	29	152 (21.8%)	175 (25.1%)	23 (3.3%)
60–74.9	80	145	64			
<60	17	55	118			

CVD risk factors include age, body mass index, previous cardiovascular disease, previous renal disease, systolic blood pressure, anti-hypertensive medications, diabetes, smoking history and treatment code. CVD indicates cardiovascular disease; eGFR estimated glomerular filtration rate and CKD-EPI - Chronic Kidney Disease Epidemiology equation.

several studies, compared with creatinine, cystatin C is more accurate in stratifying the risk of CVD and all-cause mortality in elderly individuals [21]. In a cohort of 3,075 participants aged over 70 years, each SD reduction (0.3 g/L) in cystatin C concentration was associated with an increased risk of all-cause mortality (HR 1.24, 95% CI 1.20, 1.28) and CVD mortality (HR 1.20, 95% CI 1.11, 1.30) [22]. In a population-based prospective observational cohort of 9988 individuals aged 45–64 years, cystatin C level was a much stronger predictor of all-cause mortality, coronary artery disease events, heart failure events and end-stage renal disease compared to estimates of GFR derived from CKD-EPI creatinine equation [23]. Other studies have corroborated these findings and have also shown that cystatin C level may identify the group of CKD patients that may not be identified by CKD-EPI equation as being at high risk of CVD events and all-cause mortality [24,25]. In contrast, a recent study by *Eriksen et al.* has shown that cystatin C was not superior in estimating measured GFR compared to creatinine in the general population [26] and other studies have suggested that the strong association between cystatin C and CVD or all-cause mortality may be related to other factors including body size and the presence of diabetes and inflammation [27]. The discrepant findings between studies may reflect dissimilar population of varying ages, differences in participants' characteristics such as BMI and presence of comorbidities.

Two recently developed CKD-EPI creatinine-cystatin C and CKD-EPI cystatin C equations were shown to perform better in predicting measured radionuclide GFR compared to CKD-EPI creatinine equation [14]. Although bias was similar in all three eGFR equations in predicting measured GFR, the combined CKD-EPI creatinine-cystatin C equation had greater precision and accuracy resulting in a more accurate classification of measured GFR as <60 ml/min/1.73 m^2. The use of the combined CKD-EPI creatinine-cystatin C equation was able to improve reclassification of individuals with creatinine-derived eGFR of 45–74 ml/min/1.73 m^2 (net reclassification index 19.4; 95% CI, 8.7 to 30.1; P<0.001), and also 17% of individuals with creatinine-based eGFR of 45–59 ml/min/1.73 m^2 to ≥60 ml/min/1.73 m^2. In a recent meta-analysis of 11 general population studies comprising of 90,750 participants, there was a more consistent linear association between reduced eGFR derived from CKD-EPI cystatin C and CKD-EPI creatinine-cystatin C equations and increased risks of all-cause and CVD mortality for all eGFR values below 85 mL/min/1.73 m^2 compared with CKD-EPI creatinine equation, well above the threshold of 60 mL/min/1.73 m^2 for the detection of CKD with CKD-EPI creatinine-based eGFR [12]. The NRI using either CKD-EPI cystatin C-derived equations for all-cause and CVD mortality was 0.23 (95%CI 0.18, 0.28) and 0.17 (95%CI 0.11, 0.23) respectively suggesting that cystatin C-derived eGFR equations strengthens the association between eGFR and clinical outcomes. However, in this

Table 4. Net reclassification improvement of eGFR categories for all-cause mortality and cardiovascular disease hospitalization and/or mortality using CKD-EPI creatinine-cystatin C equation compared with CKD-EPI creatinine equation.

All-cause mortality (Net reclassification improvement -1.2%, p = 0.748)

eGFR with CKD-EPI creatinine equation	eGFR with CKD-EPI creatinine-cystatin C equation			Reclassified higher eGFR	Reclassified lower eGFR	Correctly reclassified
	≥75	60–74.9	<60			
Participants who died (n = 231)						
≥75	41	19	0	30 (13.0%)	36 (15.6%)	6 (2.6%)
60–74.9	13	51	17			
<60	0	17	73			
Participants who did not die (n = 934)						
≥75	178	85	4	110 (11.8%)	146 (15.6%)	36 (3.8%)
60–74.9	52	275	57			
<60	0	58	225			

Cardiovascular disease hospitalization and/or mortality (Net reclassification improvement 3.0%, p = 0.351)

eGFR with CKD-EPI creatinine equation	eGFR with CKD-EPI creatinine-cystatin C equation			Reclassified higher eGFR	Reclassified lower eGFR	Correctly reclassified
	≥75	60–74.9	<60			
Participants with an event (n = 469)						
≥75	70	38	2	47 (10.0%)	72 (15.4%)	25 (5.4%)
60–74.9	16	128	32			
<60	0	31	152			
Participants without an event (n = 696)						
≥75	149	66	2	93 (13.4%)	110 (15.8%)	17 (2.4%)
60–74.9	49	198	42			
<60	0	44	146			

CVD risk factors include age, body mass index, previous cardiovascular disease, previous renal disease, systolic blood pressure, anti-hypertensive medications, diabetes, smoking history and treatment code. CVD indicates cardiovascular disease; eGFR estimated glomerular filtration rate and CKD-EPI - Chronic Kidney Disease Epidemiology equation.

meta-analysis, there were only two studies that have included exclusively elderly participants with mean age of over 70 years. The ULSAM study from Sweden included only men and the CHS study included 41% men and 17% participants were of Black race [28,29]. In both these studies, there was a large difference in mean eGFR across the three equations, with eGFR derived from CKD-EPI creatinine equation being much higher compared to both cystatin C equations. Our study has shown that the newly derived CKD-EPI cystatin C and CKD-EPI creatinine-cystatin C equations did not improve reclassification of eGFR categories that predicted the risk of CVD hospitalization and/or mortality or all-cause mortality compared to the commonly used CKD-EPI creatinine equation. The observed differences to the result of the meta-analysis may reflect dissimilar population characteristics with the studies included in the meta-analysis comprising men and women across all age categories and ethnicity compared to only elderly Caucasian women in our study. In addition, all elderly participants in this study were relatively healthy over the age of 70 with mild renal dysfunction, with the majority of participants within a relatively narrow range of eGFRs. In the two population cohorts of similar age (CHS and ULSAM studies), there were major differences in gender, race, BMI, comorbid status and baseline creatinine compared to this cohort, which may have contributed to the differences in study findings. There may also be potential errors in creatinine and cystatin C measurements and insufficient power in our study to detect significant differences

between the eGFR equations or to detect a significant associations between these equations and all-cause mortality, which all may have contributed to differences in the reported study findings.

The strengths of this study include the use of a large prospective cohort of subjects with complete and accurate data collection over a 10-year period. We were able to accurately examine the association between estimates of GFR using the newly developed cystatin C equations and clinical outcomes in a population with a low prevalence of CVD and renal diseases, which further strengthens this association. However, the strengths of the study must be balanced against the limitations, which include a lack of radionuclide GFR measurements and availability of single time-point measurements of creatinine and cystatin C to estimate baseline GFR. In addition, our study cohort only included white female participants with presumed adequate nutrition and muscle mass (BMI mean $\pm$ SD of 27 ± 5 kg/m^2) and therefore the applicability of our study findings to males, other ethnic minorities or racial groups and those with poor nutrition and low muscle mass remains unclear.

In conclusion, the newly developed CKD-EPI cystatin C and combined CKD-EPI creatinine-cystatin C-derived eGFR equations were not superior in predicting CVD events or all-cause mortality compared with the commonly used CKD-EPI creatinine-derived eGFR equation in older female subjects with no or early CKD and this data cannot be extrapolated to older individuals with more advanced CKD. With a substantial cost-difference between measurements of creatinine and cystatin C, together with the uncertainty of the value of cystatin C-derived eGFR equations in predicting clinical events over creatinine-derived eGFR equation, the utility and cost-effectiveness of cystatin C in the elderly must be investigated further prior to implementation in clinical practice.

Acknowledgments

The authors wish to thank the staff at the Data Linkage Branch, Hospital Morbidity Data Collection and Registry of Births, Deaths and Marriages for their work on providing the data for this study.

Disclaimer: The results presented in this paper have not been published previously in whole or part, except in abstract form.

Author Contributions

Conceived and designed the experiments: WL JL GW RP. Performed the experiments: WL JL GW. Analyzed the data: WL JL GW. Contributed reagents/materials/analysis tools: WL JL GW EL. Wrote the paper: WL JL GW RT EL PT RP.

References

1. Couser WG, Remuzzi G, Mendis S, Tonelli M (2011) The contribution of chronic kidney disease to the global burden of major noncommunicable diseases. Kidney Int 80: 1258–1270.
2. Go AS, Chertow GM, Fan D, McCulloch CE, Hsu CY (2004) Chronic kidney disease and the risks of death, cardiovascular events, and hospitalization. N Engl J Med 351: 1296–1305.
3. Levey AS, Stevens LA, Schmid CH, Zhang YL, Castro AF 3rd, et al. (2009) A new equation to estimate glomerular filtration rate. Ann Intern Med 150: 604–612.
4. Ford I, Bezlyak V, Stott DJ, Sattar N, Packard CJ, et al. (2009) Reduced glomerular filtration rate and its association with clinical outcome in older patients at risk of vascular events: secondary analysis. PLoS Med 6: e16.
5. Matsushita K, Mahmoodi BK, Woodward M, Emberson JR, Jafar TH, et al. (2012) Comparison of risk prediction using the CKD-EPI equation and the MDRD study equation for estimated glomerular filtration rate. JAMA 307: 1941–1951.
6. Wong G, Hayen A, Chapman JR, Webster AC, Wang JJ, et al. (2009) Association of CKD and cancer risk in older people. J Am Soc Nephrol 20: 1341–1350.
7. Anavekar NS, McMurray JJ, Velazquez EJ, Solomon SD, Kober L, et al. (2004) Relation between renal dysfunction and cardiovascular outcomes after myocardial infarction. N Engl J Med 351: 1285–1295.
8. Drawz P, Rosenberg M (2013) Slowing progression of chronic kidney diese. Kidney Int Suppl 3: 372–376.
9. Mathew TH, Johnson DW, Jones GR (2007) Chronic kidney disease and automatic reporting of estimated glomerular filtration rate: revised recommendations. Med J Aust 187: 459–463.
10. Cockcroft DW, Gault MH (1976) Prediction of creatinine clearance from serum creatinine. Nephron 16: 31–41.
11. Swedko PJ, Clark HD, Paramsothy K, Akbari A (2003) Serum creatinine is an inadequate screening test for renal failure in elderly patients. Arch Intern Med 163: 356–360.
12. Shlipak MG, Matsushita K, Arnlov J, Inker LA, Katz R, et al. (2013) Cystatin C versus creatinine in determining risk based on kidney function. N Engl J Med 369: 932–943.
13. Prince RL, Devine A, Dhaliwal SS, Dick IM (2006) Effects of calcium supplementation on clinical fracture and bone structure: results of a 5-year, double-blind, placebo-controlled trial in elderly women. Arch Intern Med 166: 869–875.
14. Inker LA, Schmid CH, Tighiouart H, Eckfeldt JH, Feldman HI, et al. (2012) Estimating glomerular filtration rate from serum creatinine and cystatin C. N Engl J Med 367: 20–29.
15. Britt H (1997) A new coding tool for computerised clinical systems in primary care—ICPC plus. Aust Fam Physician 26 Suppl 2: S79–82.
16. World Health Organization (1977) Manual of the international statistical classification of diseases, injuries, and causes of death: based on the recommendations of the ninth revision conference, 1975, and adopted by the Twenty-ninth World Health Assembly. Geneva: World Health Organization. 2v. p.
17. World Health Organization (2004) ICD-10: international statistical classification of diseases and related health problems: tenth revision. Geneva: World Health Organization. 3v. p.
18. Dharnidharka VR, Kwon C, Stevens G (2002) Serum cystatin C is superior to serum creatinine as a marker of kidney function: a meta-analysis. Am J Kidney Dis 40: 221–226.
19. Roos JF, Doust J, Tett SE, Kirkpatrick CM (2007) Diagnostic accuracy of cystatin C compared to serum creatinine for the estimation of renal dysfunction in adults and children—a meta-analysis. Clin Biochem 40: 383–391.
20. Laterza O, Price C, Scott M (2002) Cystatin C: an improved estimator of glomerular filtration rate? Clin Chem 48: 699–707.
21. Shlipak MG, Sarnak MJ, Katz R, Fried LF, Seliger SL, et al. (2005) Cystatin C and the risk of death and cardiovascular events among elderly persons. N Engl J Med 352: 2049–2060.
22. Shlipak MG, Wassel Fyr CL, Chertow GM, Harris TB, Kritchevsky SB, et al. (2006) Cystatin C and mortality risk in the elderly: the health, aging, and body composition study. J Am Soc Nephrol 17: 254–261.
23. Astor BC, Shafi T, Hoogeveen RC, Matsushita K, Ballantyne CM, et al. (2012) Novel markers of kidney function as predictors of ESRD, cardiovascular disease, and mortality in the general population. Am J Kidney Dis 59: 653–662.
24. Peralta CA, Katz R, Sarnak MJ, Ix J, Fried LF, et al. (2011) Cystatin C identifies chronic kidney disease patients at higher risk for complications. J Am Soc Nephrol 22: 147–155.
25. Shlipak MG, Katz R, Sarnak MJ, Fried LF, Newman AB, et al. (2006) Cystatin C and prognosis for cardiovascular and kidney outcomes in elderly persons without chronic kidney disease. Ann Intern Med 145: 237–246.
26. Eriksen BO, Mathisen UD, Melsom T, Ingebretsen OC, Jenssen TG, et al. (2010) Cystatin C is not a better estimator of GFR than plasma creatinine in the general population. Kidney Int 78: 1305–1311.
27. Stevens LA, Schmid CH, Greene T, Li L, Beck GJ, et al. (2009) Factors other than glomerular filtration rate affect serum cystatin C levels. Kidney Int 75: 652–660.
28. Shlipak M, Katz R, Kestenbaum B, Fried L, Newman A, et al. (2009) Rate of kidney function decline in older adults: a comparison using creatinine and cystatin C. Am J Nephrol 30: 171–178.
29. Ingelsson E, Sundstrom J, Lind L, Riserus U, Larsson A, et al. (2007) Low-grade albuminuria and the incidence of heart failure in a community-based cohort of elderly men. Eur Heart J 28: 1739–1745.

4

Differences in COPD Patient Care by Primary Family Caregivers: An Age-Based Study

Peng-Ching Hsiao[1], Chi-Ming Chu[2], Pei-Yi Sung[3], Wann-Cherng Perng[4], Kwua-Yun Wang[5]*

1 Graduate Institute of Medical Sciences, National Defense Medical Center, Department of Nursing, Tri-Service General Hospital, Taipei, Taiwan, 2 Section of Health Informatics, Institute of Public Health, National Defense Medical Center and University, Taipei, Taiwan, 3 Department of Nursing, Taoyuan Branch, Taipei Veterans General Hospital, Taoyuan, Taiwan, 4 Division of Pulmonary and Critical Care Medicine, Department of Internal Medicine, Tri-Service General Hospital, National Defense Medical Center, Taipei, Taiwan, 5 Graduate Institute of Medical Sciences, National Defense Medical Center, Department of Nursing, Taipei Veterans General Hospital, Taipei, Taiwan

Abstract

Background: Because Taiwan has the fastest aging rate among developed countries, care for the elderly is becoming more prominent in the country. Primary family caregivers play an important role in patient health and health promotion behavior. Chronic obstructive pulmonary disease (COPD), an age-related disease, is a major public health problem with high morbidity and mortality and can be a long-term burden for family members; however, little attention has been given to the differences in COPD care between elder caregivers and other caregivers. This study aimed to investigate the differences between elder family caregivers and non-elder family caregivers caring for COPD patients in Taiwan, including caring behavior, caregiver response, and caring knowledge.

Methods: This cross-sectional study was conducted between March 2007 and January 2008; 406 primary family caregivers of COPD patients from the thoracic outpatient departments of 6 hospitals in north-central Taiwan were recruited to answer questionnaires measuring COPD characteristics, care behavior, caregiver response, and COPD knowledge. All questionnaires, which addressed caregiver knowledge, care behaviors, and care reactions, were shown to have acceptable validity and reliability, and the data were analyzed using univariate and generalized linear model techniques.

Results: The elder caregivers group had 79 participants, and the non-elder caregivers comprised 327 participants. The COPD-related knowledge scale results were positively correlated with the family caregiver caring behavior scale, suggesting that better COPD-related knowledge among family caregivers may result in improved caring behavior. After adjusting for all possible confounding factors, the elder caregivers had significantly lower COPD-related knowledge than the non-elder caregivers (P<0.001). However, there were no significant differences in the family caregiver caring behavior scale or the caregiver reaction assessment scale between the two groups.

Conclusions: Elder family caregivers require increased education regarding medications and preventive care in COPD patient care.

Editor: Jerson Laks, Federal University of Rio de Janeiro, Brazil

Funding: This study was supported by a grant from Health Promotion Administration, Ministry of Health and Welfare, Taiwan (DOH96-HP-1101). The funders had no role in study design, data collection and analysis, decision to publish, or preparation of the manuscript.

Competing Interests: The authors have declared that no competing interests exist.

* Email: kywang7@vghtpe.gov.tw

Introduction

The aging of the population is a global phenomenon that is both inevitable and predictable [1]. There is no exception in Taiwan. The proportion of Taiwanese elders aged over 65 reached 10.7 percent in 2011 and is expected to be 14 percent in 2017 and 20 percent in 2025. The Taiwanese old-age dependency ratio $(((age>65)/(age\ 15–64))*100)$ was 7:1 in 2011 and is expected to be 4:1 in 2022 and 2:1 in 2039. Taiwan will be a super-aged society, and its aging rate will be the fastest among developed countries [2]. Thus, elder care by elders will become more common. However, with the population quickly aging and productivity rapidly declining, people in Taiwan will assume larger medical expenses and greater costs for long-term care [2]. Family caregiving represents the first and predominant source of care for 75 to 80% of people with chronic

illnesses. Family can be an entity responsible for the care of a sick person [3]. Primary caregivers, especially family caregivers, play an important role in patient health and health promotion behavior [4–7]. Caring for patients with chronic disease often exhausts caregivers and has a negative psychological impact on caregivers [8]. In people with chronic illnesses, increased knowledge can reduce the negative psychological impact on the patients or caregivers, including anxiety and depression, and can enhance care efficiency [9–11]. Therefore, knowledge may maximize the quality of caring behavior and decrease the potential negative effects on caregivers. Caregivers with negative caring behavior, overloaded caregiver burdens, and a lack of caring knowledge lead to negative patient health and health promotion behavior outcomes [6,12–14]. Therefore, the caregivers' caring behavior, caregiver burden, and caring knowledge may inevitably affect the patients. However, little is known concerning

COPD-related knowledge, caring behavior, and the burden on primary family caregivers in Taiwan. The elderly not only have higher physical and mental burdens than other age groups, but they also have higher economic burdens [15–17]. Little is known about elder family members as primary caregivers [12], especially regarding the difference between elder primary family caregivers and non-elder primary family caregivers. We hypothesized that elder primary family caregivers have different caring behavior, higher caregiver burdens, and less caring knowledge than young primary family caregivers due to the elders' physical and psychosocial development.

Chronic obstructive pulmonary disease (COPD) is a major public health problem that affects approximately 1/3 of adults and 1/5 of subjects above 65 years old; the prevalence of COPD is high and increasing [18]. Aging is associated with a marked increase in the prevalence of COPD [18,19]. Furthermore, the majority of epidemiological studies on COPD, which is usually identified as an age-related disease, have focused on the elderly population [20,21]. Additionally, respiratory symptoms, hospitalization, morbidity, mortality, depression, and anxiety have been reported to be higher in subjects with a diagnosis of COPD than in patients with other respiratory diseases [18,20,21]. As a result, COPD can become a long-term burden for family members who serve as day-to-day caregivers and may cause healthcare systems to incur substantial costs [22]. Elder caregivers who care for COPD patients may have higher caregiver burdens than other caregivers. This study aimed to investigate the differences between elder family caregivers and non-elder family caregivers in caring for COPD patients, including caring behavior, caregiver response, and caring knowledge. The results of this study may assist health practitioners in designing appropriate interventions to improve elder caregiver burden and allow elders to age actively.

Methods

Participants

This cross-sectional study was conducted between March 2007 and January 2008. Four hundred and six primary family caregivers were recruited from the thoracic outpatient departments of 3 medical centers and 3 regional hospitals in north-central Taiwan using convenience sampling. Primary family caregivers were defined as family members who provided regular, nearly daily care for a family member diagnosed with COPD as defined by the Global Initiative for Chronic Obstructive Lung Disease (GOLD) [23]. The inclusion criteria were being a primary family caregiver of a COPD patient, having normal cognitive functioning (obtaining SPMSQ scores of 8 or above) [24], and self-reporting the absence of psychiatric illness, such as anxiety, depression, bipolar, schizophrenia and dementia. Participants aged 65 years or older were classified as elder caregivers, and participants below 65 years old were classified as non-elder caregivers. A pilot study was conducted one month before the formal study. We collected data from 20 participants for the pilot study. All participants were individually administered the questionnaires in an office near the outpatient department. The participants were asked to respond to the questions either by writing their answers or by responding orally to the investigator and immediately returned the completed questionnaires on site. The participant response rate was 100 percent.

Ethics

This study was approved by the Institutional Review Board in Taiwan (IRB NO. TSGHIRB 096-05-015). Written informed consent was obtained from all participants.

Measuring instruments

Data were collected by administering 4 questionnaires, including one questionnaire on the participants' background information, the family caregiver caring behavior scale (FCCBS), the caregiver reaction assessment scale (CRAS), and the COPD-related knowledge scale (CRKS).

In terms of the participants' background information, the following data were collected: age, sex, marital status, religious status, highest educational level, socioeconomic status, sharing responsibility with family (the caregiver could share caregiving during with other family members), presence of chronic disease, residence with the patient, relationship to the patient, presence of other care-needed person(s) at home, and frequency of care.

The family caregiver caring behavior scale (FCCBS) was revised from the Family Caregivers of Cancer Patients Care-Taking Scale [25]. The scale was developed in Chinese. The scale is composed of 49 questions and divided into 4 subscales: care of companionship and monitoring, alternative care of social and general affairs, care of communication and emotion, and care of maintaining physical function. Zero points indicate no need to execute, 1 point indicates does not really need to execute, 2 points indicate sometimes needs to execute, 3 points indicate usually needs to execute, and 4 points indicate always need to execute. A higher score indicates relatively more caring behavior from the primary family caregiver. The professional validity of this score was assessed by the content validity index (CVI) [26], which was 0.98. The internal consistency was evaluated by Cronbach's α coefficient; this coefficient was 0.76 for the total scale and 0.30-0.70 for the subscales in the pilot study and 0.96 for the total scale and 0.88–0.93 for the subscales in the full study.

The caregiver reaction assessment scale (CRAS) developed by Given et al. in 1992 is used to evaluate a caregiver's perceptions of caregiving and reflects the actual workload of a caregiver [27]. We used the Chinese translation of the CRAS. The scale is composed of 24 questions. A 5-point Likert score is used, with higher scores indicating a relatively more positive reaction by the primary family caregiver and a lower actual workload. The professional validity of this score was assessed by the CVI [26], which was 1.00; the internal consistency was evaluated by Cronbach's α coefficient, which was 0.82 for the total scale in the pilot study and 0.62 for the total scale in the full study.

The COPD-related knowledge scale (CRKS) was a modified version of the Bristol COPD Knowledge Questionnaire (BCKQ), which was originally developed by White et al. in 2006 to evaluate changes in COPD patient knowledge after education [28]. In this study, we used the CRKS to represent the primary family caregivers' knowledge level about COPD. After translation and back translation, experts reviewed the scale question by question for appropriateness. According to the experts' suggestions, we added a question regarding nutrition issues with COPD and used 8 parts of the original scale, including understanding of COPD, elimination of sputum, inhaled bronchodilators, inhaled steroids, antibiotic therapy, exercise, smoking cessation, and vaccines. Each part of the scale contained 5 questions. One point was given if the primary family caregiver responded with a correct answer. In contrast, no point was given if the primary family caregiver responded with an incorrect answer or responded that he/she did not know the correct answer. A higher score indicated a higher level of COPD-related knowledge. The professional validity of this score was assessed by the CVI [26], which was 0.98; the internal consistency was evaluated by Kuder-Richardson Formula 20 and was 0.76.

Statistical analyses

Continuous and categorical variables are presented as the means ± SD and the numbers (percentage), respectively. In the univariate analysis, independent t-tests and one-way analysis of variance (ANOVA) were performed to examine differences between the categorical variables and the COPD-related knowledge scale (CRKS); the Mann-Whitney U test was performed to examine differences between the categorical variables and the family caregiver caring behavior scale (FCCBS) and the caregiver reaction assessment scale (CRAS). Spearman's rank correlation was implemented to analyze the correlation between continuous variables, as implemented by Garrod et al. [29]. Factors with P values≤0.05 in the univariate analysis were included in a generalized linear model (GLM) to control for their effects and determine the differences in the FCCBS, caregiver response scale, and CRKS between the elder family caregivers and the non-elder family caregivers. Cronbach's α coefficient was used to determine the reliability, and the CVI was used to validate the scales. All 2-sided statistics were performed with SPSS 17.0 statistical software (SPSS, Chicago, Illinois). Statistical significance was defined as a P value<0.05.

Results

Table 1 summarizes the characteristics of all 406 primary family caregivers of COPD patients. The elder caregivers group had 79 participants, and the non-elder caregivers group had 327 participants. Almost 1/4 of the primary family caregivers were elders. Both groups had more females than males. The majority of both groups was married, was religious, had low socioeconomic status, and was living with the COPD patient. In both groups, few participants reported having other care-needed person(s) at home. There were no significant differences between the two groups regarding being religious or weekly days of care. However, there were significant differences between the two groups in other background characteristics. The elder group had more females than the non-elder group. More than half of the elder caregivers were the spouses of the patients, with an elementary school education level or below; the elder caregivers had been caring for the patient for a mean of 7.3 years, 6.4 days per week, and 17.9 hours per day. Among the non-elder caregivers, more than half were the son or daughter of the patient, with an education level above senior high school; the non-elder caregivers had been caring for the patient for a mean of 5.2 years, 6.1 days per week, and 12.6 hours per day. The elder group had lower socioeconomic status and more daily hours and duration of care than the non-elder group. A higher proportion of the elder group was living with the COPD patient and had other care-needed person(s) at home compared with the non-elder group.

Three-quarters of the elder caregivers could not share caregiving responsibilities with family at home on a daily basis. However, half of the non-elder caregivers could share caregiving duties with family at home on a daily basis. Almost half of the elder group reported having a chronic illness themselves, whereas only 22.9 percent of the non-elder group reported having a chronic illness themselves.

Table 2 shows the results of the Spearman rank correlation between the caregivers' total COPD-related knowledge scale (CRKS) scores, the family caregiver caring behavior scale (FCCBS) scores, the caregiver reaction assessment scale (CRAS) scores, and the continuous characteristics. The CRKS scores were negatively correlated with daily hours of care, suggesting that high COPD-related knowledge may result in more effective daily care. The FCCBS scores were positively correlated with daily hours of care and negatively correlated with weekly days of care. Moreover,

the CRAS scores were negatively correlated with daily hours of care, suggesting that more caring behavior may result in increased daily hours of care and, thus, more negative reactions and fewer weekly days of care.

Table 3 presents the comparison of the caregivers' total COPD-related knowledge scale (CRKS) scores, the family caregiver caring behavior scale (FCCBS), and the caregiver reaction assessment scale (CRAS) among family caregivers with different categorical characteristics. The results indicate that differences in the caregivers' marital status, the presence of other care-needing person(s) at home, and the caregivers' relationship to the patient were related to the caregivers' FCCBS scores. There were significant differences in CRAS scores between male and female caregivers, and among caregivers with different highest educational levels, socioeconomic status, rotations of responsibility with family, other (chronic) disease, and other care-needed person(s) at home. In addition, differences in the caregivers' sex, marital status, educational level, socioeconomic status, rotation of responsibility with family, and relationship to the patient were related to the caregivers' CRKS scores.

Table 4, Table 5 and Table 6 show the results of a GLM controlling for confounding effects to determine differences in family caregiver caring behaviors, caregiver responses, and COPD-related knowledge between the elder family caregivers and the non-elder family caregivers. Variables that significantly correlated with the family caregiver caring behaviors scale, caregiver response scale, and COPD-related knowledge scale (CRKS) from the univariate analysis and significant subject characteristics (P<0.05) were adjusted for use in the GLM. The results of the GLM showed that after adjusting for the correlated variables, the elder group had significantly lower COPD-related knowledge scores than the non-elder group. However, there were no significant differences between the two groups in family caregiver caring behaviors scores or caregiver response scores. Furthermore, we analyzed differences in the subscales of the CRKS between the two groups using the GLM. The results indicated that after adjusting for the correlated variables, the elder group had significantly lower scores than the non-elder group in the understanding of COPD, inhaled bronchodilators, inhaled steroids, antibiotic therapy, smoking cessation, and vaccines (Table 5 and Table 6).

Discussion

In our study, most caregivers were female. With respect to the two groups, we found that the elder group had more females than the non-elder group. The majority of the elder group was spouses, while the majority of the non-elder group was sons or daughters. Most previous studies have indicated that women are the major primary family caregivers, especially in caring for the elderly or patients with chronic disease [6,8,12]. Currently, the number of females working is increasing; therefore, the caregiving duties for families with chronic disease have few gender differences in the non-elder group. In Taiwan, spouses remain the primary family caregiver due to Chinese culture, especially in the elder group [30–32]. Our data showed that a higher proportion of elder caregivers had low socioeconomic status compared with non-elder caregivers. A reason for this difference might be that the non-elder group primarily consisted of sons or daughters who were still working and saving money. Therefore, elder caregivers have greater potential physical and economic care stress than non-elder caregivers, especially elder female caregivers in Taiwan. Further policies or interventions to reduce care stress among elder caregivers demand immediate attention.

Table 1. Characteristics of study participants.

Characteristic	Elder caregivers (n = 79)	Non elder caregivers (n = 327)	P
Sex, no. (%)			0.002*
Male	17(21.5)	131(40.1)	
Female	62(78.5)	196(59.9)	
Married, no. (%)#	73(92.4)	271(82.9)	0.035*
Religious, no. (%)	68(86.1)	254(77.7)	0.098
Highest educational level, no. (%)			<0.001*
Elementary school	55(69.6)	69(21.1)	
Junior high school	8(10.1)	50(15.3)	
Senior high school	7(8.9)	100(30.6)	
College or above	9(11.4)	107(32.7)	
Social economic status, no. (%)			<0.001*
Low	67(84.8)	151(46.2)	
Moderate	5(6.3)	85(26.0)	
High	7(8.9)	91(27.8)	
Sharing responsibility with family, no. (%)	20(25.3)	185(56.6)	<0.001*
Chronic disease, no. (%)	39(49.4)	75(22.9)	<0.001*
Living with patient, no. (%)	72(91.1)	243(74.3)	0.001
Relation with patient			<0.001*
Spouse	66(83.5)	95(29.1)	
Son or daughter	79(8.9)	201(61.5)	
others	6(7.6)	31(9.5)	
Other care-needed person(s) in home, no. (%)	3(3.8)	49(15.0)	0.008*
Duration of care, mean± SD, y	7.3±6.0	5.2±3.9	<0.001*
Weekly days of care, mean ± SD	6.4±1.8	6.1±2.0	0.014*
Daily hours of care, mean ± SD	17.9±8.3	12.6±8.7	0.353

* The P value ≦0.05.
# Widow, widower, separated couple, or divorced people were not included.

Our study showed that the higher the number of daily hours of care, the higher the family caregivers' caring behaviors and the more negative the family caregivers' caring reactions. These results are consistent with the results of Alpass et al., who showed that caregivers providing higher levels of care reported a more negative psychological response and poorer mental health. The study also demonstrated that caregivers providing higher levels of care and more care across time had poorer health outcomes. Long-term and heavy daily caregiving may have detrimental effects on health status due to a lack of formal support resources and the strain of multiple roles [12].

There were no significant differences between groups in the total caregiver caring behaviors scale scores, nor were there differences in any of the caregiver caring behavior subscale scores. Our data indicate that the older caregivers had a tendency toward less caregiver caring behaviors. Elders are not as strong physically as non-elders, which may explain why the elders tended to have fewer caregiver caring behaviors than non-elders.

Our data indicate that the more caring knowledge caregivers have, the less daily hours of care they provide and, thus, the more positive caring reaction the caregivers have. Research has shown that caring for patients with chronic disease often makes caregivers feel physically and psychologically exhausted and leads to a more negative psychological impact on caregivers [8]. Friedemann et al. also indicated that patients' functional limitations yielded the strongest predictive coefficients followed by caregiver stress [33].

Table 2. Correlation between CRKS, FCCBS, CRAS, and continuous characteristics.

Variable	FCCBS (r (P))	CRAS (r (P))	CRKS (r (P))
Duration of care	−0.03(0.576)	−0.01(0.867)	0.03(0.603)
Weekly days of care	−0.11(0.033)*	0.02(0.725)	0.09(0.083)
Daily hours of care	0.13(0.011)*	−0.16(0.001)*	−0.15(0.002)*

* The P value ≦0.05.
FCCBS: Family Caregiver Caring Behaviors scale; CRAS: Caregiver Reaction Assessment scale; CRKS: COPD-related Knowledge scale.

Table 3. Comparison of CRKS, FCCBS, CRAS between different categorical characteristics.

Characteristic	FCCBS mean ± SD	P #	CRAS mean ± SD	P #	CRKS mean ± SD	P §
Age		0.563		0.032*		<0.001
Elder	97.8±33.8		74.1±6.9		21.7±4.1	
Non elder	101.9±37.6		76.0±9.1		24.8±5.5	
Sex		0.078		<0.001*		0.002*
Male	96.4±34.3		77.6±8.3		25.3±5.4	
Female	103.9±38.2		74.5±8.8		23.6±5.3	
Marriage		0.023*		0.745		0.014*
Single	114.2±45.8		75.0±10.6		23.8±6.1	
Married	98.8±34.6		75.8±8.4		24.3±5.3	
Religion		0.110		0.702		0.810
No	105.3±36.2		76.0±10.2		24.1±5.1	
Yes	100.1±37.1		75.6±8.3		24.2±5.5	
Highest educational level		0.267		<0.001*		<0.001*
Elementary school	96.0±33.0		74.3±7.9		21.9±4.8	
Junior high school	100.5±39.0		75.4±7.2		23.0±5.2	
Senior high school	107.3±40.3		74.5±8.7		24.6±5.0	
College or above	100.9±36.1		78.2±9.9		26.8±5.2	
Low social economic status		0.956		0.002*		<0.001*
No	101.2±37.9		76.9±9.5		26.1±5.2	
Yes	101.1±36.1		74.6±7.9		22.6±5.0	
Sharing responsibility with family		0.054		0.017*		<0.001*
No	97.5±34.6		74.8±8.2		22.8±5.2	
Yes	104.7±38.8		76.5±9.2		25.6±5.2	
Chronic disease		0.508		<0.001*		0.120
No	101.9±37.3		76.7±8.4		24.5±5.5	
Yes	99.1±36.1		73.0±9.2		23.5±5.0	
Living with patient		0.457		0.135		0.932
No	101.3±33.3		77.0±8.5		24.2±5.5	
Yes	101.1±38.0		75.3±8.8		24.2±5.3	
Other care-needed person(s) in home		<0.001*		0.001*		0.471
No	97.8±35.0		76.2±8.5		24.1±5.3	
Yes	123.9±41.6		71.6±9.4		24.7±5.5	
Spouse is main caregiver		0.022*		0.194		<0.001*
No	104.5±38.2		76.0±9.1		25.1±5.7	
Yes	96.0±34.4		75.2±8.1		22.8±4.5	

P # The P values were derived from Mann-Whitney U test.
P § The P values were derived from independent t-test or ANOVA.
* The P value ≦ 0.05.
FCCBS: Family Caregiver Caring Behaviors scale; CRAS: Caregiver Reaction Assessment scale; CRKS: COPD-related Knowledge scale.

In people with chronic illnesses, increased knowledge can reduce the negative psychological impact on the patients or caregivers, such as anxiety and depression, and can enhance care efficiency [9–11]. Another study demonstrated that education reduces subjective burdens, worry, and displeasure and improves intrapsychic strain, depression and all empowerment measures [32].

Our study showed that the elder caregivers' caring reaction was more negative than that of the non-elder caregivers, although this difference was not statistically significant. Most elders have at least one chronic disease and poor income due to retirement. The prevalence of frailty increases with age and is greater in women

[34]. Limpawattana et al. reported that older caregivers with poorer self-reported health status, a longer of duration of care, and a lower self-reported income had higher caregiver burdens, such as stress and depression [8]. Studies have also shown that negative care reactions by caregivers lead to negative impacts, such as caregiver depression, poor quality of care, potentially harmful behavior, and elder abuse [6,14,35]. Burdened caregivers have reported less social support, poorer quality of life, and problems with social integration [36]. Improving elder caregivers' social support systems and quality of life through respite care and education might be useful in making their caring reaction more

Table 4. Generalized linear model to analyze the difference of FCCBS, subscale of FCCBS, and CRAS in different factors.

Factors	FCCBS		Care of companionship and monitoring		Alternative care of social and general affairs		Care of communication and emotion		Care of maintaining physical function		CRAS	
	β(95%CI)	P	β(95%CI)	P	β(95%CI)	P	β(95%CI)	P	β(95%CI)	P	β(95%CI)	P
Elder vs. non elder caregivers	−4.0(−13.0~5.1)	0.388	−1.1(−4.8~2.5)	0.541	−1.8(−4.7~1.2)	0.242	−0.9(−3.4~1.6)	0.476	−0.2(−1.1~0.8)	0.743	−1.9(−4.1~0.2)	0.079
Sex (Female vs. male)	7.3(−0.1~14.7)	0.053	2.2(−0.8~5.2)	0.153	2.9(0.5~5.4)	0.017*	2.1(0.0~4.2)	0.047*	0.1(−0.7~0.9)	0.822	−3.2(−4.9~−1.4)	<0.001*
Marriage (Married vs. single)	−15.6(−25.4~−5.7)	0.002*	−6.0(−10.0~−2.0)	0.003*	−4.7(−7.9~−1.5)	0.004*	−2.5(−5.3~0.2)	0.071	−2.3(−3.3~−1.3)	<0.001*	0.8(−1.6~3.1)	0.525
Highest educational level												
Elementary school vs. college or above	−4.9(−14.1~4.4)	0.305	−1.1(−4.9~2.6)	0.553	−2.0(−5.0~1.1)	0.205	−1.4(−4.0~1.2)	0.288	−0.3(−1.3~0.6)	0.483	−3.8(−6.0~−1.7)	0.001*
Junior high school vs. college or above	−0.4(−12.0~11.1)	0.943	0.9(−3.8~5.6)	0.705	−0.4(−4.2~3.3)	0.823	−0.6(−3.8~2.6)	0.721	−0.3(−1.5~0.9)	0.614	−2.8(−5.5~−0.1)	0.042*
Senior high school vs. college or above	6.4(−3.2~16.0)	0.192	1.8(−1.1~6.7)	0.166	2.3(−0.9~5.4)	0.154	0.6(−2.1~3.3)	0.664	−0.8(−0.2~1.8)	0.137	−3.6(−5.9~−1.4)	0.002*
Low social economic status (Yes vs. no)	0.1(−7.1~7.3)	0.969	−0.3(−3.2~2.7)	0.867	0.1(−2.3~2.4)	0.947	0.5(−1.5~2.5)	0.593	−0.2(−1.0~0.5)	0.544	−2.3(−4.0~−0.6)	0.008*
Sharing responsibility with family (Yes vs. no)	7.0(−0.1~14.1)	0.055	3.9(1.0~6.8)	0.008*	1.8(−0.5~4.2)	0.130	0.2(−1.7~2.2)	0.809	1.0(0.3~1.8)	0.008*	1.2(0.0~3.4)	0.055
Chronic disease (Yes vs. no)	−2.7(−10.6~5.3)	0.513	−1.2(−4.5~2.0)	0.460	−0.8(−3.4~1.8)	0.548	0.1(−2.2~2.3)	0.965	−0.7(−1.5~0.1)	0.103	−3.7(−5.5~−1.8)	<0.001*
Other care-needed person(s) in home (Yes vs. no)	26.2(15.8~36.7)	<0.001*	7.1(2.9~11.4)	0.001*	10.2(6.8~13.6)	<0.001*	7.1(4.2~10.0)	<0.001*	1.8(0.7~2.9)	0.001*	−4.6(−7.1~−2.1)	<0.001*
Spouse is main caregiver (Yes vs. no)	−8.3(−15.6~−1.0)	0.026*	−4(−6.9~−1.0)	0.008*	−2.9(−5.2~−0.5)	0.019*	−0.5(−2.6~1.5)	0.618	−0.9(−1.7~−0.2)	0.017*	−0.8(−2.5~1.0)	0.391

*The P value ≦0.05.
FCCBS: Family Caregiver Caring Behaviors scale; CRAS: Caregiver Reaction Assessment scale.
Adjusted variable: Sex, Marriage, Highest Educational Level, Social Economic Status, Rotary, Other (chronic) disease, Living with patient, Other care-needed person(s) in home, Spouse is the main caregiver, Duration of care, Daily hours of care.

Table 5. Generalized linear model to analyze the difference of CRKS, and subscale of CRKS in different factors.

Factors	CRKS		Understanding of COPD		Elimination of sputum		Inhaled bronchodilator		Inhaled steroids	
	β(95%CI)	P	β(95%CI)	P	β(95%CI)	P	β(95%CI)	P	β(95%CI)	P
Elder vs. non elder caregivers	-3.1(-4.3~-1.8)	<0.001*	-0.7(-1.0~-0.4)	<0.001*	-0.2(-0.5~0.1)	0.232	-0.5(-0.7~-0.2)	0.002*	-0.4(-0.6~-0.1)	0.001*
Sex (Female vs. Male)	-1.7(-2.8~-0.6)	0.002*	-0.3(-0.6~-0.1)	0.012*	-0.1(-0.3~0.2)	0.606	-0.3(-0.5~-0.1)	0.007*	-0.2(-0.4~0)	0.044*
Marriage (Married vs. Single)	0.5(-1~1.9)	0.542	-0.1(-0.4~0.2)	0.574	0.2(-0.1~0.5)	0.248	0.1(-0.2~0.4)	0.677	-0.1(-0.3~0.2)	0.625
Highest educational level										
Elementary school vs. college or above	-4.9(-6.2~-3.6)	<0.001*	-0.8(-1.1~-0.5)	<0.001*	-0.5(-0.8~-0.2)	0.001*	-0.5(-0.7~-0.2)	0.002*	-0.4(-0.6~-0.1)	0.002*
Junior high school vs. college or above	-3.8(-5.4~-2.2)	<0.001*	-0.6(-1.0~-0.3)	0.001*	-0.4(-0.8~-0.1)	0.016*	-0.2(-0.6~0.2)	0.260	-0.4(-0.7~-0.1)	0.003*
Senior high school vs. college or above	-2.2(-3.5~-0.9)	0.001	-0.3(-0.6~0.1)	0.123	-0.3(-0.6~0)	0.034*	-0.19(-0.4~0.2)	0.525	0(-0.2~0.2)	0.985
Low social economic status (Yes vs. no)	-3.5(-4.5~-2.5)	<0.001*	-0.6(-0.9~-0.4)	<0.001*	-0.3(-0.5~-0.1)	0.017*	-0.4(-0.6~-0.1)	0.001*	-0.4(-0.6~-0.3)	<0.001*
Sharing responsibility with family (Yes vs. no)	2.8(1.8-3.9)	<0.001*	0.4(0.2~0.6)	0.001*	0.4(0.2~0.7)	<0.001*	0.5(0.3,0.7)	<0.001*	0.2(-0.1~0.3)	0.097
Chronic disease (Yes vs. no)	-0.9(-2.1~0.2)	0.123	-0.2(-0.4~0.1)	0.205	0(-0.2~0.3)	0.734	-0.2(-0.5~0)	0.090	-0.1(-0.3~0.1)	0.510
Other care-needed person(s) in home (Yes vs. no)	0.6(-1.0~2.2)	0.462	0.1(-0.2~0.5)	0.514	0.1(-0.2~0.4)	0.573	0(-0.4~0.3)	0.876	-0.1(-0.3~0.2)	0.540
Spouse is main caregiver (Yes vs. no)	-2.3(-3.4~-1.3)	<0.001*	-0.4(-0.6~-0.1)	0.002*	-0.1(-0.3~0.2)	0.586	-0.4(-0.7~-0.2)	<0.001*	-0.2(-0.4~-0.1)	0.008*

* The P value ≦0.05.
CRKS: COPD-related Knowledge scale.
Adjusted variable: Sex, Marriage, Highest Educational Level, Social Economic Status, Rotary, Other (chronic) disease, Living with patient, Other care-needed person(s) in home, Spouse is the main caregiver, Duration of care, Weekly days of care, Daily hours of care.

Table 6. Generalized linear model to analyze the difference of CRKS, and subscale of CRKS in different factors.

Factors	Antibiotics therapy		Exercise		Quit smoking		Nutrition		Vaccine	
	β(95%CI)	P	β(95%CI)	P	β(95%CI)	P	β(95%CI)	P	β(95%CI)	P
Elder vs. non elder caregivers	−0.9(−1.2~−0.5)	<0.001*	−0.1(−0.3~0.1)	0.593	−0.2(−0.4~0)	0.014*	−.1(−0.1~0.4)	0.300	−0.4(−0.6~−0.1)	0.005*
Sex (Female vs. male)	−0.5(−0.8~−0.2)	0.001*	−0.1(−0.2~0.1)	0.533	−0.2(−0.3~0)	0.022*	−0.1(−0.3~0.1)	0.565	0(−0.3~0.2)	0.721
Marriage (Married vs. single)	−0.3(−0.7~0.1)	0.140	0.2(0~0.4)	0.079	−0.1(−0.3~0.1)	0.430	0.5(0.3~0.8)	<0.001*	0(−0.3~0.3)	0.891
Highest educational level										
Elementary school vs. college or above	−1.4(−1.7~−1.1)	<0.001*	−0.2(−0.4~0)	0.027*	−0.4(−0.6~−0.2)	<0.001*	0(−0.2~0.3)	0.842	−0.7(−1.0~−0.5)	<0.001*
Junior high school vs. college or above	−1.0(−1.4~−0.6)	<0.001*	−0.1(−0.3~0.1)	0.589	−0.3(−0.5~−0.1)	0.008*	0(−0.4~0.3)	0.836	−0.6(−0.9~−0.3)	<0.001*
Senior high school vs. college or above	−0.8(−1.1~−0.4)	<0.001*	−0.1(−0.3~0.10)	0.571	−0.1(−0.3~0.1)	0.217	−0.1(−0.3~0.2)	0.578	−0.4(−0.7~−0.2)	0.001*
Low social economic status (Yes vs. no)	−0.8(−1.1~−0.5)	<0.001*	−0.1(−0.3~0)	0.114	−0.3(−0.5~−0.2)	<0.001*	−0.1(−0.3~0.1)	0.559	−0.4(−0.6~−0.2)	<0.001*
Sharing responsibility with family (Yes vs. no)	0.7(0.4~1.0)	<0.001*	0.1(−0.1~0.2)	0.361	0.1(0~0.3)	0.082	0(−0.2~0.2)	0.840	0.4(0.2~0.6)	<0.001*
Chronic disease (Yes vs. no)	−0.3(−0.7~0)	0.031*	−0.1(−0.3~0.1)	0.291	−0.1(−0.2~0.1)	0.292	0.1(−0.2~0.3)	0.660	0(−0.3~0.2)	0.707
Other care−needed person(s) in home (Yes vs. no)	0.3(−0.2~0.7)	0.243	0.2(0~0.5)	0.056	0(−0.2~0.2)	0.890	−0.2(−0.5~0.1)	0.168	0.2(−0.1~0.5)	0.240
Spouse is main caregiver (Yes vs. no)	−0.7(−1.0~−0.5)	<0.001*	0(−0.2~0.2)	0.980	−0.2(−0.4~−0.1)	0.002*	0.2(0~0.4)	0.119	−0.4(−0.6~−0.2)	0.001*

*The P value ≦ 0.05.

Adjusted variable: Sex, Marriage, Highest Educational Level, Social Economic Status, Rotary, Other (chronic) disease, Living with patient, Other care-needed person(s) in home, Spouse is the main caregiver, Duration of care, Weekly days of care, Daily hours of care.

positive. Our study showed that elder caregivers have a poor performance on the COPD-related knowledge scale (CRKS), which might be the result of the working memory becoming weaker with increasing age [37]. Another study also showed that the caregivers' advancing age increased the risks related to functional and cognitive impairments [38]. In addition, health professionals might not have much time to provide the caregivers with detailed information about COPD. A study showed that young men use the internet more than the elderly [39]. Younger caregivers might access COPD-related information on the internet, which might also explain the difference in the scores between older and younger participants. The results of the present study make an important contribution to the literature; elder caregivers showed poor performance on the medication-related subscales. This result might be explained by the fact that most health professionals might stereotype older persons with respect to memory and learning new concepts. Therefore, health professionals might not spend much time educating older persons, especially with respect to medication-related information. In addition, younger caregivers have greater access to medication information on the internet [39]. Elder family caregivers need more education on medications and preventive care in patients with COPD.

This study had several limitations. First, the questionnaires may have response bias due to the nature of self-reporting. Second, the subjects were recruited only from northern Taiwan, which may partially limit the generalizability of our results. However, many of these observations are likely applicable to the broader socio-cultural context of Taiwan and Southeast Asia. Third, the severity of COPD was not considered a confounder when the differences between the two groups in caregiver behavior and caregiver response were analyzed, which may somewhat restrict the interpretation of our results. Fourth, although "sharing responsi-bilities with family" is one type of "help with caregiving", we did not include the data regarding whether the primary family caregiver had assistance or other help when providing care to the COPD patient. Future studies are needed to clarify whether "help with caregiving" might affect the outcomes. Regarding possible future studies, we might develop a COPD-related knowledge education project for elder caregivers and examine the program's effects on COPD-related knowledge, care, and caregiver burden for elder caregivers. The application of these results to caregivers in the context of other chronic diseases is unknown. Further studies are needed to explore the differences in care for other age-related chronic diseases by primary family caregivers. Furthermore, research on the care needs of elder primary family caregivers caring for an elder family member with chronic disease is worth pursuing in Taiwan.

Conclusions

In conclusion, our findings indicate that there were no significant differences in family caregiver caring behavior or caregiver reaction between the elder and the non-elder caregivers. However, the elder caregivers had significantly lower COPD-related knowledge than the non-elder caregivers, especially with regard to their understanding of COPD, inhaled bronchodilators, inhaled steroids, antibiotic therapy, smoking cessation, and vaccines. Elder family caregivers need more education on COPD drugs and COPD symptom prevention.

Author Contributions

Conceived and designed the experiments: PCH. Performed the experiments: PYS. Analyzed the data: PCH CMC. Contributed reagents/materials/analysis tools: WCP CMC. Wrote the paper: PCH KYW.

References

1. World Health Organization (2012) Global brief for world Health Day. Geneva: WHO.
2. Ministry of Health and Welfare (2011) Aging tsunami struck Taiwan. Available: http://health99.hpa.gov.tw/Hot_News/h_NewsDetailN.aspx?TopIcNo=6260. Accessed 2013 Oct 7.
3. Pennacchini M, Tartaglini D (2014) The education of family caregivers as an ethical issue. Clin Ter 165: e219–e222.
4. Wu L, Chen H, Hu Y, Xiang H, Yu X, et al. (2012) Prevalence and associated factors of elder mistreatment in a rural community in People's Republic of China: A cross-sectional study. PLOS ONE 7: e33857.
5. Thielman N, Ostermann J, Whetten K, Whetten R, O'Donnell K, et al. (2012) Correlates of poor health among orphans and abandoned children in less wealthy countries: the importance of caregiver health. PLOS ONE 7: e38109.
6. Vellone E, Fida R, Cocchieri A, Sili A, Piras G, et al. (2011) Positive and negative impact of caregiving to older adults: A structural equation model. Prof Inferm 64: 237–248.
7. Dias A, Dewey ME, D'Souza J, Dhume R, Motghare DD, et al. (2008) The effectiveness of a home care program for supporting caregivers of persons with dementia in developing countries: A randomised controlled trial from Goa, India. PLOS ONE 3: e2333.
8. Limpawattana P, Theeranut A, Chindaprasirt J, Sawanyawisuth K, Pimporm J (2013) Caregivers burden of older adults with chronic illnesses in the community: A cross-sectional study. J Community Health 38: 40–45.
9. Lange JW, Mager D, Greiner PA, Saracino K (2011) The ELDER Project: educational model and three-year outcomes of a community-based geriatric education initiative. Gerontol Geriatr Educ 32: 164–181.
10. Martin P, Tamblyn R, Ahmed S, Tannenbaum C (2013) A drug education tool developed for older adults changes knowledge, beliefs and risk perceptions about inappropriate benzodiazepine prescriptions in the elderly. Patient Educ Couns 92: 81–87.
11. Lucksted A, Medoff D, Burland J, Stewart B, Fang LJ, et al. (2013) Sustained outcomes of a peer-taught family education program on mental illness. Acta Psychiatr Scand 12: 279–286.
12. Alpass F, Pond R, Stephens C, Stevenson B, Keeling S, et al. (2013) The influence of ethnicity and gender on caregiver health in older New zealanders. J Gerontol B Psychol Sci Soc Sci 68: 783–793.
13. Buurman BM, Hoogerduijn JG, de Haan RJ, Abu-Hanna A, Lagaay AM, et al. (2011) Geriatric conditions in acutely hospitalized older patients: prevalence and one-year survival and functional decline. PLOS ONE 6: e26951.

14. Wang JJ, Lin MF, Tseng HF, Chang WY (2009) Caregiver factors contributing to psychological elder abuse behavior in long-term care facilities: A structural equation model approach. Int Psychogeriatr 21: 314–320.
15. Bookman A, Kimbrel D (2011) Families and elder care in the twenty-first century. Future Child 21: 117–140.
16. Alvarenga MR, Oliveira MA, Domingues MA, Amendola F, Faccenda O (2011) Social support networks for elderly patients attended by Family Health teams. Cien Saude Colet 16: 2603–2611.
17. Woo J (2011) Nutritional strategies for successful aging. Med Clin North Am 95: 477–493, ix–x.
18. de Marco R, Pesce G, Marcon A, Accordini S, Antonicelli L, et al. (2013) The coexistence of asthma and chronic obstructive pulmonary disease (COPD): prevalence and risk factors in young, middle-aged and elderly people from the general population. PLOS ONE 8: e62985.
19. Chen J, Schooling CM, Johnston JM, Hedley AJ, McGhee SM (2011) How does socioeconomic development affect COPD mortality? An age-period-cohort analysis from a recently transitioned population in China. PLOS ONE 6: e24348.
20. Baty F, Putora PM, Isenring B, Blum T, Brutsche M (2013) Comorbidities and burden of COPD: A population based case-control study. PLOS ONE 8: e63285.
21. Coventry PA, Bower P, Keyworth C, Kenning C, Knopp J, et al. (2013) The effect of complex interventions on depression and anxiety in chronic obstructive pulmonary disease: systematic review and meta-analysis. PLOS ONE 8: e60532.
22. Najafzadeh M, Marra CA, Lynd LD, Sadatsafavi M, FitzGerald JM, et al. (2012) Future impact of various interventions on the burden of COPD in Canada: A dynamic population model. PLOS ONE 7: e46746.
23. Pauwels RA, Buist AS, Calverley PM, Jenkins CR, Hurd SS, et al. (2001) Global strategy for the diagnosis, management, and prevention of chronic obstructive pulmonary disease. NHLBI/WHO Global Initiative for Chronic obstructive Lung disease (gold) workshop summary. Am J Respir Crit Care Med 163: 1256–1276.
24. Pfeiffer E (1975) A short portable mental status questionnaire for the assessment of organic brain deficit in elderly patients. J Am Geriatr Soc 23: 433–441.
25. Yang C (2000) The development and testing of cancer caregivers' need Q-sort scale. Tao-Yuan, Taiwan: Chang Gung University.
26. Rubio DM, Berg-Weger M, Tebb SS, Lee ES, Rauch S (2003) Objectifying content validity: conducting a content validity study in social work research. Soc Work Res 27: 94–104.

27. Given CW, Given B, Stommel M, Collins C, King S, et al. (1992) The caregiver reaction assessment (CRA) for caregivers to persons with chronic physical and mental impairments. Res Nurs Health 15: 271–283.

28. White R, Walker P, Roberts S, Kalisky S, White P (2006) Bristol COPD knowledge questionnaire (BCKQ): testing what we teach patients about COPD. Chron Respir Dis 3: 123–131.

29. Garrod R, Paul EA, Wedzicha JA (2002) An evaluation of the reliability and sensitivity of the London chest activity of Daily Living Scale (LCADL). Respir Med 96: 725–730.

30. Tsai HH, Tsai YF (2013) Prevalence and factors related to depressive symptoms among family caregivers of nursing home residents in Taiwan. Soc Psychiatry Psychiatr Epidemiol 48: 1145–1152.

31. Hiyoshi K, Becker C, Siwaku K, Kinoshita A (2009) [Family caregivers' burden and marital satisfaction]. Gan To Kagaku Ryoho (Suppl 1): 30–32.

32. Chiu MY, Wei GF, Lee S, Choovanichvong S, Wong FH (2013) Empowering caregivers: impact analysis of FamilyLink Education Programme (FLEP) in Hong Kong, Taipei and Bangkok. Int J Soc Psychiatry 59: 28–39.

33. Friedemann ML, Newman FL, Buckwalter KC, Montgomery RJ (2014) Resource need and use of multiethnic caregivers of elders in their homes. J Adv Nurs 70: 662–673 doi: 10.1111/jan.12230.

34. Chen CY, Wu SC, Chen IJ, Lue BH (2010) The prevalence of subjective frailty and factors associated with frailty in Taiwan. Arch Gerontol Geriatr (Suppl 1): S43–S47.

35. Smith GR, Williamson GM, Miller LS, Schulz R (2011) Depression and quality of informal care: A longitudinal investigation of caregiving stressors. Psychol Aging 26: 584–591.

36. Gallart A, Cruz F, Zabalegui A (2013) Factors influencing burden among non-professional immigrant caregivers: A case-control study. J Adv Nurs 69: 642–654.

37. Chan RC, Xu T, Li HJ, Zhao Q, Liu HH, et al. (2011) Neurological abnormalities and neurocognitive functions in healthy elder people: A structural equation modeling analysis. Behav Brain Funct 7: 32.

38. Chau PH, Woo J, Kwok T, Chan F, Hui E, et al. (2012) Usage of community services and domestic helpers predicted institutionalization of elders having functional or cognitive impairments: A 12-month longitudinal study in Hong Kong. J Am Med Dir Assoc 13: 169–175.

39. Kernisan LP, Sudore RL, Knight SJ (2010) Information-seeking at a caregiving website: a qualitative analysis. J Med Internet Res 12: e31.

5

Saccadic Eye Movements in Depressed Elderly Patients

Nicolas Carvalho[1,2]*, Nicolas Noiret[1,4], Pierre Vandel[1,2,3], Julie Monnin[1,2,3], Gilles Chopard[1,2], Eric Laurent[4,5]*

1 Department of Clinical Psychiatry, University Hospital, Besançon, France, 2 E.A. 481, Laboratory of Neurosciences, University of Franche-Comté, Besançon, France, 3 CIC-IT 808 Inserm, Besançon University Hospital, Besançon, France, 4 E.A. 3188, Laboratory of Psychology, University of Franche-Comté, Besançon, France, 5 UMSR 3124/FED 4209 MSHE Ledoux, CNRS and University of Franche-Comté, Besançon, France

Abstract

The primary aim of this study was to characterize oculomotor performances in elderly depressed patients. The second aim was to investigate whether cognitive inhibition measured by the antisaccade task was associated with a psychomotor retardation or rather with a more specific cognitive-motor inhibition deficit. Twenty patients with a major depressive disorder and forty-seven healthy subjects performed two eye movement tasks. Saccadic reaction time and error rates were analyzed in the prosaccade task to obtain basic parameters of eye movements. Saccade latency, error rates and correction rates were evaluated in the antisaccade task to investigate inhibition capacities. Performances were impaired in patients, who exhibited a higher reaction time and error rates compared to controls. The higher time cost of inhibition suggested that the reaction time was not related to global psychomotor retardation alone. The higher time cost of inhibition could be explained by a specific alteration of inhibition processes evaluated by the antisaccade task. These changes were associated with the severity of depression. These findings provide a new perspective on cognitive inhibition in elderly depressed patients and could have important clinical implications for our understanding of critical behaviors involving deficits in inhibitory processes in the elderly.

Editor: Jan Kassubek, University of Ulm, Germany

Funding: This study was supported by a grant from the French Ministry of Health (Programme Hospitalier de Recherche Clinique: PHRC n°2009-A00942-55). The funders had no role in study design, data collection and analysis, decision to publish, or preparation of the manuscript.

Competing Interests: The authors have declared that no competing interests exist.

* Email: nic.carvalh@gmail.com (NC); eric.laurent@univ-fcomte.fr (EL)

Introduction

Cognitive inhibition, a major component of executive functioning, has been found to be impaired in depressed patients [1,2]. This function has been defined as a deletion of an automated response by the deliberate control of this response based on changes in background characteristics [3] or previously activated processes [4]. Cognitive inhibition would affect the characteristics of inputs and outputs of distracter elements to make the analysis and response processes for relevant elements available and more effective [5]. Houghton and Tipper [6] have shown that inhibition processes correspond to the cognitive function applied to the content that should be deleted.

An effective way to assess cognitive inhibition is based on oculomotor measurements particularly through the prosaccade and the antisaccade tasks [7–9]. Prosaccades are usually conceived as reflexive eye movements towards a peripherally appearing target. The prosaccade task has been used to evaluate basic characteristics of speed, latency and accuracy of saccadic eye movements. In contrast, the antisaccade task probes the ability to inhibit the automatic orientation of the eye in the direction of a peripherally appearing target in the vision fields [10]. Antisaccades are conceived as highly voluntary eye movements in the opposite direction to a peripherally appearing target. The antisaccade task is more reliable for assessing the inhibition function compared to many other tasks [11]. Antisaccade latency and error rates (ER) reflect critical cognitive abilities and can help us quantify an inhibition deficit [12].

A few reported studies have examined cognitive inhibition in depression. Sweeney et al. [13] showed that patients with depression - compared with healthy subjects - have greater difficulty in suppressing saccades towards a peripheral target in the antisaccade task. However, no difference in latency or speed was found. The study of Mahlberg et al. [14] showed that patients with depression had longer reaction times (RT) than controls in prosaccade tasks, suggesting that a psychomotor retardation affecting reflexive eye movement could characterize some depressive symptoms. The study conducted by De Lissnyder et al. [15] reported that dysphoric subjects had longer RT than controls in the antisaccade task. Globally, these results highlight the need to distinguish between basic reflexive components evaluated by prosaccade tasks and more elaborated executive processes involved in the inhibition required by the antisaccade task. A systematic distinction between these processes is critical to better characterize the kind of cognitive-motor processes that are altered in depression (i.e., global eye movement retardation vs. specific inhibitory disorder).

Moreover, all these studies only included young depressed patients. No information is available concerning oculomotor abilities in depressed elderly patients. Nevertheless, elderly depression differs from younger adult depression with a higher sadness, a psychomotor retardation, a difficulty to express their pain [16], a deficit in motor response and in response selection [17]. Depression in the elderly remains under-diagnosed [18] due to many co-morbidities such as somatic disorders [19], cerebro-vascular pathologies [20] or Alzheimer's disease [21].

The main objective of our research was to characterize oculomotor performances in elderly depressed patients. We hypothesized that depressed elderly patients would have a higher reaction time in both prosaccade and antisaccade tasks, because of global psychomotor retardation, which was previously reported in these patients. The second objective of this study was to determine whether higher antisaccade reaction time is only related to psychomotor retardation or if it is also due to a specific inhibitory problem. This is in accordance with the above mentioned alteration of response selection problems known in these patients.

Methods

1. Participants

Elderly depressed patients were recruited from the psychiatric wards of Besançon University Hospital. Non-depressed controls were mainly recruited from the open University, which welcomes many older adults. Twenty depressed patients and forty-seven controls were included and matched for age (± 5 years), sex, and education level. All patients had a major depressive disorder (MDD) according to the DSM-IV criteria [22], and a Montgom-ery-Asberg Depression Rating Scale (MADRS) [23] score higher than 25. Exclusion criteria for both groups were progressive psychiatric illness (e.g. schizophrenia, bipolar disorders), acute or chronic neurological pathologies (e.g. traumatic brain injury, brain tumors, stroke, and dementia) and presence of ophthalmic illnesses. Patients were all on stable medication at least for 4 weeks before inclusion screening. All patients were on antidepres-sants, 92% on anxiolytics, 80% benzodiazepines, 48% antipsy-chotics and 44% hypnotics. All participants gave their written informed consent to participate in the study. The research protocol was approved by the Committee for the Protection of Persons (CPP-Est-II), and was conducted in accordance with the principles laid down by the Declaration of Helsinki.

All participants underwent a complete neuropsychological battery of tests and eye movement tasks as described below. These assessments were performed within a maximum period of one month.

2. Neuropsychological assessment

The RAPID neuropsychological battery [24] was designed to ensure that no participant had cognitive impairments associated with early dementia. This battery included pencil and paper tasks assessing six cognitive domains: (1) Global cognitive function: Mini-Mental State Examination (MMSE) [25]; (2) Attention/ processing speed: Trail Making Test Part A (TMT A) [26] and Crossing-Off Test (COT) [27]; (3) Constructional praxis: part of the Signoret's battery of cognitive efficacy (BEC 96) [28]; (4) Executive function: Trail Making Test Part B (TMT B) [26] and Isaacs Set Test (IST) [29]; (5) Verbal Memory: Memory Impairment Screen (MIS) [30] and Free and Cued Selective Recall Test (FCSRT) [31,32]; (6) Language: Picture naming task (DO 30) [24]. In addition to the RAPID battery, each participant completed the Stroop test [33] in order to measure inhibitory processing.

3. Eye movement tasks

All participants were seated in a quiet room. Eye movements were recorded using video-oculography techniques based on the

corneal reflection of infra-red light. We used an ASL EYE-TRAC 6 system (ASL - Bedford, MA.) with a H6 optic camera mounted in a chin rest for stabilizing the head position. This system permits to capture data with good temporal (sampling at 120 Hz) and spatial resolution (accuracy of $0.1°$ of the visual angle). The device was calibrated for each participant at the beginning of the experimental sessions. The standard calibration of Eye-Track 6 User Interface Program (Version 1.62.1.0) with 3×3 calibration points was initially used. This was followed by an auto-calibration procedure, the 9 green points appearing one after another when the device automatically detected the subject's eye. Each participant performed a prosaccade task and then an antisaccade task. These tasks were presented in two separate blocks, the prosaccade task before the antisaccade task. In the prosaccade task, participants were instructed to fix their gaze, as quickly and accurately as possible, on the red dot appearing in the periphery of the screen. In the antisaccade task, participants were instructed to fix their gaze, as quickly and accurately as possible, on the opposite side relative to the red dot appearing in periphery of the screen, [34]. Between the two tasks, an auto-calibration was then performed again.

For both tasks, each trial began with a 2-s presentation of a central fixation dot. After this time, the peripheral red target appeared horizontally (H), on the right or left, or vertically (V), on the top or bottom, at different eccentricity levels ($4°$; $6°$; $8°$; $10°$) in a randomized order (Figure 1) and for 2-s. The number of target eccentricity levels for the antisaccade task was limited in order to reduce its duration ($4°$; $8°$). There were 4 trials in each condition of dot presentation. The central dot and the peripheral dot diameters each subtended a visual angle of $0.6°$.

Pictures were presented on a 21-in. LCD screen (ASUS LCD Monitor VH 196, 32 bits color, 1024 by 768 pixels screen resolution, refresh rate of 70 Hz) at a distance of 70 cm from the participants. The images subtended a visual angle of $32.6°$. Inquisit software (Millisecond Software, Version 3.0.3.2, Seattle, WA) was used to create the different tasks.

4. Eye Movement data analysis

Analyses were performed using the ASL-Result software. Fixations, total duration of fixation, and RT were computed on the basis of fixation detection criteria. Periods during which the eye did not vary from more than $1°$ of visual angle during at least 100 ms were considered as fixations. Accuracy zones around the red dot measured $1.8°$.

Prosaccade. Recorded data were the RT (i.e., the time between the appearance of the peripheral target and the start of the correct subsequent saccade), the gain corresponding to the ratio of the saccade amplitude divided by the target step amplitude. A gain of <1 indicated that the saccade was hypometric and a gain of >1 indicated that the saccade was hypermetric.

Antisaccade. The RT, the ER (i.e., percentage of trials with initial incorrect saccade corresponding to a saccade toward the peripheral target), and the correction factor (CF) (i.e., sequence made of a first saccade toward the peripheral dot position and a second saccade in the opposite direction) were recorded.

When the saccade RT was lower than 80 ms (typically anticipatory saccade response) [35] or higher than 600 ms (typically delayed response), trials were excluded from data analysis [36].

5. Statistical analyses

A Shapiro-Wilk test was performed to assess the normality of data. The equality of variance was controlled by a Fisher-Snedecor

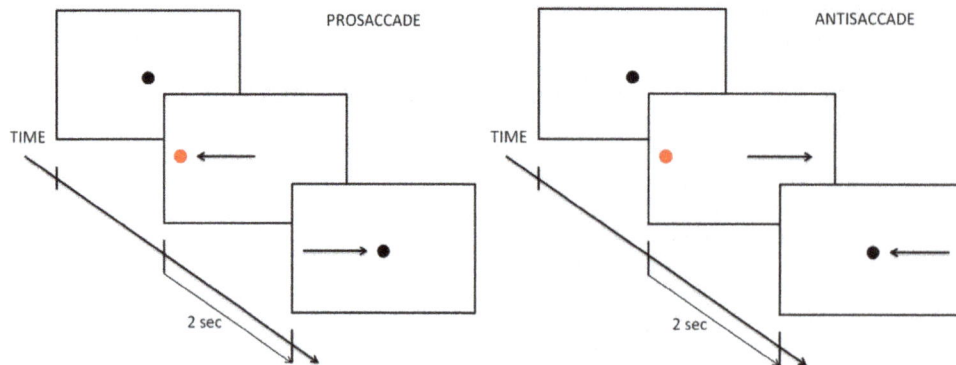

Figure 1. Eye movement tasks.

test. Categorical variables were compared using the chi-square test or the Fisher's exact test (if the sample size was less than 5). Mixed ANOVAs including the factor group (depressed patients *vs.* controls), direction (horizontal *vs.* vertical) and eccentricity (4°; 6°; 8°; 10°) were performed. Newman–Keuls post-hoc tests were applied when appropriate. The Greenhouse-Geisser correction was used when sphericity was not assumed.

Differences between both groups in the prosaccade and antisaccade tasks were evaluated using ANCOVAs including group (depressed, control) as a factor, and neuropsychological [All RAPID neuropsychological battery scores, MMSE, memory scores (free and total recall score of the FCSRT), information processing speed scores (Stroop M and C, TMT A, COT), executive functions scores (TMT B-A, IST, Stroop INT)] and psychiatric (MADRS) scores, as covariates.

The significance alpha level was fixed to 0.05. Effect sizes were measured by partial Eta squared (η^2_p), with small, medium and large effects defined as 0.01, 0.06 and 0.14 respectively [37]. All computations were performed using Stata Software release 10.1 (StataCorp, College Station, TX).

Results

Demographic, psychiatric and neuropsychological data of the two groups are presented in table 1. There was no significant differences in age (depressed mean = 70.4, SD = 9.62; control mean = 66.72, SD = 5.48; $W_{67} = 0.81$, $p = 0.41$), gender ($\chi^2_{(1)} = 1.10$, $p = 0.29$) or educational level ($\chi^2_{(3)} = 5.25$, $p = 0.21$) between patients and controls. Scores on the MADRS were significantly higher in the patient group (MADRS: $W_{67} = 6.36$, $p < 0.001$). Though patients with depression performed significantly worse than controls on most neuropsychological tests (Table 1), none of them had cognitive impairment sufficiently severe to constitute early dementia. As mentioned earlier, ANCOVAs were applied in order to control potential effects of neuropsychological performances on eye movements.

1. Differences in parameters of saccadic eye movements

1.1. Prosaccade reaction time. Depressed patients had a significantly higher RT than controls [$F(1,65) = 24.71$, $p < 0.001$, $\eta^2_p = 0.27$, d = 1.3] (Table 2). There was no effect of direction [$F(1,65) = 2.27$, $p = 0.14$, $d_s < 0.76$], eccentricity [$F(1,65) = 2.5$, $p = 0.11$, $d_s < 0.77$] and no interaction between direction and eccentricity [$F(1,65) = 0.91$, $p = 0.34$, $d_s < 0.43$].

1.2. Prosaccade gain. The accuracy of prosaccade was not reduced in depressed group in comparison with the control group [$F(1,65) = 0.02$, $p = 0.89$, $\eta^2_p < 0.001$, d = 0.04] (Table 2).

1.3. Antisaccade reaction time. Depressed subjects had longer mean reaction times than controls [$F(1,65) = 22.11$, $p < 0.001$, $\eta^2_p = 0.26$, d = 1.33] (Table 2). There was a significant effect of direction [$F(1,65) = 10.98$, $p < 0.01$, $d_s > 0.28$]. Horizontal RT was significantly higher for depressed patients (M = 420 ms, SD = 152) than healthy controls (M = 272 ms, SD = 52) ($p < 0.05$; d = 1.30) but there was no difference in vertical direction ($M_{depressed} = 326$ ms, $SD_{depressed} = 138$; $M_{controls}$ mean = 296 ms, $SD_{controls} = 63$; $p = 0.22$; d = 0.27). There was no effect of eccentricity [$F(1,65) = 0.59$, $p = 0.44$, $d_s < 0.99$] and no interaction between direction and eccentricity [$F(1,65) = 0.05$, $p = 0.82$, $d_s < 0.04$].

1.4. Antisaccade error rate. Depressed patients had higher ER than controls [$F(1,65) = 23.68$, $p < 0.001$, $\eta^2_p = 0.27$, d = 1.22] (Table2). There was no significant effect of direction [$F(1,65) = 0$, $p = 1$, $d_s < 1.15$], eccentricity [$F(1,65) = 0.001$, $p = 0.97$, $d_s < 0.99$] and no interaction between direction and eccentricity [$F(1,65) = 0.02$, $p = 0.87$, $d_s < 0.85$].

1.5. Antisaccade correction factor. Depressed patients and controls had a similar correction rate of antisaccade errors [$F(1,65) = 0.99$, $p = 0.32$, $\eta^2_p = 0.01$, d < 0.001] (Table 2).

2. Time cost of inhibition

In addition to direct measures of RT, the time cost of inhibition (antisaccade RT minus prosaccade RT) was calculated in order to control global eye movement retardation and provide a more reliable evaluation of the cognitive inhibition function (required in the antisaccade task). The time cost of inhibition was significantly higher in depressed patients (M = 114 ms, SD = 89) than in controls (M = 53 ms, SD = 42) [$F(1,65) = 30.69$; $p < 0.001$].

3. Analysis of confounding variables (ANCOVA)

Due to the significant disparity in cognitive performances of the depressed patients and controls, we reanalyzed the eye movement performances explored in the two tasks using neuropsychological tests as predictor variables. All RAPID neuropsychological scores, MMSE, memory scores, information processing scores and executive function scores were not found to be significant predictors for eye movement performance differences ($F_s > 0.01$; $p_s > 0.05$).

With a MADRS score of 31.7 for the depressed patients and 2.3 for the healthy controls, our data were reanalyzed using MADRS as a predictor variable of eye movement differences. As reported above, a mixed ANOVA had indicated that depressed patients had significantly lower eye movements performances than controls except for prosaccade gain and antisaccade CF. After adjustment

Table 1. Demographic and clinical data.

Characteristic	MDD(N = 20)	HC(N = 47)	p
Age	70.4±9.6	66.7±5.5	N.S.
Female	15(75)	29(61.7)	N.S.
Education (%)			N.S.
Low	25	21	N.S.
Medium	30	32	N.S.
High	45	47	N.S.
MADRS, (range 0–60)	31.7±5.6	2.3±2.3	<0.001
MIS Score, (range 0–8)	7.4±0.6	7.8±0.5	<0.001
IST Score,	31.3±5.3	43.3±5.8	<0.001
MMSE score, (range 0–30)	26.1±3.2	29.1±0.9	<0.001
FCSRT score, (range 0–48)			
Free recall	20.4±7.1	26.3±4.4	0.02
Total recall	43.4±6.8	45.7±2.5	N.S.
COT score,	145.6±48.4	213.7±42.1	<0.001
TMT score,			
Part A (range 0–150)	73.1±49.3	34.6±9.1	<0.001
Part B (range 0–300)	236.7±133.8	105.6±47.2	<0.001
BEC 96, (range 0–6)	5.6±1.1	6±0.2	0.03
DO 30, (range 0–30)	29.5±0.8	29.8±0.5	N.S.
Stroop Task score,			
Word	100±22.2	110.9±13.7	N.S.
Color	71.1±11.5	82.1±11.3	<0.001
Incompatible color-word	33.8±12.5	44±9	0.006
Interference	-8.3±9.5	-3.2±7.4	0.02

Legend: MDD, Major Depressive Disorder; HC, Healthy Controls; MADRS, Montgomery Asberg Depression Rating Scale; MIS, Memory Screen Impairment; IST, Isaacs Set Test; MMSE, Mini Mental State Examination; FCSRT, Free and Cued Selective Recall Test; COT, Crossing Off Test; TMT, Trail Making Test; BEC 96, Bec 96 figure Copy; DO 30, Picture naming task with 30 items; N.S., not significant.
Values given as n (%) or mean ± SD.

by the MADRS, the oculomotor performances between the two groups did not differ significantly except for prosaccade gain and antisaccade CF. These results confirmed an effect of MADRS score on eye movements (Table 3).

Discussion

In this study, oculomotor impairments were found in elderly depressed patients. In the prosaccade and antisaccade tasks, depressed patients had higher RT and ER than controls.

Table 2. Means and standard deviations for the saccadic reaction time, gain, error and correction rates.

Oculomotor parameter	MDD(N = 20)	HC(N = 47)	p	η^2_p
Prosaccades				
RT (ms)	291±59	231±28	<0.001	0.27
Gain	0.97±0.3	0.98±0.03	N.S.	<0.001
Antisaccades				
RT (ms)	405±116	284±54	<0.001	0.26
ER (%)	62±28.6	31±21.5	<0.001	0.27
CF (%)	83±17.6	83±24.9	N.S.	0.01

Legend: MDD, Major Depressive Disorder; HC, Healthy Controls; RT, Reaction time; ER, Error Rates; CF, Correction Factor; N.S., not significant.
Values given as mean ± SD.

Table 3. Eye movement performances×MADRS interaction between the 2 groups.

| Covariable | Dependent variable | Group | | |
		$F_{1,65}$	p	η^2_p
MADRS	Pro RT	3.68	N.S.	0.05
	Pro gain	7.97	<0.01	0.11
	Anti RT	0.02	N.S.	<0.001
	Anti ER	0.5	N.S.	<0.01
	Anti CF	2.79	N.S.	<0.01
	Anti - Pro RT	0.96	N.S.	0.06

Legend: MADRS, Montgomery Asberg Depression Rating Scale; Pro, Prosaccade; Anti, Antisaccade; RT, Reaction time; ER, Error Rates; CF, Correction Factor; η^2_p: effect size; N.S., not significant.

For both groups, the RT was longer in the antisaccade task than in the prosaccade task due to the incompatibility between the target position and the target-directed movement. This result was consistent with those found in other studies [38,39]. Moreover, patients with depression had higher RT in both prosaccade and antisaccade task compared to controls.

We cannot deny the effect of global eye movement retardation, since we found significant differences in RT even in the prosaccade task. Many studies have shown altered cortical structures such as the cerebellum [40,41], the dorsolateral prefrontal cortex [42,43] and frontal eye fields [44] in depression that could play a role in the RT of eye saccade [45–47]. In our study, depressed patients also had higher ER in the antisaccade task. Alteration of motor adjustment could have played a role in the antisaccade task as well as in the prosaccade task [48].

However, we ensured that differences found in the antisaccade task were not only due to psychomotor retardation. First, we controlled neuropsychological performances. Second, we computed the time cost of inhibitory processes. Inhibitory processing is altered in patients with depression, which affects saccade latency. Inhibitory processing may be changed at the selection stage of the motor response [49] that is sent to the oculomotor system. Indeed, it has been suggested that an alteration of this function could be related to attentional biases observed in depression through its involvement in the selective attention process. It is also noteworthy that all differences that were reported concerning RT, gain and ER, in prosaccades, antisaccades, and in the differential measures specific to inhibition cost, were dependent on the MADRS scores, but globally not predicted by classic neuropsychological tests. Therefore, depression seems to be at the heart of the changes in eye movements, and not the result of more generic neuropsychological alterations. The relative independency of neuropsychological scores and eye movement performances in elderly depression constitutes eye tracking as a complementary tool for inhibitory capacity evaluation in depressive disorders.

However, our analyses suggest that psychomotor retardation was not the major cause of patients' worse performances in the antisaccade task. The depressed elderly also exhibited reduced performances on the interference score of the Stroop test. These results suggest an inhibition deficit in depressed patients affecting interference performance. However, it may be questioned whether this is the same deficit that causes impairment on the antisaccade task. Indeed, the lack of correlation between the Stroop interference score and antisaccade minus prosaccade RT ($rho = -0.34$, $p = 0.16$), prosaccade gain ($rho = 0.35$, $p = 0.15$) or antisaccade error rates ($rho = 0.32$, $p = 0.19$) suggests that there

could be an additional specific alteration of the inhibition mechanism at the level of the movement planning process [50]. The antisaccade task requires a motor response at the opposite of the target whereas the Stroop test requires an incongruent motor response [51]. In the Stroop test, inhibition corresponds to both the interference (the mechanism that prevents irrelevant information entered in memory) and inhibition (active suppression process). Several studies using different tasks to assess the inhibition showed that the correlations between the scores of these tasks were low or nonexistent [52,53]. Several studies have reported a link between cognitive impairment and an inhibition deficit in depression [54–56] associated with pre-frontal cortex dysfunctions [57,58], especially when executive functions were scrutinized [59,60]. Other cognitive functions may also be linked to inhibition such as working memory [61,62]. However, these results remain controversial [54]. Methodological differences regarding the sample size and the heterogeneity of inclusion criteria could explain these disparities. Generally, the involvement of executive functions and inhibition mechanisms would be most important but this not only depends on the different types of depression [63–65], but also on their severity [56] and the age at the first depressive episode [66,67]. Additional efforts are needed to identify precise processes than underlie the changes in inhibitory capacities. For example, Crawford *et al.* [68] found that the RT in prosaccade and antisaccade tasks did not differ between patients with Alzheimer disease (AD) and control subjects. However, patients with AD had more ER in the antisaccade task. Moreover, these performances were correlated with the severity of cognitive impairment in AD patients [68,69]. In our study, elderly depressed patients had an inhibition deficit characterized by an higher ER in the antisaccade task, although the difference between depressed patients and controls in prosaccade and antisaccade RT seems to be related both to the effect of inhibition impairment and psychomotor retardation. These results were correlated with severity of the depression but not with cognitive impairment. Therefore, the current results may open new windows on specific moderation of the prefrontal cortex by affective circuits, possibly through amygdala-prefrontal cortex connections [70], even when stimuli are not emotional in nature. Current research also provides us with information about the specificity of motor inhibition impairment in elderly depressive patients, since this impairment is relatively independent from more cognitive-verbal processes measured by classic neuropsychological tests (e.g., Stroop test).

Inhibition deficit has been shown to be related to suicide risk in elderly depressed patients [71]. Cognitive inhibition is involved in decision-making and could help the depressed patient in preventing late-life suicide [72]. Cognitive inhibition could also reduce the intrusion of suicidal ideation and rumination [71]. Alexopoulos [73] suggested that the presence of cognitive inhibition alteration could be predictive of a lack of therapeutic response to antidepressants in the depressed elderly. Moreover, Malsert et al. [74] reported that the RT and ER performances in antisaccade task were associated with the severity of depression and could predict response to transcranial magnetic stimulation over the dorsolateral prefrontal cortex. Our results suggest that the oculomotor performances evaluated by the RT and the ER could be useful measurements of cognitive inhibition in elderly depressed patients. These performances are *complementary* to classical neuropsychological measurements since they seem to be at least partially independent. Further research would be required in order to confirm the interest of using eye movement measurements to predict treatment response or suicidal risks in elderly patients.

A possible limitation of this study, which is common to many experiments in the field, is related to the effect of drugs. Various studies have shown that drugs can affect eye movements [75]. Fafrowicz et al. [76] have highlighted an increase in saccadic RT in healthy volunteers treated by anxiolytic drugs. Green et al. [77] have also demonstrated an increase in antisaccade errors in schizophrenic patients treated by benzodiazepine. However, other series did not show any treatment effects on eye movements [78] or latency and ER for antisaccade in schizophrenic and depressed patients [79]. To reduce intervening effects, we ensured that all patients were in a stable phase of their disease and were not showing any clinical signs of drug side effects.

In conclusion, the results of this study have offered a new insight into the cognitive-motor inhibition impairment of elderly depressed patients. We used two simple eye movement tasks and additional data analysis focusing on the cost of inhibitory processes. Elderly depression was never previously studied based on this methodology. From a theoretical point of view, this questions the validity of a monolithic approach to cognitive inhibition. More specific conceptual categories are needed in order to account for the multiplicity of inhibitory processes and behaviors. From a clinical point of view, implications may include a more precise evaluation of inhibitory capacities in patients. Complementary research is needed in order to measure the predictive power of the manipulated variables on ecologically-relevant behaviors (i.e., suicidal risk, therapeutic response to treatment).

Acknowledgments

The authors are grateful to Richard Medeiros, Medical Editor of Medical Editing International for editing the manuscript, Emmanuel Haffen, Djamila Bennabi, Laurianne Vuillez for psychiatric assessments and Gregory Tio for their useful suggestions.

Author Contributions

Conceived and designed the experiments: EL PV JM. Performed the experiments: NC NN PV GC. Analyzed the data: NC NN. Contributed reagents/materials/analysis tools: NC EL PV GC NN JM. Contributed to the writing of the manuscript: NC EL PV GC JM NN.

References

1. Austin MP, Ross M, Murray C, O'Carroll RE, Ebmeier KP, et al. (1992) Cognitive function in major depression. Journal of Affective Disorders 25: 21–29.
2. Foster SM, Davis HP, Kisley MA (2013) Brain responses to emotional images related to cognitive ability in older adults. Psychology and Aging 28: 179–190.
3. Nigg JT (2000) On inhibition/disinhibition in developmental psychopathology: views from cognitive and personality psychology and a working inhibition taxonomy. Psychol Bull 126: 220–246.
4. Harnishfeger KK (1995) The development of cognitive inhibition : theories, definitions and research evidence. In: Dempster FN, Brainerd CJ, editors. Interference and inhibition in cognition. San Diego: Academic Press. pp. 175–204.
5. Harnishfeger KK, Bjorklund DF (1994) A developmental perspective on individual differences in inhibition. Learning and Individual Differences 6: 331–355.
6. Houghton G, Tipper SP (1994) A model of inhibitory mechanisms in selective attention. Inhibitory processes in attention, memory, and language. In: Dagenbach D, Carr TH, editors. Inhibitory processes in attention, memory, and language. San Diego, CA, US: Academic Press. pp. 53–112.
7. Everling S, Munoz DP (2000) Neuronal correlates for preparatory set associated with pro-saccades and anti-saccades in the primate frontal eye field. The Journal of Neuroscience 20: 387–400.
8. Leigh RJ, Kennard C (2004) Using saccades as a research tool in the clinical neurosciences. Brain 127: 460–477.
9. Hutton SB (2008) Cognitive control of saccadic eye movements. Brain and Cognition 68: 327–340.
10. Rafal R, Henik A (1994) The neurology of inhibition: Integrating controlled and automatic processes. In: Dagenbach D, Carr TH, editors. Inhibitory processes in attention, memory, and language. San Diego: Academic Press. pp. 1–51.
11. Currie J, Ramsden B (1991) Validation of a clinical antisaccadic eye movements test in the assessment of dementia. Archive Neurology 48: 949.
12. Miyake A, Friedman NP, Emerson MJ, Witzki AH, Howerter A, et al. (2000) The unity and diversity of executive functions and their contributions to complex "Frontal Lobe" tasks: a latent variable analysis. Cognitive Psychology 41: 49–100.
13. Sweeney JA, Strojwas MH, Mann JJ, Thase ME (1998) Prefrontal and cerebellar abnormalities in major depression: evidence from oculomotor studies. Biological Psychiatry 43: 584–594.
14. Mahlberg R, Steinacher B, Mackert A, Flechtner KM (2001) Basic parameters of saccadic eye movements–differences between unmedicated schizophrenia and affective disorder patients. European Archive of Psychiatry and Clinical Neuroscience 251: 205–210.
15. De Lissnyder E, Derakshan N, De Raedt R, Koster EH (2011) Depressive symptoms and cognitive control in a mixed antisaccade task: specific effects of depressive rumination. Cognition & Emotion 25: 886–897.
16. Fiske A, Wetherell JL, Gatz M (2009) Depression in older adults. Annual Review of Clinical Psychology 5: 363–389.
17. Joormann J, Yoon KL, Zetsche U (2007) Cognitive inhibition in depression. Applied and preventive psychology 12: 128–139.
18. Mecocci P, Cherubini A, Mariani E, Ruggiero C, Senin U (2004) Depression in the elderly: new concepts and therapeutic approaches. Aging Clinical and Experimental Research 16: 176–189.
19. Gallagher D, O'Regan C, Savva GM, Cronin H, Lawlor BA, et al. (2012) Depression, anxiety and cardiovascular disease: Which symptoms are associated with increased risk in community dwelling older adults? Journal of Affective Disorders.
20. Alexopoulos GS (2006) The vascular depression hypothesis: 10 years later. Biological Psychiatry 60: 1304–1305.
21. Thorpe L, Groulx B (2001) Depressive syndromes in dementia. Canadian Journal of Neurological Sciences 28: S83–95.
22. APA (2000) Diagnostic and Statistical Manual of Mental Disorders, Fourth Edition: DSM-IV®. Paris: American Psychiatric Association.
23. Montgomery SA, Asberg M (1979) A new depression scale designed to be sensitive to change. The British Journal of Psychiatry 134: 382–389.
24. Ferreira S, Vanholsbeeck G, Chopard G, Pitard A, Tio G, et al. (2010) [Comparative norms of RAPID neuropsychological battery tests for subjects aged between 50 and 89 years]. Revue Neurologique 166: 606–614.
25. Folstein MF, Folstein SE, McHugh PR (1975). "Mini-mental state". A practical method for grading the cognitive state of patients for the clinician. The Journal of Psychiatric Research 12: 189–198.
26. Reitan RM (1958) Validity of the Trail Making Test as an indicator of organic brain damage. Perceptual and Motor Skills 8: 271–276.
27. Goldman WP, Baty JD, Buckles VD, Sahrmann S, Morris JC (1999) Motor dysfunction in mildly demented AD individuals without extrapyramidal signs. Neurology 53: 956–962.
28. Signoret J-L (1989) Evaluation des troubles de la mémoire et des désordres cognitifs associés. Paris, France: Ipsen.
29. Isaacs B, Kennie AT (1973) The Set test as an aid to the detection of dementia in old people. The British Journal of Psychiatry 123: 467–470.
30. Buschke H, Kuslansky G, Katz M, Stewart WF, Sliwinski MJ, et al. (1999) Screening for dementia with the memory impairment screen. Neurology 52: 231–238.
31. Grober E, Buschke H (1987) Genuine memory deficits in dementia Developmental Neuropsychology 3: 13–36.

32. Van der Linden M, Coyette F, Poitrenaud J, Kalafat M, Calicis F, et al. (2004) L'épreuve de rappel libre/rappel indicé à 16 items (RL/RI-16). L'évaluation des troubles de la mémoire Présentation de quatre tests de mémoire épisodique (avec leur étalonnage). Marseille, France: Solal. pp. 25–44.

33. Stroop JR (1935) Studies of interference in serial verbal reactions. Journal of Experimental Psychology 18: 643–662.

34. Everling S, Fischer B (1998) The antisaccade: a review of basic research and clinical studies. Neuropsychologia 36: 885–899.

35. Fischer B, Weber H (1992) Characteristics of "anti" saccades in man. Experimental Brain Research 89: 415–424.

36. Nijboer T, Vree A, Dijkerman C, Van der Stigchel S (2010) Prism adaptation influences perception but not attention: evidence from antisaccades. Neuroreport 21: 386–389.

37. Cohen J (1988) Statistical power analysis for the behavioral sciences. Hillsdale, NJ: Erlbaum.

38. Godijn R, Kramer AF (2007) Antisaccade costs with static and dynamic targets. Perception & Psychophysics 69: 802–815.

39. Gooding DC, Mohapatra L, Shea HB (2004) Temporal stability of saccadic task performance in schizophrenia and bipolar patients. Psychological Medicine 34: 921–932.

40. Liu Z, Xu C, Xu Y, Wang Y, Zhao B, et al. (2010) Decreased regional homogeneity in insula and cerebellum: a resting-state fMRI study in patients with major depression and subjects at high risk for major depression. Psychiatry Research 182: 211–215.

41. Robinson FR, Fuchs AF (2001) The role of the cerebellum in voluntary eye movements. Annual Review of Neuroscience 24: 981–1004.

42. Baxter LR, Schwartz JM, Phelps ME, Mazziotta JC, Guze BH, et al. (1989) Reduction of prefrontal cortex glucose metabolism common to three types of depression. Archives of General Psychiatry 46: 243–250.

43. Crevits L, Van den Abbeele D, Audenaert K, Goethals M, Dierick M (2005) Effect of repetitive transcranial magnetic stimulation on saccades in depression: a pilot study. Psychiatry Research 135: 113–119.

44. Gaymard B, Ploner CJ, Rivaud S, Vermersch AI, Pierrot-Deseilligny C (1998) Cortical control of saccades. Experimental Brain Research 123: 159–163.

45. Pierrot-Deseilligny C, Muri RM, Ploner CJ, Gaymard B, Demeret S, et al. (2003) Decisional role of the dorsolateral prefrontal cortex in ocular motor behaviour. Brain 126: 1460–1473.

46. Pierrot-Deseilligny C, Muri RM, Ploner CJ, Gaymard B, Rivaud-Pechoux S (2003) Cortical control of ocular saccades in humans: a model for motricity. Progress in Brain Research 142: 3–17.

47. Pierrot-Deseilligny C, Milea D, Muri RM (2004) Eye movement control by the cerebral cortex. Current Opinion in Neurology 17: 17–25.

48. Munoz DP, Everling S (2004) Look away: the anti-saccade task and the voluntary control of eye movement. Nature Review Neuroscience 5: 218–228.

49. Bonin-Guillaume S, Hasbroucq T, Blin O (2008) [Psychomotor retardation associated to depression differs from that of normal aging]. Psychologie & Neuropsychiatrie du Vieillissement 6: 137–144.

50. Hamilton AC, Martin RC (2005) Dissociations among tasks involving inhibition: a single-case study. Cognitive, Affective & Behavioral Neuroscience 5: 1–13.

51. Unsworth N, Spillers GJ, Brewer GA, McMillan B (2011) Attention control and the antisaccade task: a response time distribution analysis. Acta Psychologica 137: 90–100.

52. Gallo JJ, Coyne JC (2000) The challenge of depression in late life: bridging science and service in primary care. JAMA 284: 1570–1572.

53. Kramer AF, Humphrey DG, Larish JF, Logan GD, Strayer DL (1994) Aging and inhibition: beyond a unitary view of inhibitory processing in attention. Psychol Aging 9: 491–512.

54. Austin MP, Mitchell P, Goodwin GM (2001) Cognitive deficits in depression: possible implications for functional neuropathology. The British Journal of Psychiatry 178: 200–206.

55. Baudic S, Tzortzis C, Barba GD, Traykov L (2004) Executive deficits in elderly patients with major unipolar depression. Journal of Geriatric Psychiatry and Neurology 17: 195–201.

56. Boone KB, Lesser IM, Miller BL, Wohl M, Berman N, et al. (1995) Cognitive functioning in older depressed outpatients: Relationship of presence and severity of depression to neuropsychological test scores. Neuropsychology 9: 390–398.

57. Funahashi S (2001) Neuronal mechanisms of executive control by the prefrontal cortex. Neuroscience Research 39: 147–165.

58. Naismith SL, Norrie LM, Mowszowski L, Hickie IB (2012) The neurobiology of depression in later-life: clinical, neuropsychological, neuroimaging and pathophysiological features. Progress in Neurobiology 98: 99–143.

59. Baudic S, Benisty S, Dalla Barba G, Traykov L (2007) [Impairment of executive function in elderly patients with major unipolar depression: influence of psychomotor retardation]. Psychologie & Neuropsychiatrie du Vieillissement 5: 65–71.

60. Marazziti D, Consoli G, Picchetti M, Carlini M, Faravelli L (2010) Cognitive impairment in major depression. European Journal of Pharmacology 626: 83–86.

61. Eenshuistra RM, Ridderinkhof KR, van der Molen MW (2004) Age-related changes in antisaccade task performance: inhibitory control or working-memory engagement? Brain and Cognition 56: 177–188.

62. Gohier B, Ferracci L, Surguladze SA, Lawrence E, El Hage W, et al. (2009) Cognitive inhibition and working memory in unipolar depression. Journal of Affective Disorders 116: 100–105.

63. Basso MR, Bornstein RA (1999) Neuropsychological deficits in psychotic versus nonpsychotic unipolar depression. Neuropsychology 13: 69–75.

64. Palmer BW, Boone KB, Lesser IM, Wohl MA, Berman N, et al. (1996) Neuropsychological deficits among older depressed patients with predominantly psychological or vegetative symptoms. Journal of Affective Disorders 41: 17–24.

65. Winograd-Gurvich C, Georgiou-Karistianis N, Fitzgerald PB, Millist L, White OB (2006) Ocular motor differences between melancholic and non-melancholic depression. Journal of Affective Disorders 93: 193–203.

66. Alexopoulos GS (2003) Role of executive function in late-life depression. Journal of Clinical Psychiatry 64: 18–23.

67. Lockwood KA, Alexopoulos GS, Kakuma T, Van Gorp WG (2000) Subtypes of cognitive impairment in depressed older adults. The American Journal of Geriatric Psychiatry 8: 201–208.

68. Crawford TJ, Higham S, Renvoize T, Patel J, Dale M, et al. (2005) Inhibitory control of saccadic eye movements and cognitive impairment in Alzheimer's disease. Biol Psychiatry 57: 1052–1060.

69. Shafiq-Antonacci R, Maruff P, Masters C, Currie J (2003) Spectrum of saccade system function in Alzheimer disease. Arch Neurol 60: 1272–1278.

70. Townsend JD, Torrisi SJ, Lieberman MD, Sugar CA, Bookheimer SY, et al. (2013) Frontal-amygdala connectivity alterations during emotion downregulation in bipolar I disorder. Biol Psychiatry 73: 127–135.

71. Richard-Devantoy S, Jollant F, Kefi Z, Turecki G, Olie JP, et al. (2012) Deficit of cognitive inhibition in depressed elderly: a neurocognitive marker of suicidal risk. Journal of Affective Disorders 140: 193–199.

72. Dombrovski AY, Butters MA, Reynolds CF, 3rd, Houck PR, Clark L, et al. (2008) Cognitive performance in suicidal depressed elderly: preliminary report. The American Journal of Geriatric Psychiatry 16: 109–115.

73. Alexopoulos GS (2005) Depression in the elderly. Lancet 365: 1961–1970.

74. Malsert J, Guyader N, Chauvin A, Polosan M, Poulet E, et al. (2012) Antisaccades as a follow-up tool in major depressive disorder therapies: a pilot study. Psychiatry Research 200: 1051–1053.

75. Ball DM, Glue P, Wilson S, Nutt DJ (1991) Pharmacology of saccadic eye movements in man. 1. Effects of the benzodiazepine receptor ligands midazolam and flumazenil. Psychopharmacology 105: 361–367.

76. Fafrowicz M, Unrug A, Marek T, van Luijtelaar G, Noworol C, et al. (1995) Effects of diazepam and buspirone on reaction time of saccadic eye movements. Neuropsychobiology 32: 156–160.

77. Green JF, King DJ (1998) The effects of chlorpromazine and lorazepam on abnormal antisaccade and no-saccade distractibility. Biological Psychiatry 44: 709–715.

78. Flechtner KM, Steinacher B, Sauer R, Mackert A (2002) Smooth pursuit eye movements of patients with schizophrenia and affective disorder during clinical treatment. European Archive of Psychiatry and Clinical Neuroscience 252: 49–53.

79. Katsanis J, Kortenkamp S, Iacono WG, Grove WM (1997) Antisaccade performance in patients with schizophrenia and affective disorder. Journal of Abnormal Psychology 106: 468–472.

6

Lack of Involvement of CEP Adducts in TLR Activation and in Angiogenesis

John Gounarides[1], Jennifer S. Cobb[1], Jing Zhou[1], Frank Cook[1], Xuemei Yang[1], Hong Yin[1], Erik Meredith[2], Chang Rao[1], Qian Huang[3], YongYao Xu[3], Karen Anderson[4], Andrea De Erkenez[4], Sha-Mei Liao[4], Maura Crowley[4], Natasha Buchanan[4], Stephen Poor[4], Yubin Qiu[4], Elizabeth Fassbender[4], Siyuan Shen[4], Amber Woolfenden[4], Amy Jensen[4], Rosemarie Cepeda[4], Bijan Etemad-Gilbertson[4], Shelby Giza[4], Muneto Mogi[2], Bruce Jaffee[4], Sassan Azarian[4]*

1 Analytical Sciences, Novartis Institutes for Biomedical Research, Cambridge, MA, United States of America, 2 Global Discovery Chemistry, Novartis Institutes for Biomedical Research, Cambridge, MA, United States of America, 3 Developmental and Metabolic Pathways, Novartis Institutes for Biomedical Research, Cambridge, MA, United States of America, 4 Ophthalmology, Novartis Institutes for Biomedical Research, Cambridge, MA, United States of America

Abstract

Proteins that are post-translationally adducted with 2-(ω-carboxyethyl)pyrrole (CEP) have been proposed to play a pathogenic role in age-related macular degeneration, by inducing angiogenesis in a Toll Like Receptor 2 (TLR2)-dependent manner. We have investigated the involvement of CEP adducts in angiogenesis and TLR activation, to assess the therapeutic potential of inhibiting CEP adducts and TLR2 for ocular angiogenesis. As tool reagents, several CEP-adducted proteins and peptides were synthetically generated by published methodology and adduction was confirmed by NMR and LC-MS/MS analyses. Structural studies showed significant changes in secondary structure in CEP-adducted proteins but not the untreated proteins. Similar structural changes were also observed in the treated unadducted proteins, which were treated by the same adduction method except for one critical step required to form the CEP group. Thus some structural changes were unrelated to CEP groups and were artificially induced by the synthesis method. In biological studies, the CEP-adducted proteins and peptides failed to activate TLR2 in cell-based assays and in an in vivo TLR2-mediated retinal leukocyte infiltration model. Neither CEP adducts nor TLR agonists were able to induce angiogenesis in a tube formation assay. In vivo, treatment of animals with CEP-adducted protein had no effect on laser-induced choroidal neovascularization. Furthermore, in vivo inactivation of TLR2 by deficiency in Myeloid Differentiation factor 88 (Myd88) had no effect on abrasion-induced corneal neovascularization. Thus the CEP-TLR2 axis, which is implicated in other wound angiogenesis models, does not appear to play a pathological role in a corneal wound angiogenesis model. Collectively, our data do not support the mechanism of action of CEP adducts in TLR2-mediated angiogenesis proposed by others.

Editor: Michael E. Boulton, Indiana University College of Medicine, United States of America

Funding: This study was funded by the Novartis Institutes for Biomedical Research. The funder provided support in the form of salaries for all authors, but did not have any additional role in the study design, data collection and analysis, decision to publish, or preparation of the manuscript. The specific roles of these authors are articulated in the 'author contributions' section.

Competing Interests: The authors were all full-time employees of the Novartis Institutes of Biomedical Research, which funded this study, at the time this work was completed. There are no patents, products in development or marketed products to declare.

* Email: Sassan.Azarian@novartis.com

Introduction

Age-related macular degeneration (AMD) is a major cause of legal blindness in the elderly. The macula is a specialized area of the central retina that is enriched in photoreceptor cells and is responsible for high acuity vision. In AMD, progressive macular degeneration can impair critical daily functions such as reading, driving, and face recognition. Thus AMD can have a profound impact on quality of life. There are two forms of advanced AMD: dry and wet (neovascular) AMD [1]. AMD is thought to be a disease of the retinal pigment epithelium (RPE) cells, which provide critical support functions to adjacent photoreceptors [1]. In the early stage of disease, AMD retinas show progressive accumulation of extracellular deposits, drusen, as well as intracellular deposits, lipofuscin, at the level of the RPE. These deposits initially tend to accumulate in the macular area. Over time, RPE cells show pigmentary changes and begin to degenerate. In advanced stages, dry AMD patients exhibit substantial delineated areas of RPE atrophy, or geographic atrophy. Advanced wet AMD patients exhibit leaky blood vessels in the macula, in many cases emanating from the choriocapillaris [1].

Currently there are no treatments for dry AMD. In the Age-Related Eye Disease Study 1 (AREDS 1), dietary supplements comprised of anti-oxidants and select minerals reduced the risk of progression to advanced AMD by 25% [1]. Several therapeutic approaches are being tested in clinical trials [2] but there are no FDA-approved treatments in practice at this point. For wet AMD, anti-angiogenic treatments have been clinically proven to be efficacious [3]. However, not all patients respond to treatment and the burden of treatment is still relatively high. Thus there is a great medical need for novel treatments for AMD. The molecular details of pathogenesis in AMD are not fully established but several pathogenic mechanisms have been implicated [1]. For example, human molecular genetic data indicate the involvement of the alternative complement pathway. Another potential cause is proposed to be cumulative oxidative stress, based on preclinical studies and on the AREDS1 trial. One manifestation of oxidative stress is proposed to be the formation of CEP adducts, which are a type of advanced glycation end products [4].

Photoreceptor cells are highly enriched in docosahexaenoic acid (DHA), a labile fatty acid that is susceptible to breakdown by photo-oxidation and other forms of oxidative stress. The breakdown products include a reactive aldehyde, 4-hydroxy-7-oxohept-5-enoic acid, which can condense with primary amines to form a Schiff base. In the case of proteins, 4-hydroxy-7-oxohept-5-enoic acid condenses with lysineε-amines. Subsequent reactions result in a covalently attached CEP moiety, yielding a stable CEP adduct [4]. In previous reports, antibodies raised against synthetic CEP reagents were used to identify, localize, and quantify CEP adducts by various immunological assays [5]. Elevated levels of CEP adducts were initially reported in proteomic studies of AMD donor eyes [5] and subsequently in AMD plasma [6,7]. Thus CEP adducts were implicated in AMD [5–7]. In later studies CEP adducts were reported to be pro-angiogenic, both *in vitro* and *in vivo*. These *in vivo* studies utilized the micropocket corneal neovascularization (CoNV) and the laser-induced choroidal neovascularization (CNV) models [8]. More recently, Toll-like receptor 2 (TLR2) was reported to mediate the CEP adduct-induced angiogenesis [9]. The angiogenic activity was reported to be independent of the vascular endothelial growth factor (VEGF) pathway [8,9].

There is a medical need for novel treatments for both wet and dry AMD. CEP adducts are implicated in both forms of AMD and represent an attractive potential target for drug discovery. Thus we initiated validation studies to assess the therapeutic potential of inhibiting CEP adducts.

Results

Synthesis of Tool Reagents

Several synthetic CEP adducts were generated according to reported procedures [10]. These tool reagents included protein (e.g. human serum albumin-CEP, or HSA-CEP), peptide (e.g. Ac-Gly-Lys-OMe-CEP, or dipeptide-CEP), and phospholipid (e.g. phosphatidyl ethanolamine-CEP, or PE-CEP) adducts, as listed in **Table S1**. The presence of CEP adducts and the stoichiometry of adduction was confirmed by ^{1}H-NMR and LC-MS/MS (**Figure S1 and Figure S2**). Invariably the presence of CEP moiety was established in the adducted samples and was never detected in the controls. CEP adduction was deemed successful by several measures. For example, ^{1}H-NMR analysis indicated the expected molecular signature of the CEP group in dipeptide-CEP but not the untreated dipeptide (**Figure S1B**). Likewise, LC-MS/MS analysis of enzymatic hydrolyzed adducted proteins detected lysine-CEP in HSA-CEP and MSA-CEP (mouse serum albumin-CEP) but not the respective controls (**Figure S1C**). For protein adducts, two controls were used: CTL1, which represents untreated protein; and CTL2, which represents treated unadducted protein. The latter control was treated exactly the same way as the corresponding CEP adduct except for one step, to prevent adduction (see Materials and Methods). No CEP moiety was detected in HSA-CTL2 or MSA-CTL2. There are a total of 59 lysines in HSA (UnitPro P02768) and 50 lysines in MSA

(UnitPro P07724). We identified 14 lysine-CEP sites in HSA-CEP and 40 lysine-CEP sites in MSA-CEP (**Figure S2**). These values are in fair agreement with the reported stoichiometries: 6 or 17 CEP-modified lysines for HSA-CEP [10,11], and 15 for MSA-CEP [10].

Does CEP-Adduction Affect Protein Structure?

When we analyzed HSA-CEP, HSA-CTL2, and HSA-CTL1 in structural studies we observed significant structural alterations in HSA-CEP in comparison with HSA-CTL1. However, HSA-CTL2 also incurred significant alterations, similar to but less extensive than HSA-CEP. On SDS-PAGE gels HSA-CEP and HSA-CTL2 but not HSA-CTL1 appeared to form oligomers in a ladder-like fashion (**Figure 1A**). Comparison of size exclusion chromatography (SEC) profiles indicated progressive loss of the HSA monomer in the order of HSA-CTL1 > HSA-CTL2 > HSA-CEP (**Figure 1B**). Circular dichroism (CD) also indicated a significant loss in secondary structure in HSA-CTL2 and HSA-CEP compared to HSA-CTL1 (**Figure 1C**).

Collectively these data show that our synthetic CEP adducts can incur two kinds of structural changes: a) CEP-independent changes and b) CEP-dependent changes. Comparison of our HSA-CTL1 and HSA-CTL2 illustrates the CEP-independent changes in protein structure, which indicate artificial changes introduced by the procedure for generating synthetic adducts. Comparison of our HSA-CTL2 and HSA-CEP illustrates the CEP-dependent changes that occur as a result covalent CEP groups in HSA-CEP, beyond the CEP-independent changes in HSA-CTL2.

Is TLR2 Activated By CEP Adducts?

We tested several CEP adducts in a cell-based TLR2 assay, essentially as described [9]. Pam3CSK4, a known TLR2 agonist, showed dose-dependent activation of TLR2 as monitored by production of NF-κB or IL-8 in cellular assays (**Figure 2**, top and middle panels). However, no TLR2 activation was detected by HSA-CEP (**Figure 2**), or several other CEP adducts tested: MSA-CEP, dipeptide-CEP, or PE-CEP (not shown). None of these adducts showed any cytotoxicity, as measured with CellTiter-Glo (CTG) kit (**Figure 2**). Next we used THP-1 cells, which naturally express several TLRs, including TLR2. While positive controls showed specific activation of the corresponding TLR, CEP adducts failed to activate TLR2 or any other TLR that was monitored (**Figure 2,** bottom panel). *In vivo*, CEP adducts did not induce biological effects that are mediated by TLR2. As **Figure 3A** shows, treatment of mice with Pam3CSK4 induced infiltration of neutrophils and macrophages in the retina. However, neither dipeptide-CEP nor MSA-CEP (not shown) induced retinal infiltration in the same assay. Representative images of this experiment are shown in **Figure 3B**. These results suggest that CEP adducts do not activate TLRs, including TLR2.

Are CEP Adducts or TLR2 Involved in Angiogenesis?

We used the tube formation *in vitro* assay to determine if CEP adducts are angiogenic, similar to a previously reported assay [9]. VEGF induced significant tube formation; however, neither CEP adducts nor Pam3CSK4 affected tube formation (**Table 1**). In addition, poly (I:C) (a TLR3 agonist) and LPS (a TLR4 agonist) failed to show any effect. Representative images of the tube formation assay are shown in **Figure 4**.

The CEP adducts were further evaluated in the laser-induced choroidal neovascularization (CNV) model, as was reported earlier [8]. Initial laser CNV studies were performed with C57BL/6N mice, which showed no effect of MSA-CEP (**File S1**). In light of

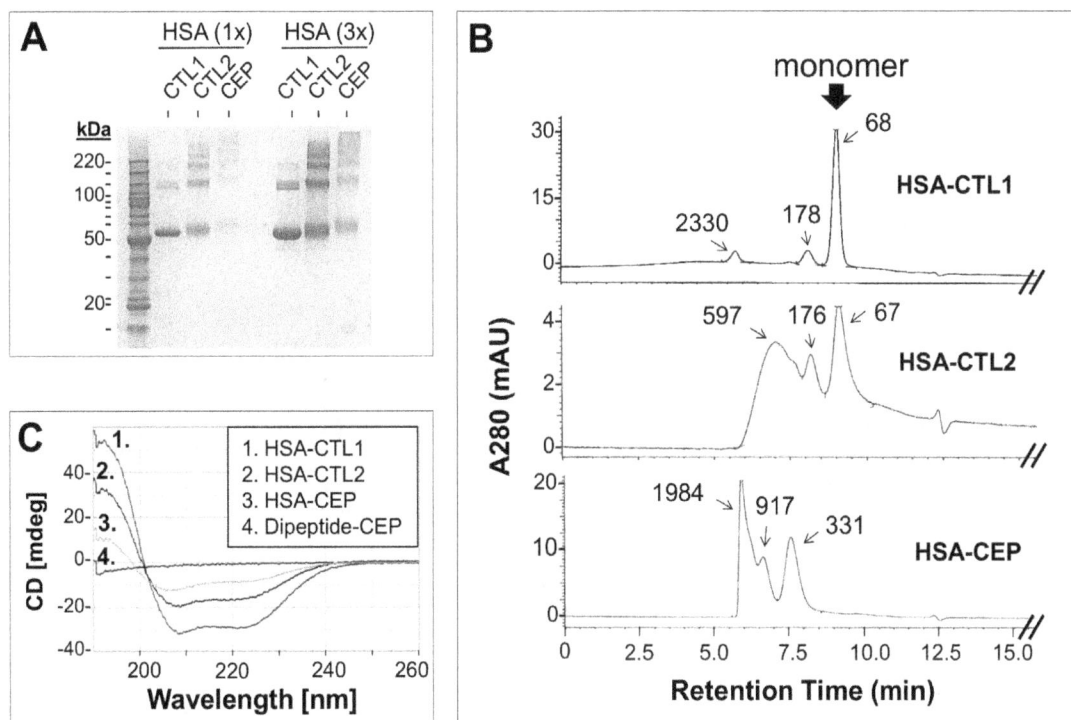

Figure 1. Structural Analyses of CEP Adducts. A) *SDS-PAGE analysis.* Aliquots of HSA-CTL1 (untreated), HSA-CTL2 (treated but unadducted) and HSA-CEP were subjected to reducing SDS-PAGE on 4–10% gels. Compared to HSA-CTL1, both HSA-CTL2 and HSA-CEP showed an increase in high-MW bands. B) *Size exclusion chromatography.* SEC under non-denaturing conditions indicated an increase in faster-eluting peaks in HSA-CTL2 and HSA-CEP compared to HSA-CTL1. C) *Circular dichroism.* CD analysis revealed a loss of secondary structure in HSA-CTL2 and HSA-CEP compared to HSA-CTL1.

the *rd8* mutation in the *Crb1* gene reported in this strain [12], we repeated the study with C57BL/6J mice which are wildtype for *Crb1* [12] and were used in the previously reported study [8]. We observed the same results with 2 experiments in each strain. Subretinal injection of VEGF significantly exacerbated CNV, while a VEGF-neutralizing antibody inhibited CNV (**Figure 5A and File S1**). This is consistent with VEGF being a major pro-angiogenic factor in CNV. However, subretinally administered MSA-CEP, at a dose nearly identical to that used in the previous report [8], had no effect in this model (**Figure 5A and File S1**). Representative images of the experiments in Figure 5A are shown in **Figure 5B**.

In studies with a corneal neovascularization (CoNV) mouse model, we observed that *Myd88*-deficiency had no significant effect on CoNV (**Figure 6**) when compared with similarly treated wild-type mice. Since *Myd88* deficiency abolishes TLR2 activity, this indicates that TLR2 is not required for angiogenesis in the abrasion-induced CoNV model. In contrast, CoNV is greatly dependent on VEGF-A: a) qPCR analysis showed a 30-fold increase in *VEGF-A* mRNA expression and b) treatment of abraded mice with VEGF-A neutralizing antibody showed significant reduction in CoNV area (**Figure S3**).

Discussion

Summary

Here we performed validation studies for the proposed CEP-TLR2 axis to assess the therapeutic potential for wet AMD treatment. Following a published procedure we generated synthetic CEP adducts and confirmed the presence of covalent

CEP groups. Structural analyses of a CEP adduct indicated changes in tertiary structure that were not observed in the naïve protein; however, similar structural changes were observed in the treated, unadducted control. Thus the physiological relevance of the observed structural changes is uncertain. Next we attempted to reproduce some of the reported biological effects of synthetic CEP adducts. When we tested our synthetic CEP adducts in *in vitro* and *in vivo* assays, we observed neither TLR2 activation nor pro-angiogenic activity. We conclude that our data do not support the CEP-TLR2 hypothesis.

Structural Changes in CEP Adducts

In our hands the published protocol for generating CEP adducts worked successfully, by the criterion of the presence of covalently-linked CEP groups in the adduct. This protocol worked robustly with all classes of reagents tested, including proteins, dipeptide, and lipid. Furthermore, the stoichiometry of adduction of each reagent was in fair agreement with the corresponding published stoichiometry.

In our attempt to understand the biological consequences of CEP adduction we initiated protein structural studies with HSA-CEP. Since the conversion of a significant number of positively-charged lysine side chains to negatively charged CEP groups (from the carboxylate group) would greatly alter its surface electrostatic potential, we anticipated and indeed observed structural changes in HSA-CEP in comparison to untreated HSA control (HSA-CTL1). We were surprised, however, to detect similar changes in HSA-CTL2, the treated unadducted control (**Figure 1**). Our interpretation is that two kinds of structural alterations can occur in synthetic CEP adducts: a) alterations that do not involve the

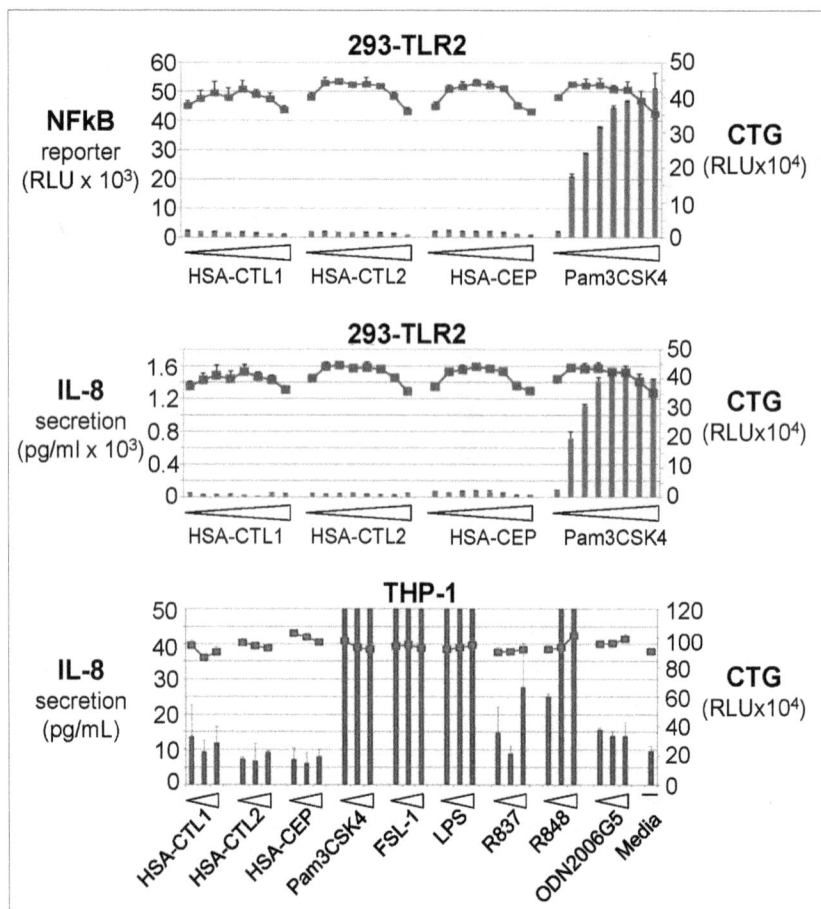

Figure 2. Cell-Based TLR Activation Assays. Various CEP adducts and TLR agonists were tested in HEK293 or THP-1 cells. Readouts were NFkB reporter signal or IL-8 secretion (columns), as indicated. In addition, the same wells were analyzed for viability with the CellTiter-Glo kit (axis on right; square symbols) to ensure that any lack of activation was not due to cell toxicity. HEK293 cells were treated with the following reagents: HSA-CTL1, HSA-CTL2, or HSA-CEP: 0, 3.9, 7.8, 15.6, 32.6, 62.5, and 125 and 250 µg/ml; Pam3CSK4: 0, 1.5, 3.2, 6.3, 12.5, 25, 50, 100 ng/mL. THP-1 cells were treated with the following reagents: HSA-CTL1, HSA-CTL2, or HSA-CEP: 62.5, 125, and 250 µg/mL; Pam3CSK4: 4, 20, and 100 ng/mL; FSL-1:0.4, 2, and 10 ng/mL; LPS: 4, 20, and 100 ng/mL; R837 or R848:0.4, 2, and 10 µM; ODN2006G5:0.2, 1, and 5 µM.

CEP group and were observed when comparing HSA-CTL2 to HSA-CTL1; and b) alterations that occur as a result of covalently-linked CEP groups and were observed when comparing HSA-CEP to HSA-CTL2. It is not clear which step(s) or reagents in the published adduction procedure led to the CEP-independent changes in HSA-CTL2. A candidate culprit is the organic solvent, dimethylformamide; organic solvents are known to affect the structure of some proteins. The adduction procedure entails exposure of protein to 30% dimethylformamide/PBS solution for 4 days at 37°C [10]. In searching the literature we found similar significant structural alteration in a CEP adduct published by another laboratory. A synthetic MSA-CEP adduct appeared to migrate as a continuous smear on denaturing SDS-PAGE and immunoblot, whereas the untreated MSA (the equivalent of MSA-CTL1) migrated as one predominant electrophoretic band (Figure 1 in [13]). A treated unadducted control, the equivalent of our MSA-CTL2, was not included in the report [13]. However since we used similar procedures for generating CEP adducts, in all likelihood the published MSA-CEP incorporated both CEP-independent and -dependent changes.

Thus far, no endogenous CEP adducts have been isolated directly from any biological sources and none have been characterized in the literature. For example, the stoichiometry of

CEP adduction (moles CEP per mole protein) and structural properties have not been reported for any endogenous CEP adducts. Hence at this point it would not be possible to verify that any synthetic CEP adduct is representative of endogenous ones with respect to protein structure. This caveat notwithstanding, we proceeded with biological studies to see if we could reproduce the biological effects of CEP adducts with regards to TLR2 activation and angiogenesis. In our approach we included HSA-CTL2 and MSA-CTL2 in the biological assays of the corresponding CEP adducts, so we might discern biological effects that are specific to the CEP group.

TLR2 Activation by CEP Adducts

We tested CEP-adducted protein or dipeptide in two cell-based assays: a) HEK293-TLR2 cells that specifically expressed TLR2 and, b) THP-1 cells that express multiple TLRs, including TLR2. In both assays, TLR2 activation was observed with a synthetic TLR2 agonist, Pam3CSK4, but not with synthetic CEP adducts. Specifically, we did not detect any effect of HSA-CEP in TLR2-expressing HEK293 cells, as was reported (Figure S14 in [9]). Not surprisingly the controls for our CEP adducts did not have any effects, either. Our cellular assays also did not register any effect of

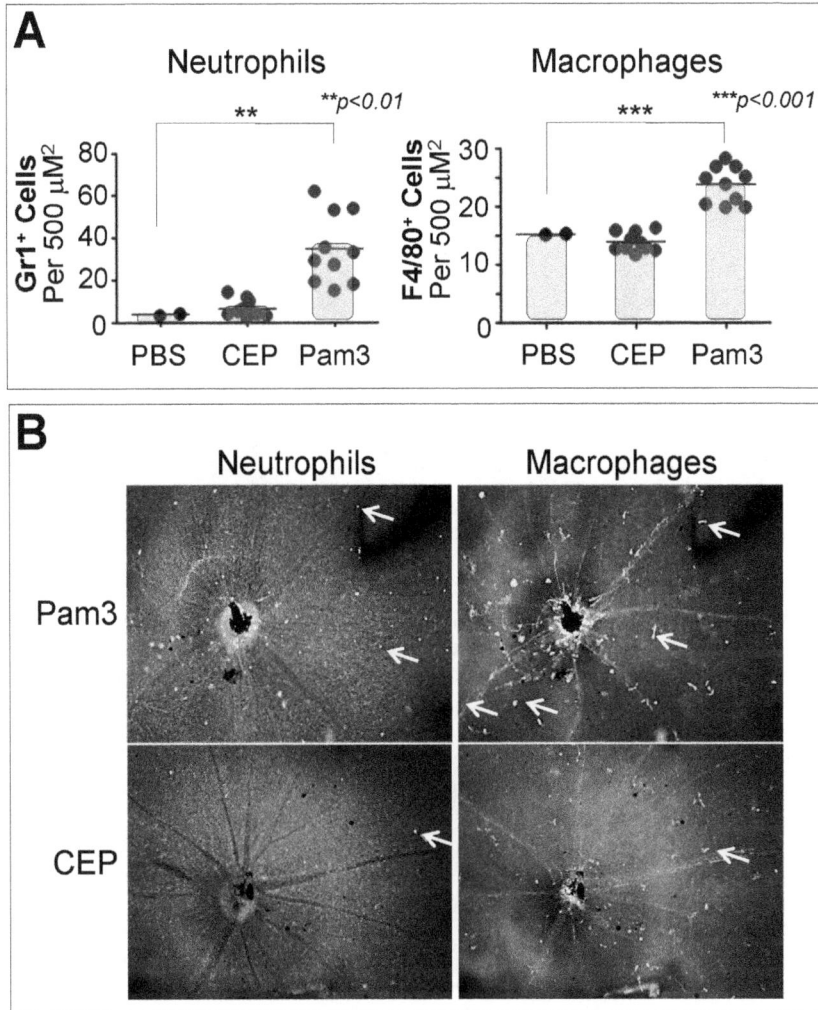

Figure 3. Retinal Leukocyte Infiltration Assay. A) Mice were injected intraperitoneally with either PBS, Pam3CSK4 (25 µg per animal, in PBS), or dipeptide-CEP (400 µg per animal, in PBS) and the retinas were analyzed 8 hours later. Retinal infiltration by neutrophils (Gr1+ cells) or macrophages (F4/80+ cells) was assessed by immunostaining with the respective markers and quantitated with Axiovision, as described in Materials and Methods. Statistical analysis was performed using the Student t-test. Only statistically significant differences are indicated in the graph. B) Shown are representative images of the experiment in **Figure 3A**. Arrows indicate examples of macrophages or neutrophils in the corresponding images. *CEP*, Dipeptide-CEP; *Pam3*, Pam3CSK4.

the dipeptide-CEP, which was reported to be pro-angiogenic in several cellular and *in vivo* assays in a TLR2-dependent manner [9]. However, this dipeptide-CEP was not tested in the same cell-based TLR assay used for HSA-CEP [9], so a direct comparison with our cell-based data is not possible.

We also evaluated CEP adducts in an *in vivo* model for TLR2 activation. In this model, treatment with Pam3CSK4 induced retinal leukocyte infiltration in wild-type mice, but not in *Myd88*−/− nor *TLR2*−/− mice (not shown). However, treatment of wild-type mice with CEP adducts did not result in measurable retinal leukocyte infiltration, indicating that TLR2 was not activated by CEP adducts *in vivo*.

CEP-TLR2 in Angiogenesis Assays

In vitro, neither HSA-CEP nor Pam3CSK4 (TLR2 agonist) showed any pro-angiogenic effect in the tube formation assay with human umbilical vein endothelial cells (HUVECs). Likewise, agonists to other TLRs (LPS, poly (I:C)) were not pro-angiogenic, whereas VEGF was.

In vivo, synthetic MSA-CEP did not exacerbate laser-induced CNV in a mouse model as reported [8]. This was the case with two substrains of C57BL/6 mice. In the initial two laser CNV studies we used C57BL/6N mice. Subsequently, it was reported that this substrain carries the *rd8* mutation in the *Crb1* gene [12]. We then performed two additional laser CNV studies with the C57BL/6J substrain, which has the wild-type *Crb1* gene [12]. The C57BL/6J substrain is the same one used in the previously published laser CNV study [8]. We observed similar results in all four laser CNV studies: CNV was exacerbated with exogenous VEGF, ameliorated with a VEGF-neutralizing antibody, and unaffected with MSA-CEP. Collectively, these data are consistent with a major angiogenic role for the VEGF pathway, but not for CEP adducts, in the laser-induced CNV model.

As an alternative *in vivo* model of ocular angiogenesis for exploring the CEP-TLR2 hypothesis, we used an abrasion-induced corneal neovascularization model (CoNV). This CoNV model is different from that used earlier with CEP adducts: in the corneal pocket CoNV model, a pellet containing synthetic HSA-

Table 1. Evaluation of CEP Adducts and TLR Agonists in the Tube Formation Assay.

	Reagent	Concentration	Average Tube Length (mm/mm^2)	Std Dev	P value[a]
Experiment 1	untreated	–	1.97	+/−0.35	–
	LPS	10 ng/mL	3.38	+/−0.59	0.0072
	Poly (I:C)	10 μg/mL	0.16	+/−0.09	0.0005
	Pam3CSK4	500 nM	2.13	+/−0.24	0.9997
	VEGF[b]	3.1 ng/mL	10.61	–	<0.0001
Experiment 2	untreated	–	1.85	+/−0.27	–
	HSA-CEP	2 μg/mL	1.18	+/−0.32	0.1079
	HSA-CTL2	2 μg/mL	2.32	+/−0.45	0.3594
	VEGF	4 ng/mL	9.00	+/−1.64	<0.0001

GFP-transfected HUVEC, co-cultured with human fibroblasts, were treated on days 1, 2, 5, 7 and 9 with VEGF, TLR agonists, HSA-CEP, or HSA-CTL2. Control wells ("untreated") received media alone. Average tube length (mm/mm^2) was determined by fluorescence measurements as described in Materials and Methods. Representative images from these two experiments are shown in **Figure 3**.
[a]One way ANOVA with Dunnett's multiple comparison test, compared to untreated sample.
[b]This VEGF control was measured in duplicate and not in triplicate, therefore no Std Dev is presented.

CEP was implanted in the cornea [8]. Since our synthetic CEP adducts were biologically inactive in all assays so far, we aimed to use a model where endogenous -not synthetic- CEP adducts might play a role. In the abrasion-induced CoNV model, angiogenesis occurs as part of the wound healing process, induced by mechanical abrasion of the cornea. Furthermore, it has been shown that macrophages are recruited to the cornea during early stages of neovascularization [14]. This resembles the back punch model, in which wound angiogenesis entails recruitment of macrophages [9]. CEP adducts were reported to be transiently present during this time, detected by immunocytochemistry with an antibody against synthetic CEP adducts. By immunolabeling, a substantial portion of CEP adducts was present in the recruited F4/80+ macrophages [9]. Treatment with dipeptide-CEP in this model accelerated wound closure and vascularization in a TLR2-dependent manner, as shown by the comparison of *TLR2−/−* and *TLR2+/+* mice. In the same vein, we used the abrasion-induced CoNV model and compared littermate *Myd88−/−* and *Myd88+/+* mice. (Myd88 is required for TLR2 function.) We found no difference in CoNV area between the two groups. This indicates that, in the abrasion-induced CoNV model, TLR2 and other Myd88-dependent TLRs are not involved in angiogenesis. It is not known whether endogenous CEP adducts are present in the abrasion-induced CoNV model. We also tested topical treatment with synthetic HSA-CEP, but observed no effect on CoNV (not shown). It seems therefore the CEP-TLR2 axis proposed for other wound angiogenesis models [9] does not apply to corneal abrasion-induced wound angiogenesis model tested here.

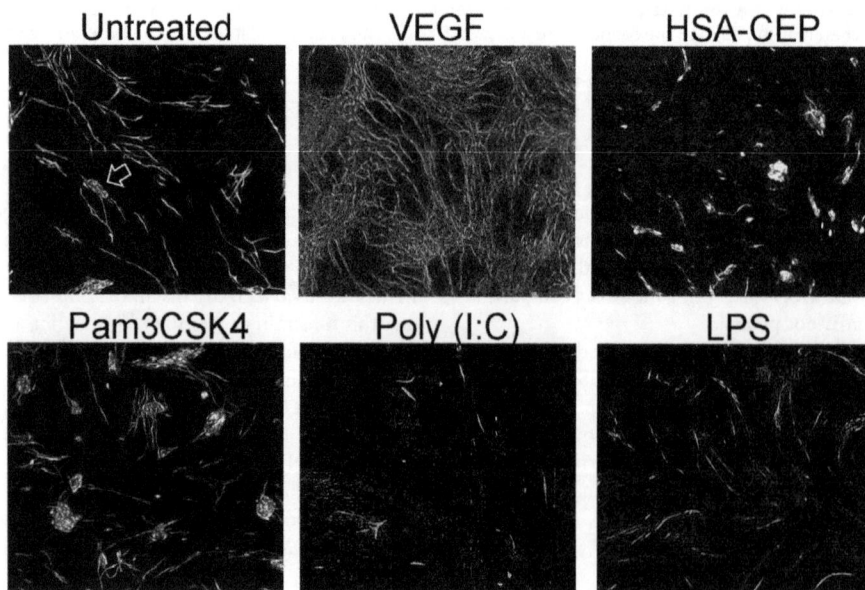

Figure 4. Tube Formation Assay. Shown are representative images of the experiments in presented numerically in **Table 1.** The figure shows images for untreated negative control (untreated), positive control (VEGF 165, 4 ng/mL), HSA-CEP (2 μg/mL), Pam3CSK4 (500 nM), LPS (10 ng/mL), poly (I:C) (10 μg/mL). The arrow in the untreated image shows an example of an island of unmigrated HUVEC cells, which is also seen in other images.

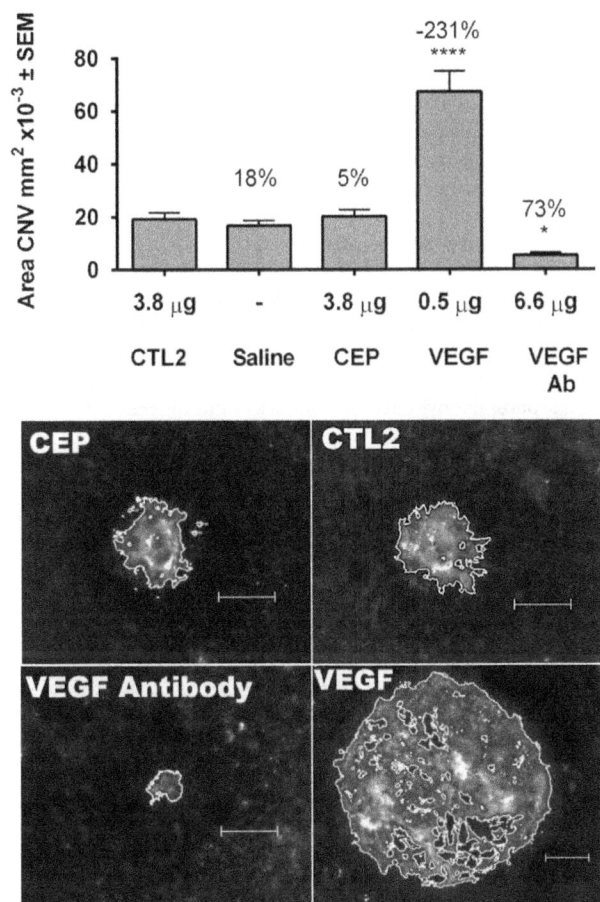

Figure 5. Mouse Laser-Induced CNV Assay. (A) Subretinal injection of MSA-CEP does not increase CNV area compared to mice injected with saline or MSA-CTL2. Bar graph shows mean area of CNV +/− SEM from first experiment evaluating the effect of subretinal injection of saline, 0.5 µg of rhVEGF165, 3.8 µg of MSA-CTL2, 3.8 µg of MSA-CEP, or 6.6 µg of 4G3 (an anti-mVEGF antibody) on laser-induced CNV in C57BL/6J mice. The number above each bar is the percentage inhibition relative to average CNV area in mice injected with MSA-CTL2. Subretinal injection of VEGF increases CNV area and subretinal injection of an anti-mVEGF antibody inhibits CNV area. * p<0.05, **** p<0.0001 by ANOVA with a Dunnett's post hoc analysis. (B) Representative fluorescent images of CNV lesions 7 days after laser from mice injected in the subretinal space with MSA-CEP, MSA-CTL2, VEGF or a VEGF Antibody as described above. Scale bar = 100 microns. *CTL2*, MSA-CTL2; *CEP*, MSA-CEP.

Synthetic vs. Endogenous CEP Adducts

It has been proposed that the biological effects of CEP adducts depend solely on the presence of CEP groups and not the host carrier [9]. This was not the case in our study: neither protein CEP adducts nor dipeptide CEP adducts produced any of the published biological effects [8,9] that were tested here. Our synthetic reagents were verified for the presence of covalently-attached CEP groups. There is no obvious explanation for these discrepancies. As innate immune receptors, TLRs recognize structures and patterns so it is conceivable that changes in structure, even if artificial, could elicit TLR activation. Thus one possibility is that there are structural differences between our synthetic CEP adducts and those used in previous studies, as the reagents were prepared at different laboratories.

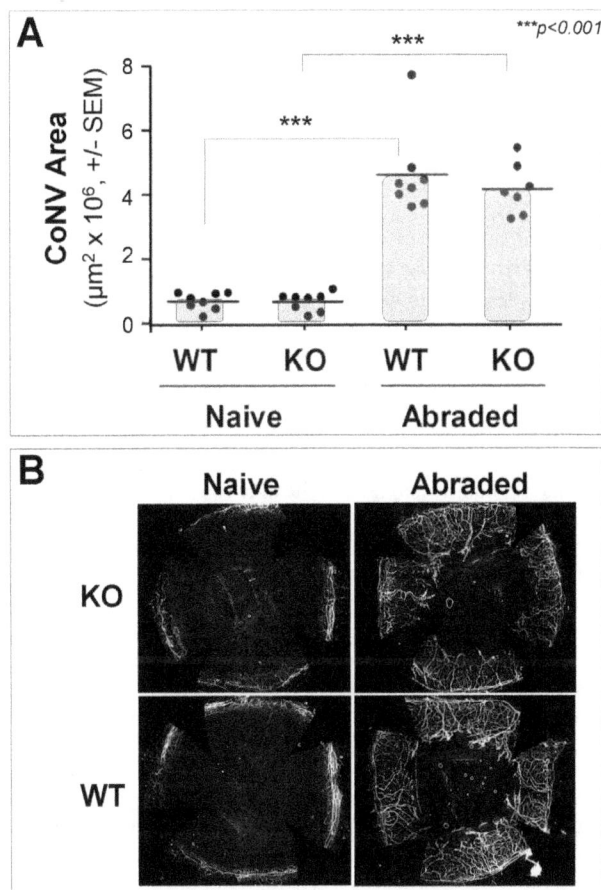

Figure 6. Mouse CoNV Assay. A) Adult *Myd88−/−* (KO) and littermate *Myd88+/+* (WT) mice (N = 7 to 8 animals/group) were subjected to corneal abrasion on Day 0. On Day 21 post-abrasion animals were euthanized and CoNV area (+/− SEM) was measured by fluorescence microscopy, as described in Materials and Methods. Statistical analysis was performed using two-way ANOVA. Within each genotype, the abraded group was significantly different from the naïve group (p<0.0001). However, comparison between the two genotypes showed no significant effect of the *Myd88* deficiency on CoNV area in response to abrasion. B) Representative images of the 4 groups shown in **Figure 6A**.

So far endogenous CEP adducts from any biological systems have not been isolated and therefore none have been characterized in structural studies. Furthermore, the abnormal electrophoretic patterns seen with synthetic CEP adducts reported here or by others [13] do not seem to resemble those of *in vivo* CEP adducts detected on immunoblots, reported either in human donor material (e.g. Figure 3 in [5]) or in the light-induced rat retinal degeneration model (e.g. Figure 1 in [15]). It is therefore uncertain which synthetic CEP adducts are representative of endogenous ones; perhaps none. The final answer awaits the isolation of endogenous CEP adducts and their characterization.

By extension, the biological effects reported with synthetic CEP adducts also need to be confirmed with endogenous CEP adducts. Our HSA-CTL2 did not show any biological activity, but neither did our HSA-CEP; hence in our study there was no concern about non-physiological biological effects, which HSA-CTL2 was intended for as a control. However, a treated unadducted control would be critically important when biological activity with a synthetic CEP adduct is observed. This is exemplified in a recent publication where the unadducted control, "sham-MSA", showed biological activity in some assays. In BALB/c macrophages, sham-MSA induced the upregulation of M1 markers and of an inflammatory gene, *KC*, 2 to 5 fold above that of control levels (Figures 1A and S2, respectively, in [16]). In some cases the sham-MSA effect represented 30%–40% in magnitude of the MSA-CEP effect: (*IL-1β*, *TNFα*, and *KC*), despite the absence of CEP groups in sham-MSA [16].

Treated unadducted controls were not used in earlier studies that reported a role for synthetic CEP adducts in TLR2 activation and in angiogenesis [8,9]. If it is possible that our CEP adducts are different from those used by others, it is also possible that our treated unadducted controls are different. The fact that our treated, unadducted controls (HSA-CTL2, MSA-CTL2) were biologically inactive does not necessarily apply to other studies in literature, as the example above illustrates. Thus the physiological relevance of synthetic CEP adducts is unclear, especially when untreated proteins were used as the only controls in the biological assays.

Polyclonal and monoclonal antibodies raised to synthetic CEP adducts have been reported to immunolabel biological samples from AMD patients in Western blots, immunohistochemical sections, and ELISAs [5–7,11]. The same antibodies reportedly immunolabelled biological samples in animal studies, e.g. [15,17]. However, the immunolabelled proteins were not confirmed to have any CEP moieties, by other independent assays that do not use antibodies (e.g. LC-MS/MS); i.e. the immunolabelled proteins were not confirmed to be bona fide CEP adducts. For example, several candidate CEP adducts were immunolabelled on Western blots of patient donor material and subsequently identified by LC-MS/MS analysis, however the presence of covalently-linked CEP groups was not confirmed by LC-MS/MS or other assays [5]. The fact that a synthetic CEP adduct (used a control) was immuno-labelled on the same western blot is not a surprise, as CEP antibodies were raised against a synthetic CEP adduct. At this point, the antibodies against synthetic CEP adducts [5] have not yet been validated for detection of endogenous CEP adducts. This is underscored by the electrophoretic changes in synthetic CEP adducts that do not seem to resemble those of endogenous CEP adducts, as explained above. Data generated by other (non-immunological) assays is needed to validate CEP antibodies.

Arguably the *in vivo* existence of CEP adducts requires confirmation, as well, since all evidence so far has been generated with these antibodies. For example, a proteomics study of AMD patient samples identified and quantified hundreds of proteins by LC-MS/MS [18]. Yet the same study reported that CEP adducts were below detection limits and "none were reliably identified" (supplemental information in [18]). On a promising note, an improved LC-MS/MS assay has been reported, with a sensitivity of 1 pmol or less of CEP-lysine in enzymatically-digested patient plasma samples [19]. According to ELISA data [7] the average levels of CEP adducts in AMD plasma is 37 pmol/mL, thus hopefully the improved LC-MS/MS assay can confirm the presence of CEP adducts *in vivo*.

In conclusion, our studies of synthetic CEP adducts did not validate the CEP-TLR2 axis in angiogenesis as proposed [8,9]. While the cause of the discrepancies is not clear, it does seem clear that the mere presence of CEP groups is not sufficient to elicit the reported biological responses. More data, ideally with endogenous CEP adducts, is needed to understand what properties of CEP adducts, if any, can lead to TLR2 activation and to angiogenesis. In light of the prevalence of AMD and the unmet medical needs, more research into the pathophysiology of CEP adducts is warranted.

As a postscript, after submission of our manuscript an independent report [20] also showed that CEP adducts alone do not induce TLR2 signalling nor related biological effects (e.g. Figures 1A and 1B), as we have reported here. Rather, the report claims that CEP adducts potentiate the effect of a synthetic TLR2 agonist, Pam3CSK4, in cultured murine bone-marrow derived macrophages [20].

Materials and Methods

Synthesis and Verification of CEP Adducts

Synthesis. All CEP adducts were synthesized as described [10]. The dipeptide, Ac-Gly-Lys-OMe, was obtained from BACHEM; HSA from AlbuminBio; MSA from AlbuminBio or Sigma; phosphatidyl ethanolamine was from Sigma. Controls for protein CEP adducts included untreated protein (CTL1) and treated unadducted protein (CTL2). The latter control was processed in the same synthesis procedure as that for CEP adducts, except 4,7-dioxoheptanoic acid 9-fluorenylmethyl ester was left out to avoid the covalent addition of CEP moiety. Protein CEP adducts, after final dialysis in PBS, were quantified by the Bradford assay and tested for endotoxins with the Endosafe-PTS kit (Charles River). For storage, samples were filtered through 0.2 μm, divided aseptically in 1-mL aliquots, and stored at −80 C.

Amino acids complete digestion. Enzymatic hydrolysis was adapted from [21]. An aliquot of 100 μg of protein is dissolved in 25 μl of PBS buffer (pH 7.4). Pronase E (Sigma, Cat. # P5147) (2 mg/ml in 10 mM potassium phosphate buffer, pH 7.4, 5 μl) was added. The sample was incubated at 37°C for 24 hours. Prolidase (Sigma, Cat. # P6675) and aminopeptidase (Sigma, Cat. # A8200) (both 2 mg/ml in 10 mM potassium phosphate buffer, pH 7.4, 5 μl) were added. The sample was incubated at 37°C for 48 hours. Amino acids from enzymatic hydrolysate (10 μl) was derivatized by Waters AccQ•Fluor (Waters, Cat.# WAT052880). Then 2 μl of derivatized samples was analyzed by Xevo-G2QTOF with Waters BEH C18 2.1 × 50 mm 1.7 μm column at 50°C at 1.0 mL/min, 0.1% formic acid in water, 0.04% formic acid in acetonitrile, 3–98% B in 9 min. An aliquot of 100 μg of protein is dissolved in 25 μl of PBS buffer (pH 7.4). Pronase E (Sigma, Cat. # P5147) (2 mg/ml in 10 mM potassium phosphate buffer, pH 7.4, 5 μl) was added. The sample was incubated at 37°C for 24 hours. Aminopeptidase (Sigma, Cat. # P6675) and prolidase (Sigma, Cat. # A9934) (both 2 mg/ml in 10 mM potassium phosphate buffer, pH 7.4, 5 μl) were added. The sample was incubated at 37°C for 48 hours. Amino acids from enzymatic hydrolysate (10 μl) was derivatized by Wasters AccQ Fluor (Waters, Cat.# Wat052880). Then 2 μl of derivatized samples was analyzed by Xevo-G2QTOF with Waters BEH C18 2.1 × 50 mm 1.7 μm column at 50°C at 1.0 mL/min, 0.1% formic acid in water, 0.04% formic acid in acetonitrile, 3–98% B in 9 min.

NMR of protein hydrolysate samples. Hydrolyzed protein samples were prepared for NMR analysis by the addition of 5 μL of D2O (CIL) to 15 μL of Hydrolysate solutions. Sodium 3-trimethylsilyl [2,2,3,3-d4]propionate (TMSP) as added as an internal chemical shift and quantitation reference. High-resolution ^{1}H-NMR spectra were acquired at 300 ± 1 K, using a standard (D-90°-acquire) pulse sequences on a Bruker-600 Avance spectrometer (^{1}H frequency of 600.26 MHz). ^{1}H-NMR spectra were acquired with 256 free induction decays, 65,536 complex data points, a spectral width of 7.2 kHz, and a relaxation delay of 5 s. All spectra were processed by multiplying the FID by an exponential weighting function corresponding to a line broadening of 0.3 Hz. The CEP pyrrole resonances at ^{1}H$_δ$ 6.8 ppm, ^{1}H$_δ$

6.1 ppm and $^1H_\delta$ 5.9 ppm were integrated relative to the aromatic resonance of phenylalanine and tyrosine using the ACD 10.0 package (Advanced Chemistry Development, Toronto, Canada).

LC-MS/MS confirmation of CEP-lysine adduct. Carboxyethylpyrrole (CEP) adduct presence in CEP-conjugated murine serum albumin (MSA) and human serum albumin (HSA) has been confirmed by LC-MS/MS methodologies. CEP-MSA and CEP-HSA were hydrolyzed using protease cocktails (descriptions in above, AA complete digestion), followed by Accq-Tag Ultra derivatization (Catalog number 186003836, Waters Corporation, Milford, MA). Accq-Tagged CEP-lysine ionizes in electrospray positive mode and gives a protonated molecular ion of 439.1981, which can fragment and gives a characteristic 171.1 daughter ion from the Accq-Tag and a daughter ion of 206.1 from the carboxyethylpyrrole moiety. We employed multiple reaction monitoring, 206.1 precursor scan on a Triple Quadrupole mass spectrometer. Strong signal of 439.2 → 171.1 and 439.2 → 206.1 were observed using AB Sciex API4000 Triple Quad. Precursor ion of 439.2 was observed for 206.1 daughter ion in a precursor ion scan on the same API4000. Waters Xevo G2 Q-TOF mass spectrometer was employed for its high resolution power to further confirm the presence of CEP-lysine adducts. The molecular species of 439.1981 was observed in MS scan with 5 ppm mass accuracy across the chromatographic peak; the daughter ion 206.1181 was observed in the MS/MS scan with 10 ppm mass accuracy in the MSE approach.

Peptide Mapping for CEP Modification Location

Sample preparation. All solvents (HPLC grade) and chemicals were purchased from Sigma-Aldrich (St. Louis, MO) unless otherwise stated. MSA-CEP and MSA-CTL2 (50 ug each) were denatured with 6 M guanidine hydrochloride (GuHCl), reduced with 25 mM dithiothreitol (DTT), alkylated with 50 mM iodoacetamide, dialyzed against 50 mM ammonium bicarbonate using 10 kDa MWCO Slide-A-Lyzer cassettes (Thermo Scientific, Rockford, IL). Protein was digested 1 to 50 enzyme to protein with trypsin, chymotrypsin, and trypsin/Glu-C overnight at 37°C; note all enzymes purchased from Roche Diagnostics GMBH, Germany. For HSA-CEP and HSA-CTL1 digestions, 125 μg protein was denatured using ProteaseMAX surfactant (Promega, Madison, WI), reduced with 5 mM DTT, alkylated with 15 mM iodoacetamide and digested with 1 to 50 trypsin to protein overnight at 37°C.

Reverse phase LC-MS/MS analysis. Resulting peptides from MSA-CEP and MSA-CTL2 were analyzed by LC-ESI MS/MS on a Thermo Velos Orbitrap coupled to a Waters nanoACQUITY UPLC (Milford, MA). 70 pmol of digested MSA-CEP and MSA-CTL2 were HPLC separated on column (Waters Acquity HSS T3 1.8 μm beads, 1 × 100 mm at 40°C) at 15 μL/min. The 55 min gradient started 0–3 min, 3% B (B = acetonitrile, 0.1% formic acid), increased to 97% B at 35 min, then 95% B at 37 min, followed by washing and column equilibration. Mass spectrometer parameters included a full scan event using the FTMS analyzer at 100000 resolution from m/z 300–2000 for 10 ms. Collision induced dissociation (CID) MS/MS was conducted on the top seven intense ions (excluding 1+ ions) in the ion trap analyzer, activated at 500 (for first event) and 2000 (for remaining events) signal intensity for 10 ms.

For HSA-CEP and HSA-CTL1 digestion, resulting peptides were analyzed by LC-ESI MS/MS on a Thermo LTQ Orbitrap Discovery coupled to Agilent CapLC (Santa Clara, CA). 10 pmol of digested HSA-CEP and HSA-CTL1 were HPLC separated on column (Waters Acuity BEH C18, 1.7 μm, 1 × 100 mm column at 40°C) at 10 μL/min. The 80 min gradient started 0–1 min, 4%

B, increased to 7% B at 1.1 min, 45% B at 55 min, then 95% B at 63 min, followed by washing and column equilibration. Mass spectrometer parameters included a full scan event using the FTMS analyzer at 30000 resolution from m/z 300–2000 for 30 ms. CID MS/MS was conducted on the top seven intense ions (excluding 1+ ions) in the ion trap analyzer, activated at 500 (for all events) signal intensity for 30 ms.

Data analysis and database searching. All mass spectra were processed in Qual Browser V 2.0.7 (Thermo Scientific). Mascot generic files (mgf) were generated with MS DeconTools (R.D. Smith Lab, PPNL) and searched using Mascot V2.3.01 (Matrix Science Inc., Boston, MA) database search against the SwissProt database, V57, with 513,877 sequences. Search parameters included: enzyme: semitrypsin, chymotrypsin, none, or trypsin/Glu-C, allowed up to two missed cleavages; fixed modification carbamidomethyl on cysteines (when applicable); variable modifications searched: Arg-CEP on arginines, Gln-> pyro-Glu (at N-term glutamine), Lys-CEP on lysines, oxidation on methionine; peptide tolerance: ±25 ppm; MS/MS tolerance: ±0.6 Da. Sequence coverage and CEP modification assessments were evaluated on peptide scores with >95% confidence. High-scoring peptide ions were then selected for manual MS/MS analysis using Qual Browser.

Structural Analyses of CEP Adducts

SDS-PAGE analysis. After boiled for 5 min, 5 μg of total protein mixed with 4X sample buffer (Invitrogen, cat. # NP0007) was loaded on 4–12% NuPAGE Bis-Tris gel (Invitrogen, Cat. # NP0321BOX) with NuPAGE MOPS running buffer (Invitrogen, Cat. # NP0001). SeeBlue Plus2 Protein Ladder (Invitrogen, cat. # LC5925) or BenchMark Protein Ladder (Invitrogen, Cat. # 10747-012) was used to estimate the protein size. Gel was stained with SimpleBlue SafeStain (Invitrogen, Cat. # LC6060) for overnight at 4°C and destained with HPLC water. The gel image was taken by Bio-Rad ChemiDoc XRS+ Imaging System.

Size exclusion chromatography (SEC). Human Serum Albumin (HSA) samples (20 μg) were injected on Shodex KW-803 column with 1 mL/min flow rate, 20 mM Tris, 200 mM NaCl, 0.25 mM TCEP, 3 mM NaN3, pH 7.5 as mobile phase on Agilent 1200 HPLC. UV signal was recorded at 280 nm by Agilent 1260 DAD detector. Mouse Serum Albumin (MSA) samples (50 μg) were injected on a Large S200 Column with GE Superdex 200 10/300GL and at 500 μL/min flow rate, 150 mM NaCl and 0.02% NaN3 in Dulbecco's PBS as mobile phase on Agilent 1260 BioInert HPLC. UV signal was measured at 280 nm by Wyatt TREOS/OptiLab Rex.

Circular dichroism (CD). Protein samples were diluted in 10X diluted PBS (pH 7.4) to achieve similar concentration. Baseline was blanked by 10X diluted PBS (pH 7.4). The CD spectra (average of five scans) of protein samples were collected from 260 nm to 190 nm on a Jasco J-815 CD Spectrometer with 0.02-cm path length quartz cell at 10°C.

In Vitro Assays

Cell-based TLR assays. HEK293 cells expressing TLR2 and NFKB luciferase reporter (gift from Novartis Vaccine, Siena, Italy) were seeded at 30000 per well the night before. HSA-CEP was added and incubated for either 6 hr or 24 hr. Supernatant was collected for IL-8 ELISA (R&D, cat# DY208). NFkB luciferase activity was assayed on remaining cells, using Bright-Glo (Promega, cat# E2610). HEK293 cells in a separate plate with the same treatment were used for cell viability measurement using CellTiter-Glo (Promega, cat# G7570), according to manufacturer's instruction.

Thp1 (ATCC, cat# TIB-202) was primed with 0.5% DMSO for overnight, at 100,000/well, then incubate with HSA-CEP for 24 hr, with TLR ligands (Pam3CSK4, FSL1, R837 and R848 were all from Invivogen; LPS was purchased from Sigma) as controls. Supernatant was collected for IL-8 ELISA (R&D), and the remaining cells were used for cell viability measurement using CellTiter-Glo.

In vitro tube formation assay. The CellPlayer GFP Angiokit-96 by Essen BioScience (Ann Arbor, MI) was used to measure tube formation in vitro. Briefly, GFP-transfected HU-VEC were co-cultured with human fibroblasts in a specially designed medium for 11 days in a 96-well format. Cells were treated on days 1, 2, 5, 7 and 9 with VEGF, TLR agonists, or CEP-adducted or control-treated proteins. Fluorescence measurements (IncuCyte, Essen BioScience) were taken kinetically every 12 hours for the duration of the experiment and average tube length (mm/mm^2) was quantified on the last day of the experiment according to the manufacturer's instructions. Control wells received media alone. Reagents were obtained from the following sources: Human VEGF 165– Peprotech; Pam3CSK4– InvivoGen; LPS -Sigma-Aldrich; Poly (I:C) –InVivoGen.

In Vivo Assays

Animals. All animal experiments were approved by the Animal Care and Use Committee at the Novartis Institutes for Biomedical Research. Upon arrival at the vivarium, mice were acclimated for at least 4 days before any studies were initiated. The animals were fed standard laboratory chow and sterile water ad libitum. Genotyping was performed on genomic DNA obtained from tail snips by standard procedures. All mouse strains were genotyped for the *Crb1* gene, to determine if they carried the *rd8* mutation.

C57BL/6N mice were obtained from Taconic; the *rd8* mutation was present in these mice. C57BL/6J mice were obtained from Jackson; the *rd8* mutation was absent in these mice. *Myd88*-deficient mice lacking exons 2–5 were generated at Novartis Institutes for Biomedical Research. Mice were back-crossed to C57BL/6J mice for at least 10 generations; the *rd8* mutation was absent in these mice. Heterozygous breeding generated littermate pups of each genotype, identified by PCR genotyping. *Myd88* deficiency was also functionally confirmed by the *in vivo* retinal infiltration assay below: mutant vs. littermate *wt* mice with treated with either TLR2 agonists and with TLR4 agonists and the retinal infiltration was measured as described (not shown).

Laser-induced choroidal neovascularization (CNV). CNV was induced by laser injury in age and sex matched on a) C57BL/6N mice and b) C57BL/6J mice. Two in vivo experiments were performed with each mouse strain. After pupil dilation with 1% cylate and 10% phenylephrine, the mice were anesthetized and the retinas were visualized with a slit lamp microscope and a cover slip. The laser (Iridex Oculight GLx 532 nm green laser) was applied at 3 locations with a successful laser shot inducing a vaporization bubble. Laser pulses are applied to both eye yielding 6 CNV area data points per mouse and with 10 mice per group yielding 60 CNV area data points per test condition. Immediately after laser 2.0 µl of test article was injected into the subretinal space of both eyes. A sclerotomy was first made with a 30 gauge needle, and then the test article was injected through the same incision with a 33 gauge blunt tipped needle and a 10 µl Hamilton syringe. Injections were visualized under a surgical microscope with direct observation of a small retinal detachment. 7 days post laser, mice were injected i.v. with a vascular label and then euthanized. Mouse eyes were fixed in 4%

paraformaldehyde; RPE-choroid-scleral complexes were isolated and mounted on microscope slides. Fluorescent images of each laser-induced CNV were captured using a Axiocam MR3 camera on a Axio.Image M1 microscope (Zeiss). The CNV lesion sizes were quantified with Axiovision software (Version 4.5 Zeiss). Inter-group differences were analyzed with an ANOVA with a Dunnett's multiple comparison test on GraphPad Prism 6 for Windows software. Data was masked during image acquisition and data analysis.

Recombinant human VEGF165 (Peprotech), IgG2A (R&D, MAB006) and a proprietary anti-mouse VEGF antibody (4G3) were reconstituted in sterile saline (Hospira) to a concentration of 0.05, 0.5, 2.5 or 3.3 mg/ml respectively. 1.4 or 1.9 mg/ml of CEP-MSA and MSA-CTL2 (control 2, mouse serum albumin treated but not adducted) or the other reagents were injected in to the subretinal space on day 0 immediately after a laser as described. After the application of laser burns and subretinal injections of test reagents, antibiotic ointment (Tobramycin or Neomycin ophthalmic ointment depending on availability) was applied to both eyes. The anti-VEGF antibody, 4G3, is a mouse anti-VEGF IgG1 antibody. It binds to mouse VEGF with an EC50 of 0.047 nM in a sandwich ELISA and neutralizes mouse VEGF binding to human VEGFR-2 with an EC50 of 0.15 nM in a binding assay (ELISA MSD).

Corneal neovascularization (CoNV). Acute CoNV was induced in 7- to 9- week old anesthetized mice by complete removal of the corneal epithelium with mechanical abrasion, as detailed [14]. At the end of the studies, mice were humanely euthanized and the area of CoNV was quantitated as described [14]. Animals were randomized prior to treatment and analysis was performed in a masked fashion. N = 5–10 mice/group.

In studies using *Myd88*−/− mice (**Figure 6**), male knockout (KO) and male wild-type littermate controls (WT) were abraded on day 0 and euthanized at the end of the study on day 21 for analysis. *Myd88*-deficient and littermate wild-type mice are on the C57BL6/J background and are described above.

For other CoNV studies (**Figure S3**), C57BL6/N mice were used. The *Crb1* gene product is expressed in the retina, but not in the cornea [22]. In the study presented in **Figure S3C**, animals (N = 10–12 mice/group) were injected i.p. with PBS (200 µl), control antibody (IgG1, 0.5 mg/kg) or anti-VEGF antibody (4G3, 0.5 mg/kg) on days 0, 3 and 5 post-abrasion and eyes were collected on day 6 for analysis.

In vivo TLR2-mediated retinal leukocyte infiltration. TLR2 ligand, Pam3CSK4, was purchased from Invivogen. Female C57BL/6N mice (7 weeks old, Taconic) were treated with either dipeptide-CEP (400 µg per animal, in PBS) or Pam3CSK4 (25 µg per animal, in PBS) via intraperitoneal injection. Control animals received an intraperitoneal injection of sterile PBS. Eight hours after injection, mice were euthanized. Eyes were enucleated and were fixed in 4% paraformaldehyde. For immunostaining, retinas were dissected out. Macrophages was stained using the F4/80-Alexa 488 conjugated antibody (AbD serotec, Oxford, UK). Neutrophils were stained using a biotinylated-Gr-1 antibody (San Diego, CA) and an Alexa Fluor 594 conjugated streptavidin secondary antibody (Molecular Probes, Eugene, OR). After retinas were flat mounted onto glass slides, fluorescent images were taken. And F4/80 and Gr-1 positive cells on the retina were counted using Zeiss AxioVision program.

Supporting Information

Figure S1 Confirmation of CEP Adduction By ^{1}H-NMR and LC-MS/MS. A) *Structure for Dipeptide-CEP*. B) *^{1}H-NMR* *of Dipeptide-CEP*. The signature peaks for CEP, lysine, and glycine are indicated. The CEP peaks were not detected in the unadducted dipeptide (not shown). C) *LC-MS/MS of completely hydrolyzed MSA-CEP*. MSA-CEP was enzymatically hydrolyzed and processed for LC-MS/MS analysis. Only MSA-CEP showed a peak corresponding to lysine-CEP; untreated MSA-CTL1 (not shown) and treated but unadducted MSA-CTL2 (lower panel) did not have the CEP peak. D) *^{1}H-NMR of completely hydrolyzed HSA-CEP*. The signature peaks for CEP, Tyr, and Phe are indicated. The resonances corresponding to CEP were absent in HSA-CTL1 and HSA-CTL2 (not shown).

Figure S2   Peptide Mapping of CEP Adduction by LC-MS/MS. A) *LC-MS/MS Analysis of Trypsinized HSA-CEP*. LC-MS/MS of trypsin digested HSA-CEP showed sequence coverage of 65% where bold residues represent observed peptides. In HSA-CEP 14 sites of CEP adduction were identified by this analysis (shown as underlined amino acids). B) *LC-MS/MS Analysis of Trypsinized MSA-CEP*. MSA-CEP was digested with trypsin, chymotrypsin, and trypsin-gluC yielding a sequence coverage of 92% with bold residues representing observed peptides. In MSA-CEP 40 sites of CEP adduction were identified by this analysis (shown as underlined amino acids). The initial signal and propeptides are not observed in the mature, processed protein sequence for HSA and MSA and are shown as italicized residues.

Figure S3   CoNV Model is VEGF-Driven. A) *Progression of Neovascularization*. Adult C57BL/6N mice (N = 5 animals/group) were subjected to corneal abrasion on Day 0 and dissected corneas were analyzed for neovascularization area at different timepoints after abrasion. Neovascularization area progressively increased and plateaued around 2 weeks after abrasion. Statistical analysis was performed using one-way ANOVA with Dunnet's post-test, comparing each time point to Naïve. Only the statistically significant differences between groups are indicated. B) *Upregulation of VEGFA Transcript*. Total RNA was prepared from dissected corneas from naïve mice and or cornea-abraded mice that were euthanized on Day 1 and Day 6 post-abrasion as indicated (N = 5 to 6 animals/group). First-strand cDNA was generated using the High Capacity RNA-to-cDNA Master Mix (Applied Biosystems). Pre-amplification products were generated using the Taqman PreAmp Master Mix Kit (Applied Biosystems)

and a pool of FAM-labelled Taqman assays on demand (Applied Biosystems). qPCR was performed on diluted pre-amplification products using the same Taqman assays on demand in qPCR singleplex reactions. Relative quantification (RQ) performed using $\Delta\Delta$Ct method and data presented as RQ median with error bars as RQ min and RQ max. *VEGFA, PECAM-1*(expressed by vascular endothelial cells), and *β-actin* mRNA expression was normalized by expression of *β-actin* gene and expressed relative to naïve animals. Statistical analysis was performed using one-way ANOVA with Dunnett's post-test. C) *VEGF Ab inhibits CoNV*. Adult C57BL/6N mice (N = 10–12 animals/group) were subjected to corneal abrasion on Day 0 and injected intraperitoneally with the reagents as indicated on Days 0, 3, and 5 post-abrasion. Reagents included PBS (vehicle), control IgG1 Ab, and anti-VEGF antibody (4G3). The antibodies were dosed at 0.5 mg/kg. On Day 6 the animals were euthanized and CoNV area was measured by fluorescence microscopy as described in Materials and Methods. Statistical analysis was performed using one-way ANOVA with Dunnett's post-test.

Acknowledgments

Myd88−/− mice were generated by Mueller M, Wirsching J, Lemaistre M, Doll T, Isken A, Kinzel B (Developmental & Molecular Pathways, NIBR, Basel, Switzerland). Littermate *Myd88−/−* and *Myd88+/+* mice were bred and genotyped by Vanessa Davis and John Halupowski (Transgenic Services, NIBR, Cambridge, USA). Shawn Hanks (Ophthalmology, NIBR, Cambridge, USA) helped with some of the statistical analyses.

Author Contributions

Conceived and designed the experiments: JG EM QH KA S-ML SP BEG MM BJ SA. Performed the experiments: JG JSC JZ FC XY HY EM CR YX ADE MC NB YQ EF SS AW AJ RC SG. Analyzed the data: JG JSC JZ EM QH KA S-ML SP BEG MM BJ SA. Contributed reagents/materials/analysis tools: JG EM QH KA S-ML SP BEG SA. Wrote the paper: JG EM QH KA S-ML SP BEG MM BJ SA.

References

1. Miller JW (2013) Age-related macular degeneration revisited–piecing the puzzle: the LXIX Edward Jackson memorial lecture. Am J Ophthalmol 155: 1–35 e13.
2. Kuno N, Fujii S (2011) Dry age-related macular degeneration: recent progress of therapeutic approaches. Curr Mol Pharmacol 4: 196–232.
3. Nguyen DH, Luo J, Zhang K, Zhang M (2013) Current therapeutic approaches in neovascular age-related macular degeneration. Discov Med 15: 343–348.
4. Salomon RG, Hong L, Hollyfield JG (2011) Discovery of carboxyethylpyrroles (CEPs): critical insights into AMD, autism, cancer, and wound healing from basic research on the chemistry of oxidized phospholipids. Chem Res Toxicol 24: 1803–1816.
5. Crabb JW, Miyagi M, Gu X, Shadrach K, West KA, et al. (2002) Drusen proteome analysis: an approach to the etiology of age-related macular degeneration. Proc Natl Acad Sci U S A 99: 14682–14687.
6. Gu X, Meer SG, Miyagi M, Rayborn ME, Hollyfield JG, et al. (2003) Carboxyethylpyrrole protein adducts and autoantibodies, biomarkers for age-related macular degeneration. J Biol Chem 278: 42027–42035.
7. Gu J, Pauer GJ, Yue X, Narendra U, Sturgill GM, et al. (2009) Assessing susceptibility to age-related macular degeneration with proteomic and genomic biomarkers. Mol Cell Proteomics 8: 1338–1349.
8. Ebrahem Q, Renganathan K, Sears J, Vasanji A, Gu X, et al. (2006) Carboxyethylpyrrole oxidative protein modifications stimulate neovascularization: Implications for age-related macular degeneration. Proc Natl Acad Sci U S A 103: 13480–13484.
9. West XZ, Malinin NL, Merkulova AA, Tischenko M, Kerr BA, et al. (2010) Oxidative stress induces angiogenesis by activating TLR2 with novel endogenous ligands. Nature 467: 972–976.
10. Lu L, Gu X, Hong L, Laird J, Jaffe K, et al. (2009) Synthesis and structural characterization of carboxyethylpyrrole-modified proteins: mediators of age-related macular degeneration. Bioorg Med Chem 17: 7548–7561.
11. Gu J (2009) Biomarkers for Age-Related Macular Degeneration [Electronic Thesis or Dissertation.]. Cleveland, Ohio: Case Western Reserve University. 223 p.
12. Mattapallil MJ, Wawrousek EF, Chan CC, Zhao H, Roychoudhury J, et al. (2012) The Rd8 mutation of the Crb1 gene is present in vendor lines of C57BL/6N mice and embryonic stem cells, and confounds ocular induced mutant phenotypes. Invest Ophthalmol Vis Sci 53: 2921–2927.
13. Hollyfield JG, Bonilha VL, Rayborn ME, Yang X, Shadrach KG, et al. (2008) Oxidative damage-induced inflammation initiates age-related macular degeneration. Nat Med 14: 194–198.
14. Sivak JM, Ostriker AC, Woolfenden A, Demirs J, Cepeda R, et al. (2011) Pharmacologic uncoupling of angiogenesis and inflammation during initiation of pathological corneal neovascularization. J Biol Chem 286: 44965–44975.
15. Renganathan K, Gu J, Rayborn ME, Crabb JS, Salomon RG, et al. (2013) CEP Biomarkers as Potential Tools for Monitoring Therapeutics. PLoS One 8: e76325.
16. Cruz-Guilloty F, Saeed AM, Duffort S, Cano M, Ebrahimi KB, et al. (2014) T cells and macrophages responding to oxidative damage cooperate in

pathogenesis of a mouse model of age-related macular degeneration. PLoS One 9: e88201.

17. Organisciak DT, Darrow RM, Rapp CM, Smuts JP, Armstrong DW, et al. (2013) Prevention of retinal light damage by zinc oxide combined with rosemary extract. Mol Vis 19: 1433–1445.

18. Yuan X, Gu X, Crabb JS, Yue X, Shadrach K, et al. (2010) Quantitative proteomics: comparison of the macular Bruch membrane/choroid complex from age-related macular degeneration and normal eyes. Mol Cell Proteomics 9: 1031–1046.

19. Jang G-F, Zhang L, Hong L, Wang H, Salomon RG, et al. (2012) Quantification Of CEP By LC MS/MS. Investigative Ophthalmology & Visual Science 53: 6478.

20. Saeed AM, Duffort S, Ivanov D, Wang H, Laird JM, et al. (2014) The Oxidative Stress Product Carboxyethylpyrrole Potentiates TLR2/TLR1 Inflammatory Signaling in Macrophages. PLoS One 9: e106421.

21. Ahmed N, Argirov OK, Minhas HS, Cordeiro CA, Thornalley PJ (2002) Assay of advanced glycation endproducts (AGEs): surveying AGEs by chromato-graphic assay with derivatization by 6-aminoquinolyl-N-hydroxysuccinimidyl-carbamate and application to Nepsilon-carboxymethyl-lysine- and Nepsilon-(1-carboxyethyl)lysine-modified albumin. Biochem J 364: 1–14.

22. Alves CH, Pellissier LP, Wijnholds J (2014) The CRB1 and adherens junction complex proteins in retinal development and maintenance. Prog Retin Eye Res 40: 35–52.

7

Relative Deprivation, Poverty, and Subjective Health: JAGES Cross-Sectional Study

Masashige Saito[1]*, Katsunori Kondo[2], Naoki Kondo[3], Aya Abe[4], Toshiyuki Ojima[5], Kayo Suzuki[6] and the JAGES group[¶]

1 Department of Social Welfare, Nihon Fukushi University, Aichi, Japan, 2 Center for Preventive Medical Science, Chiba University, Chiba, Japan, 3 Department of Health Economics and Epidemiology Research, The University of Tokyo, Tokyo, Japan, 4 Department of Empirical Social Security Research, National Institute of Population and Social Security Research, Tokyo, Japan, 5 Department of Community Health and Preventive Medicine, Hamamatsu University School of Medicine, Shizuoka, Japan, 6 Department of Social Studies, Aichi Gakuin University, Aichi, Japan

Abstract

To evaluate the association between relative deprivation (lacking daily necessities) and subjective health in older Japanese adults, we performed a cross-sectional analysis using data from the Japan Gerontological Evaluation Study (JAGES). The data were obtained from functionally independent residents aged ≥65 years from 24 municipalities in Japan (n = 24,742). Thirteen items in three dimensions were used to evaluate relative deprivation of material conditions. Approximately 28% of older Japanese people indicated that they lacked some daily necessities (non-monetary poverty). A two-level Poisson regression analysis revealed that relative deprivation was associated with poor self-rated health (PR = 1.3–1.5) and depressive symptoms (PR = 1.5–1.8) in both men and women, and these relationships were stronger than those observed in people living in relative poverty (monetary poverty). The interaction effect between relative deprivation and relative poverty was not associated with poor health. As a dimension of the social determinants of health, poverty should be evaluated from a multidimensional approach, capturing not only monetary conditions but also material-based, non-monetary conditions.

Editor: Takeru Abe, Waseda University, Japan

Funding: This study was supported in part by Grant-in-Aid for Scientific Research (KAKENHI 26285138 and 23243070) from the Japan Society for the Promotion of Science, and Health Labour Sciences Research Grant, Comprehensive Research on Aging and Health (H25-Choju-ippan-003) from the Japanese Ministry of Health, Labour and Welfare. This survey data was supported by MEXT Supported Program for the Strategic Research Foundation at Private Universities 2009–2013, Health Labour Sciences Research Grant, Comprehensive Research on Aging and Health (H22-Choju-shitei-008), JSPS KA-KENHI Grant Number 22330172, 22119506, 22390400, 22592327, 22700694, 23590786, 23700819 & 23243070, and Japan Foundation for Aging and Health. The funders had no role in study design, data collection and analysis, decision to publish, or preparation of the manuscript.

Competing Interests: The authors have declared that no competing interests exist.

* Email: masa-s@n-fukushi.ac.jp

¶ Membership of the JAGES project is provided in the Acknowledgments.

Introduction

The association between poverty and health has been established. A number of studies have revealed that relative income poverty is significantly related to poor health [1–3]. However, this approach has limitations when attempting to capture the diverse and complex aspects of poverty. In reality, older people tend to have comparatively high-quality living conditions due to savings and property ownership, even if their income is low [4]. To overcome this limitation, poverty research has proposed the concept of relative deprivation in material conditions to reflect the multidimensional non-monetary aspects of poverty [5–15]. Townsend [5] developed 60 relative deprivation indices within 12 dimensions composed of items such as "Household does not have a refrigerator" and "Has not had a week's holiday away from home in the last 12 months," and found that poverty in the United Kingdom was more extensive than generally believed or officially reported. The Europe 2020 strategy has adopted the concept of relative deprivation as a material dimension of social exclusion and has set the elimination of severe material deprivation as a goal for the next decade [16].

In investigating relationships between poverty and health, some studies have applied a social indicator approach, such as the Carstairs deprivation score or Townsend deprivation index, to include unemployment rate or proportion of non-car ownership. These previous studies found that relatively deprived areas were associated with standardized mortality rates [17–20], cancer mortality rates [21], suicide rates [22], coronary heart disease [23], dental caries [24], number of sound teeth remaining [25], and depression symptoms [26]. However, there have been few studies analyzing the relationship between an individual's relative deprivation and his or her health. Some studies have shown an association between deprivation in living conditions and poor health [14], low levels of satisfaction with life [27], and poor social support [28]. Furthermore, no studies investigating the different associations between relative deprivation, relative poverty, and health have been conducted, although it has been suggested that people who live in relative deprivation have different character-

Table 1. Distribution of control variable.

Variable	Category	Total	Men	Women
Individual (n = 24,742)				
Sex	men	45.9	-	-
	women	54.1	-	-
Age	65–69	25.4	26.9	24.0
	70–74	29.1	29.5	28.7
	75–79	23.3	23.2	23.4
	80–84	14.1	13.5	14.7
	85 -	8.1	6.8	9.2
Education	>9	47.6	51.8	44.1
	= <9	49.9	46.5	52.9
	unknown	2.4	1.7	3.0
Marital status	married	69.0	84.0	56.0
	divorced	22.6	8.6	34.5
	separated	3.2	2.6	3.8
	never married	2.1	1.9	2.3
	unknown	3.1	2.9	3.4
Disease and/or impairment	no	22.4	24.1	20.8
	yes	68.5	67.6	69.3
	unknown	9.1	8.3	9.9
Self recognition of forgetfulness	no	79.3	79.5	79.1
	yes	16.8	16.5	17.1
	unknown	3.9	4.1	3.8
Social supports	present	85.6	84.4	86.7
	absent	8.1	9.9	6.5
	unknown	6.3	5.7	6.8
Municipality (n = 24)				
Proportion of older people	mean (SD)	24.4 (5.2)	-	-
Population density [1000 p/km²]	mean (SD)	1.70 (1.36)	-	-
Proportion of person receiving public assistance[‰]	mean (SD)	8.5 (10.7)	-	-

istics than those living in relative poverty [9,13,15]. In order to clarify the relationships between poverty and health, it is important to identify the aspects of poverty that are the strongest predictors of health.

In addition, there have been few studies focusing on relative deprivation among older adults [8,15]. Previous studies comparing younger and older people found that both the prevalence and depth of deprivation were more severe in younger people or single parents of working age [4,13,29]. However, from a life course perspective, the impact of relative deprivation on health should be evidenced in older people because the influence of poverty on health may accumulate over time. Finally, with the exception of a study that analyzed 131,335 people in 11 countries [10], most of the previous related research has been conducted on a relatively small scale. Analysis of relative deprivation should be performed with a large sample in order to derive robust findings, as few cases fall into each of the deprivation indices.

The present study posed three research questions: (1) is relative deprivation associated with poor health, even after monetary poverty is controlled for; (2) is the interaction effect between

relative deprivation and relative poverty significantly associated with poor health, and (3) do older people with social support have good health, even if they are relatively deprived? In social psychology and sociology, the concept of relative deprivation has also been used to measure psychosomatic stress related to complaints or dissatisfaction based on comparisons with their reference groups [30–38]. However, our focus on relative deprivation is based on Townsend's definition used in the poverty and social policy research described above.

Methods

Study samples

We used data from the Japan Gerontological Evaluation Study (JAGES), which was cross-sectional in design. JAGES was a postal survey of 112,123 people aged ≥65 who were randomly selected from the older residents of 31 municipalities in Japan. Data were collected from August 2010 to January 2012, with a response rate of 66.3%. For our study, we included 24,742 respondents from 24 municipalities who answered a relative deprivation questionnaire. The average age of the respondents was 74.6 years [standard

Table 2. Distribution of relative deprivation index.

Dimension	Item	Category	n	%	Crude odds ratio (95% CI) self-rated health (1 = fair/poor)	depressive symptom (1 = present)
Lack of daily necessities due to economic reasons	no television	no	23,594	97.6	1.00	1.00
		yes (+)	592	2.4	1.47 (1.22–1.77)	2.25 (1.87–2.72)
	no refrigerator	no	23,781	98.3	1.00	1.00
		yes (+)	405	1.7	1.32 (1.05–1.66)	1.67 (1.32–2.11)
	no air conditioner	no	22,823	94.4	1.00	1.00
		yes (+)	1,363	5.6	1.62 (1.44–1.83)	2.23 (1.97–2.52)
	no microwave oven	no	23,315	96.4	1.00	1.00
		yes (+)	871	3.6	1.62 (1.40–1.88)	1.88 (1.61–2.19)
	no water heater	no	23,213	96.0	1.00	1.00
		yes (+)	973	4.0	1.63 (1.41–1.87)	2.14 (1.85–2.48)
Lack in living environment	private WC	yes	22,606	93.5	1.00	1.00
		no (+)	1,580	6.5	1.40 (1.24–1.57)	1.78 (1.58–2.01)
	private kitchen	yes	22,260	92.0	1.00	1.00
		no (+)	1,926	8.0	1.43 (1.29–1.59)	1.79 (1.60–2.00)
	private bathroom	yes	22,153	91.6	1.00	1.00
		no (+)	2,033	8.4	1.40 (1.27–1.56)	1.83 (1.64–2.04)
	dining room separated from bedroom	yes	20,585	85.1	1.00	1.00
		no (+)	3,601	14.9	1.48 (1.37–1.61)	1.81 (1.67–1.97)
Lack of social life due to economic reasons	no telephone	no	23,229	96.0	1.00	1.00
		yes (+)	957	4.0	1.52 (1.32–1.76)	2.25 (1.94–2.60)
	no ceremonial dress	no	23,644	97.8	1.00	1.00
		yes (+)	542	2.2	1.53 (1.27–1.85)	1.92 (1.58–2.34)
	absence from relative's ceremonial occasions	no	21,952	93.4	1.00	1.00
		yes (+)	1,549	6.6	2.47 (2.22–2.76)	3.27 (2.91–3.67)
	cut-off of essential services in the past year	no	23,509	98.4	1.00	1.00
		yes (+)	388	1.6	2.09 (1.70–2.59)	4.10 (3.27–5.14)
Number of relative deprivation index		none	16,812	72.0	1.00	1.00
		1	3349	14.3	1.61 (1.48–1.75)	1.93 (1.77–2.10)
		2	916	3.9	2.01 (1.74–2.32)	2.68 (2.31–3.12)
		3	480	2.1	2.04 (1.67–2.48)	2.89 (2.36–3.52)
		4	1109	4.8	1.61 (1.40–1.85)	2.04 (1.77–2.36)
		5	271	1.2	2.30 (1.77–2.98)	3.49 (2.66–4.58)
		>=6	401	1.7	1.75 (1.40–2.19)	2.92 (2.33–3.67)
		>=2	3177	13.6	1.86 (1.70–2.02)	2.57 (2.35–2.81)

(+) is related to relative deprivation.

deviation (SD) = 6.4] and 54.1% were women. Our study protocol and questionnaire procedures were approved by the Ethics Committee in Research of Human Subjects at Nihon Fukushi University. Written informed consent was assumed with voluntary return of the questionnaire.

Dependent variables

We used self-rated health and depressive symptoms as indicators of subjective health. Self-rated health and depressive symptoms have been found to be highly valid predictors of mortality, regardless of other medical, behavioral, or psychosocial factors [39,40]. Self-rated health was measured using the question "How do you feel about your current health status: excellent, good, fair, or poor?" Responses were recoded into dichotomous response variables (excellent/good or fair/poor). Depressive symptoms were assessed using the short version of the Geriatric Depression Scale (GDS-15), which was developed for self-administration in the community using a simple yes/no format [41,42]. The validity and

Table 3. Combination of relative deprivation and poverty.

	n (%)	Self-rated health		Depressive symptom	
		fair/poor %	Crude OR (95%CI)	present %	Crude OR (95%CI)
No deprivation or poverty	10,241 (53.7)	16.9	1.00	21.0	1.00
Poverty only	3,987 (20.9)	23.3	1.50 (1.37–1.64)	29.0	1.54 (1.41–1.68)
Deprivation only (=1)	1,334 (7.0)	23.1	1.48 (1.29–1.70)	32.1	1.78 (1.56–2.03)
Deprivation only (>=2)	893 (4.7)	25.4	1.68 (1.43–1.97)	36.4	2.16 (1.85–2.52)
Poverty and deprivation (=1)	1,305 (6.8)	31.4	2.26 (1.98–2.57)	43.2	2.86 (2.51–3.26)
Poverty and deprivation (>=2)	1,300 (6.8)	33.8	2.51 (2.21–2.86)	48.4	3.53 (3.10–4.02)

reliability of this scale have also been confirmed for Japanese older people, and it is often used in Japanese surveys [43,44]. According to Sheikh et al. [42], scores of ≥5 on the GDS-15 indicated the presence of depressive symptoms of mild to severe depression. Our data showed approximately 30% of respondents had depressive symptoms. It is consistent with preceding Japanese studies [43,44].

Independent variables: relative deprivation and relative poverty

The indicators of relative deprivation used in preceding studies differ, because the standard living condition or decent life varies by culture and times. In reference to preceding research including Japanese studies [5–8,10–12,14], we evaluated thirteen indices that equated "lack of daily necessities," "lack of living environment," and "lack of social life due to economic reasons" with a low standard of living. Although lack of access to medical and health care services is another important element of standard of living, this was excluded from our deprivation indices because we assumed it to be directly reflected in poor health. On the other hand, we included experience of cutoff of essential services as a typical condition of lacking decent life, which is also used as a measure of social exclusion in a Japanese study [45].

Indicators of "lack of daily necessities" included having no television, refrigerator, air conditioner, microwave oven, or water heater. "Lack of living environment" indicators included having no private toilet, kitchen, or bathroom in the house and having a dining room that was not separate from the bedroom. "Lack of social life due to economic reasons" indicators included having no telephone or formal dress, being absent from family celebrations and events during the previous year due to economic reasons, and having essential services such as water, electricity or gas, cut off in the previous year (except in cases of forgetting to make a payment).

Relative poverty was defined as an income of less than half of the median annual equivalent income in the National Survey of Family Income and Expenditure in Japan [46]; the threshold was 1.49 million Japanese yen. This is the definition of relative poverty accepted by the Organisation for Economic Co-operation and Development and is conceptually based on the relative approach of the Luxembourg Income Study [47]. We used annual pre-tax household income. For each response, we calculated the equivalent household income by dividing income by the square root of the number of household members. Responses were categorized

into three groups: poverty (28.2%), non-poverty (51.7%), and unknown (20.1%).

Covariates

We used several control variables at the individual level: sex, age, educational attainment (to represent ascribed and achieved statuses), medical treatment (to represent recent physical condition), self-recognition of forgetfulness (to represent prodrome of dementia), and social support (to represent a buffer between poverty and health). Medical treatment was determined by asking "Are you currently receiving any medical treatment?" Self-recognition of forgetfulness was measured by asking "Do people around you notice your forgetfulness, for example, by telling you that you often ask the same thing?" Social support was measured using two questions representing emotional and institutional support: "Do you have someone who listens to your concerns and complaints?" and "Do you have someone who looks after you when you are sick and have to stay in bed for a few days?" Responses of "no" or "nobody" to both questions indicated an absence of social support.

In our data set, individuals were nested within each municipality. Previous studies reported significant associations between individual health and regional characteristics such as social capital and income inequality [48,49]. We used the proportion of older people residing in the area (%), population density in inhabitable areas (1,000 person/km2), and the proportion of persons receiving public assistance (‰) for characteristics at the municipal level. These variables were based on 2010 census and government data for Japan. The distribution of these variables is shown is Table 1.

Statistical analysis

First, we confirmed the distribution of the relative deprivation index and calculated crude odds ratios for subjective health. Second, we applied two-level Poisson regression analysis of random-intercept and fixed-slope models to assess the relationship between relative deprivation and self-rated health and depressive symptoms, adjusting for individual factors and municipal-level covariates (level 1: 24,742 individuals, level 2: 24 municipalities). We adopted multilevel modeling in order to control for intraclass (municipal level) cluster correlation. We also examined the interaction effect of relative deprivation and relative poverty. Individual and municipality fixed parameters were converted to prevalence ratios (PR) with a 95% confidence interval (95%CI).

Table 4. Association of subjective health and relative deprivation by two-level Poisson regression analysis[a].

	Self-rated health (fair/poor)				Depressive symptom (present)			
	Men		Women		Men		Women	
	PR	(95%CI)	PR	(95%CI)	PR	(95%CI)	PR	(95%CI)
FIXED EFFECTS								
Individual level								
Age (ref.: 65–69)								
70–74	1.06	(0.94–1.19)	1.09	(0.97–1.23)	0.92	(0.83–1.02)	1.00	(0.90–1.11)
75–79	1.24***	(1.11–1.40)	1.29***	(1.15–1.46)	1.03	(0.93–1.15)	0.98	(0.88–1.10)
80–84	1.31***	(1.15–1.49)	1.49***	(1.31–1.70)	0.95	(0.84–1.08)	1.02	(0.90–1.15)
85 -	1.23*	(1.05–1.45)	1.54***	(1.33–1.79)	0.95	(0.81–1.13)	1.15*	(1.00–1.33)
Education (ref.: >9 years)								
= <9 years	1.07	(0.98–1.16)	1.19***	(1.09–1.29)	1.16***	(1.07–1.25)	1.09*	(1.01–1.18)
Marital status (ref.: married)								
divorced	0.99	(0.86–1.13)	0.83***	(0.76–0.90)	1.23**	(1.09–1.39)	1.03	(0.95–1.12)
separated	1.22	(0.99–1.51)	0.91	(0.75–1.10)	1.37**	(1.14–1.65)	1.10	(0.92–1.31)
never married	1.17	(0.90–1.53)	0.92	(0.72–1.19)	1.29*	(1.03–1.62)	0.98	(0.77–1.26)
Disease and/or impairment (ref.: no)								
yes	4.76***	(4.05–5.60)	3.90***	(3.34–4.56)	1.33***	(1.21–1.46)	1.28***	(1.16–1.41)
Self recognition of forgetfulness (ref.: no)								
yes	1.47***	(1.34–1.61)	1.65***	(1.52–1.79)	1.71***	(1.57–1.86)	1.83***	(1.69–1.98)
Social supports (ref.: present)								
absent	1.37***	(1.21–1.54)	1.58***	(1.39–1.79)	1.57***	(1.41–1.75)	1.84***	(1.64–2.07)
Relative poverty (ref.: non-poverty)								
poverty (< ¥ 1.49 million)	1.25***	(1.11–1.40)	1.13*	(1.01–1.26)	1.34***	(1.20–1.50)	1.24***	(1.11–1.37)
Relative deprivation score (ref.: none)								
1	1.19*	(1.03–1.37)	1.31***	(1.15–1.50)	1.45***	(1.27–1.65)	1.36***	(1.19–1.55)
>=2	1.34***	(1.16–1.54)	1.27*	(1.10–1.46)	1.62***	(1.42–1.85)	1.43***	(1.25–1.64)
Interaction Effect								
poverty×deprivation (1)	1.08	(0.87–1.34)	0.95	(0.78–1.17)	1.03	(0.84–1.26)	1.00	(0.84–1.26)
poverty×deprivation (>=2)	1.01	(0.82–1.25)	1.06	(0.86–1.31)	0.94	(0.77–1.14)	1.01	(0.82–1.23)
Municipal level								
Proportion of older people [1%]	1.00	(0.99–1.01)	0.99	(0.98–1.00)	1.01*	(1.00–1.02)	1.02**	(1.01–1.03)
Population density [1000 p/km²]	0.96**	(0.94–0.99)	0.94***	(0.92–0.97)	1.03*	(1.00–1.06)	1.01	(0.99–1.04)
Prop. of receiving public assistance [5‰]	1.03*	(1.00–1.06)	1.04**	(1.01–1.07)	0.96**	(0.93–0.99)	0.95**	(0.93–0.98)

Table 4. Cont.

| | Self-rated health (fair/poor) | | | | Depressive symptom (present) | | | |
| | Men | | Women | | Men | | Women | |
	PR	(95%CI)	PR	(95%CI)	PR	(95%CI)	PR	(95%CI)
RANDOM EFFECTS[b]								
Municipality level variance (standard error)	.039 (.050)		.046 (.042)		.045 (.031)		.035 (.031)	

***p<.001 **p<.01 *p<.05 PR: Prevalence ratio.
[a]Each estimated coefficient of "unknown" category was omitted in above table.
[b]Random effect in null model:
SRH(men) = .147(SE = .034), SRH(women) = .197(SE = .037), GDS(men) = .093(SE = .027), GDS(women) = .101(SE = .026).

Finally, we calculated the proportion of poor health among deprived people with social support. We used the computer software, STATA 12.1 for all analyses.

Results

Table 2 showed that 1.6% to 8.4% of respondents lived in deprived conditions, as defined by the study parameters. A higher percentage of respondents did not have a dining room separate from the bedroom (14.9%). Univariate analysis showed that ORs for respondents living in deprived conditions, according to each relative deprivation index, were approximately 1.3–2.5 times higher for fair/poor self-rated health and 1.7–4.1 times higher for depressive symptoms than respondents who did not live in relative deprivation. In particular, the crude ORs for having essential services cut off and absence from family celebrations and events were relatively high. Relative deprivation scores also showed that respondents who were deprived of one item (14.3%) and two or more items (13.6%) were more likely to report fair/poor self-rated health [OR = 1.61 (95%CI: 1.48–1.75) and OR = 1.86 (95%CI: 1.70–2.02), respectively] and depressive symptoms [OR = 1.93 (95%CI: 1.77–2.10) and OR = 2.57 (95%CI: 2.35–2.81), respectively].

Table 3 shows the associations between subjective health and a combination of relative deprivation and relative poverty. The proportion of respondents with poor health was high with respect to "poverty and deprivation," "deprivation only," "poverty only," and "no deprivation or poverty." Odds ratios for respondents living in poverty and deprivation (two or more deprivation items) were 2.51 (95%CI: 2.21–2.86) and 3.53 (95%CI: 3.10–4.02) times higher for fair/poor self-rated health and depressive symptoms, respectively, than ORs for respondents with no deprivation or poverty.

Table 4 shows the results of a two-level Poisson regression analysis. Random effects showed that municipal-level variance in each model was smaller than that in the null model. This means that part of the municipal-level variance was explained by the individual- and municipal-level variables in the model. Fixed effects showed similar associations for both genders. Respondents with low educational attainment, no social support, under medical treatment, and prodrome of dementia tended to have poor subjective health, although relationships between age and municipal level variables were not consistent.

Relative deprivation was significantly associated with poor health, regardless of the status of relative poverty and other individual- and municipal-level characteristics. In male respondents with two or more deprivation items, rates of fair/poor self-rated health were 1.34 times (95%CI: 1.16–1.54) higher and rates of depressive symptoms were 1.62 times (95%CI: 1.42–1.85) higher than those observed in non-deprived individuals. Similarly, relative deprivation was associated with fair/poor self-rated health [PR = 1.27 (95%CI: 1.10–1.46)] and depressive symptoms [PR = 1.43 (95%CI: 1.25–1.64)] in women. Relative poverty was also related to self-rated health [men: PR = 1.25 (95%CI: 1.11–1.40); women: PR = 1.13 (95%CI: 1.01–1.26)] and depressive symptoms [men: PR = 1.34 (95%CI: 1.20–1.50); women: PR = 1.24 (95%CI: 1.11–1.37)]. The PRs for relative deprivation were comparatively higher than those for relative poverty. The interaction effect between relative poverty and relative deprivation for subjective health was not statistically significant.

Figure 1 shows different associations between subjective health and relative deprivation according to social support. The proportion of respondents with poor health was remarkably lower in those with social support relative to those without. However,

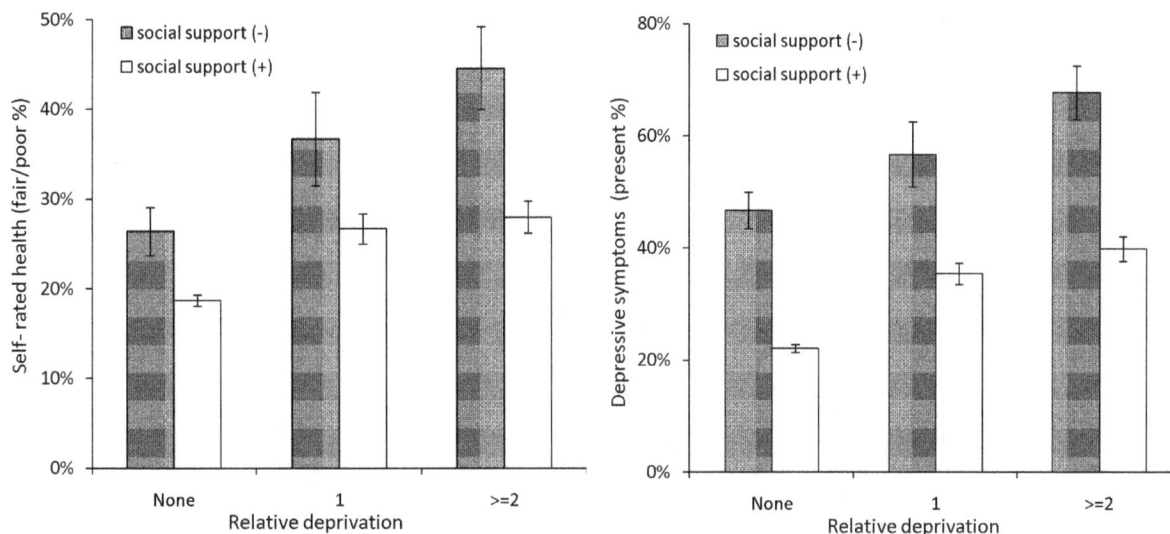

Figure 1. Proportion (95% Confidence Interval) of poor health in relation to relative deprivation and social support. Both figures show a low proportion of poor health in the presence of social support. Meanwhile, the proportion of those with poor health increases as the relative deprivation index score increases even with social support, indicating that social support does not fully cancel out the negative impacts of relative deprivation on health.

relative to non-deprived respondents with any level of social support, the proportions of respondents with poor/fair subjective health were remarkably higher in the relative deprivation groups (1 and ≤2, respectively).

Discussion

It was previously thought that all Japanese people were middle class. However, recent surveys have shown that intergenerational inequality exists in Japan [50], and the number of older people on public assistance is increasing [51]. The World Health Organization stated that poverty and relative deprivation have a major impact on health and premature death [52]. On the other hand, most poverty research has been based solely on the concept of relative poverty (monetary poverty) since data on material and environmental poverty was severely limited in Japan.

The present study addressed the concepts of both relative poverty and relative deprivation through a large survey of older Japanese and analyzed the association between health and relative poverty and deprivation. Our results showed that relative deprivation and relative poverty were related to poor health, even after other variables were controlled for. Our results were consistent with preceding findings; Abe [14] found that relative deprivation is closely associated with poor self-rated health and the presence of depressive symptoms using national Japanese representative cross-sectional data of participants aged ≥20 years. In particular, our results suggest that the concept of relative deprivation could address a different aspect of poverty that is related to health but is not addressed by the concept of relative poverty. People who have overlapping multidimensional disadvantages are more likely to be socially excluded [9] and to experience premature death [53]. Our results also showed that the negative effects of relative poverty and deprivation on health are additive; people with both relative deprivation and poverty were more disadvantaged with respect to health, but the relationship was not multiplicative.

Our study adds new evidence regarding which elements of poverty have strong impacts on the health of older adults. An

important finding is that relative deprivation has a stronger association with subjective health than relative poverty for both sexes. Some studies have revealed that people living in relatively deprived conditions experienced long-term, severe poverty throughout their life course [10,11]. For example, Whelan et al. [10] reported that approximately 40% of persistent income poverty overlapped with lifestyle deprivation in a broadly uniform manner. Consequently, the concept of relative deprivation could capture severe and absolute poverty better than relative poverty, which is based on the distribution of income in society. This could mean that relatively deprived older people might tend to be more disadvantaged, even in good health.

Finally, similar to a preceding study using cross-sectional data from 5,624 women aged 2059 [28], our data confirmed that relative deprivation was associated with the absence of social support [15]. Moreover, our results showed that having social support of any form could mitigate some of the negative impacts of relative deprivation on health. However, it is important to note that even with social support, relatively deprived people have more disadvantages with respect to health than non-deprived people. Therefore, the effects of material and environmental deprivation on poor health cannot be explained only by the absence of social support. As shown in preceding study [30–38], relative deprivation might increase social stresses and anxieties while lowering self-efficacy by depriving a living standard most people in the society enjoy. Furthermore, unlike monetary poverty, poor standard of living such as relative deprivation might closely be related to unhealthy lifestyles including poor eating habit and nutrition and lack of access to healthcare and welfare services.

Compared to relative poverty, which is based on a simple indicator and is often used in international comparative studies, relative deprivation is composed of complex indicators and has limitations for use in comparative studies. In fact, most preceding studies have applied a consensual approach based on public opinion in creating and selecting daily necessities and basic needs indices [4,6,7,10,12–14]. As a result, each relative deprivation indicator was different among preceding studies, although they often reflected the characteristics of that nation and culture.

However, relative deprivation could more accurately represent the phenomenon of poverty due to multidimensional living conditions than it does relative poverty. Although measurements of relative deprivation have been made in order to establish the poverty line, our results suggest that relative deprivation is also important for public health policy as it represents a dimension of the social determinants of health.

Study limitations

The present study has some limitations. First, our relative deprivation indicators did not cover the full range of daily resources among older people in Japan. Although we included indicators used in preceding studies, the indicators should be more sophisticated. Second, while the overall response rate for our data was relatively high, the response rates among the lower income categories were comparatively lower [54]. Therefore, our findings may be underestimated because people living in serious poverty and deprivation may have been less likely to participate in our survey. Third, there is a possibility of selection bias at the municipal level since our data are not representative of the whole country. On the other hand, our subjects were randomly selected in each municipality, and it is important to note that we did perform a large-scale survey concerning non-monetary poverty among older people in more than one municipality. Further research should include longitudinal surveys to reveal whether a causal relationship between relative deprivation and health exits.

Conclusion

Relative deprivation (non-monetary poverty) is an important element in poverty. To the best of our knowledge, this is the first study to investigate the association between health conditions and relative deprivation and poverty among older Asian adults. The

results showed that relative deprivation has stronger associations with self-rated health and depressive symptoms than with relative poverty. There was an independent and additive association between relative deprivation and poverty with respect to subjective health, and the presence of social support may not fully mitigate the negative association between relative deprivation and health. Our results suggest that relative deprivation is one social determinant of health that the concept of relative poverty cannot address.

Acknowledgments

The JAGES project (2014) comprises a coordinating group and collaborating investigators in each of the following field centers: Prof. K. Kondo (lead investigator; BZH12275@nifty.ne.jp), Dr H. Hikichi, Mr Y. Miyaguni, Dr Y. Sasaki, Dr Y Nagamine, Dr M. Hanazato, Chiba University; Dr N. Kondo, Dr T. Ashida, Dr D. Takagi, Dr Y. Tani, Tokyo University; Prof. T. Ojima, Dr E. Okada, Hamamatsu University School of Medicine; Prof. K. Osaka, Dr J. Aida, Dr T. Tuboya, Tohoku University; Dr M. Saito, Nihon Fukushi University; Dr H. Hirai, Iwate University; Dr Y. Shobugawa, Niigata university; Dr K. Suzuki, Aichi Gakuin University; Dr Y. Ichida, Doctoral Institute for Evidence Based Policy; Dr T. Yamamoto, Kanagawa Dental University; Prof. C. Murata, Dr T. Saito, Dr S. Jeong, National Institute for Longevity Sciences; Dr M. Nakade, Tokai Gakuen University; Prof. T Takeda, Seijo University; Prof. N Cable, University College London; Prof. H. Todoroki, Dr K Shirai, University of the Ryukyuus; Mr T Hayashi, Tokai College of Medical Science. Dr A. Tamakoshi, Hokkaido University; Dr J Misawa, Rikkyo University; Dr Y Fujino, University of Occupational and Environmental Health.

Author Contributions

Conceived and designed the experiments: MS NK KK. Performed the experiments: KK the JAGES group. Analyzed the data: MS. Contributed to the writing of the manuscript: MS KK NK AA TO KS.

References

1. Lynch J, Kaplan G (2000) Socioeconomic position. In: Berkman LF, Kawachi I, editors. *Social epidemiology*. New York: Oxford University Press, 13–35.
2. Claussen B, Davey Smith G, Thelle D (2003) Impact of childhood and adulthood socio-economic position on cause specific mortality: the Oslo Mortality Study. Journal of Epidemiology and Community Health, 2003, 57: 40–45.
3. Shaw M, Dorling D, Davey Smith G (2006) Poverty, social exclusion, and minorities. In: Marmot M, Wilkinson R, editors. *Social determinants of health; second edition*. New York: Oxford university press, 196–223.
4. Abe A (2006) Empirical analysis of relative deprivation in Japan using Japanese micro-data. The Journal of Social Policy and Labor Studies (Shakai-seisaku Gakkai Shi). 16: 251–275 (in Japanese with English abstract).
5. Townsend P (1979) *Poverty in the United Kingdom; a survey of household resources and standards of living*. Harmondsworth: Penguin Books.
6. Mack J, Lansley S (1985) *Poor Britain. London*, George Allen and Unwin.
7. Gordon D, Adelman L, Ashworth K, Bradshaw J, Levitas R, et al. (2000) *Poverty and social exclusion in Britain*. Rowntree Foundation.
8. Hiraoka K (2002) *Social inequalities among elderly people in Japan*. Tokyo: University of Tokyo Press. (in Japanese).
9. Bradshaw J, Finch N (2003) Overlaps in dimensions of poverty. Journal of Social Policy, 32(4): 513–525.
10. Whelan CT, Layte R, Maitre B (2003) Persistent income poverty and deprivation in the European Union; an analysis of first three waves of the European Community Household Panel. International Social Policy, 32(1): 1–18.
11. Iwata M, Hamamoto C (2004) Experience of poverty in deflationary depression. In: Higuchi Y, Ota K, the institute for research on household economics, editors. *Women in Heisei depression (Jyosei tachi no Heisei fukyo)*. Nikkei INC, 203–233. (in Japanese).
12. Saunders P (2008) Measuring well-being using non-monetary indicators; deprivation and social exclusion. Family Matters, 78: 8–17.
13. Saunders P, Abe A (2010) Poverty and deprivation in young and old: a comparative study of Australia and Japan. Poverty & Public Policy, 2(1): 67–97.
14. Abe A (2014). Constructing a deprivation scale for Japan; an index to supplement the relative poverty rate. the Quarterly of Social Security Research. 49(4): 360–371. (in Japanese).

15. Saito M, Kondo K, Kondo N, Ojima T, Suzuki K, et al. (2014) Prevalence and characteristics of relative deprivation among older people; from cross-sectional data in JAGES project. the Quarterly of Social Security Research. 50(3): in press. (in Japanese).
16. European Commission (2011) *The social dimension of the Europe 2020 strategy; A report of the social protection committee*. Directorate-General for Employment, Social Affairs and Inclusion.
17. Eames M, Ben-Shlomo Y, Marmot MG (1993) Social deprivation and premature mortality: regional comparison across England. British Medical Journal, 307(6912), 1097–1102.
18. Mac Loon P, Boddy FA (1994) Deprivation and mortality in Scotland, 1981 and 1991. British Medical Journal, 309(6967): 1465–1470.
19. Langford IH, Bentham G (1996) Regional variations in mortality rates in England and Wales: an analysis using multilevel modeling. Social Science & Medicine, 42(6): 897–908.
20. O'Reilly D (2002) Standard indicators of deprivation; Do they disadvantage older people? Age and Ageing, 31(3): 197–202.
21. Nakaya T (2011) Evaluation socio-economic inequalities in cancer mortality by using areal statistics in Japan: a note on the relation between municipal cancer mortality and areal deprivation index. Proceedings of Institute of Statistical Mathematics. 59(2): 239–265. (in Japanese with English abstract).
22. Mac Loon P (1996) Suicide and deprivation in Scotland. British Medical Journal. 312(7030): 543–544.
23. Lawlor DA, Davey Smith G, Patel R, Ebrahim S (2005) Life-course socioeconomic position, area deprivation, and coronary heart disease; findings from the British Women's Heart and Health Study. American Journal of Public Health. 95(1): 91–97.
24. Ellwood RP, Davies GM, Worthington HV, Blinkhorn AS, Taylor GO, et al. (2004) Relationship between area deprivation and the anticaries benefit of an oral health programme providing free fluoride toothpaste to young children. Community Dentistry and Oral Epidemiology, 32(3): 159–165.
25. Bower E, Gulliford M, Steele J, Newton T (2007) Area deprivation and oral health in Scottish adults: a multilevel study. Community Dentistry and Oral Epidemiology, 35(2): 118–129.
26. Walters K, Breeze E, Wilkinson P, Price GM, Bulpitt CJ, et al. (2004) Local area deprivation and urban-rural differences in anxiety and depression among people

older than 75 years in Britain. American Journal of Public Health. 94(10): 1768–1774.

27. Carp FM, Carp A (1981) Age, deprivation, and personal competence; effects on satisfaction. Research on Aging. 3(3): 279–298.

28. Sacker A, Bartley M, Firth D, Fitzpatrick R (2001) Dimensions of social inequality in the health of women in England: occupational, material and behavioral pathways. Social Science and Medicine, 52(5): 763–781.

29. Golant S, La Greca A (1995) The relative deprivation of U.S. elderly households as judged by their housing problems. Journal of Gerontology, 50B(1): S13–S23.

30. Stouffer SA, Suchman EA, Devinney LC, Star SA, Williams RM (1949) *The American Soldier. Volume 1.: Adjustment During Army Life*. Princeton University Press.

31. Runciman WG (1966) *Relative deprivation and social justice: a study of attitudes to social inequality in twentieth century England*. London: Routledge & Kegan Paul.

32. Scase R (1974) Relative deprivation: a comparison of English and Swedish manual workers. Wedderburn.D (eds) *Poverty, inequality, and class structure*. London: Syndics of cambridge university press. 197–216.

33. Crosby FJ (1982) *Relative deprivation and working women*. New York: Oxford University Press.

34. Kosaka K (1986) A model of relative deprivation. Journal of Mathematical Sociology, 12(1): 35–48.

35. Turley RNL (2002) Is relative deprivation beneficial? the effects of richer and poorer neighbors on children's outcomes. Journal of Community Psychology, 30(6): 671–686.

36. Walker I, Smith HJ (2002) *Relative deprivation: specification, development, and integration*. Cambridge: Cambridge University Press.

37. Tougas F, Lagace M, Sablonniere R, Kocum L (2004) A new approach to the link between identity and relative deprivation in the perspective of ageism and retirement. International Journal of Aging and Human Development, 59(1): 1–23.

38. Kondo N, Kawachi I, Hirai H, Kondo K, Subramanian SV, et al. (2009b) Relative deprivation and incident functional disability among older Japanese women and men: prospective cohort study. Journal of Epidemiology & Community Health, 63(6): 461–467.

39. Idler EL, Benyamini Y (1997) Self-rated health and mortality: a review of twenty-seven community studies. Journal of Health Social Behaviour, 38(1): 21–37.

40. Royall DR, Schillerstrom JE, Piper PK, Chiodo LK (2007) Depression and mortality in elders referred for geriatric psychiatry consultation. Journal of the American Medical Directors Association, 8(5): 318–321.

41. Yesavage JA, Brink TL, Rose TL, Lum O, Huang V, et al. (1983) Development and validation of a geriatric depression screening scale: A preliminary report. Journal of Psychiatric Research, 17: 37–49.

42. Sheikh JI, Yesavage JA (1986) Geriatric Depression Scale (GDS): Recent evidence and development of a shorter version. Clinical Gerontologist, 5: 165–173.

43. Murata C, Saito Y, Kondo K, Hirai H (2011) Social support and depression among community living older people. Japanese Journal of Gerontology, 33(1): 15–21. (in Japanese with English abstract).

44. Watanabe M, Imagawa T (2013) Factor structure of short form of the geriatric depression scale (GDS): reliability, validity and cutoff points. the Japanese Journal of Personality, 22(2): 193–197. (in Japanese with English abstract).

45. Abe A (2007) Measuring Social Exclusion in Japan. the Quarterly of Social Security Research. 43(1): 27–40. (in Japanese).

46. Ministry of internal affairs and communications (2009) National Survey of Family Income and Expenditure. (in Japanese). (http://www.stat.go.jp/data/zensho/2009/index.htm. Accessed 2014 Oct 3.).

47. Förster MF (1994) Measurement of low incomes and poverty. OECD labour market and social policy occasional papers, no. 14. doi:10.1787/112854878327.

48. Ichida Y, Kondo K, Hirai H, Hanibuchi T, Yoshikawa G, et al. (2009) Social capital, income inequality and self-rated health in Chita peninsula, Japan: a multilevel analysis of older people in 25 communities. Social Science & Medicine, 69(4): 489–499.

49. Aida J, Hanibuchi T, Nakade M, Hirai H, Osaka K, et al. (2009) The different effects of vertical social capital and horizontal social capital on dental status; A multilevel analysis. Social Science & Medicine, 69(4): 512–518.

50. Krueger AB, Abraham KG, Shapiro C (2012) *Economic report of the president, transmitted to the congress February 2012; together with the annual report of the council of economic advisors*. United States government printing office.

51. National Institute of Population and Social Security Research (2013) *Japanese public statistics data base concerning public assistance* (in Japanese). (http://www.ipss.go.jp/s-info/j/seiho/seiho.asp. Accessed 2014 Oct 3.).

52. Wilkinson R, Marmot M (2003) Social determinants of health: The solid facts (2nd ed.). WHO Regional Office for Europe.

53. Saito M, Kondo N, Kondo K, Ojima T, Hirai H (2012) Gender differences on the impacts of social exclusion on mortality among older Japanese: AGES cohort study. Social Science and Medicine, 75(5): 940–945.

54. Kondo K (2010) *Health inequalities in Japan: An empirical study of the older people*. Melbourne: Trans Pacific Press.

8

Diabetes Mellitus and Risk of Age-Related Macular Degeneration

Xue Chen[1,2], **Shi Song Rong**[2], **Qihua Xu**[1,3], **Fang Yao Tang**[2], **Yuan Liu**[1], **Hong Gu**[2,4], **Pancy O. S. Tam**[2], **Li Jia Chen**[2], **Mårten E. Brelén**[2], **Chi Pui Pang**[2]*, **Chen Zhao**[1]*

1 Department of Ophthalmology, The First Affiliated Hospital of Nanjing Medical University and State Key Laboratory of Reproductive Medicine, Nanjing Medical University, Nanjing, China, 2 Department of Ophthalmology & Visual Sciences, The Chinese University of Hong Kong, Hong Kong, China, 3 Department of Ophthalmology, The Affiliated Jiangyin Hospital of Southeast University Medical College, Jiangyin, China, 4 Department of Ophthalmology, Ningbo Medical Treatment Center Lihuili Hospital, Ningbo, China

Abstract

Age-related macular degeneration (AMD) is a major cause of severe vision loss in elderly people. Diabetes mellitus is a common endocrine disorder with serious consequences, and diabetic retinopathy (DR) is the main ophthalmic complication. DR and AMD are different diseases and we seek to explore the relationship between diabetes and AMD. MEDLINE, EMBASE, and the Cochrane Library were searched for potentially eligible studies. Studies based on longitudinal cohort, cross-sectional, and case-control associations, reporting evaluation data of diabetes as an independent factor for AMD were included. Reports of relative risks (RRs), hazard ratios (HRs), odds ratio (ORs), or evaluation data of diabetes as an independent factor for AMD were included. Review Manager and STATA were used for the meta-analysis. Twenty four articles involving 27 study populations were included for meta-analysis. In 7 cohort studies, diabetes was shown to be a risk factor for AMD (OR, 1.05; 95% CI, 1.00–1.14). Results of 9 cross-sectional studies revealed consistent association of diabetes with AMD (OR, 1.21; 95% CI, 1.00–1.45), especially for late AMD (OR, 1.48; 95% CI, 1.44–1.51). Similar association was also detected for AMD (OR, 1.29; 95% CI, 1.13–1.49) and late AMD (OR, 1.16; 95% CI, 1.11–1.21) in 11 case-control studies. The pooled ORs for risk of neovascular AMD (nAMD) were 1.10 (95% CI, 0.96–1.26), 1.48 (95% CI, 1.44–1.51), and 1.15 (95% CI, 1.11–1.21) from cohort, cross-sectional and case-control studies, respectively. No obvious divergence existed among different ethnic groups. Therefore, we find diabetes a risk factor for AMD, stronger for late AMD than earlier stages. However, most of the included studies only adjusted for age and sex; we thus cannot rule out confounding as a potential explanation for the association. More well-designed prospective cohort studies are still warranted to further examine the association.

Editor: Yuk Fai Leung, Purdue University, United States of America

Funding: This work was supported by National Key Basic Research Program of China (2013CB967500); National Natural Science Foundation of China (No. 81222009 and 81170856); Thousand Youth Talents Program of China (to C.Z.); Jiangsu Outstanding Young Investigator Program (BK2012046); Jiangsu Province's Key Provincial Talents Program (RC201149); Jiangsu Province's Scientific Research Innovation Program for Postgraduates (CXZZ13_0590 to X.C.); an Endowment Fund for the Lim Por-Yen Eye Genetics Research Centre; the General Research Fund from the Research Grants Council of Hong Kong (No. 473410); and A Project Funded by the Priority Academic Program Development of Jiangsu Higher Education Institutions (PAPD). The sponsor or funding organization had no role in the design or conduct of this research.

Competing Interests: The authors have declared that no competing interests exist.

* Email: dr.zhaochen@gmail.com (CZ); cppang@cuhk.edu.hk (CP)

Background

Age-related macular degeneration (AMD) has become a major cause of irreversible visual impairments in elderly people around the world, casting a heavy socio-economic burden on eye care [1,2,3]. AMD can be classified into the early and late stages. Patients with early AMD are usually asymptomatic, while severe vision loss frequently occurs in its late stage. Late AMD can be further categorized into two main subtypes: neovascular AMD (nAMD) and geographic atrophy (GA) [3]. The estimated prevalence is 6.8% for early AMD and 1.5% for late AMD in Caucasians over the age of 40 years [3]. It is estimated that 5% of early AMD patients will progress to late AMD over a 5-year period, increasing to nearly 15% over a 15-year period [4,5].

Similar prevalence has been identified in Asians but not in the black population [6,7].

The pathogenesis of AMD is complicated with multiple risk factors, including age, ocular dysfunctions, systemic diseases, diet, smoking, genetic, and environmental factors [8]. As a modifiable personal factor, whether diabetes play a role in the development and progression of AMD has been vigorously studied. While several reports presented positive correlations between diabetes and AMD [9,10,11,12,13,14], some other reports showed no such effect [15,16]. Even inversed relationship has been reported [17]. To gain a clear insight into the relationship between AMD and diabetes, we conducted a meta-analysis to assess whether diabetes is a risk factor for AMD.

Methods

Eligibility Criteria for Considering Studies for This Review

Included studies were: (1) studies evaluating diabetes as an individual risk factor for AMD; (2) prospective or retrospective cohort study, or study of cross-sectional or case-control design; (3) studies using predefined criteria and procedures for diabetes diagnosis and AMD grading; and (4) relative risks (RRs), hazard ratios (HRs), and odds ratio (ORs) have been reported, or data provided that enabled calculations of these outcomes. Case reports, reviews, abstracts, conference proceedings, editorials, reports with incomplete data, and non-English articles were excluded. For serial publications from the same research team using overlapped subjects, we included those: (1) with the latest follow-up information; and (2) providing adjusted RRs, HRs, or ORs with 95% CIs. To come up with a more precise insight into whether diabetes is an independent risk factor for AMD, only studies investigating diabetes as the main exposure, or provides adjusted RRs, HRs, or ORs with 95% CIs were included. This study was approved and reviewed by the institutional ethics committee of The First Affiliated Hospital of Nanjing Medical University and adhered to the tenets of the Declaration of Helsinki.

Search Methods for Identifying Studies

We searched MEDLINE, EMBASE, and the Cochrane Library for all relevant articles starting from year 1946 to March 18, 2014. We followed the Cochrane Handbook for Systematic Reviews of Interventions [18] and Meta-analysis of Observational Studies in Epidemiology (MOOSE) guideline [19] in designing and reporting the current study. Our search strategies were detailed in **Appendix S1**. No language filters was applied. Additional studies were identified from reference lists of the retrieved reports. Retrieved records and eligibility status were managed using EndNote X5 software (http://endnote.com/).

Study Selection

Two investigators (X.C. and S.S.R.) independently screened all retrieved citations based on title, abstract, and complete document if necessary. All relevant full-text articles were obtained and reviewed to determine the eligibility of each study. Disagreements were resolved via consensus with a senior reviewer (C.Z.).

Data Collection and Risk of Bias Assessment

The two reviewers (X.C. and S.S.R.) extracted outcomes from each study separately with a customized datasheet. Data obtained included: first author, year of publication, title of the study (if any), duration of the study, country or region, races, study design, sample size, estimated ORs, RRs, or HRs, adjusted factors in multiple regression analysis, and clinical examinations and diagnostic criteria for AMD and diabetes. We used the Newcastle Ottawa Scale (NOS, accessed via http://www.ncbi.nlm.nih.gov/books/NBK35156/) [20] and the criteria recommended by Agency for Healthcare Research and Quality (AHRQ, accessed via http://www.ncbi.nlm.nih.gov/books/NBK35156/) [21] to evaluate the risk of biases for prospective cohorts or case-control studies, and cross-sectional studies, respectively. All data from these two reviewers were compared. Agreement among the reviewers was sought after completion of grading.

Data Synthesis and Analysis

We assessed the association between diabetes and AMD by combining ORs from case-control and cross-sectional studies, and RRs or HRs from cohort studies. Heterogeneity between studies were tested by Cochran's Q statistic, and evaluated by the proportion of variation attributable to among-study heterogeneity, I^2. Heterogeneity among studies was considered no, low, moderate, and high when I^2 equals to 0% to 24%, 25% to 49%, 50% to 74%, and more than 75%, respectively. If p for Q< 0.1 or I^2>50%, a random-effects model (the DerSimonian and Laird method) was used [22], otherwise we used a fixed-effects model(the Mantel-Haenszel method) [23]. Subgroup analysis was conducted by the study designs, AMD stages and clinical subtypes, and ethnic groups. The Asians were further divided into subgroups, including the East Asians (Japan, China, Taiwan, and Korea), Southeast Asians (Singapore), West Asians (Israel, Iran, and Turkey), and South Asians (Nepal, and India). As to the subgroup analysis concerning different AMD stages, we applied the widely accepted clinical classification system as described by the Age-Related Eye Disease Study Research Group [24,25]. Briefly, early AMD was defined by the appearance of drusen and pigmentary alterations within 2 disc diameters of the fovea. Late AMD was featured by the presence of large drusen (soft and/or indistinct) together with pigmentary abnormalities, or can be generally recognized as nAMD and/or GA. Moreover, sensitivity analysis was conducted to affirm the estimated association by removing studies with poor quality or prone to introducing biases. Publication bias and small-study effects were assessed with funnel plots [26] and Egger's test [27]. All analyses were conducted with Review Manager version 5.2 (Cochrane Collaboration, Oxford, UK; http://ims.cochrane.org/revman) and STATA software (version 12.0; StataCorp LP, College Station, TX). Alpha was set to 0.05 for two-sided test.

Results

Literature

A total of 3205 records were yielded from digital search and manual screen of reference list. Thirty-eight articles, published from 1986 to 2013, were included for the systematic review. Workflow of literature screen and review was shown in **Figure 1**. In addition, to provide a better understanding in diabetes as an independent risk factor for AMD, fourteen studies that presented diabetes as a covariate and provided ORs/RRs/HRs from baseline data without any adjustment were excluded, involving 12 cross-sectional [11,15,17,28,29,30,31,32,33,34,35,36] and 2 case-control studies [37,38]. The 24 articles included 1858350 participants in 27 independent study populations, comprising 7 cohort studies [39,40,41,42,43], 9 cross-sectional studies [9,14,16,44,45,46,47,48], and 11 case-control studies [12,13,36,49,50,51,52,53,54,55,56]. Among the 27 study populations, 10 were in Asia, 9 in North America (United States), 6 in Europe, 1 in Oceania (Australia), and 1 in South America (Barbados). Most studies used predefined criteria for AMD diagnosis and adopted standard grading system [57,58]. Samples sizes varied widely, from less than 50 to over 1.5 million (**Table 1**). Only two of the earliest studies, in 1986 [49] and 1998 [50], had sample sizes less than 100. Risk of bias assessments for cohort, cross-sectional, and case-control studies has been performed (**Tables S1–S3**). Tan et al [59] and Tomany et al [42] both involved the Blue Mountain Eye Study cohort, we included latter one in the analysis. The ORs/RRs/HRs with 95% CI and the corresponding adjusted variables for each study were listed in overall AMD, early AMD or late AMD (**Table 2**).

Meta-Analysis

The effects of diabetes on the risk of AMD in all these studies were found to be essentially consistent (**Figure 2 and Table 3**).

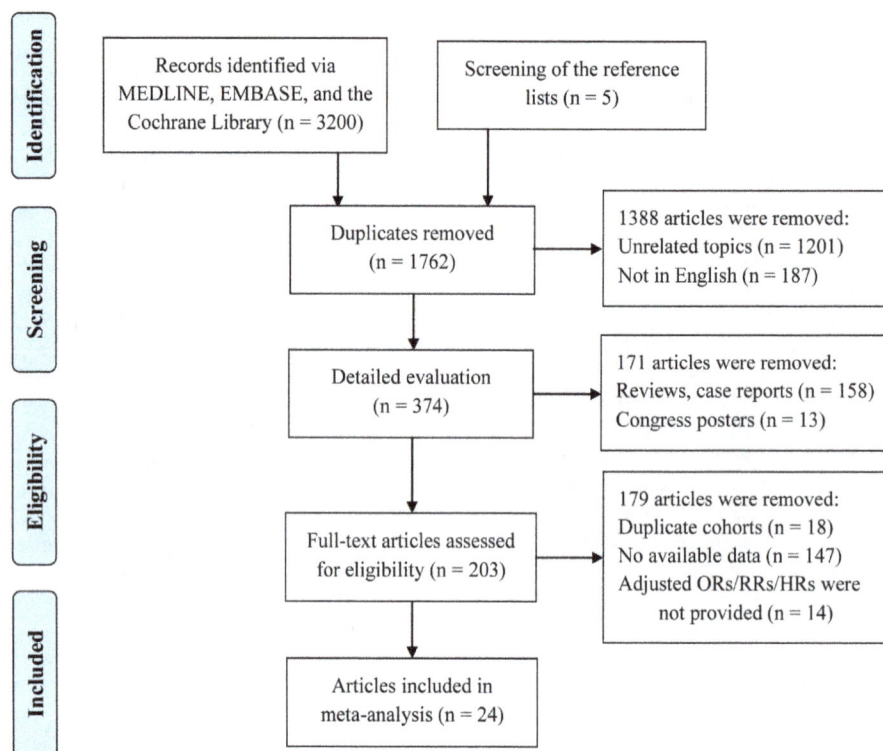

Figure 1. Flow chart depicting the screening process for inclusion in the meta-analysis.

According to the meta-analysis of 7 cohort studies, diabetes was associated with AMD (OR, 1.05; 95% CI, 1.00–1.11). Subgroup analysis based on AMD stages revealed diabetes as a marginal risk factor for late AMD (OR, 1.05; 95% CI, 0.99–1.10), but not for its early form (OR, 0.83; 95% CI, 0.60–1.15). Subgroup analysis by AMD subtypes showed that the pooled OR of diabetes for risk of nAMD was 1.10 (95% CI, 0.96–1.26), for risk of GA was 1.63 (95% CI, 0.51–5.21). In the 9 cross-sectional study populations, diabetes was found increasing AMD risk (OR, 1.21; 95% CI, 1.00–1.45). Subgroup analysis confirmed this effect for late AMD (OR, 1.48; 95% CI, 1.44–1.51), and nAMD (OR, 1.48; 95% CI, 1.44–1.51), but not for early AMD (OR, 0.99; 95% CI, 0.88–1.12) or GA (OR, 1.58; 95% CI, 0.63–3.99). The results kept consistent in the analysis of 11 case-control studies. The pooled OR of diabetes for AMD was 1.29 (95% CI, 1.13–1.49). The pooled OR was 1.16 (95% CI, 1.11–1.21) for late AMD, and 1.15 (95% CI, 1.11–1.21) for nAMD. To reduce the methodological heterogeneity and the potential effect led by other risk factors, we also conducted meta-analysis solely using multivariate-adjusted outcomes. Only 3 cohort studies and 2 cross-sectional were included, and the results varied from the overall data, which was probably due to the limited number of included studies. However, in both groups, diabetes was found as a marginal risk factor for nAMD in cross-sectional studies (OR, 1.04; 95% CI, 0.99–1.10) and a solid risk factor for late AMD in cohort studies (OR, 1.81; 95% CI, 1.10–2.98). No association between diabetes and early AMD or GA was found in both groups (**Table 4**). Subgroup analyses by ethnic group were further performed. The associations of diabetes and overall and early AMD were similar between the Asian and Caucasian populations (**Table 5**), while associations between diabetes and all subtypes of late AMD were suggested only for the Caucasian group, but not for the overall Asian population or any of its subgroups. No indication of any obvious asymmetry was observed according to the shapes of Begg's funnel plots and Egger's test for all groups as detailed in **Tables 3–5**.

Risk of Bias Assessment and Sensitivity Analysis

In our assessment, we found most studies have a robust design and reported in a clear manner, thus have lower risks in introducing bias (**Tables S1–S3**). However, we did identify one cross-sectional study which had relative higher risk to introduce biases when used to evaluate risk-modifying effect of diabetes for AMD [14] (**Tables S2**), thus were subjected to sensitivity analysis. In sensitivity analysis, we sequentially omitted one study at a time and removed studies of higher risk of introducing bias to affirm the associations. Sensitivity analyses revealed that the study conducted by Alexander et al [52] contributed to the heterogeneity in the subgroup analysis of case-control studies, but did not alter the results in each subgroup. When removing the studies conducted by Shalev et al and Hahn et al in the subgroup analysis of cohort studies, respectively, although the p values for diabetes and AMD became insignificant, the direction of ORs was kept and associations of marginal significance were revealed (removing study by Shalev et al: OR, 1.04; 95% CI, 0.99–1.10; Hahn et al: OR, 1.12; 95% CI, 0.98–1.29). Similar findings were revealed by subgroup analyses involving cross-sectional and case-control studies. In the analysis of cross-sectional studies, the removal of studies by Vaičaitienė et al [14], Duan et al [45], Xu et al [16], and Choi et al [47] would also lead to borderline results (removing study by Vaičaitienė et al: OR, 1.10; 95% CI, 0.98–1.23; Duan et al: OR, 1.30; 95% CI, 0.97–1.73; Xu et al: OR, 1.21; 95% CI, 0.99–1.47; Choi et al: OR, 1.16; 95% CI, 0.96–1.41). In addition, in the subgroup analysis of case-control studies, an association of borderline significance between diabetes and AMD (OR, 1.23;

Table 1. Characteristics of Included Cohorts.

First Author (Publication Year)	Study	Study Period	Region	Race	Sample Size	Diagnostic Criteria AMD	Diabetes
Cohort Studies (Prospective & Retrospective)							
Tomany et al (2004)	BDES	1993–1995	US	Caucasian	3562	I & W	PGL & S
	BMES	1997–1999	Australia	Caucasian	2330	I & W	PGL & S
	RS	1997–1999	Netherlands	Caucasian	3631	I & W	PGL & S
Leske et al (2006)	BISED II	1987–1992	Barbados	Mixed	2793	W	M & S
Yasuda et al (2009)	Hisayama Study	2007	Japan	East Asian	1401	I & W	M & PGL
Shalev et al (2011)	MHS	1998–2007	Israel	West Asian	108973	ICD9	M
Hahn et al (2013)	NA	1995–2005	US	Caucasian	16510	ICD9	ICD9
Cross-sectional Studies							
Delcourt et al (2001)	POLA	1995–1997	France	Caucasian	2584	I & W	Interview
Vaičaitienė et al (2003)	NA	1995–1997	Lithuania	Caucasian	438	NA	NA
Duan et al (2007)	NA	2000–2001	US	Caucasian	1519086	ICD9	ICD9
Klein et al (2007)	WHISE	1993–2002	US	Caucasian	4288	W	M
Topouzis et al (2009)	EUREYE study	2000–2003	Europe¶	Caucasian	4722	I	S
Xu et al (2009)	Beijing Eye Study	2006	China	East Asian	2960	W	PGL & S
Choi et al (2011)	NA	2006–2008	Korea	East Asian	3008	W	M & PGL
Cheung et al (2013)	SIES	2007–2009	Singapore	Southeast Asian	3337	W	PGL & S
	CIEMS	2006–2008	India	South Asian	3422	W	PGL & S
Case-control Studies							
Blumenkranz et al (1986)	NA	NA	US	Caucasian	49	NA	PGL
Ross et al (1998)	NA	NA	US	Caucasian	94	Detailed in paper.	M
McGwin et al (2003)	NA	1997–2001	US	Caucasian	6050	ICD9	ICD9
Moeini et al (2005)	NA	2001	Iran	West Asian	130	NA	PGL
Alexander et al (2007)	NA	2001–2003	US	Caucasian	62179	ICD9	ICD9
Kim et al (2008)	NA	1998–2003	US	Caucasian	204	W	Questionnaire
Lin et al (2008)	NA	2002–2006	Taiwan	East Asian	280	I	NA
Nitsch et al (2008)	GPRD	1987–2002	UK	Caucasian	104176	Readcodes & OXMIS	M
Cackett et al (2011)	NA	2007–2008	Singapore	Southeast Asian	1617	W	Questionnaire
Sogut et al (2013)	NA	NA	Turkey	West Asian	280	W	ADA
Torre et al (2013)	NA	2011	Italy	Caucasian	246	NA	Questionnaire

¶ Europe: Estonia, France, Greece, Italy, Norway, Spain, UK;

Abbreviation: BDES: Beaver Dam Eye Study; BMES: Blue Mountains Eye Study; RS: Rotterdam Study; BISED II: Barbados Incidence Study of Eye Diseases; MHS: Maccabi Healthcare Services; NA: not available; POLA: Pathologies Oculaires Liées àl'Age Study; WHISE: Women's Health Initiative Sight Examination; SIES: Singapore Indian Eye Study; CIEMS: Central India Eye and Medical Study; GPRD: General Practice Research Database; AMD: Age Related Macular Degeneration; &: represents a combination of two diagnostic methods; I: International Classification and Grading System for AMD; W: Wisconsin Age-Related Maculopathy Grading System; ICD9: International Classification of Diseases with Clinical Modifications, Ninth Revision; PGL: Plasma Glucose Level; S: Self-reported diabetic history or medications; M: Medical recorded diabetic history or medications; ADA: American Diabetes Association diagnostic criteria.

Table 2. Detailed Analytical Information for Included Cohorts.

First Author(Publication Year)	OR/RR/HR$^\Delta$ [95% CI]					Adjusted Variables
	Early AMD	Late AMD			AMD	
		nAMD	GA	Total		
Cohort Studies (Prospective & Retrospective)						
Tomany (2004)	—	0.67 [0.24, 1.86]	2.05 [0.84, 4.99]	1.21 [0.62, 2.36]	1.21 [0.62, 2.36]	Age, Sex
BDES	—	—	0.79 [0.10, 6.31]	—	—	Age, Sex
BMES	—	—	8.31 [2.34, 29.50]	—	—	Age, Sex
RS	—	—	0.79 [0.10, 6.19]	—	—	Age, Sex
Leske (2006)	0.88 [0.60, 1.30]	—	—	2.70 [1.00, 7.30]	1.02 [0.71, 1.47]	Age
Yasuda (2009)	0.70 [0.37, 1.31]	—	—	0.69 [0.16, 2.95]	0.69 [0.39, 1.24]	Multiple Factors$^\#$
Shalev (2011)	—	—	—	—	1.18 [1.01, 1.38]	Mutually adjusted
Hahn (2013)	—	1.11 [0.97, 1.27]	1.03 [0.97, 1.09]	1.04 [0.99, 1.10]	1.04 [0.99, 1.10]	Multiple Factors*
Cross-sectional Studies						
Delcourt (2001)	—	—	—	1.22 [0.45, 3.29]	1.22 [0.45, 3.29]	Age, Sex
Vaičaitienė (2003)	—	—	—	—	4.61 [2.45, 8.67]	Age, Sex
Duan (2007)	—	1.48 [1.44, 1.51]	—	1.48 [1.44, 1.51]	1.18 [1.16, 1.19]	Age, Sex, Race
Klein (2007)	0.87 [0.67, 1.12]	2.49 [1.17, 5.31]	2.28 [0.63, 8.28]	2.43 [1.26, 4.70]	0.94 [0.74, 1.20]	Age
Topouzis (2009)	0.98 [0.83, 1.17]	1.81 [1.10, 2.98]	1.06 [0.28, 4.04]	1.38 [0.90, 2.12]	1.01 [0.85, 1.19]	Multiple Factors‡
Xu (2009)	1.30 [0.69, 2.43]	—	—	1.13 [0.14, 9.40]	1.28 [0.70, 2.34]	None
Choi (2011)	1.87 [1.07, 3.28]	—	—	—	1.87 [1.07, 3.28]	Multiple Factors†
Cheung (2013)						
SIES	0.93 [0.68, 1.28]	—	—	—	0.93 [0.68, 1.28]	Age, Sex
CIEMS	1.14 [0.47, 2.77]	—	—	—	1.14 [0.47, 2.77]	Age, Sex
Case-control Studies						
Blumenkranz (1986)	—	—	—	0.53 [0.06, 4.71]	0.53 [0.06, 4.71]	Use siblings
Ross (1998)	—	—	—	—	1.09 [0.21, 5.59]	Age
McGwin Jr (2003)	—	—	—	—	1.78 [1.43, 2.20]	Age, Sex
Moeini (2005)	—	—	—	—	1.29 [0.52, 3.21]	Age, Sex, Risk factors
Alexander (2007)	—	1.16 [1.11, 1.21]	—	1.16 [1.11, 1.21]	1.16 [1.11, 1.21]	Age, Sex, Race, Database length
Kim (2008)	—	0.61 [0.27, 1.39]	—	0.61 [0.27, 1.39]	0.61 [0.27, 1.39]	Use siblings
Lin (2008)	—	1.20 [0.44, 3.26]	0.97 [0.36, 2.63]	1.07 [0.45, 2.57]	1.07 [0.45, 2.57]	Age, Sex
Nitsch (2008)	—	—	—	—	1.36 [1.29, 1.43]	Age, Sex, Practice, Consultation Rate
Cackett (2011)	—	0.92 [0.50, 1.70]	—	0.92 [0.50, 1.70]	0.92 [0.50, 1.70]	Age, Sex
Sogut (2013)	—	—	—	1.68 [0.76, 3.69]	1.68 [0.76, 3.69]	Age, Sex
Torre (2013)	—	—	—	—	0.80 [0.08, 8.07]	Age, Sex, Smoking

$^\Delta$OR is for cross-sectional and case-control studies, RR is for prospective cohort studies, HR is for retrospective cohort studies;
$^\#$Age, Sex, Smoking habit, White blood cells;
*Age, Sex, Race, History of hypertension, Atherosclerosis, Stroke, Coronary heart disease, Hyperlipidemia, Charlson index;
‡Age, Sex, Smoking, Education, BMI, Alcohol consumption, Cardiovascular disease, Aspirin use, Systolic blood pressure, Alpha-tocopherol ratio, Vitamin C, Lutein;
†Age, Sex, Current smoking, Obesity, Hypertension.
Abbreviations: OR: odds ratio; RR: risk ratio; HR: hazard ratio; CI: confidence interval; AMD: Age-related macular degeneration; nAMD: neovascular AMD; GA: geographic atrophy; WBC: white blood cell.

95% CI, 0.97–1.56) was presented if the study by Nitsch et al [13] was excluded.

Discussion

Diabetes is a major concern in ophthalmic care. Whether it contributes to the prevalence of AMD has been an unsolved dilemma targeted by a large number of studies. However, obvious inconsistencies between studies, including a few large cohorts, suggest the necessity to conduct an exhaustive review and quantitative analysis on all the evidences to determine its effect. In the present systemic review and meta-analysis, we reviewed 3205 published reports and completed analysis on 1858350 participants of 27 study populations from 24 original studies. We found that diabetes is a risk factor for AMD, especially for nAMD. To our knowledge, this is the first meta-analysis addressing the

A

Study or Subgroup	Weight	Risk Ratio IV, Fixed, 95% CI
Tomany 2004	0.5%	1.21 [0.62, 2.36]
Leske 2006	1.8%	1.02 [0.71, 1.47]
Yasuda 2009	0.7%	0.70 [0.39, 1.24]
Shalev 2011	9.9%	1.18 [1.01, 1.38]
Hahn 2013	87.0%	1.04 [0.99, 1.10]
Total (95% CI)	100.0%	1.05 [1.00, 1.11]

Heterogeneity: Chi² = 4.34, df = 4 (P = 0.36); I² = 8%
Test for overall effect: Z = 2.09 (P = 0.04)

Risk Ratio IV, Fixed, 95% CI — 0.5 0.7 1 1.5 2 — Non-Diabetes / Diabetes

B

Study or Subgroup	Weight	Odds Ratio IV, Random, 95% CI
Delcourt 2001	3.0%	1.22 [0.45, 3.29]
Vaičaitienė 2003	6.3%	4.61 [2.45, 8.67]
Duan 2007	23.2%	1.17 [1.16, 1.19]
Klein 2007	16.6%	0.94 [0.74, 1.20]
Topouzis 2009	19.4%	1.01 [0.85, 1.19]
Xu 2009	6.7%	1.28 [0.70, 2.34]
Choi 2011	7.4%	1.87 [1.07, 3.28]
Cheung 2013 SIES	13.8%	0.93 [0.68, 1.28]
Cheung 2013 CIEMS	3.7%	1.14 [0.47, 2.77]
Total (95% CI)	100.0%	1.21 [1.00, 1.45]

Heterogeneity: Tau² = 0.04; Chi² = 29.20, df = 8 (P = 0.0003); I² = 73%
Test for overall effect: Z = 2.00 (P = 0.05)

Odds Ratio IV, Random, 95% CI — 0.5 0.7 1 1.5 2 — Non-Diabetes / Diabetes

C

Study or Subgroup	Weight	Odds Ratio IV, Random, 95% CI
Blumenkranz 1986	0.4%	0.53 [0.06, 4.71]
Ross 1998	0.7%	1.09 [0.21, 5.59]
McGwin Jr 2003	18.7%	1.78 [1.43, 2.20]
Moeini 2005	2.1%	1.29 [0.52, 3.21]
Alexander 2007	33.0%	1.16 [1.11, 1.21]
Kim 2008	2.6%	0.61 [0.27, 1.39]
Lin 2008	2.3%	1.08 [0.45, 2.57]
Nitsch 2008	32.5%	1.36 [1.29, 1.43]
Cackett 2011	4.4%	0.92 [0.50, 1.70]
Torre 2013	0.4%	0.80 [0.08, 8.07]
Sogut 2013	2.8%	1.67 [0.76, 3.69]
Total (95% CI)	100.0%	1.29 [1.13, 1.49]

Heterogeneity: Tau² = 0.01; Chi² = 37.39, df = 10 (P < 0.0001); I² = 73%
Test for overall effect: Z = 3.67 (P = 0.0002)

Odds Ratio IV, Random, 95% CI — 0.05 0.2 1 5 20 — Non-Diabetes / Diabetes

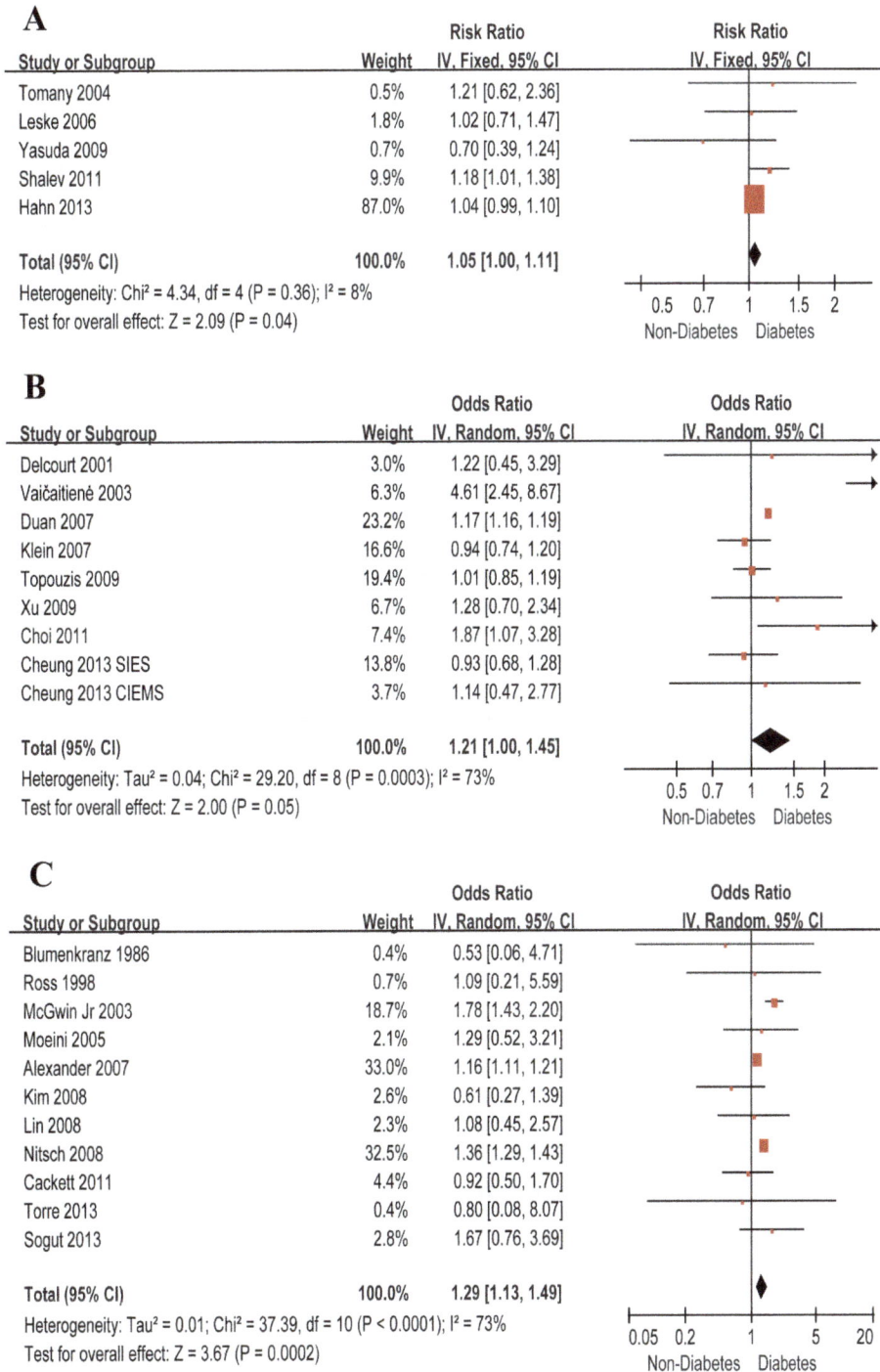

Figure 2. Effects of diabetes on AMD risks. Graphs showing the effects of diabetes on the risk of Age-related Macular Degenerations in longitudinal cohort studies (A), cross-sectional studies (B), and case-control studies (C). IV: inverse variance, CI: confidence interval.

topic for AMD and all its subtypes, and by using data from a comprehensive collection of prospective and retrospective cohort, cross-sectional, and case-control studies.

Clinically, AMD can be classified based on drusen features and retinal pigment epithelial abnormalities, we found most included studies follow the Wisconsin Age-related Maculopathy Grading Scheme, according to 4 levels: level 1 (no AMD), level 2 and 3 (early AMD), and level 4 (late AMD) [57,60]. The contribution of diabetes to early AMD is inconsistent in studies. Diabetic patients have increased occurrence of early AMD in a cross-sectional study of a Korean cohort of 3008 adults [47]. No similar association has been observed in other studies. An inverse relationship is observed in the Age-Related Eye Disease Study (AREDS) [17]. In the Beaver Dam Eye Study (BDES), diabetes was found to be a protective factor for incident reticular drusen based on a 15-year cumulative incidence [61]. In this meta-analysis, no clear

Table 3. Analysis of Diabetes as a Risk Factor for AMD in Different AMD Types.

Study Design	No. of Cohorts	Sample Size	Overall Effect OR/RR* [95% CI]	Z score	p value	Heterogeneity I² (%)	Q (p)	Egger's Test
Cohort Studies								
AMD	7	139200	1.05 [1.00, 1.11]	2.09	0.037	8	0.361	0.961
Early AMD	2	4194	0.83 [0.60, 1.15]	1.12	0.261	0	0.529	NA
Late AMD	6	30227	1.05 [0.99, 1.10]	1.70	0.088	25	0.260	0.504
nAMD	4	26033	1.10 [0.96, 1.26]	1.40	0.160	0	0.335	NA
GA	4	26033	1.63 [0.51, 5.21]†	0.83	0.407	72	0.014	0.523
Cross-sectional Studies								
AMD	9	1543845	1.21 [1.00, 1.45]†	2.00	0.045	73	0.000	0.813
Early AMD	6	21737	0.99 [0.88, 1.12]	0.15	0.883	28	0.224	0.205
Late AMD	5	1533640	1.48 [1.44, 1.51]	32.20	0.000	0	0.642	0.774
nAMD	3	1528096	1.48 [1.44, 1.51]	32.23	0.000	20	0.287	0.154
GA	2	9010	1.58 [0.63, 3.99]	0.97	0.333	0	0.419	NA
Case-control Studies								
AMD	11	175305	1.29 [1.13, 1.49]†	3.67	0.000	73	0.000	0.976
Late AMD	6	64609	1.16 [1.11, 1.21]	6.65	0.000	0	0.520	0.334
nAMD	4	62179	1.15 [1.11, 1.21]	6.55	0.000	0	0.416	0.257
GA	1	280	0.97 [0.36, 2.63]	0.06	0.954	NA	NA	NA

* OR is for cross-sectional and case-control studies, RR is for cohort studies.
† Studies using random effect model.
Abbreviations: OR: odds ratio; RR: risk ratio; CI: confidence interval; AMD: age related macular degeneration; nAMD: neovascular AMD; GA: geographic atrophy; NA: not available.

Table 4. Analysis of Diabetes as a Risk Factor for AMD in Different AMD Types with Multivariate-adjusted ORs/RRs/HRs.

Study Design	No. of Cohorts	Sample Size	Overall Effect			Heterogeneity		Egger's Test
			OR/RR* [95% CI]	Z score	p value	I² (%)	Q (p)	
Cohort Studies								
AMD	3	126884	1.07 [0.93, 1.22]†	0.96	0.339	52	0.125	0.904
Early AMD	1	1401	0.70 [0.37, 1.31]	1.12	0.262	NA	NA	NA
Late AMD	2	17911	1.04 [0.99, 1.10]	1.56	0.118	0	0.574	NA
nAMD	1	16510	1.11 [0.97, 1.27]	1.52	0.129	NA	NA	NA
GA	1	16510	1.03 [0.97, 1.09]	0.94	0.349	NA	NA	NA
Cross-sectional Studies								
AMD	2	7730	1.29 [0.71, 2.35]†	0.85	0.397	77	0.038	NA
Early AMD	2	7730	1.28 [0.69, 2.39]†	0.78	0.640	78	0.031	NA
Late AMD	1	4722	1.38 [0.90, 2.12]	1.46	0.145	NA	NA	NA
nAMD	1	4722	1.81 [1.10, 2.98]	2.34	0.020	NA	NA	NA
GA	1	4722	1.06 [0.28, 4.04]	0.09	0.928	NA	NA	NA

* OR is for cross-sectional and case-control studies, RR is for cohort studies.
† Studies using random effect model.
Abbreviations: OR: odds ratio; RR: risk ratio; CI: confidence interval; AMD: age related macular degeneration; nAMD: neovascular AMD; GA: geographic atrophy; NA: not available.

Table 5. Analysis of Diabetes as a Risk Factor for AMD in Different Ethnic Groups.

Ethnic Group	No. of cohorts	Sample Size	Overall Effect OR/RR* [95% CI]	Z score	p value	Heterogeneity I² (%)	Q (p)	Egger's Test
AMD								
Caucasian	16	1730149	1.20 [1.12, 1.29]†	4.86	0.000	84	0.000	0.733
Asian	10	125408	1.14 [1.01, 1.29]	2.11	0.035	2	0.423	0.978
East Asian	4	7649	1.18 [0.86, 1.61]	1.03	0.301	49	0.115	0.856
West Asian	3	109383	1.20 [1.03, 1.39]	2.35	0.019	0	0.688	0.385
Southeast Asian	2	4954	0.93 [0.70, 1.23]	0.50	0.616	0	0.973	NA
South Asian	1	3422	1.14 [0.47, 2.77]	0.29	0.771	NA	NA	NA
Total	27	1858350	1.18 [1.11, 1.26]†	5.11	0.000	74	0.000	0.909
Early AMD								
Caucasian	2	9010	0.95 [0.82, 1.09]	0.77	0.442	0	0.422	NA
Asian	5	14128	1.06 [0.85, 1.34]	0.54	0.588	40	0.152	0.626
East Asian	3	7369	1.21 [0.68, 2.14]†	0.65	0.517	62	0.070	0.385
Southeast Asian	1	3337	0.93 [0.68, 1.28]	0.43	0.667	NA	NA	NA
South Asian	1	3422	1.14 [0.47, 2.77]	0.29	0.771	NA	NA	NA
Total	8	25931	0.97 [0.86, 1.09]	0.53	0.595	16	0.303	0.478
Late AMD								
Caucasian	11	1619145	1.25 [1.05, 1.49]†	2.50	0.013	96	0.000	0.479
Asian	5	6538	1.09 [0.73, 1.63]	0.44	0.663	0	0.770	0.882
East Asian	3	4641	0.97 [0.48, 1.97]	0.07	0.941	0	0.865	0.800
Southeast Asian	1	1617	0.92 [0.50, 1.70]	0.26	0.795	NA	NA	NA
West Asian	1	280	1.68 [0.76, 3.69]	1.28	0.200	NA	NA	NA
Total	17	1628476	1.25 [1.07, 1.46]†	2.74	0.006	92	0.000	0.454
Neovascular AMD								
Caucasian	9	1616512	1.29 [1.09, 1.54]†	2.92	0.003	94	<0.001	0.524
Asian	2	1897	0.99 [0.59, 1.67]	0.04	0.970	0	0.662	NA
East Asian	1	280	1.20 [0.44, 3.26]	0.35	0.724	NA	NA	NA
Southeast Asian	1	1617	0.92 [0.50, 1.70]	0.26	0.795	NA	NA	NA
Total	11	1618409	1.27 [1.07, 1.50]†	2.81	0.005	93	<0.001	0.429
Geographic Atrophy								
Caucasian	6	24408	1.97 [1.07, 3.64]	2.17	0.030	35	0.172	0.178
Asian	1	280	0.97 [0.36, 2.63]	0.06	0.954	NA	NA	NA
East Asian	1	280	0.97 [0.36, 2.63]	0.06	0.954	NA	NA	NA
Total	7	24688	1.62 [0.96, 2.74]	1.82	0.069	34	0.166	0.687

* OR is for cross-sectional and case-control studies, RR is for prospective cohort studies.
† Studies using random effect model.
Abbreviations: OR: odds ratio; RR: relative risk; CI: confidence interval; AMD: age related macular degeneration.

association was detected between diabetes and early AMD based on 16 relevant cohorts.

The associations of diabetes with late AMD are also inconsistent among previous reports. According to analysis from 5 cross-sectional and 6 case-control studies, diabetes is significantly correlated with late AMD, especially with nAMD, but not for GA. Temporal relationships revealed by 7 cohort studies further supports diabetes as a potential risk factor for late AMD, only for nAMD but not for GA. However, an association between diabetes and GA was identified in Caucasians. Also, the Blue Mountains Eye Study (BMES) has revealed diabetes as a predictor of incident GA, but not incident nAMD. This is consistent with a cross-sectional baseline report [62,63], to 5-year [42] and 10-year [59] incident reports, providing evidence for a diabetes and GA association.

In the current meta-analysis, we found no obvious ethnic divergence regarding the association between the diabetes and risk of overall AMD and its early form. The results obtained from different Asian groups are consistent in all types of AMD. However, the association between diabetes and late AMD in the Caucasian population differs from that in the Asian population, which is probably due to the large variation of genetic factors among different ethnic groups [64], and the differences in dietary habits and lifestyles.

The biological interplay between diabetes and AMD is complicated and has not been fully elucidated. First, diabetic conditions may lead to the accumulation of the highly stable advanced glycation end products (AGEs) in multiple tissues, including the retinal pigment epithelium (RPE) cell layers and photoreceptors [51,65]. These AGEs would first contribute to the modification of molecules, leading to the activation of NFκB, NFκB nuclear translocation, and up-regulation in the expression of the receptor for AGEs (RAGE) [66]. Further, the up-regulated RAGE, which usually localized to the neuroglia in the inner retina [67], would integrate with AGE, thus leading to high levels of the nondegradable aggregates AGE-RAGE ligands in retina [65]. Therefore, accumulated AGEs would reduce the dosage dependent RAGE-mediated activation of RPE/photoreceptor cells [68]. AGEs and RAGE were found in the RPE or both RPE and photoreceptors in the maculas of human donor retina from patients with AMD, but not in normal eyes [66,68], indicating that AGE deposition and RAGE up-regulation in diabetic conditions are implicated in the pathogenesis of AMD.

Second, hyperglycemia and dyslipidemia in diabetic patients will disturb homeostasis of the retina by inducing inflammatory responses in tissue cells, including oxidative stress [69]. Significantly elevated oxidative stress markers and total oxidative stress (TOS), as well as decreased total anti-oxidant capacity (TAC), are found in the serum of AMD patients when compared with age-matched controls free of AMD [70,71]. Meanwhile, anti-oxidants and omega-3 fatty acids have been shown to help with the preservation of RPE health and prevent retinal degeneration in animal models [72,73]. Therefore, oxidative stress is recognized as one of the principle pathogenic elements in AMD [74]. Oxidative stress may further activate NF-κB regulated inflammatory genes and lead to inflammation, which would in turn generate reactive oxygen species and aggregate oxidative stress. Inflammation disrupts the NF-κB, JUN N-terminal kinase (JNK), and the NADPH oxidase pathways, consequently dysregulations of many inflammatory cytokines and chemokines, involving the tumor necrosis factor (TNF), interleukin-6 (IL-6), IL-1β, C-reactive protein (CRP), CC-chemokine ligand 2 (CCL2), and adipokines [75]. These inflammatory activations would lead to the dysfunction and even death of the RPE/photoreceptor cells [69]. Thus,

oxidative stress and inflammations in the retina are pre-requites for development of AMD [74].

Meanwhile, diabetic microangiopathy shares common pathogenic pathways with AMD. Hyperglycemia and dyslipidemia in diabetic patients will lead to multiple microvascular complications, including diabetic retinopathy (DR). AMD and DR share some common features in pathogenesis and treatment. In a longitudinal study over 10 years, individuals with DR, including both the nonproliferative and proliferative form, were at higher risk for nAMD when compared to diabetic patients without DR or normal controls [39]. Vascular endothelial growth factor (VEGF) seems to play an important role in both DR and AMD, and anti-VEGF treatment are useful for both [76,77]. Apolipoproteins are also involved. Lower apoAI and higher apoB and apoB/AI levels, biomarkers for diabetic retinopathy [78], are involved in the pathogenesis of cardiovascular diseases [79], which is a risk factor for AMD [8,59]. Meanwhile, mitochondrial dysfunctions have been reported to contribute to metabolic disorders as well as AMD [74,80,81]. All these suggested that hyperglycemia probably affects the function and structure of the retinal pigment epithelium, Bruch membrane, and the choroidal circulation [47], thus increase the risk of AMD. Our study indicates a potential relationship between diabetes and late AMD, but further evidences from more epidemiological and biological investigations are required.

To enhance the reliability of our results, we adopted quality assessment tools recommended by the AHRQ and NOS for observational studies. Only studies discussing diabetes as the main exposure or providing adjusted ORs/HRs/RRs were included in the present meta-analysis for a more precise association of diabetes as a relatively independent risk factor for AMD. In addition, for studies reporting duplicated cohorts, only those with the latest follow-up information or provides better adjusted results were included. Subgroup analysis was performed to affirm the association and to explorer the sources of the heterogeneity. Meanwhile, our study entailed some limitations. Data obtained from prospective cohort studies would be more convincing. But the number of prospective cohort studies was quite limited. Retrospective cohort, cross-sectional, and case-control studies were also included in the present study, which may partly help to reflect the association between diabetes and AMD. However, these studies have limitation. Retrospective cohort studies use healthcare databases and have inherent methodological limitations, which may obscure the association between diabetes and AMD [82]. Cross-sectional does not establish temporality and case-control studies may introduce selection bias and established temporality [82]. Early AMD can be further classified into more specific categories. Herein, we could only judge the relationship between diabetes and early AMD. Other than diabetic status, plenty of other risk factors have been suggested for AMD. Although we have tried to narrow down the influence of other risk factors by selecting studies with adjusted data, some included studies only reported data adjusted for age and sex, and the number of studies providing multivariate-adjusted data was quite limited. With the limited information provided by each individual study, therefore, this present meta-analysis only deals with the relationship between diabetic disease status and risk of AMD, but not the specific type of diabetes, the disease course, and blood glucose levels.

In conclusion, results of this meta-analysis indicate diabetes as a potential risk factor for AMD, especially for its late form. No clear association between diabetes and early AMD is identified. More longitudinal studies are needed to ascertain the association between diabetes and AMD. And biological studies involving the inflammatory pathways might help understand the molecular basis behind this association.

Author Contributions

Conceived and designed the experiments: CP CZ. Performed the experiments: XC SR. Analyzed the data: XC SR QX FT YL HG. Contributed reagents/materials/analysis tools: PT LC MB. Wrote the paper: XC SR CP CZ.

References

1. Bressler NM (2004) Age-related macular degeneration is the leading cause of blindness. JAMA 291: 1900–1901.
2. Jager RD, Mieler WF, Miller JW (2008) Age-related macular degeneration. N Engl J Med 358: 2606–2617.
3. Lim LS, Mitchell P, Seddon JM, Holz FG, Wong TY (2012) Age-related macular degeneration. Lancet 379: 1728–1738.
4. Cheung N, Shankar A, Klein R, Folsom AR, Couper DJ, et al. (2007) Age-related macular degeneration and cancer mortality in the atherosclerosis risk in communities study. Arch Ophthalmol 125: 1241–1247.
5. Mitchell P, Wang JJ, Foran S, Smith W (2002) Five-year incidence of age-related maculopathy lesions: the Blue Mountains Eye Study. Ophthalmology 109: 1092–1097.
6. Kawasaki R, Yasuda M, Song SJ, Chen SJ, Jonas JB, et al. (2010) The prevalence of age-related macular degeneration in Asians: a systematic review and meta-analysis. Ophthalmology 117: 921–927.
7. Friedman DS, Katz J, Bressler NM, Rahmani B, Tielsch JM (1999) Racial differences in the prevalence of age-related macular degeneration: the Baltimore Eye Survey. Ophthalmology 106: 1049–1055.
8. Chakravarthy U, Wong TY, Fletcher A, Piault E, Evans C, et al. (2010) Clinical risk factors for age-related macular degeneration: a systematic review and meta-analysis. BMC Ophthalmol 10: 31.
9. Topouzis F, Anastasopoulos E, Augood C, Bentham GC, Chakravarthy U, et al. (2009) Association of diabetes with age-related macular degeneration in the EUREYE study. Br J Ophthalmol 93: 1037–1041.
10. Borger PH, van Leeuwen R, Hulsman CA, Wolfs RC, van der Kuip DA, et al. (2003) Is there a direct association between age-related eye diseases and mortality? The Rotterdam Study. Ophthalmology 110: 1292–1296.
11. Karesvuo P, Gursoy UK, Pussinen PJ, Suominen AL, Huumonen S, et al. (2013) Alveolar bone loss associated with age-related macular degeneration in males. J Periodontol 84: 58–67.
12. McGwin G Jr, Owsley C, Curcio CA, Crain RJ (2003) The association between statin use and age related maculopathy. Br J Ophthalmol 87: 1121–1125.
13. Nitsch D, Douglas I, Smeeth L, Fletcher A (2008) Age-related macular degeneration and complement activation-related diseases: a population-based case-control study. Ophthalmology 115: 1904–1910.
14. Vaicaitiene R, Luksiene DK, Paunksnis A, Cerniauskiene LR, Domarkiene S, et al. (2003) Age-related maculopathy and consumption of fresh vegetables and fruits in urban elderly. Medicina (Kaunas) 39: 1231–1236.
15. Fraser-Bell S, Wu J, Klein R, Azen SP, Hooper C, et al. (2008) Cardiovascular risk factors and age-related macular degeneration: the Los Angeles Latino Eye Study. Am J Ophthalmol 145: 308–316.
16. Xu L, Xie XW, Wang YX, Jonas JB (2009) Ocular and systemic factors associated with diabetes mellitus in the adult population in rural and urban China. The Beijing Eye Study. Eye (Lond) 23: 676–682.
17. Clemons TE, Rankin MW, McBee WL (2006) Cognitive impairment in the Age-Related Eye Disease Study: AREDS report no. 16. Arch Ophthalmol 124: 537–543.
18. (2011) Cochrane Handbook for Systematic Reviews of Interventions. In: Julian PT Higgins, Green S, editors: The Cochrane Collaboration.
19. Stroup DF, Berlin JA, Morton SC, Olkin I, Williamson GD, et al. (2000) Meta-analysis of observational studies in epidemiology: a proposal for reporting. Meta-analysis Of Observational Studies in Epidemiology (MOOSE) group. JAMA 283: 2008–2012.
20. Yuan D, Yuan S, Liu Q (2013) The age-related maculopathy susceptibility 2 polymorphism and polypoidal choroidal vasculopathy in Asian populations: a meta-analysis. Ophthalmology 120: 2051–2057.
21. Rostom A, Dubé C, Cranney A, Saloojee N, Sy R, et al. (2004) Evidence Reports/Technology Assessments, No. 104.Celiac Disease: Rockville (MD): Agency for Healthcare Research and Quality (US).
22. DerSimonian R, Laird N (1986) Meta-analysis in clinical trials. Control Clin Trials 7: 177–188.
23. Kuritz SJ, Landis JR, Koch GG (1988) A general overview of Mantel-Haenszel methods: applications and recent developments. Annu Rev Public Health 9: 123–160.
24. Davis MD, Gangnon RE, Lee LY, Hubbard LD, Klein BE, et al. (2005) The Age-Related Eye Disease Study severity scale for age-related macular degeneration: AREDS Report No. 17. Arch Ophthalmol 123: 1484–1498.
25. Ferris FL, Davis MD, Clemons TE, Lee LY, Chew EY, et al. (2005) A simplified severity scale for age-related macular degeneration: AREDS Report No. 18. Arch Ophthalmol 123: 1570–1574.
26. Begg CB, Mazumdar M (1994) Operating characteristics of a rank correlation test for publication bias. Biometrics 50: 1088–1101.
27. Egger M, Davey Smith G, Schneider M, Minder C (1997) Bias in meta-analysis detected by a simple, graphical test. BMJ 315: 629–634.
28. Wong TY, Klein R, Sun C, Mitchell P, Couper DJ, et al. (2006) Age-related macular degeneration and risk for stroke. Ann Intern Med 145: 98–106.
29. Jeganathan VS, Kawasaki R, Wang JJ, Aung T, Mitchell P, et al. (2008) Retinal vascular caliber and age-related macular degeneration: the Singapore Malay Eye Study. Am J Ophthalmol 146: 954–959 e951.
30. Baker ML, Wang JJ, Rogers S, Klein R, Kuller LH, et al. (2009) Early age-related macular degeneration, cognitive function, and dementia: the Cardiovascular Health Study. Arch Ophthalmol 127: 667–673.
31. Pokharel S, Malla OK, Pradhananga CL, Joshi SN (2009) A pattern of age-related macular degeneration. JNMA J Nepal Med Assoc 48: 217–220.
32. Hu CC, Ho JD, Lin HC (2010) Neovascular age-related macular degeneration and the risk of stroke: a 5-year population-based follow-up study. Stroke 41: 613–617.
33. Weiner DE, Tighiouart H, Reynolds R, Seddon JM (2011) Kidney function, albuminuria and age-related macular degeneration in NHANES III. Nephrol Dial Transplant 26: 3159–3165.
34. Cheung CM, Tai ES, Kawasaki R, Tay WT, Lee JL, et al. (2012) Prevalence of and risk factors for age-related macular degeneration in a multiethnic Asian cohort. Arch Ophthalmol 130: 480–486.
35. Yang K, Zhan SY, Liang YB, Duan X, Wang F, et al. (2012) Association of dilated retinal arteriolar caliber with early age-related macular degeneration: the Handan Eye Study. Graefes Arch Clin Exp Ophthalmol 250: 741–749.
36. La Torre G, Pacella E, Saulle R, Giraldi G, Pacella F, et al. (2013) The synergistic effect of exposure to alcohol, tobacco smoke and other risk factors for age-related macular degeneration. Eur J Epidemiol 28: 445–446.
37. Mattes D, Haas A, Renner W, Steinbrugger I, El-Shabrawi Y, et al. (2009) Analysis of three pigment epithelium-derived factor gene polymorphisms in patients with exudative age-related macular degeneration. Mol Vis 15: 343–348.
38. Vine AK, Stader J, Branham K, Musch DC, Swaroop A (2005) Biomarkers of cardiovascular disease as risk factors for age-related macular degeneration. Ophthalmology 112: 2076–2080.
39. Hahn P, Acquah K, Cousins SW, Lee PP, Sloan FA (2013) Ten-year incidence of age-related macular degeneration according to diabetic retinopathy classification among medicare beneficiaries. Retina 33: 911–919.
40. Shalev V, Sror M, Goldshtein I, Kokia E, Chodick G (2011) Statin use and the risk of age related macular degeneration in a large health organization in Israel. Ophthalmic Epidemiol 18: 83–90.
41. Leske MC, Wu SY, Hennis A, Nemesure B, Yang L, et al. (2006) Nine-year incidence of age-related macular degeneration in the Barbados Eye Studies. Ophthalmology 113: 29–35.
42. Tomany SC, Wang JJ, Van Leeuwen R, Klein R, Mitchell P, et al. (2004) Risk factors for incident age-related macular degeneration: pooled findings from 3 continents. Ophthalmology 111: 1280–1287.
43. Yasuda M, Kiyohara Y, Hata Y, Arakawa S, Yonemoto K, et al. (2009) Nine-year incidence and risk factors for age-related macular degeneration in a defined Japanese population the Hisayama study. Ophthalmology 116: 2135–2140.
44. Delcourt C, Michel F, Colvez A, Lacroux A, Delage M, et al. (2001) Associations of cardiovascular disease and its risk factors with age-related macular degeneration: the POLA study. Ophthalmic Epidemiol 8: 237–249.
45. Duan Y, Mo J, Klein R, Scott IU, Lin HM, et al. (2007) Age-related macular degeneration is associated with incident myocardial infarction among elderly Americans. Ophthalmology 114: 732–737.
46. Klein R, Deng Y, Klein BE, Hyman L, Seddon J, et al. (2007) Cardiovascular disease, its risk factors and treatment, and age-related macular degeneration:

Women's Health Initiative Sight Exam ancillary study. Am J Ophthalmol 143: 473–483.

47. Choi JK, Lym YL, Moon JW, Shin HJ, Cho B (2011) Diabetes mellitus and early age-related macular degeneration. Arch Ophthalmol 129: 196–199.

48. Gemmy Cheung CM, Li X, Cheng CY, Zheng Y, Mitchell P, et al. (2013) Prevalence and risk factors for age-related macular degeneration in Indians: a comparative study in Singapore and India. Am J Ophthalmol 155: 764–773, 773 e761–763.

49. Blumenkranz MS, Russell SR, Robey MG, Kott-Blumenkranz R, Penneys N (1986) Risk factors in age-related maculopathy complicated by choroidal neovascularization. Ophthalmology 93: 552–558.

50. Ross RD, Barofsky JM, Cohen G, Baber WB, Palao SW, et al. (1998) Presumed macular choroidal watershed vascular filling, choroidal neovascularization, and systemic vascular disease in patients with age-related macular degeneration. Am J Ophthalmol 125: 71–80.

51. Monnier VM, Sell DR, Genuth S (2005) Glycation products as markers and predictors of the progression of diabetic complications. Ann N Y Acad Sci 1043: 567–581.

52. Alexander SL, Linde-Zwirble WT, Werther W, Depperschmidt EE, Wilson LJ, et al. (2007) Annual rates of arterial thromboembolic events in medicare neovascular age-related macular degeneration patients. Ophthalmology 114: 2174–2178.

53. Kim IK, Ji F, Morrison MA, Adams S, Zhang Q, et al. (2008) Comprehensive analysis of CRP, CFH Y402H and environmental risk factors on risk of neovascular age-related macular degeneration. Mol Vis 14: 1487–1495.

54. Lin JM, Wan L, Tsai YY, Lin HJ, Tsai Y, et al. (2008) Pigment epithelium-derived factor gene Met72Thr polymorphism is associated with increased risk of wet age-related macular degeneration. Am J Ophthalmol 145: 716–721.

55. Cackett P, Yeo I, Cheung CM, Vithana EN, Wong D, et al. (2011) Relationship of smoking and cardiovascular risk factors with polypoidal choroidal vasculopathy and age-related macular degeneration in Chinese persons. Ophthalmology 118: 846–852.

56. Sogut E, Ortak H, Aydogan L, Benli I (2013) Association of Paraoxonase 1 L55m and Q192r Single-Nucleotide Polymorphisms with Age-Related Macular Degeneration. Retina.

57. Klein R, Davis MD, Magli YL, Segal P, Klein BE, et al. (1991) The Wisconsin age-related maculopathy grading system. Ophthalmology 98: 1128–1134.

58. Bird AC, Bressler NM, Bressler SB, Chisholm IH, Coscas G, et al. (1995) An international classification and grading system for age-related maculopathy and age-related macular degeneration. The International ARM Epidemiological Study Group. Surv Ophthalmol 39: 367–374.

59. Tan JS, Mitchell P, Smith W, Wang JJ (2007) Cardiovascular risk factors and the long-term incidence of age-related macular degeneration: the Blue Mountains Eye Study. Ophthalmology 114: 1143–1150.

60. (2001) The Age-Related Eye Disease Study system for classifying age-related macular degeneration from stereoscopic color fundus photographs: the Age-Related Eye Disease Study Report Number 6. Am J Ophthalmol 132: 668–681.

61. Klein R, Meuer SM, Knudtson MD, Iyengar SK, Klein BE (2008) The epidemiology of retinal reticular drusen. Am J Ophthalmol 145: 317–326.

62. Mitchell P, Wang JJ (1999) Diabetes, fasting blood glucose and age-related maculopathy: The Blue Mountains Eye Study. Aust N Z J Ophthalmol 27: 197–199.

63. Smith W, Mitchell P, Leeder SR, Wang JJ (1998) Plasma fibrinogen levels, other cardiovascular risk factors, and age-related maculopathy: the Blue Mountains Eye Study. Arch Ophthalmol 116: 583–587.

64. Klein R, Li X, Kuo JZ, Klein BE, Cotch MF, et al. (2013) Associations of Candidate Genes to Age-Related Macular Degeneration Among Racial/Ethnic Groups in the Multi-Ethnic Study of Atherosclerosis. Am J Ophthalmol.

65. Stitt AW (2010) AGEs and diabetic retinopathy. Invest Ophthalmol Vis Sci 51: 4867–4874.

66. Hammes HP, Hoerauf H, Alt A, Schleicher E, Clausen JT, et al. (1999) N(epsilon)(carboxymethyl)lysin and the AGE receptor RAGE colocalize in age-related macular degeneration. Invest Ophthalmol Vis Sci 40: 1855–1859.

67. Soulis T, Thallas V, Youssef S, Gilbert RE, McWilliam BG, et al. (1997) Advanced glycation end products and their receptors co-localise in rat organs susceptible to diabetic microvascular injury. Diabetologia 40: 619–628.

68. Howes KA, Liu Y, Dunaief JL, Milam A, Frederick JM, et al. (2004) Receptor for advanced glycation end products and age-related macular degeneration. Invest Ophthalmol Vis Sci 45: 3713–3720.

69. Zhang W, Liu H, Al-Shabrawey M, Caldwell RW, Caldwell RB (2011) Inflammation and diabetic retinal microvascular complications. J Cardiovasc Dis Res 2: 96–103.

70. Totan Y, Yagci R, Bardak Y, Ozyurt H, Kendir F, et al. (2009) Oxidative macromolecular damage in age-related macular degeneration. Curr Eye Res 34: 1089–1093.

71. Venza I, Visalli M, Cucinotta M, Teti D, Venza M (2012) Association between oxidative stress and macromolecular damage in elderly patients with age-related macular degeneration. Aging Clin Exp Res 24: 21–27.

72. Cao X, Liu M, Tuo J, Shen D, Chan CC (2010) The effects of quercetin in cultured human RPE cells under oxidative stress and in Ccl2/Cx3cr1 double deficient mice. Exp Eye Res 91: 15–25.

73. Tuo J, Ross RJ, Herzlich AA, Shen D, Ding X, et al. (2009) A high omega-3 fatty acid diet reduces retinal lesions in a murine model of macular degeneration. Am J Pathol 175: 799–807.

74. Ardeljan D, Chan CC (2013) Aging is not a disease: distinguishing age-related macular degeneration from aging. Prog Retin Eye Res 37: 68–89.

75. Donath MY, Shoelson SE (2011) Type 2 diabetes as an inflammatory disease. Nat Rev Immunol 11: 98–107.

76. Ho AC, Scott IU, Kim SJ, Brown GC, Brown MM, et al. (2012) Anti-vascular endothelial growth factor pharmacotherapy for diabetic macular edema: a report by the American Academy of Ophthalmology. Ophthalmology 119: 2179–2188.

77. Rofagha S, Bhisitkul RB, Boyer DS, Sadda SR, Zhang K (2013) Seven-Year Outcomes in Ranibizumab-Treated Patients in ANCHOR, MARINA, and HORIZON: A Multicenter Cohort Study (SEVEN-UP). Ophthalmology 120: 2292–2299.

78. Sasongko MB, Wong TY, Nguyen TT, Kawasaki R, Jenkins AJ, et al. (2012) Serum apolipoproteins are associated with systemic and retinal microvascular function in people with diabetes. Diabetes 61: 1785–1792.

79. Di Angelantonio E, Sarwar N, Perry P, Kaptoge S, Ray KK, et al. (2009) Major lipids, apolipoproteins, and risk of vascular disease. JAMA 302: 1993–2000.

80. Turner N, Robker RL (2014) Developmental programming of obesity and insulin resistance: does mitochondrial dysfunction in oocytes play a role? Mol Hum Reprod.

81. Sorriento D, Pascale AV, Finelli R, Carillo AL, Annunziata R, et al. (2014) Targeting mitochondria as therapeutic strategy for metabolic disorders. ScientificWorldJournal 2014: 604685.

82. Wu J, Uchino M, Sastry SM, Schaumberg DA (2014) Age-related macular degeneration and the incidence of cardiovascular disease: a systematic review and meta-analysis. PLoS One 9: e89600.

9

Resistant Hypertension, Patient Characteristics, and Risk of Stroke

Chen-Ying Hung[1,2], Kuo-Yang Wang[1,3]*, Tsu-Juey Wu[1,3,4], Yu-Cheng Hsieh[1,4], Jin-Long Huang[1,3,4], El-Wui Loh[5], Ching-Heng Lin[6]*

1 Cardiovascular Center, Taichung Veterans General Hospital, Taichung, Taiwan, 2 Department of Internal Medicine, Taipei Veterans General Hospital, Hsinchu Branch, Hsinchu County, Taiwan, 3 School of Medicine, Chung Shan Medical University, Taichung, Taiwan, 4 Department of Internal Medicine, Faculty of Medicine, Institute of Clinical Medicine, Cardiovascular Research Center, National Yang-Ming University School of Medicine, Taipei, Taiwan, 5 Kaohsiung Municipal Kai-Syuan Psychiatric Hospital, Kaohsiung, Taiwan, 6 Department of Medical Research, Taichung Veterans General Hospital, Taichung, Taiwan

Abstract

Background: Little is known about the prognosis of resistant hypertension (RH) in Asian population. This study aimed to evaluate the impacts of RH in Taiwanese patients with hypertension, and to ascertain whether patient characteristics influence the association of RH with adverse outcomes.

Methods and Results: Patients aged ≥45 years with hypertension were identified from the National Health Insurance Research Database. Medical records of 111,986 patients were reviewed in this study, and 16,402 (14.6%) patients were recognized as having RH (continuously concomitant use of ≥3 anti-hypertensive medications, including a diuretic, for ≥2 years). Risk of major adverse cardiovascular events (MACE, a composite of all-cause mortality, acute coronary syndrome, and stroke [included both fatal and nonfatal events]) in patients with RH and non-RH was analyzed. A total of 11,856 patients experienced MACE in the follow-up period (average 7.1±3.0 years). There was a higher proportion of females in the RH group, they were older than the non-RH (63.1 vs. 60.5 years) patients, and had a higher prevalence of cardiovascular co-morbidities. Overall, patients with RH had higher risks of MACE (adjusted HR 1.17; 95%CI 1.09–1.26; p<0.001). Significantly elevated risks of stroke (10,211 events; adjusted HR 1.17; 95%CI 1.08–1.27; p<0.001), especially ischemic stroke (6,235 events; adjusted HR 1.34; 95%CI 1.20–1.48; p<0.001), but not all-cause mortality (4,594 events; adjusted HR 1.06; 95%CI 0.95–1.19; p = 0.312) or acute coronary syndrome (2,145 events; adjusted HR 1.17; 95%CI 0.99–1.39; p = 0.070) were noted in patients with RH compared to those with non-RH. Subgroup analysis showed that RH increased the risks of stroke in female and elderly patients. However, no significant influence was noted in young or male patients.

Conclusions: Patients with RH were associated with higher risks of MACE and stroke, especially ischemic stroke. The risks were greater in female and elderly patients than in male or young patients.

Editor: Yan Li, Shanghai Institute of Hypertension, China

Funding: This study was supported in part by grants from Taichung Veterans General Hospital, Taiwan (TCVGH-1027308C) (Registered number NHIRD-101-560). The funders had no role in study design, data collection and analysis, decision to publish, or preparation of the manuscript.

Competing Interests: The authors have declared that no competing interests exist.

* Email: wky@vghtc.gov.tw (KYW); epid@vghtc.gov.tw (CHL)

Introduction

Hypertension is one of the most important cardiovascular problems and is associated with an increased risk of stroke, myocardial infarction, and mortality [1,2]. It is also one of the most important modifiable risk factors for cardiovascular diseases [2]. Resistant hypertension (RH) represents a potentially higher risk subset of the disease and is associated with higher cardiovascular morbidity and mortality. A recent scientific statement from the American Heart Association and the European Society of Cardiology defined RH as uncontrolled blood pressure (BP) despite patient adherence to 3 anti-hypertensive drugs (including a diuretic), or controlled BP when using ≥4 anti-hypertensive drugs [3,4].

Previous studies indicated that 12% to 30% of patients with hypertension in Western countries may have RH [3,5,6], but the exact prevalence of RH in Asian population has not been

examined in advanced. The observation that many patients with hypertension have high BP despite the use of multiple anti-hypertensive drugs, has led to an increased interest in the independent role of RH [3]. A greater understanding of the prevalence and prognosis of RH is important to improve the management of these patients. Therefore, RH has been defined as a major current focus of hypertension research by the American Heart Association [3].

In this study, we investigated the prognosis of RH in an Asian population. The purpose of the present study was to evaluate the association of RH with major adverse cardiovascular events (MACE) in a large cohort of hypertensive patients in Taiwan. We compared the risk of all-cause mortality, acute coronary syndrome, and stroke between patients with RH and non-RH. We also wanted to determine if demographic data or cardiovascular co-morbidity could predict the influence of RH.

Methods

Research database

The National Health Insurance program, which was implemented in Taiwan in 1995, covers about 99% of the island's population. The National Health Research Institute (NHRI) has established the National Health Insurance Research Database. We used a systemic sampling of patient data, which was released by the NHRI (from 2000 to 2011 with a total of 1,000,000 subjects), for the current analysis. The development of the research database has been described in detail elsewhere [7,8]. In brief, the random samples have been confirmed by the NHRI to be representative of the general population. The NHRI made data available at the individual level in an anonymous format, and safeguarded the privacy of individuals. This study was approved by the Institutional Review Board of Taichung Veterans General Hospital.

Study population

Patients aged ≥45 years with hypertension were identified according to the International Classification of Diseases, Ninth Revision, Clinical Modification (ICD-9-CM) code 401–405. Since the lack of BP data in our research database, we use medication using information to avoid misclassifications and ensure the diagnostic validity. Only patients who had a diagnosis of hypertension and were treated with anti-hypertensive drugs in the period 2000–2010 were selected. Patients were not eligible for enrollment in this cohort study if they had a history of atrial fibrillation, atrial flutter, heart failure, stroke, or acute coronary syndrome. This dynamic cohort included 111,986 patients for analysis. According to the guidelines of the Taiwan Society of Cardiology for the management of hypertension, hypertension was defined as systolic BP ≥140 mmHg or diastolic BP ≥90 mmHg, with lower cutoffs of systolic BP ≥130 mmHg or diastolic BP ≥ 80 mmHg for high-risk patients, such as those with chronic kidney disease, diabetes, stroke, coronary artery disease or its equivalents [9].

Definition of RH

Anti-hypertensive medication records were retrieved from ambulatory and inpatient claims data. Medications were identified based on drug class, such as angiotensin-converting enzyme inhibitors (ACEIs) or angiotensin receptor blockers (ARBs), alpha blockers, beta blockers, calcium channel blockers, diuretics, spironolactone, aspirin, clopidogrel, warfarin, statins, oral hypoglycemic agents, and insulins. Each medication in combination anti-hypertensive pills was counted as a separate class of drug. Patients were divided into a RH and a non-RH group according to their medication use in the period 2000–2010. RH was defined as a hypertension with continuously concomitant use of ≥3 anti-hypertensive medications, including a diuretic, for ≥2 years (at any time during 2001–2010). Hypertensive patients who did not meet our criteria for RH were classified into the non-RH group.

Definition of Outcomes

The primary outcome of this study was defined as MACE, which was a composite of all-cause mortality, acute coronary syndrome, and stroke (included both fatal and nonfatal events), whichever occurred first. Other outcomes included all-cause mortality, acute coronary syndrome, overall stroke, ischemic stroke and hemorrhagic stroke. The study endpoint was defined as any events after patients being classified into RH or non-RH groups during the 11-year follow-up period (2001–2011). To ensure the diagnostic validity, only patients with at least 1 inpatient hospitalization diagnosis of acute coronary syndrome or stroke

were identified. Other co-morbidities were identified by ICD-9-CM diagnostic code (at least 1 inpatient hospitalization diagnosis or at least 3 consensus diagnoses at an outpatient department) when inclusive: diabetes mellitus, hyperlipidemia, ischemic heart disease, peripheral vascular disease, valvular heart disease, pulmonary disease, and renal disease. Charlson co-morbidity index was also calculated for each patient.

Statistical analysis

The data are presented as the mean values and standard deviations (SD) for continuous variables, and proportions for categorical variables. The differences between values were analyzed by using t test for continuous variables, and chi-square test for categorical variables. The MACE-free survival curves were plotted via the Kaplan–Meier method with statistical significance examined by the log-rank test. Multivariable Cox proportional hazards regression models were used to identify independent factors contributing to MACE occurrence (adjusted for age, sex, co-morbidities, Charlson co-morbidity index, and medications). For further controlling the potential confounding bias, we performed multivariable analyses by using a Cox proportional hazards regression model that adjusting for age, sex, co-morbidities, Charlson co-morbidity index, and medications. All statistical analyses were carried out by SAS software version 9.2 (SAS Institute, Inc., Cary, NC, USA). A p value of <0.05 was considered statistically significant.

Results

Clinical characteristics

A total of 111,986 hypertensive patients aged ≥45 years were enrolled in this study, of whom 16,402 (14.6%) patients met our definition of RH. All patients were followed up for a maximum period of 11 years (average 7.1±3.0 years). The mean age of the study population was 60.9±10.6 years, with 34.5% of them aged ≥65 years. Females accounted for 49.6% of the population. The average Charlson co-morbidity index of the cohort was 1.1±1.5. Among patients with RH, 36.8% were on 4 anti-hypertensive agents, and 7.4% on ≥5 agents. Anti-hypertensive drugs used by patients with RH included ACEIs or ARBs (82.6%), alpha blockers (15.6%), beta blockers (62.1%), calcium channel blockers (87.4%), and spironolactone (4.4%); by definition, all patients with RH used diuretics.

Table 1 summarizes the baseline characteristics of the patients with RH and non-RH. Patients with RH were older (63.1 vs. 60.5 years; p<0.001), more likely to be female (50.9% vs. 49.4%; p< 0.001), and had a higher prevalence of co-morbidities, such as diabetes mellitus, hyperlipidemia, ischemic heart disease, peripheral vascular disease, valvular heart disease, pulmonary disease, and renal disease, when compared to those with non-RH (p values <0.001). The RH group had higher rates of drug use, including anti-hypertensives, aspirin, clopidogrel, warfarin, statins, oral hypoglycemic agents, and insulins than the non-RH group (p values <0.001). Patients with RH also has a higher Charlson co-morbidity index than those with non-RH (1.4 vs.1.0; p<0.001).

Outcomes

The Kaplan-Meier survival plot presented in Figure 1 shows the MACE-free survival rate between RH and non-RH group. The non-RH group had a higher survival probability than the RH group (log rank p<0.001). Table 2 demonstrates the adjusted hazard ratio (HR) for the development of MACE in the cohort. During the follow-up period, 11,856 patients (10.6% of the study population) developed MACE. MACE occurred more frequently

Table 1. Baseline characteristics.

Variables	Original cohort (n = 111,986)		
	RH	Non-RH	P value
	(n = 16,402, 14.6%)	(n = 95,584, 85.4%)	
	No. (%)	No. (%)	
Age at entry, years			
mean ± SD	63.1±10.5	60.5±10.5	<0.001
45–54	4,610 (28.1)	36,126 (37.8)	<0.001
55–64	4,604 (28.1)	27,938 (29.2)	
65–74	4,743 (28.9)	21,284 (22.3)	
≥75	2,445 (14.9)	10,236 (10.7)	
Female	8,344 (50.9)	47,167 (49.4)	<0.001
Co-morbidities			
Diabetes mellitus	4,686 (28.6)	14,851 (15.5)	<0.001
Hyperlipidemia	3,656 (22.3)	11,495 (12.0)	<0.001
Ischemic heart disease	3,288 (20.1)	9,102 (9.5)	<0.001
Peripheral vascular disease	333 (2.0)	1,012 (1.1)	<0.001
Valvular heart disease	619 (3.8)	1,637 (1.7)	<0.001
Pulmonary disease	1,729 (10.5)	7,573 (7.9)	<0.001
Renal disease	718 (4.4)	2,176 (2.3)	<0.001
Charlson co-morbidity index			
mean ± SD	1.4±1.6	1.0±1.5	<0.001
Medications			
ACEIs or ARBs	13,555 (82.6)	40,633 (42.5)	<0.001
Alpha blockers	2,552 (15.6)	5,459 (5.7)	<0.001
Beta blockers	10,180 (62.1)	32,601 (34.1)	<0.001
Calcium channel blockers	14,337 (87.4)	43,896 (45.9)	<0.001
Diuretics	16,402 (100.0)	16,999 (17.8)	<0.001
Spironolactone	723 (4.4)	934 (1.0)	<0.001
Aspirin	5,224 (31.9)	10,879 (11.4)	<0.001
Clopidogrel	333 (2.0)	957 (1.0)	<0.001
Warfarin	138 (0.8)	499 (0.5)	<0.001
Statins	2,901 (17.7)	5,459 (5.7)	<0.001
Oral hypoglycemic agents	4,176 (25.5)	8,169 (8.6)	<0.001
Insulins	887 (5.4)	1,125 (1.2)	<0.001

ACEI = angiotensin-converting enzyme inhibitor; ARB = angiotensin receptor blocker; RH = resistant hypertension; SD = standard deviations.

in RH group when compared with non-RH group before and after adjustment (13.9 vs. 10.0%; adjusted HR 1.17; 95% confidence interval [CI] 1.09–1.26; p<0.001). Patients with RH had a 17% higher risk of the primary endpoint (all-cause mortality, acute coronary syndrome, or stroke) when compared to patients with non-RH. The rise was likely to be caused by frequent stroke events in RH group (10,211 events; 11.8 vs. 8.7%; adjusted HR 1.17; 95% CI 1.08–1.27; p<0.001), especially ischemic stroke (6,235 events; 7.4 vs. 5.3%; adjusted HR 1.34; 95% CI 1.20–1.48; p< 0.001). Rates of all-cause mortality (4,594 events; adjusted HR 1.06; 95% CI 0.95–1.19; p = 0.312), acute coronary syndrome (2,145 events; adjusted HR 1.17; 95% CI 0.99–1.39; p = 0.070), and hemorrhagic stroke (1,967 events; adjusted HR 0.96; 95% CI 0.80–1.15; p = 0.634) were similar.

Sensitivity analysis

When a strict definition (patients on ≥4 agents, including a diuretic) was used for RH, the overall prevalence of the disease decreased from 14.6% to 6.5% (Table not shown). The strictly defined RH was still associated with a significant hazard for the primary endpoint in these patients on multivariate adjusted analyses (adjusted HR 1.26; 95% CI 1.15–1.39; p<0.001) when compared to pure non-RH group (patients on <3 agents or without a diuretic). There was a significant association between RH and all-cause mortality (adjusted HR 1.21; 95% CI 1.04–1.41; p = 0.012), and between RH and acute coronary syndrome (adjusted HR 1.35; 95% CI 1.09–1.68; p = 0.007); all other outcomes were similar to the primary definition (For stroke: adjusted HR 1.24; 95% CI 1.11–1.37; p<0.001. For ischemic and hemorrhagic stroke, the adjusted HR were 1.40 [95% CI 1.22–1.61; p<0.001] and 1.13 [95% CI 0.89–1.42; p = 0.313]).

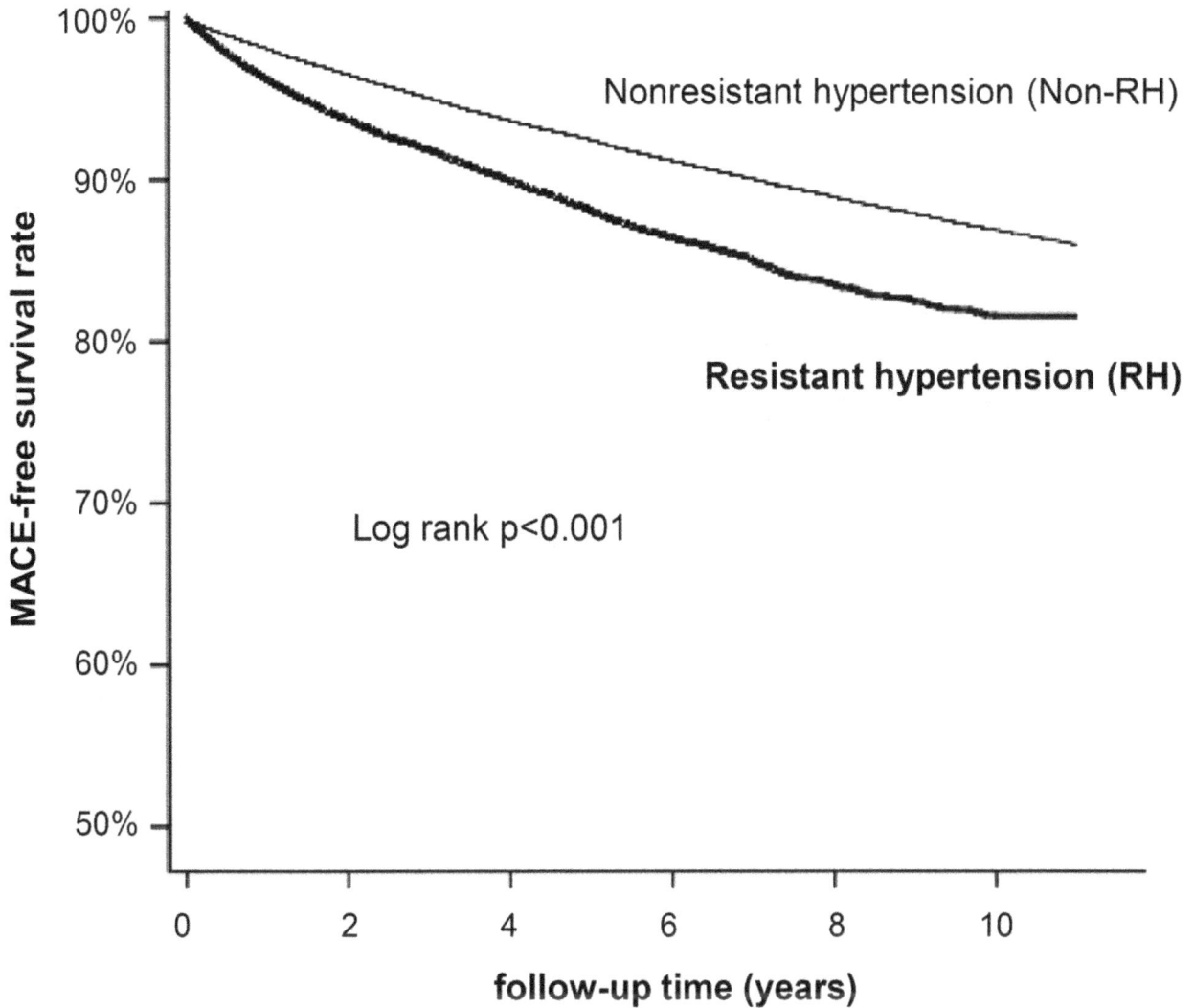

Number at risk

Non-RH	95,584	83,523	67,988	53,242	37,316	16,538
RH	16,402	15,381	10,954	7,122	3,622	25

Figure 1. Major adverse cardiovascular events (MACE)-free survival rate between resistant hypertension (RH) and non-RH groups.

When we recruited only those with diagnosis of essential hypertension (ICD-9-CM code 401), a total of 105,277 patients were enrolled in analysis. The overall prevalence of RH was similar (13.8%) to the original model. The new model revealed that RH was still associated with a significant hazard for the primary endpoint in these patients on multivariate adjusted analyses (adjusted HR 1.12; 95% CI 1.05–1.19; p = 0.001) when compared to non-RH group (see model 2 of table 2). There was a significant association between RH and acute coronary syndrome (adjusted HR 1.16; 95% CI 1.00–1.35; p = 0.047), and other outcomes were similar to the primary definition (For stroke: adjusted HR 1.11; 95% CI 1.03–1.19; p = 0.004. For ischemic and hemorrhagic stroke, the adjusted HR were 1.24 [95% CI 1.14–1.36; p<0.001] and 0.98 [95% CI 0.83–1.15; p = 0.794]).

Subgroup analysis

Figure 2 displays the subgroup analysis for MACE and stroke occurrence based on Cox proportional hazards analysis with RH as a covariate. The relationships of baseline characteristics and co-morbidities and the risk of MACE and stroke were evaluated in patients with RH and with non-RH. Female (adjusted HR 1.38; 95% CI 1.23–1.55; p<0.001) and elderly (adjusted HR 1.20; 95% CI 1.09–1.33; p<0.001) RH patients had significantly worse outcome than non-RH patients. A borderline significance was noted in developing MACE in younger patients (aged 45–64 years; adjusted HR 1.12; 95% CI 1.00–1.26; p = 0.048). However, no significant elevated risk was found in male patients (adjusted HR 1.05; 95% CI 0.95–1.15; p = 0.375). No significant difference in developing stroke was found between RH and non-RH groups in male (adjusted HR 1.05; 95% CI 0.95–1.17; p = 0.337) and

Table 2. Adjusted HR for MACE.

| Outcomes | Model 1: original cohort (n = 111,986)*** | | | | Model 2 (n = 105,277)**** | |
| | RH | Non-RH | Adjusted HR (95% CI)** | P value | Adjusted HR (95% CI)** | P value |
	No. (%)	No. (%)				
MACE	2,283 (13.9)	9,573 (10.0)	1.17 (1.09–1.26)	<0.001	1.12 (1.05–1.19)	0.001
All-cause mortality	882 (5.4)	3,712 (3.9)	1.06 (0.95–1.19)	0.312	1.05 (0.95–1.17)	0.299
Acute coronary syndrome*	459 (2.8)	1,686 (1.8)	1.17 (0.99–1.39)	0.070	1.16 (1.00–1.35)	0.047
Stroke*	1,933 (11.8)	8,278 (8.7)	1.17 (1.08–1.27)	<0.001	1.11 (1.03–1.19)	0.004
Ischemic stroke*	1,209 (7.4)	5,026 (5.3)	1.34 (1.20–1.48)	<0.001	1.24 (1.14–1.36)	<0.001
Hemorrhagic stroke*	345 (2.1)	1,622 (1.7)	0.96 (0.80–1.15)	0.634	0.98 (0.83–1.15)	0.794
Unclassified stroke*	379 (2.3)	1,630 (1.7)	0.96 (0.80–1.14)	0.625	1.00 (0.86–1.16)	0.976

* Included both fatal and nonfatal events.
** Adjusted for age, sex, co-morbidities, Charlson co-morbidity index, and medications.
*** Model 1: original cohort recruited patients with diagnosis of hypertension (ICD-9-CM code 401–405) for analysis.
**** Model 2: recruited only patients with diagnosis of essential hypertension (ICD-9-CM code 401) for analysis.
CI = confidence interval; HR = hazard ratio; MACE = major adverse cardiac events; RH = resistant hypertension.

younger patients (adjusted HR 1.12; 95% CI 0.99–1.26; p = 0.080). On the other hand, there was a significant difference between RH and non-RH groups in female (adjusted HR 1.35; 95% CI 1.20–1.53; p<0.001) and elderly (adjusted HR 1.20; 95% CI 1.08–1.33; p = 0.001). Meanwhile, patients with and without any cardiovascular co-morbidities had similar hazards of these outcomes (HR ranged from 1.12 to 1.38).

Discussion

Main findings

This nationwide cohort study is one of the largest studies (enrolled 111,986 subjects) with the longest follow-up period (from 2001 to 2011) for analysis the prognosis of RH patients in Asian population. The main results of this study were that the risk of MACE was higher in RH patients than non-RH patients, especially for female and elderly patients. RH was associated with a significant increase in the risk of MACE and stroke, especially ischemic stroke. Our study also showed that female gender and old

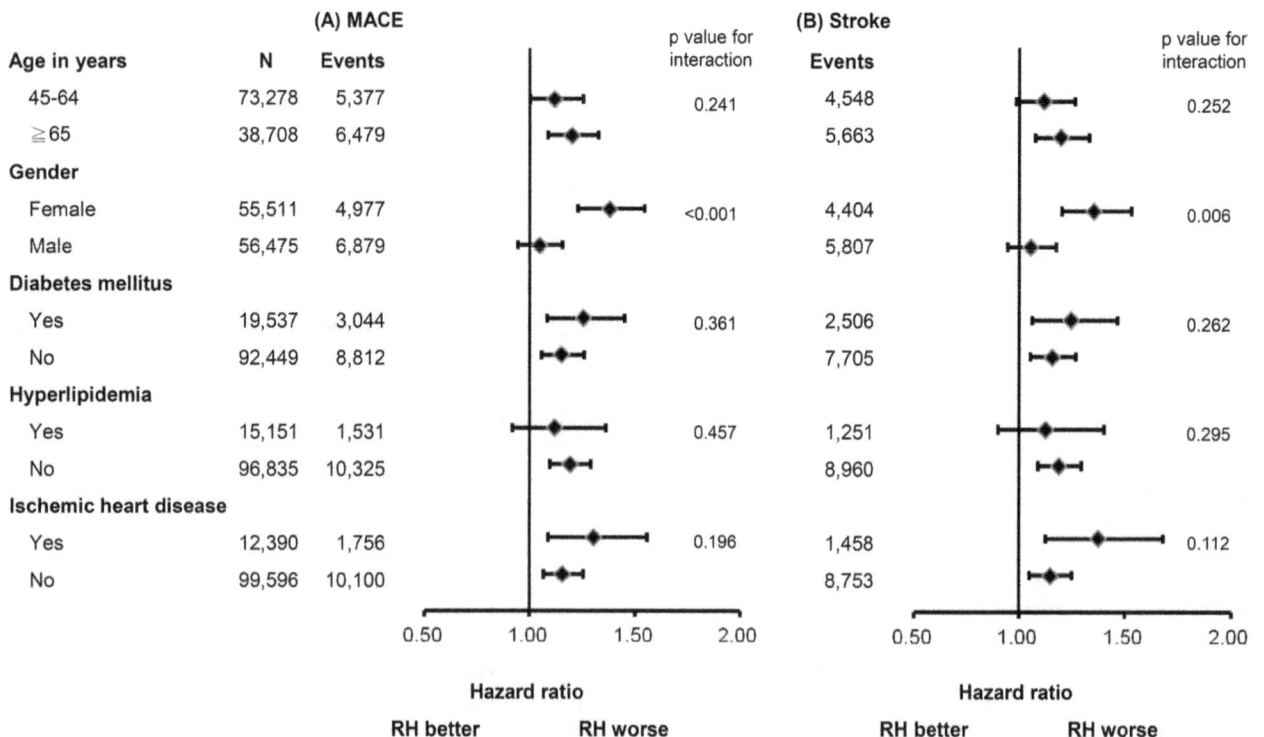

Figure 2. Subgroup analysis for (A) major adverse cardiovascular events (MACE), and (B) stroke.

age predicts the influence of RH. Female patients with RH were 35% more likely to experience a stroke event when comparing to those with non-RH, while no such difference was noted in male patients.

The association of RH with MACE

Our study found that RH was associated with long-term MACE, especially stroke, independent of other factors known to influence the long-term outcomes. An USA registry, which followed 205,750 patients for 3.8 years, found that RH was associated with a higher risk of cardiovascular events [6]. The international Reduction of Atherothrombosis for Continued Health (REACH) registry followed 53,530 hypertensive patients for 4 years found an 11% increased risk of the adverse long-term outcomes (a composite of cardiovascular death, myocardial infarction, or stroke), especially the non-fatal stroke risk [10]. Our study showed similar results and is consistent with current understanding on stroke risk and elevated BP [11]. This finding is especially critical in Asian population since few studies have directly compared cardiovascular outcomes between RH and non-RH patients in this population. Furthermore, the increase in cardiovascular events in this cohort was probably due to a 34% increase in the risk of ischemic stroke.

Age, Gender, and MACE

Herein, we demonstrated that age and gender were convenient and useful characteristics for predicting the influence of RH. Female and elderly patients were associated with a 35% and 20% increased risk of stroke, respectively. On the other hand, male and young patients had no significantly increased stroke risk from RH. This implies that the gender and age can be used to predict the cardiovascular risk in patients with RH. Although male with hypertension in general had a higher cardiovascular risk than female [12–14], limited information was available regarding the impact of RH on male and female separately. In a recent analysis of the Women's Ischemia Syndrome Evaluation (WISE) study [15], female with RH had a greater long-term risk of adverse events when compared to female with non-RH. This result partially supports our findings: RH was associated with increase risks of MACE in female.

Male and female had different clinical characteristics and diverse results of treatment in the aspect of resistant hypertension. There was a higher proportion of female in RH populations than non-RH populations in our cohort as well as other studies [10,16]. Female is more likely to be prescribed antihypertensive medications, but has a lower rate of BP control than male, especially in the elderly [16–19]. Our study further revealed that female with RH was associated with a profoundly increased risk of stroke compared with female with non-RH. Some studies may support these findings. Tang et al indicated a heterogeneous contribution of risk factors for stroke between male and female in a Chinese cohort [20]; obesity and hypertension were risk factors for stroke in female, whereas dyslipidemia were associated with stroke in male. Another study conducted by Kim et al further supported the findings that risk factors for cerebral atherosclerosis differ between genders. Hypertension was the most important risk factor for females to develop cerebral atherosclerosis, while diabetes and hypercholesterolemia for males [21]. While this is the first study to explore the relationship between gender, age, and MACE in patients with RH, further research is needed to confirm this relationship and to identify the exact mechanisms involved.

Prevalence of RH in Taiwan

A recent report suggests that the prevalence of hypertension was around 10.5% to 13.3%, with only slightly increased in recent years, in a Southern Chinese population [22]. Meanwhile, current RH prevalence estimates vary between studies. Data from large clinical trials suggest that a third of hypertensive patients were on ≥3 BP controlling agents [3,5]. The estimated prevalence of RH was around 8.9% in the hypertensive population in the period 2003–2008 in a recent analysis of the USA National Health and Nutrition Examination Survey data [23], and RH became 20.7% in the period 2005–2008. A Spanish registry [24] and a USA cross-sectional study [25] found around 12% of hypertensive patients met the criteria for RH. In Asian, the Japanese J-HOME study reported a prevalence of RH of 13% [26]. Our cohort showed a similar finding that 14.6% of the hypertensive patients in Taiwan met the definition of RH.

Strength and limitations

The major strength of this study is that the research subjects were sampled from a large community cohort. Importantly, we showed that the risk of MACE was significantly higher in those with RH than with non-RH in an Asian population. Several limitations should be considered when interpreting the present study. First, the study population included mainly Taiwanese people, and we did not have the details of ethnic data for further analysis. Second, information regarding levels of BP and duration of hypertension were not available in the research database. Therefore, we cannot clarify the BP levels or the BP control rate of RH and non-RH groups. In order to address this limitation, we conducted sensitivity analyses by varying the definition of RH. Using a strict definition (patients on ≥4 agents) or recruiting only patients with essential hypertension resulted in similar HRs for the primary endpoint. Third, anti-hypertensive drug use was defined at baseline when these patients were divided into RH or non-RH groups. Patient adherence to drugs also could not be assessed. Fourth, some patients labeled as having RH in our study had either white-coat or pseudo-resistant hypertension, and were thus misclassified. Conversely, we likely misclassified some patients with uncontrolled hypertension on fewer than 3 medications who would remain uncontrolled on ≥3 medications as non-RH patients. Pierdomenico SD et al. have showed that patients with pseudo-resistant hypertension are at lower risk than those with true RH, and those with masked hypertension are at higher risk than those with responder hypertension [27]. Our study design may therefore underestimate the hazards of RH. Finally, the present study did not account for optimal dosing of each medication. However, medication use in the present study represents real-world management choices.

Conclusions

Our study showed that patients with RH were associated with higher risks for cardiovascular events than those with non-RH. The elevated risks mainly contribute to increasing stroke events, especially ischemic stroke. Combining the clinical diagnosis of RH with the analysis of patient characteristics (gender and age) allows better risk stratification.

Acknowledgments

This study is based in part on data obtained from the National Health Insurance Research Database provided by the Bureau of National Health Insurance, Department of Health, Taiwan, and managed by the National Health Research Institutes (Registered number NHIRD-101-560). The interpretation and conclusions contained herein do not represent those of the Bureau of National Health Insurance, Department of Health, or National Health Research Institutes, Taiwan.

Author Contributions

Conceived and designed the experiments: CYH KYW CHL. Performed the experiments: CYH KYW CHL. Analyzed the data: CYH CHL. Wrote the paper: CYH KYW. Discussed results and provided critical review: CYH KYW TJW YCH JLH EWL CHL.

References

1. Lawes CM, Vander Hoorn S, Rodgers A, International Society of H (2008) Global burden of blood-pressure-related disease, 2001. Lancet 371: 1513–1518.
2. Yusuf S, Hawken S, Ounpuu S, Dans T, Avezum A, et al. (2004) Effect of potentially modifiable risk factors associated with myocardial infarction in 52 countries (the INTERHEART study): case-control study. Lancet 364: 937–952.
3. Calhoun DA, Jones D, Textor S, Goff DC, Murphy TP, et al. (2008) Resistant hypertension: diagnosis, evaluation, and treatment: a scientific statement from the American Heart Association Professional Education Committee of the Council for High Blood Pressure Research. Circulation 117: e510–526.
4. Mancia G, Fagard R, Narkiewicz K, Redon J, Zanchetti A, et al. (2013) 2013 ESH/ESC guidelines for the management of arterial hypertension: the Task Force for the Management of Arterial Hypertension of the European Society of Hypertension (ESH) and of the European Society of Cardiology (ESC). Eur Heart J 34: 2159–2219.
5. Sarafidis PA, Bakris GL (2008) Resistant hypertension: an overview of evaluation and treatment. J Am Coll Cardiol 52: 1749–1757.
6. Daugherty SL, Powers JD, Magid DJ, Tavel HM, Masoudi FA, et al. (2012) Incidence and prognosis of resistant hypertension in hypertensive patients. Circulation 125: 1635–1642.
7. Hung CY, Lin CH, Loh el W, Ting CT, Wu TJ (2013) CHADS(2) score, statin therapy, and risks of atrial fibrillation. Am J Med 126: 133–140.
8. Hung CY, Lin CH, Wang KY, Huang JL, Hsieh YC, et al. (2013) Dosage of statin, cardiovascular comorbidities, and risk of atrial fibrillation: A nationwide population-based cohort study. Int J Cardiol 168: 1131–1136.
9. Chiang CE, Wang TD, Li YH, Lin TH, Chien KL, et al. (2010) 2010 guidelines of the Taiwan Society of Cardiology for the management of hypertension. J Formos Med Assoc 109: 740–773.
10. Kumbhani DJ, Steg PG, Cannon CP, Eagle KA, Smith SC Jr, et al. (2013) Resistant hypertension: a frequent and ominous finding among hypertensive patients with atherothrombosis. Eur Heart J 34: 1204–1214.
11. Chobanian AV, Bakris GL, Black HR, Cushman WC, Green LA, et al. (2003) The Seventh Report of the Joint National Committee on Prevention, Detection, Evaluation, and Treatment of High Blood Pressure: the JNC 7 report. JAMA 289: 2560–2572.
12. De Nicola L, Gabbai FB, Agarwal R, Chiodini P, Borrelli S, et al. (2013) Prevalence and prognostic role of resistant hypertension in chronic kidney disease patients. J Am Coll Cardiol 61: 2461–2467.
13. Daugherty SL, Masoudi FA, Zeng C, Ho PM, Margolis KL, et al. (2013) Sex differences in cardiovascular outcomes in patients with incident hypertension. J Hypertens 31: 271–277.
14. Quan H, Chen G, Walker RL, Wielgosz A, Dai S, et al. (2013) Incidence, cardiovascular complications and mortality of hypertension by sex and ethnicity. Heart 99: 715–721.
15. Smith SM, Huo T, Delia Johnson B, Bittner V, Kelsey SF, et al. (2014) Cardiovascular and mortality risk of apparent resistant hypertension in women with suspected myocardial ischemia: a report from the NHLBI-sponsored WISE Study. J Am Heart Assoc 3: e000660.
16. Brambilla G, Bombelli M, Seravalle G, Cifkova R, Laurent S, et al. (2013) Prevalence and clinical characteristics of patients with true resistant hypertension in central and Eastern Europe: data from the BP-CARE study. J Hypertens 31: 2018–2024.
17. McDonald M, Hertz RP, Unger AN, Lustik MB (2009) Prevalence, awareness, and management of hypertension, dyslipidemia, and diabetes among United States adults aged 65 and older. J Gerontol A Biol Sci Med Sci 64: 256–263.
18. Gu Q, Burt VL, Paulose-Ram R, Dillon CF (2008) Gender differences in hypertension treatment, drug utilization patterns, and blood pressure control among US adults with hypertension: data from the National Health and Nutrition Examination Survey 1999–2004. Am J Hypertens 21: 789–798.
19. Daugherty SL, Masoudi FA, Ellis JL, Ho PM, Schmittdiel JA, et al. (2011) Age-dependent gender differences in hypertension management. J Hypertens 29: 1005–1011.
20. Tang X, He L, Cao Y, Wang JW, Li N, et al. (2011) Gender-specific differences in relative effects of cardiovascular risk factors among rural population. Beijing Da Xue Xue Bao 43: 379–385.
21. Kim YS, Hong JW, Jung WS, Park SU, Park JM, et al. (2011) Gender differences in risk factors for intracranial cerebral atherosclerosis among asymptomatic subjects. Gend Med 8: 14–22.
22. Lao XQ, Xu YJ, Wong MC, Zhang YH, Ma WJ, et al. (2013) Hypertension Prevalence, Awareness, Treatment, Control and Associated Factors in a Developing Southern Chinese Population: Analysis of Serial Cross-Sectional Health Survey Data 2002–2010. Am J Hypertens.
23. Roberie DR, Elliott WJ (2012) What is the prevalence of resistant hypertension in the United States? Curr Opin Cardiol 27: 386–391.
24. de la Sierra A, Segura J, Banegas JR, Gorostidi M, de la Cruz JJ, et al. (2011) Clinical features of 8295 patients with resistant hypertension classified on the basis of ambulatory blood pressure monitoring. Hypertension 57: 898–902.
25. Sim JJ, Bhandari SK, Shi J, Liu IL, Calhoun DA, et al. (2013) Characteristics of Resistant Hypertension in a Large, Ethnically Diverse Hypertension Population of an Integrated Health System. Mayo Clin Proc 88: 1099–1107.
26. Nishikawa T, Omura M, Saito J, Matsuzawa Y (2013) The possibility of resistant hypertension during the treatment of hypertensive patients. Hypertens Res 36: 924–929.
27. Pierdomenico SD, Lapenna D, Bucci A, Di Tommaso R, Di Mascio R, et al. (2005) Cardiovascular outcome in treated hypertensive patients with responder, masked, false resistant, and true resistant hypertension. Am J Hypertens 18: 1422–1428.

10

Distribution and Determinants of Non Communicable Diseases among Elderly Uyghur Ethnic Group in Xinjiang, China

Lei Feng[1,2◎], **Ping Li**[2◎], **Xihua Wang**[2], **Zhi Hu**[1], **Ying Ma**[1], **Weiming Tang**[3,4], **Yanli Ben**[2], **Tanmay Mahapatra**[5], **Xiaolin Cao**[2], **Sanchita Mahapatra**[5], **Min Ling**[2], **Anshuan Gou**[2], **Yanmei Wang**[2], **Jiangqin Xiao**[2], **Ming Hou**[2], **Xiuli Wang**[2], **Bo Lin**[2], **Faxing Wang**[2*]

1 Department of health service management, School of Health Service Administration, Anhui medical university, Hefei, Anhui, China, 2 Medical Department, The people's hospital of Xinjiang Uighur autonomous region, Urumqi, Xinjiang, China, 3 Project-China, University of North Carolina, Guangzhou, China, 4 Department of STI Control, Guangdong Center for Skin Diseases and STI Control, Guangzhou, China, 5 Department of Epidemiology, Fielding School of Public Health, University of California Los Angeles, Los Angeles, California, United States of America

Abstract

Background: Non-communicable diseases (NCDs) are showing an increasing trend globally as well as in China. Elderly population are more prone to these NCDs. Situation in China is worse owing to the higher proportion of geriatric population. Burden of NCDs and the role of their socio-demographic and behavioral predictors among these elderly and more so among the ethnic minority groups among them, need to be investigated specifically, owing to their distinct genetic background, lifestyles and behavior.

Methods: A cross-sectional study was conducted among 1329 randomly selected persons of Uyghur ethnicity, aged 60 years or more in Xinjiang, the largest administrative division in China to measure the burden of NCDs, understand the distribution of socio-demographic, behavioral and life event-related potential correlates of them and to estimate the association of the NCDs with these correlates.

Results: Among these participants 54.2% were female, 86.8% were married and more than half had only attended elementary school or less. 41.46% was suffering from at least one NCD. 20.22% had one NCD, 12.11% had two and 8.58% had three or more. 27.3% had hypertension, 4.06% had diabetes, 6.02% had hyperlipidemia, 7.37% had angina, 14.52% had cardiovascular diseases, 11.59% had any kind of cancers and 9.78% had chronic obstructive pulmonary diseases. Rural residents (OR = 1.45, 95% CI: 1.17–1.80, AOR = 2.00, 95% CI: 1.53–2.61) and current smokers had higher odds of having more NCDs (AOR = 1.53, 95% CI: 1.00–2.34). Additionally not being satisfied with current life, not being able to take care of self in daily life, currently not being involved in farm work, less intake of fresh vegetables, fruits and garlic, too less or too much salt intake, not having hobbies were found to be positively associated with having more NCDs.

Conclusion: Implementation of effective intervention strategies to promote healthy life styles among the Uyghur elderly population of China seems urgent.

Editor: Renate B. Schnabel, University Heart Center, Germany

Funding: This work was supported by the Natural Science Fund Regional Fund of China (8126212) and Science and Technology Project of Xinjiang Autonomous Region (201242178) and National Institutes of Health (NIH) program (1D43TW009532-01). The funders had no role in study design, data collection and analysis, decision to publish, or preparation of the manuscript.

Competing Interests: The authors have declared that no competing interests exist.

* Email: wfx116@126.com

◎ These authors contributed equally to this work.

Introduction

Non-communicable diseases (NCDs) have culminated into a major public health challenge worldwide, killing more than 35 million people each year and accounting for two-thirds of the cumulative global deaths [1]. Rapid urbanization, environmental pollution, economic transition and higher exposure to different behavioral risk factors like unhealthy diet, physical inactivity, addiction to tobacco and alcohol abuse have resulted into a progressive worldwide rise in the burden of NCDs and China, world's most populous country, is no exception [2–4].

Over the past few decades, NCDs have emerged at a much faster rate in China than in western countries [2,4]. As per the estimates provided by the Centers for Disease Control and

Prevention (CDCs), about 82% of total disease burden was attributable to NCDs in China [5]. Compared to other leading G-20 countries, mortality rates due to NCDs like stroke, cancers, chronic obstructive pulmonary diseases (COPD) in this country were also quite high [6]. Based on the current trend, it is predicted that over next two decades, number of NCDs among people over 40 will become double or even triple in this country [6]. Evidences from recent surveys strongly suggested that the estimated prevalence of hypertension, high blood glucose, overweight/ obesity and high blood cholesterol have increased alarmingly among Chinese adults [4,6–11]. In a nationwide population based survey among residents aged 50 years or more, during 2010, self-reported prevalence of hypertension, diabetes, angina and stroke were estimated to be 27%, 7%, 8% and 3%, respectively [9].

It was estimated that during 2010, about 580 million citizens of China were exposed to at least one of the modifiable behavioral and nutritional risk factors known to be associated with NCDs [6]. There are current evidences in favor of a notable shift in the burden of disease from infectious to NCDs and gradually progressive aging of the population is probably worsening the scenario in this country [6,9]. According to World Bank projections, in China there will be at least 40% increase in the burden of NCDs owing to this population aging by 2030 [6]. However, the NCDs services in the local area of China were very limited (community based clinics only could offer routinely hypertension test), particular among minority people like Uygur population. Hence a comprehensive understanding of the distribution and determinants of NCDs among elderly seems to be the need of the hour for designing effective public health interventions and prioritization of public health policies targeting those determinants so that the preventable burden of morbidity and mortality due to NCDs can be reduced substantially.

Although available evidences clearly suggested that burden of NCDs among elderly is growing rapidly in different regions of China resulting in serious social and economic consequences and the correlates of NCDs in this population may well be different than other age groups, efforts to identify definite action points for controlling the modifiable risk factors in this population have been slow and inadequate [3].

Xinjiang Autonomous Region is the largest administrative division of China and mainly inhabited by the Uyghur, one of the ethnic minority groups in this country [12]. Because of their different genetic backgrounds, customs, culture and food consumption, predictors of NCDs among elderly Uyghur might be quite distinct and evidences in this regard were limited [13].

Thus a detailed evaluation was called for to identify the distribution and determinants of NCDs among Uyghur elderly in Xinjiang, where alike other parts of the country, prevalence of NCDs also demonstrated a persistent upward trend during 1998 to 2008 and aging of population was identified as the main contributor [11,14].

The objective of the current study was thus to measure the burden of NCDs, understand the distribution of their socio-demographic, behavioral and life event-related potential correlates and to estimate the association of the NCDs with these correlates among elderly population in Xinjiang Uyghur Autonomous Region of China.

Methods

Recruitment

This cross-sectional study was conducted, between the months of March and December, 2011. Stratified random sampling was used to select a diverse and representative sample of Uygur people

in Xinjiang. Based on the ethnic, demographic, economic and cultural factors, Xinjiang was divided into three regions (southern, eastern and northern). In each of these regions, a specific unique identification number (UID) was assigned to every administrative unit. Next using a computer based random selection procedure, two UIDs were randomly chosen from the list of UIDs in each region. Thus, two units per region were selected randomly making a total of six overall sampling areas (Hotan, Lop, Hami, Huicheng, Urumqi County and Tianshan District). In each sampling area, the aforementioned random selection method was repeated, and one community/village was next selected randomly to have six randomly selected study sites altogether.

The inclusion criteria included 1) Age 60 years or more; 2) Uyghur ethnicity and 3) Agreeing to participate by providing written informed consent. From the population database (Chinese population registration system, which is maintained and held by the police department and can be assessed by submitting application form to the local/state government) of the residents of the selected communities, 2033 persons with Uyghur ethnicity who were aged 50 years or more were identified. Among them, 1766 had their residential address and other contact information correctly recorded in the population database. After contacting them, to minimize non-participation, all these 1766 seniors were screened by visiting them at their residence and 1455 of them met the inclusion criteria and 1329 agreed to participate and completed the survey.

Structured Interview

A face-to-face interview using an interviewer-administered, structured questionnaire was conducted for each participant to collect information on demographics, behaviors, medical history and important events of life. Several PhD students who were trained for conducting the interviews using the same training modules and protocol conducted the interviews. In order to reduce the bias due to non-response, all the interviews were conducted at the residence of the participants.

The demographic information included age (continuous, and further categorized into 60–63/64–67/68–71/71–75/>75), gender (male/female), education level (elementary school or less/ junior or senior high school/college and higher), marital status (never married/married/divorced or widowed), residency (urban/ rural), occupation before retirement (officer/worker/farmer/others) and average annual income per person in the family [less than 2000 Yuan/2001–8000 Yuan/more than 8000 Yuan (while 1 US dollar = 6.05 Yuan)]. Ethnicity of each participant was determined based on the recorded ethnicity in the population registration system of China.

Behaviors were assessed by collecting information (yes/no) on smoking, alcohol drinking, religious belief, farm work and pesticide use. The participants were also asked whether they were satisfied with their current life (Very satisfied/satisfied/dis-satisfied/very much dis-satisfied), whether they had the ability to take care of themselves in daily life, what were their hobbies (watching TV, listening to radios, watching opera or films, reading books or papers, calligraphy, planting flowers, having pets, fishing, playing cards, playing Mahjong, playing chess, doing exercise, walking and travelling in a group). Negative events in the past two years were also enquired (significant deterioration in health status, serious economic difficulties, death of someone with intimate relation and important thing being lost or stolen). Besides these, we also asked the frequency of vegetables, fruits and garlic consumptions (two times or more per day/one time per day/less than one time per day but more than two times per week/one time per week or less). Average salt intake per day was estimated for each participant (3

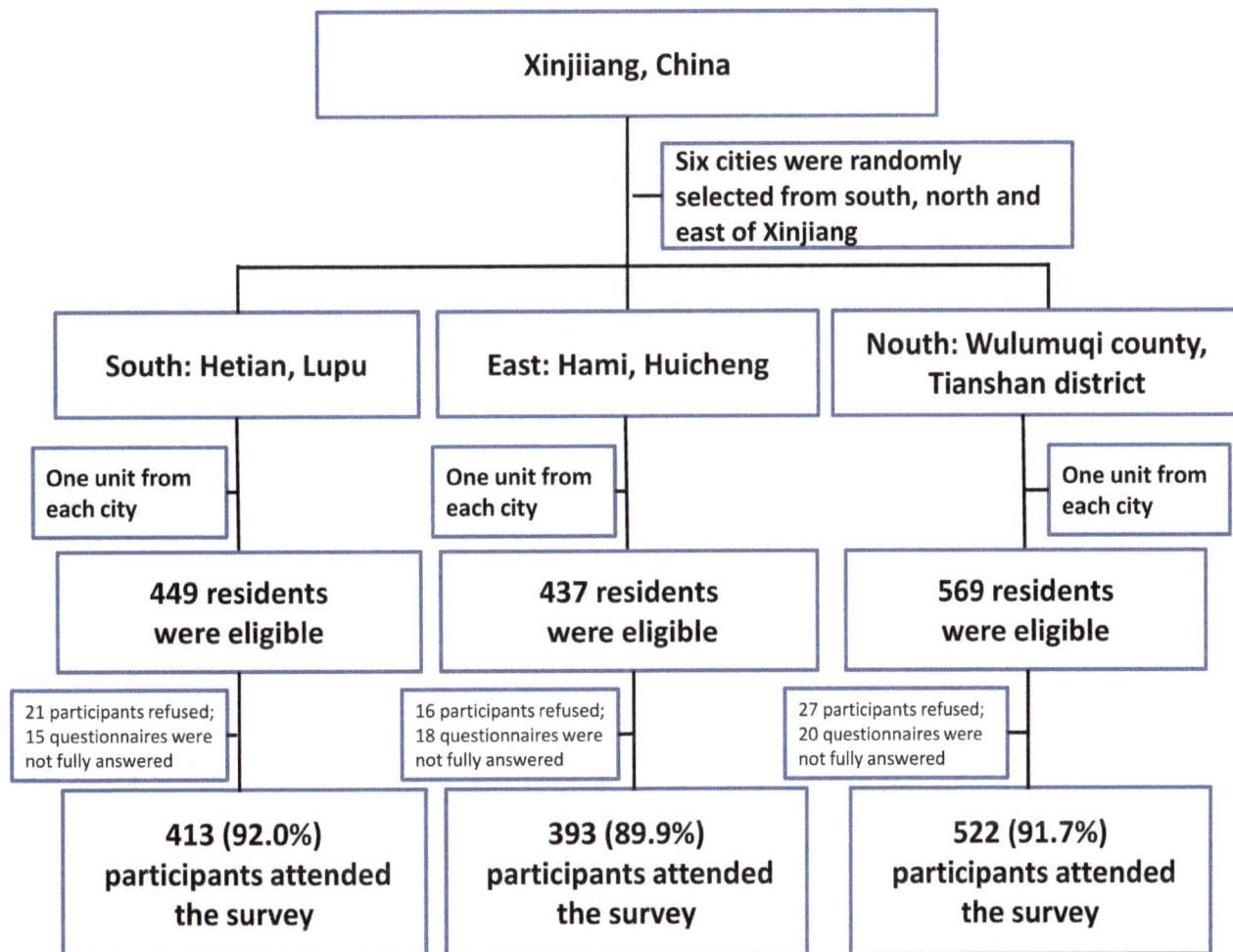

Figure 1. Flow Chart of the recruitment of the elderly Uyghur in Xinjiang Uyghur Autonomous Religion, China (N = 1329), 2011.

grams or less per day/4–6 grams per day/7 grams or more per day). Chili consumption was enquired and categorized as often/sometimes/never.

Disease assessment

Blood pressure of each of the participants was checked before and after the interview. In our study, hypertensives were defined as those who had prior diagnosis of hypertension or met any of following criteria 1) systolic blood pressures (SBP) in both readings being ≥140 mm of Hg; 2) the diastolic blood pressure (DBP) in both readings being ≥90 mmg.

Prior diagnosis of diabetes, hyperlipidemia, coronary heart disease/valvular heart disease (CHD), stroke, angina, cancers, and chronic obstructive pulmonary disease (COPD) were also enquired and recorded (yes/no). If the participant had any of the above mentioned NCDs, she/he was categorized as a subject having NCD. The total number of NCDs for each participant were calculated and categorized into four groups (0/1/2/≥3). Data on geriatric depression was also measured but findings were reported elsewhere (PONE-D-14-17995, Weiming Tang, "Burden and correlates of geriatric depression among Uygur elderly, observation from Xinjiang, China").

Data Analysis

Data was double-entered using the software EpiData 3.0 [15] and multiple logic checks were used to ensure the data quality. SAS version 9.1 [16] was used for all statistical analyses. Descriptive analyses were conducted to determine the distribution of the demographic factors, behaviors, life events and to calculate the prevalence proportions of different kind of NCDs. In addition, to assess the strength and direction of the association between NCDs and their potential correlates, ordinal logistic regressions were performed for univariate analysis [Odds ratio (OR) and 95% CI]. In the ordinal logistic regression, we categorized the participants into four groups based on the numbers of NCDs they had: having no NCDs/having one NCD/having two NCDs/having three or more NCDs. Since the principal dependent variable (number of NCDs) had 4 clearly defined categories (suffering from no NCD/1 NCD/2 NCDs/≥3 NCDs) with a typical order (0<1<2<3 or more) hence to have increased efficiency of analyses, to determine the association of the independent variables with the odds of having higher number of NCDs, we used ordinal logistic regression [17]. We further performed multivariate ordinal logistic regression adjusting for gender, education and occupation in model 1, and gender, education, occupation, age (continuous) and marital status in model 2. For each of the regression analyses we used appropriate model diagnostics and the models that we used did fit well (P<

Table 1. Sociodemographic characteristics and prevalence of diseases among Uyghur elderly (60 or older) in Xinjiang Uyghur Autonomous Region, China (N = 1329), 2011.

Variables		Female (n = 720)			Male (n = 609)			Total (N = 1329)	
		Frequency	Percent	95% CI	Frequency	Percent	95% CI	Frequency	Percent
Age	60–63	307	42.64	39.02,46.26	226	37.23	33.38,41.09	533	40.17
	64–67	157	21.81	18.78,24.83	134	22.08	18.77,25.38	291	21.93
	68–71	103	14.31	11.74,16.87	94	15.49	12.60,18.37	197	14.85
	72–75	65	9.03	6.93,11.13	78	12.85	10.18,15.52	143	10.78
	More than 75	88	12.22	9.82,14.62	75	12.36	9.73,14.98	163	12.28
Residence	Urban	471	65.42	61.93,68.90	358	58.78	54.86,62.70	829	62.38
	Rural	249	34.58	31.10,38.06	251	41.22	37.29,45.14	500	37.62
Marital Status	Married	594	82.50	79.72,85.28	559	91.79	89.60,93.98	1153	86.76
	Never married	22	3.06	1.80,4.32	21	3.45	2.00,4.90	43	3.24
	Divorced or widowed	104	14.44	11.87,17.02	29	4.76	3.06,6.46	133	10.01
Education	Elementary school or less	423	58.75	55.14,62.35	301	49.43	45.44,53.41	724	54.48
	Junior or senior high school	152	21.11	18.12,24.10	145	23.81	20.42,27.20	297	22.35
	College or above	145	20.14	17.20,23.08	163	26.77	23.24,30.29	308	23.18
Occupation	Officer	111	15.42	12.77,18.07	135	22.17	18.86,25.48	246	18.51
	Worker	132	18.33	15.50,21.17	108	17.73	14.69,20.78	240	18.06
	Farmer	325	45.14	41.50,48.78	295	48.44	44.46,52.42	620	46.65
	Others	152	21.11	18.12,24.10	71	11.66	9.10,14.21	223	16.78
Income	0–2000	458	63.61	60.09,67.13	335	55.01	51.05,58.97	793	59.67
	2001–8000	167	23.19	20.10,26.28	176	28.90	25.29,32.51	343	25.81
	8001 and above	95	13.19	10.72,15.67	98	16.09	13.16,19.02	193	14.52
Hypertension	No	503	69.86	66.50,73.22	463	76.03	72.63,79.43	966	72.69
	Yes	217	30.14	26.78,33.50	146	23.97	20.57,27.37	363	27.31
CHD	No	601	83.47	80.75,86.19	535	87.85	85.25,90.45	1136	85.48
	Yes	119	16.53	13.81,19.25	74	12.15	9.55,14.75	193	14.52
Hyperlipidemia	No	676	93.89	92.14,95.64	573	94.09	92.21,95.97	1249	93.98
	Yes	44	6.11	4.36,7.86	36	5.91	4.03,7.79	80	6.02
Angina	No	654	90.83	88.72,92.95	577	94.75	92.97,96.52	1231	92.63
	Yes	66	9.17	7.05,11.28	32	5.25	3.48,7.03	98	7.37
Stoke	No	698	96.94	95.68,98.20	597	98.03	96.92,99.14	1295	97.44
	Yes	22	3.06	1.80,4.32	12	1.97	0.86,3.08	34	2.56
Diabetes	No	680	94.44	92.77,96.12	595	97.70	96.51,98.89	1275	95.94
	Yes	40	5.56	3.88,7.23	14	2.30	1.10,3.49	54	4.06
Cancers	No	613	85.14	82.53,87.74	562	92.28	90.16,94.41	1175	88.41
	Yes	107	14.86	12.26,17.46	47	7.72	5.59,9.84	154	11.59

Table 1. Cont.

Variables		Female (n=720)			Male (n=609)			Total (N=1329)	
		Frequency	Percent	95% CI	Frequency	Percent	95% CI	Frequency	Percent
COPD	No	632	87.78	85.38,90.18	567	93.10	91.08,95.12	1199	90.22
	Yes	88	12.22	9.82,14.62	42	6.90	4.22,8.92	130	9.78
NCDs	No	381	52.92	49.26,56.57	397	65.19	61.39,68.98	778	58.54
	1	168	23.33	20.24,26.43	108	17.73	14.69,20.78	276	20.77
	2	94	13.06	10.59,15.52	67	11.00	8.51,13.49	161	12.11
	3 or more	77	10.69	8.43,12.96	37	6.08	4.17,7.98	114	8.58

0.001) while the proportional odds assumptions for ordinal logistic regressions were also met in each of them.

Ethics statement

The study process and content were approved by the Ethics Committee of Xinjiang Autonomous Region. Signed written informed consent was obtained from each participant prior to the interviews. Each of the participants had the discretion to freely decline or withdraw from this survey at any point of time. The filled-in questionnaires, written consent documents and computerized data were properly secured.

Results

Demographics and behaviors

In this comprehensive cross-sectional study, overall 1329 elderly persons of Uyghur ethnicity were recruited in Xinjiang, China. Figure 1 presented the response rate in each selected region of Xinjiang. Among these participants, 720 were female (about 54.2%), 41% (42.6% among female and 37.2% among male) were aged between 60 and 63 years old, majority (86.8%) were married (82.5% and 91.8% among female and male respectively) and more than half had only attended elementary school or less (58.8% for female and 49.4% for male) (Table 1).

Prevalence of NCDs

Out of 1329 participants, 363 were either previously diagnosed with hypertension or met the diagnosis criteria of hypertension, with an overall hypertension prevalence of 27.3% (30.1% in female and 24.0% in male). Fifty-four participants (4.06%) reported that they were diagnosed with diabetes before (5.56% among female and 2.30% among male), 80 participants had hyperlipidemia (6.02%). Besides these, the participants reported that 98 of them had angina (7.37%), 34 suffered from stroke (2.32%), 193 (14.52%) had CHD, 154 (11.59%) had any kind of cancers and 130 had COPD (9.78%) (Table 1).

Overall, 20.22% of the participants had one NCD (23.33% among female and 17.73% among male), 12.11% had two NCDs and 8.58% had three or more NCDs. In total, 551 participants had at least one kind of NCDs, with an overall NCD prevalence of 41.46% (47.08% for female and 34.81% for male).

Figure 2 demonstrated that the participants who were aged 70 years or more had higher prevalence of hypertension, CHD, cancer, diabetes and angina than those who were aged between 60 and 69 years.

Behaviors and life events

The results did show that only about 18% of the participating population were not satisfied with their current life (19.0% among female and 17.1% among male), 7% were current smokers (2.5% among female and 11.5% among male), and 2–3% percent were current drinkers (0.7% among female and 4.6% among male). Majority (81.4%) had religious belief (80.0% among female and 82.3% among male). Overall, only about 18% did not have any hobbies (18.1% and 18.7% for female and male, respectively). More than 96% (95.4% for female and 97.0% for male) of the participants reported that they could take care of themselves in their daily life. About 39% of the participated elderly reported that they experienced at least one of the listed negative events in the past two years. In addition, about 13%, 16% and 40% of the participants reported that they consumed fresh vegetables, fruits and garlic two or more times per day, respectively. Only about 8% participants consumed more than 7 grams salt per day, 12% often ate chili, and 21% were still involved in farming work (Table 2).

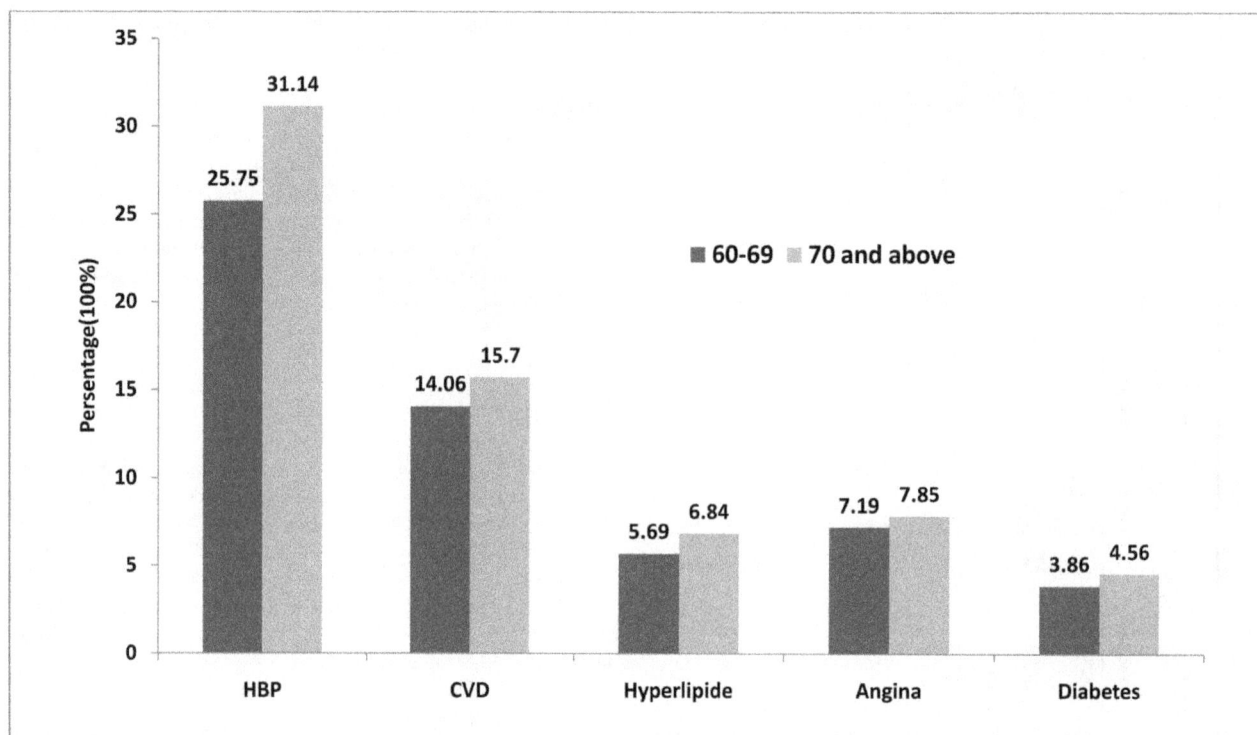

Figure 2. Prevalence of different kind of NCDs among different age among Uyghur elderly in Xinjiang Uyghur Autonomous Region, China (N = 1329), 2011.

Correlates of NCDs

Both crude and adjusted models (adjusted for gender, education and occupation) indicated that compared to the participants who were living in urban area, the rural residents were more likely to suffer from increased no. NCDs (unadjusted Odds Ratio: OR = 1.45, 95% CI: 1.17–1.80 while adjusted Odds Ratio: AOR = 2.00, 95% CI: 1.53–2.61). In addition, both in crude and adjusted analyses, compared to those who were not satisfied with their daily life, the participants who were satisfied or very satisfied with their life had significantly lower chance of having more NCDs. Compared to those who had no religious beliefs, participants who were religious had higher odds of having more NCDs (OR = 2.75, 95% CI: 2.01–3.75; AOR in model one = 3.07, 95% CI: 2.22–4.25). Model one did also show that compared to current non-smokers, current smokers had significantly higher odds of having more NCDs (AOR = 1.53, 95% CI: 1.00–2.34) (Table 3).

The crude and adjusted model one demonstrated that not being able to take care of themselves in daily life was also positively associated with having more NCDs (OR = 4.36, 95% CI: 2.63–7.24; AOR = 4.64, 95% CI: 2.78–7.74). Not being involved in farm work currently was also found to be positively associated with suffering from more NCDs in both crude (OR = 1.45, 95% CI 1.11–1.90) and adjusted model one (AOR = 1.41, 95% CI 1.05–1.90). Both crude and adjusted model one also demonstrated that compared to those who consumed fresh vegetables more than two times per week, participants who consumed less fresh vegetables had significantly higher (for One time per day: AOR = 4.81, 95% CI 2.47–9.35; for Two or more times per week: AOR = 9.45, 95% CI 5.48–16.32 and for One time per week or less AOR = 12.82, 95% CI 7.23–22.75) chance of developing more NCDs. Similar results were observed for less fruits and garlic consumptions.

Crude and adjusted model one further pointed out that compared to those who consumed salt between 4 and 6 grams per day, participants who consumed less or more salt had higher odds of having more NCDs (AOR = 1.99 for 3 grams or less, 95% CI 1.58–2.50, and AOR = 1.98 for 7 grams or more, 95% CI 1.35–2.91).

Having one (AOR = 0.33, 95% CI 0.23–0.47), three or more (AOR = 0.75, 95% CI 0.58–0.98) hobbies were found to be negatively associated with having more NCDs, compared to these who had no hobbies (Table 3).

After further adjustment for age and marital status (model two, table 3), the results did not change much, compared to model one.

Discussion

In this cross-sectional survey involving a comprehensive sample of Uyghur elderly residents (60 years old or more) of Xinjiang district of China, the prevalence of NCDs like hypertension (27.31%), cancers (11.59%), COPD (9.78%) and CHD (14.52%) were measured. 8.58% participants reported that they had three or more kinds of listed NCDs. Overall, the prevalence of at least one NCD among the participants was 41.46%, which was lower than the figure reported in SAGE-China Wave 1 study [9].

Corroborating with prior observations, our study also found that with increasing age, the prevalence of NCDs also increased. One potential mechanism behind this phenomenon could be that aging process might have lead to the change of hormone secretion, which in turn resulted in decline in physical and cognitive functions [18].

The participants who were aged 70 years or more had significantly higher prevalence of hypertension and this finding was similar to the result of a meta-analysis which summarized hypertension prevalence among Chinese Han population [19].

Table 2. Behaviors and life events of Uyghur elderly (60 or older) in Xinjiang Uyghur Autonomous Region, China (N = 1329), 2011.

Variables		Female (n = 720)			Male (n = 609)			Total (N = 1329)	
		Frequency	Percent	95% CI	Frequency	Percent	95% CI	Frequency	Percent
Satisfaction regarding life events	Very satisfied	131	18.19	15.37,21.02	113	18.56	15.46,21.65	244	18.36
	satisfied	452	62.78	59.24,66.32	392	64.37	60.55,68.18	844	63.51
	Not satisfied	137	19.03	16.15,21.90	104	17.08	14.08,20.07	241	18.13
Smoking	No	702	97.50	96.36,98.64	539	88.51	85.96,91.05	1241	93.38
	Yes	18	2.50	1.36,3.64	70	11.49	8.95,14.03	88	6.62
Alcohol drinking	No	715	99.31	98.70,99.91	581	95.40	93.73,97.07	1296	97.52
	Yes	5	0.69	0.09,1.30	28	4.60	2.93,6.26	33	2.48
Religion belief	No	144	20.00	17.07,22.93	108	17.73	14.69,20.78	252	18.96
	Yes	576	80.00	77.07,82.93	501	82.27	79.22,85.31	1077	81.04
Number of hobbies	0	130	18.06	15.24,20.87	114	18.72	15.61,21.82	244	18.36
	1	126	17.50	14.72,20.28	105	17.24	14.23,20.25	231	17.38
	2	232	32.22	28.80,35.64	197	32.35	28.62,36.07	429	32.28
	3 or more	232	32.22	28.80,35.64	193	31.69	27.98,35.40	425	31.98
Have the ability to take care of themselves in daily life	Yes	687	95.42	93.88,96.95	591	97.04	95.70,98.39	1278	96.16
	No	33	4.58	3.05,6.11	18	2.96	1.61,4.30	51	3.84
Total negative events in the past two years	No	423	58.75	55.14,62.35	384	63.05	59.21,66.90	807	60.72
	1	156	21.67	18.65,24.68	114	18.72	15.61,21.82	270	20.32
	2	82	11.39	9.06,13.71	77	12.64	10.00,15.29	159	11.96
	3 or more	59	8.19	6.19,10.20	34	5.58	3.75,7.41	93	7.00
Fresh Vegetables consumption	Two or more times per day	108	15.00	12.38,17.61	68	11.17	8.66,13.67	176	13.24
	One time per day	66	9.17	7.05,11.28	41	6.73	4.74,8.73	107	8.05
	Two or more times per week	392	54.44	50.80,58.09	380	62.40	58.54,66.26	772	58.09
	One time per week or less	154	21.39	18.39,24.39	120	19.70	16.54,22.87	274	20.62
Fruits consumption	Two or more times per day	131	18.19	15.37,21.02	79	12.97	10.30,15.65	210	15.80
	One time per day	84	11.67	9.32,14.02	62	10.18	7.77,12.59	146	10.99
	Two or more times per week	376	52.22	48.56,55.88	362	59.44	55.53,63.35	738	55.53
	One time per week or less	129	17.92	15.11,20.72	106	17.41	14.38,20.42	235	17.68
Garlic Consumption	Two or more times per day	282	39.17	35.59,42.74	240	39.41	35.52,43.30	522	39.28
	One time per day	102	14.17	11.61,16.72	90	14.78	11.95,17.60	192	14.45
	Two or more times per week	255	35.42	31.92,38.92	220	36.12	32.30,39.95	475	35.74
	One time per week or less	81	11.25	8.94,13.56	59	9.69	7.33,12.04	140	10.53
Salt consumption	3 grams or less per day	284	39.44	35.87,43.02	216	35.47	31.66,39.28	500	37.62
	4-6 grams per day	378	52.50	48.84,56.16	340	55.83	51.87,59.78	718	54.03
	7 grams or more per day	58	8.06	6.06,10.05	53	8.70	6.458,10.95	111	8.35

Table 2. Cont.

Variables		Female (n = 720)			Male (n = 609)			Total (N = 1329)	
		Frequency	Percent	95% CI	Frequency	Percent	95% CI	Frequency	Percent
Involved in farm work currently	No	606	84.17	81.49,86.84	442	72.58	69.02,76.13	1048	78.86
	Yes	114	15.83	13.16,18.51	167	27.42	23.87,30.98	281	21.14

The observed overall proportion of hypertension in our study was higher than the findings of another study conducted in Xinjiang Uyghur autonomous region, which sampled participants aged between 20 and 84 in 2007 [4]. This prevalence was also higher than the age-standardized prevalence rate of hypertension among Chinese reported in 2002, which was 17.7% [20]. As hypertension was a disease associated with aging [21], the age difference may explain part of the disparity between this presented study and others. However, the reported hypertension prevalence was still very high, which could also have increased the risk of stroke, ischemic heart disease, hypertensive disease and other cardiovascular diseases [22,23].

Several studies reported that China is experiencing an increasing epidemic of cardiovascular diseases, and CHD already became a leading cause of morbidity and mortality among Han adults in China [24,25]. Similar to Han population, Uyghur elderly population also seemed to be under serious threat of CHD, since 14.52% participants had CHD, 7.37% experienced angina and 2.56% had stroke before. These results pointed out that targeted intervention strategies to control these diseases should be tailored for Uyghur population.

Global cancer statistics pointed out that under the effect of aging and growth of the world population, both developing and developed countries were having increasing burdens of cancers [26]. This was also true for China, since China has the world's largest population and meets the largest challenge of aging [27]. In this presented study, 11.59% of the participating Uyghur elderly population reported that they were suffering from cancers, which further pointed out that ethnic minority populations in China are experiencing the same situation as Han population.

In addition to CVD and cancers, the participants also reported higher prevalence of diabetes and COPD. The higher prevalence of NCDs were likely to further increase the health and economic burden on the society and the risk of related complications and death [8].

Overall, 41.46% participants reported that they had at least one of the listed NCDs, 12.11% of them were suffering from two of these diseases, and 8.58% of them had three or more NCDs. Such worsening epidemic of NCDs among Uyghur elderly population seemed to be a warning signal, as NCDs already accounted for around 60% of all deaths worldwide [28]. Urgent intervention strategies need to be designed and implemented in this ethnic minority population in China.

Our results indicated that rural participants had higher chances of developing more NCDs, which corroborated with the results of another study conducted among Chinese and Indian population [29]. One study that summarized the chronic non-communicable diseases of China also reported that rural residents had higher age-standardized death rate of NCDs, particularly for CVD and COPD [4]. Lack of education, lower life standard, lack of awareness and poor access to health care could be potential reasons for this disparity. In addition, female participants had higher NCDs prevalence than male. The female partners were older could be the main reason for this phenomenon, as older age is highly related to NCDs.

Both crude and adjusted models indicated that consuming less fruits, and fresh vegetables could significantly increase the risk of developing more NCDs. Similar findings were also reported before, which revealed that low consumption of fresh fruits and vegetables and thus the lack of their nutrient biomarkers were associated with increased risk of CVD, cancer and other NCDs [30,31]. The mechanism behind this phenomenon was probably that fresh fruits and vegetables being rich sources of dietary fiber

Table 3. Factors correlated with more NCDs in ordinal logistic regression among Uyghur Elderly in Xinjiang Uyghur Autonomous Region, China (N=1329), 2011.

Variables		Crude Model		Model 1*		Model 2#	
		OR	95% CI	OR	95% CI	OR	95% CI
Residence	Urban	Ref		Ref		Ref	
	Rural	1.45	1.17,1.80	2.00	1.53,2.61	1.99	1.51,2.62
Life satisfaction	Not satisfy	Ref		Ref		Ref	
	Satisfy	0.82	0.63,1.08	0.84	0.64,1.11	0.84	0.64,1.11
	Very satisfy	0.59	0.41,0.84	0.61	0.43,0.88	0.62	0.43,0.89
Alcohol Drinking	No	Ref		Ref		Ref	
	Yes	1.14	0.59,2.21	1.36	0.69,2.67	1.32	0.67,2.60
Smoking	No	Ref		Ref		Ref	
	Yes	1.30	0.86,1.95	1.53	1.00,2.34	1.55	1.02,2.37
Religion belief	No	Ref		Ref		Ref	
	Yes	2.75	2.01,3.75	3.07	2.22,4.25	3.08	2.23,4.26
Number of hobbies	No	Ref		Ref		Ref	
	1	0.33	0.23,0.46	0.33	0.24,0.47	0.33	0.23,0.46
	2	0.84	0.62,1.14	0.89	0.65,1.22	0.85	0.62,1.17
	3 or more	0.74	0.57,0.96	0.75	0.58,0.98	0.74	0.56,0.96
Have the ability to take care of themselves in daily life	Yes	Ref		Ref		Ref	
	No	4.36	2.63,7.24	4.64	2.78,7.74	4.45	2.64,7.51
Total negative events in the past two years	No	Ref		Ref		Ref	
	1	1.24	0.94,1.61	1.28	0.97,1.67	1.29	0.98,1.68
	2	1.25	0.90,1.74	1.37	0.98,1.91	1.39	0.99,1.94
	3 or more	1.63	1.09,2.44	1.59	1.06,2.39	1.59	1.05,2.39
Fresh Vegetables consumption	Two or more times per day	Ref		Ref		Ref	
	One time per day	4.66	2.40,9.03	4.81	2.47,9.36	4.83	2.48,9.40
	Two or more times per week	8.75	5.09,15.04	9.45	5.48,16.32	9.45	5.47,16.34
	One time per week or less	12.72	7.20,22.48	12.82	7.23,22.75	12.84	7.23,22.78
Fruit consumption	Two or more times per day	Ref		Ref		Ref	
	One time per day	4.13	2.58,6.61	4.44	2.76,7.14	4.47	2.78,7.19
	Two or more times per week	3.57	2.44,5.23	3.76	2.55,5.53	3.75	2.54,5.53
	One time per week or less	5.43	3.54,8.32	5.40	3.50,8.34	5.42	3.51,8.37
Garlic consumption	Two or more times per day	Ref		Ref		Ref	
	One time per day	1.28	0.92,1.77	1.32	0.95,1.84	1.32	0.94,1.84
	Two or more times per week	1.52	1.19,1.94	1.55	1.19,2.01	1.56	1.20,2.02
	One time per week or less	1.83	1.28,2.61	1.80	1.25,2.60	1.84	1.27,2.66

Table 3. Cont.

Variables	Crude Model		Model 1*		Model 2#	
	OR	95% CI	OR	95% CI	OR	95% CI
Salt consumption						
Less than 4 grams per day	1.91	1.53,2.39	1.99	1.58,2.50	2.00	1.59,2.51
4-7 grams per day	Ref		Ref		Ref	
More than 7 grams per day	1.91	1.31,2.80	1.98	1.35,2.91	1.97	1.34,2.90
Involving farm work currently						
Yes	Ref		Ref		Ref	
No	1.45	1.11,1.90	1.41	1.05,1.90	1.38	1.03,1.86

Note: *model 1 adjusted for gender, education and occupation;
#model 2 adjusted for gender, education, occupation, age and marital status.

and other human body essential elements, could lower the risk of having NCDs [31].

Alike fresh fruits and vegetables, our study also found that less garlic consumption was also highly correlated with having more NCDs. Previous studies also demonstrated that raw garlic consumption could lower the risk of cancers [9], hypertension [32] and other NCDs, while it also could bring down the cholesterol levels, in turn reducing the risk of hyperlipidemia [33].

Previous studies demonstrated that reduced salt intake could reduce the risk of hypertension, CVD and other chronic diseases [34,35]. However, the results of our study indicated that both too much and too less salt intake could increase the risk of developing more NCDs. The detailed mechanism behind this phenomenon for low salt intake was unknown, while reverse causation could be one potential explanation for this.

Active smoking was also correlated with more NCDs acquisition, which was similar with the findings of prior studies [36]. These findings probably emphasized on the need for tobacco control programs, although Uyghur elderly population had a lower smoking rate (6.62% in our study).

Lacking the ability of taking care of themselves in daily life and not involving in farm work were also positively correlated with having more NCDs. Reverse causation could be a potential reason for this, as NCDs might have limited the mobility of the participants, which could have prevented them from farm work and taking care of themselves. Having three or more negative events in the past two years was also positively associated with development of more NCDs. One potential reason for this could be the possibility that negative events may be correlated with psychological dysfunction, and such psychological dysfunction may influence on the secretion of hormones, which may lead to or facilitate the development of NCDs [37].

Being satisfied with current life and having three or more hobbies were negatively associated with having more NCDs. These correlations may share the same reason for the negative events, but on the other side of the coin.

One study conducted in other cities in Xinjiang [38] also reported that BMI was highly correlated with blood lipids, which suggests that we should include it in our future studies.

According to our knowledge this was the first comprehensive study in Xinjiang Uyghur Autonomous Region to determine the association of NCDs with their potential predictors. By virtue of its sampling design this study was able to recruit a representative population of Uyghur elderly. The measured prevalence of NCDs as well as the observed associations of NCDs with their potential predictor can thus be extrapolated by the policy-makers for the purpose of designing appropriate targeted interventions. Large sample size, higher response rate (91.34%) and the use of ordinal logistic regression were the strengths of this presented study.

As an observational study, our study had several limitations. Because of the cross-sectional design, temporal ambiguity prevented us from drawing causal inferences based on our results and we recommend that any such interpretation should be made with caution. Vulnerability of the self-reported information, particularly for the NCDs, might lead to misclassification for both exposure and outcome. To check the problem of miss-reporting of NCDs, we used the hypertension as a surrogate, and the sensitivity and specificity for hypertension reporting were 0.84 and 0.87, respectively. Although the non-response rate was very low in our study, a small potential for selection bias still remained, which can be in either directions. In addition, the possibility of having residual confounding due to uncontrolled or unmeasured confounders was there. Also, the multiple categories of the outcome limited our ability to calculate the overall changes in absolute risk for the major risk factors for NCDs. In addition, even the social-demographic information of the participants of our study were similar to the overall Xinjiang Uygur population, we could not general our findings to other populations in China, since majority of the Uygur population in China are living in Xinjiang.

tion, too less or too much salt consumption and smoking. In addition, rural area participants were more likely to develop more NCDs. To reduce the burden of NCDs, the policy makers need to implement effective intervention strategies to promote healthy life styles among the Uyghur elderly population of China.

Conclusion

Even with these limitations, we can still conclude that the prevalence of NCDs, particular for hypertension, CVD and cancers were high among Uyghur elderly population (aged 60 or more) in Xinjiang, China. More importantly, these NCDs were highly correlated with negative life events, unhealthy life styles like less fresh fruits and vegetable consumption, less garlic consump-

Author Contributions

Conceived and designed the experiments: LF PL FW. Performed the experiments: Xihua Wang ZH YB XC ML AG YW JX MH Xiuli Wang BL. Analyzed the data: YM WT TM SM. Contributed reagents/materials/analysis tools: LF YM WT TM SM PL FW. Wrote the paper: LF YM WT TM SM PL FW.

References

1. USCDC (2011) The problem of noncommunicable diseases and CDC's role in combating them, Global Health, Noncommunicable Diseases, Overview, Centers for Disease Control and Prevention (CDC).
2. Wu Y (2011) Chronic diseases in China. Sick Societies: Responding to the Global Challenge of Chronic Disease: 241.
3. Tang S, Ehiri J, Long Q (2013) China's biggest, most neglected health challenge: Non-communicable diseases. Infect Dis Poverty 2: 7.
4. Yang G, Kong L, Zhao W, Wan X, Zhai Y, et al. (2008) Emergence of chronic non-communicable diseases in China. The Lancet 372: 1697–1705.
5. Cappuccio FP, Cooper D, D'Elia L, Strazzullo P, Miller MA (2011) Sleep duration predicts cardiovascular outcomes: a systematic review and meta-analysis of prospective studies. European heart journal 32: 1484–1492.
6. The World Bank (2011) Toward a Healthy and Harmonious Life in China, Stemming the rising tide of noncommunicable diseases, Human Development Unit, East Asia and Pacific Region, The World Bank.
7. Xu Y, Wang L, He J, Bi Y, Li M, et al. (2013) Prevalence and control of diabetes in Chinese adults. JAMA 310: 948–959.
8. Yang W, Lu J, Weng J, Jia W, Ji L, et al. (2010) Prevalence of diabetes among men and women in China. New England Journal of Medicine 362: 1090–1101.
9. Jin Z-Y, Wu M, Han R-Q, Zhang X-F, Wang X-S, et al. (2013) Raw Garlic Consumption as a Protective Factor for Lung Cancer, a Population-Based Case–Control Study in a Chinese Population. Cancer Prevention Research.
10. Alcorn T, Ouyang Y (2012) Diabetes saps health and wealth from China's rise. The Lancet 379: 2227–2228.
11. Qin J, Wang G, Yin T, Tang J, Deng D, et al. (2010) [Analysis on the changing trends of non-communicable diseases in Xinjiang Production and Construction Corps, from 1998 to 2008]. Article in Chinese 31: 430–433.
12. Cai W, Song JM, Zhang B, Sun YP, Yao H, et al. (2014) The prevalence of nonalcoholic Fatty liver disease and relationship with serum uric Acid level in uyghur population. ScientificWorldJournal 2014: 393628.
13. Li N, Wang H, Yan Z, Yao X, Hong J, et al. (2012) Ethnic disparities in the clustering of risk factors for cardiovascular disease among the Kazakh, Uygur, Mongolian and Han populations of Xinjiang: a cross-sectional study. BMC Public Health 12: 499.
14. Qin J, Deng D-J, Wang G-J (2010) Influencing factors of chronic diseases in a population of Xinjiang Production and Construction Corps. Chinese Journal of Public Health 7: 055.
15. Lauritsen J, Bruus M (2003) A comprehensive tool for validated entry and documentation of data. EpiData (version 3) Odense: EpiData Association.
16. Institute S (1996) The SAS system for Windows. SAS Institute Cary, NC.
17. Bender R, Grouven U (1997) Ordinal logistic regression in medical research. J R Coll Physicians Lond 31: 546–551.
18. Chapman IM, Hartman ML, Pezzoli SS, Harrell Jr FE, Hintz RL, et al. Effect of Aging on the Sensitivity of Growth Hormone Secretion to Insulin-Like Growth Factor-I Negative Feedback1; 2013. Endocrine Society.
19. Chen X, Wang Y (2008) Tracking of Blood Pressure From Childhood to Adulthood A Systematic Review and Meta–Regression Analysis. Circulation 117: 3171–3180.
20. Li L-L, Liu X-Y, Ran J-X, Wang Y, Luo X, et al. (2008) Analysis of prevalence and risk factors of hypertension among Uygur adults in Tushala and Hetian Xinjiang Uygur Autonomous Region. Cardiovascular Toxicology 8: 87–91.
21. Varagic J, Susic D, Frohlich ED (2001) Heart, aging, and hypertension. Current opinion in cardiology 16: 336–341.
22. Lawes CM, Hoorn SV, Rodgers A (2008) Global burden of blood-pressure-related disease, 2001. The Lancet 371: 1513–1518.
23. MacMahon S, Alderman MH, Lindholm LH, Liu L, Sanchez RA, et al. (2008) Blood-pressure-related disease is a global health priority. American journal of hypertension 21: 843–844.
24. Zhang X, Lu Z, Liu L (2008) Coronary heart disease in China. Heart 94: 1126–1131.
25. Wu Z, Yao C, Zhao D, Wu G, Wang W, et al. (2001) Sino-MONICA project A collaborative study on trends and determinants in cardiovascular diseases in China, part I: morbidity and mortality monitoring. Circulation 103: 462–468.
26. Jemal A, Bray F, Center MM, Ferlay J, Ward E, et al. (2011) Global cancer statistics. CA: a cancer journal for clinicians 61: 69–90.
27. Gavrilov LA, Heuveline P (2003) Aging of population. The encyclopedia of population 1: 32–37.
28. Daar AS, Singer PA, Persad DL, Pramming SK, Matthews DR, et al. (2007) Grand challenges in chronic non-communicable diseases. Nature 450: 494–496.
29. Popkin BM, Horton S, Kim S, Mahal A, Shuigao J (2001) Trends in diet, nutritional status, and diet-related noncommunicable diseases in China and India: The economic costs of the nutrition transition. Nutrition reviews 59: 379–390.
30. Peasey A, Bobak M, Kubinova R, Malyutina S, Pajak A, et al. (2006) Determinants of cardiovascular disease and other non-communicable diseases in Central and Eastern Europe: rationale and design of the HAPIEE study. BMC Public Health 6: 255.
31. Steinmetz KA, Potter JD (1996) Vegetables, fruit, and cancer prevention: a review. Journal of the American Dietetic Association 96: 1027–1039.
32. Silagy CA, Neil HAW (1994) A meta-analysis of the effect of garlic on blood pressure. Journal of hypertension 12: 463–468.
33. Harenberg J, Giese C, Zimmermann R (1988) Effect of dried garlic on blood coagulation, fibrinolysis, platelet aggregation and serum cholesterol levels in patients with hyperlipoproteinemia. Atherosclerosis 74: 247–249.
34. Asaria P, Chisholm D, Mathers C, Ezzati M, Beaglehole R (2007) Chronic disease prevention: health effects and financial costs of strategies to reduce salt intake and control tobacco use. The Lancet 370: 2044–2053.
35. Beaglehole R, Bonita R, Horton R, Adams C, Alleyne G, et al. (2011) Priority actions for the non-communicable disease crisis. The Lancet 377: 1438–1447.
36. Dowse GK, Gareeboo H, Alberti KGM, Zimmet P, Tuomilehto J, et al. (1995) Changes in population cholesterol concentrations and other cardiovascular risk factor levels after five years of the non-communicable disease intervention programme in Mauritius. Bmj 311: 1255–1259.
37. Barouki R, Gluckman PD, Grandjean P, Hanson M, Heindel JJ (2012) Developmental origins of non-communicable disease: implications for research and public health. Environ Health 11.
38. Cong L, Zhan JQ, Yang L, Zhang W, Li SG, et al. (2014) Overweight and Obesity among Low-Income Muslim Uyghur Women in Far Western China: Correlations of Body Mass Index with Blood Lipids and Implications in Preventive Public Health. PloS one 9: e90262.

11

Alterations to the Frequency and Function of Peripheral Blood Monocytes and Associations with Chronic Disease in the Advanced-Age, Frail Elderly

Chris P. Verschoor[1], Jennie Johnstone[2], Jamie Millar[1], Robin Parsons[1], Alina Lelic[1], Mark Loeb[1,2,3,4], Jonathan L. Bramson[1,4], Dawn M. E. Bowdish[1,4]*

1 Department of Pathology and Molecular Medicine, McMaster University, Hamilton, Ontario, Canada, 2 Department of Clinical Epidemiology and Biostatistics, McMaster University, Hamilton, Ontario, Canada, 3 Department of Medicine, McMaster University, Hamilton, Ontario, Canada, 4 Institute for Infectious Diseases Research, McMaster University, Hamilton, Ontario, Canada

Abstract

Background: Circulating myeloid cells are important mediators of the inflammatory response, acting as a major source of resident tissue antigen presenting cells and serum cytokines. They represent a number of distinct subpopulations whose functional capacity and relative concentrations are known to change with age. Little is known of these changes in the very old and physically frail, a rapidly increasing proportion of the North American population.

Design: In the following study the frequency and receptor expression of blood monocytes and dendritic cells (DCs) were characterized in a sample of advanced-age, frail elderly (81–100 yrs), and compared against that of adults (19–59 yrs), and community-dwelling seniors (61–76 yrs). Cytokine responses following TLR stimulation were also investigated, as well as associations between immunophenotyping parameters and chronic diseases.

Results: The advanced-age, frail elderly had significantly fewer CD14(++) and CD14(+)CD16(+), but not CD14(++)CD16(+) monocytes, fewer plasmacytoid and myeloid DCs, and a lower frequency of monocytes expressing the chemokine receptors CCR2 and CX$_3$CR1. At baseline and following stimulation with TLR-2 and -4 agonists, monocytes from the advanced-age, frail elderly produced more TNF than adults, although the overall induction was significantly lower. Finally, monocyte subset frequency and CX$_3$CR1 expression was positively associated with dementia, while negatively associated with anemia and diabetes in the advanced-age, frail elderly.

Conclusions: These data demonstrate that blood monocyte frequency and phenotype are altered in the advanced-age, frail elderly and that these changes correlate with certain chronic diseases. Whether these changes contribute to or are caused by these conditions warrants further investigation.

Editor: Serge Nataf, University of Lyon, France

Funding: Funding provided by Canadian Institutes of Health Research: http://www.cihr-irsc.gc.ca/; MOP123404. Ontario Lung Association: www.on.lung.ca/; No grant number provided. The funders had no role in study design, data collection and analysis, decision to publish, or preparation of the manuscript.

Competing Interests: The authors have declared that no competing interests exist.

* Email: bowdish@mcmaster.ca

Introduction

Age-related changes in circulating immune cell composition and levels of circulating pro-inflammatory cytokines have been associated with longevity [1], frailty [2] and age-related diseases such as Alzheimer's and Parkinson's disease [3], and rheumatoid arthritis [4]. Although the original description of the "immune risk phenotype" (a constellation of immunological markers that is predictive of survival in the aged) consisted primarily of T cell markers and levels of circulating pro-inflammatory cytokines [5], recent studies have begun to investigate age-related changes in myeloid cells such as monocytes and dendritic cells [6–11]. In the peripheral blood, monocytes can be subdivided into the classical (CD14++HLA-DR+), intermediate (CD14++CD16+HLA-DR+) and non-classical (CD14+/dimCD16+HLA-DR+) subsets, and dendritic cells can be subdivided into myeloid CD1c+HLA-DR+ or CD141++HLA-DR+ subsets and the plasmacytoid (pDCs, CD303+HLA-DR+ or CD123++HLA-DR+) subset [12]. For individuals that are particularly susceptible to developing infectious or chronic disease, such as the advanced-age, frail elderly, alterations to these cellular populations may be a sensitive biomarker in determining their level of risk. These markers could include the frequency of a given cellular subset in the circulation, the expression of receptors that are critical for the migration to tissues via chemokine gradients or the innate response to pathogens, or potentially the *ex vivo* response to an exogenous stimuli.

In the following study, we characterized the frequency of blood monocytes and DCs, as well as their expression of the innate signalling receptors toll-like receptor (TLR) -2 and -4, and the chemokine receptors CCR2 and CX_3CR1. Furthermore, we sought to test the hypothesis that monocytes from the advanced-age, frail elderly are immunosenescent, and therefore are likely to be less responsive to innate ligands for TLR-2 (Pam3CSK4) and -4 (lipopolysaccharide, LPS), compared to adults. To investigate whether monocyte and DC frequency and phenotype associate with chronic diseases common to the very old, we recruited a second, larger cohort of the advanced-age, frail elderly.

Methods

Participants

Young and middle-aged adults (19–59 years old, median = 34, n = 35 (42% female)) and community-dwelling seniors (61–76 years old, median = 69, n = 45 (67% female)) were recruited from Hamilton, Ontario between January and May in 2012. The advanced-age, frail elderly (defined as having a score of at least 4 on the Clinical Frailty Scale [13]) were recruited from five local nursing homes in 2010 and 2012. Participants were excluded if they were currently on immunosuppressive medication and pre-existing diseases were established by review of each participant's medical chart (Table 1). Participants recruited between January and May in 2012 (81–100 years old, median = 89, n = 49, 88% female) were compared against adults and community-dwelling seniors with regards to monocyte and DC frequency and phenotype, while participants recruited between September and December in 2010 (68–99 years old, median = 88, n = 136, 85% female) were examined for associations between those immuno-phenotyping variables and pre-existing diseases. The latter, second cohort was deemed necessary in order to have sufficient statistical power to perform the desired association tests. For all participants venous blood was collected from all donors by sodium heparin vacutainer (BD Biosciences, NJ, USA). Written informed consent was obtained from all participants or their legally appointed guardian in the event they were not competent to provide consent themselves. These studies and consent procedures and documents were approved by the McMaster Research Ethics Board (#13-05-14).

Immunophenotyping procedure

Antibody staining was performed as described previously [14]. For the comparison of young adults, community-dwelling seniors and advanced-age, frail elderly, fluorochrome conjugated antibodies included: CD2-PE, CD3-PE, CD16-PE, CD19-PE, CD56-PE, NKp46-PE, CCR2-Alexa647 (BD Biosciences, NJ, USA); CD15-PE, CD1c-FITC, CD141-APC (Miltenyi Biotec, CA, USA); CD14-APC-Alexa750 (Invitrogen, ON, CAN); CX_3CR1-FITC (Biolegend, CA, USA); CD16-PE-Cy7, HLADR-PerCp-Cy5.5, CD45-eFluor605NC, CD123-PE-Cy7, TLR-4-Alexa700, TLR-2-eFluor450 (eBioscience, CA, USA). For monocyte staining, lineage cells were defined as CD2, CD3, CD15, CD19, CD56 and NKp46 positive, and CD16 thresholds were defined using a fluorescent-minus-one (FMO) with isotype control (Figure 1). For DC staining, lineage cells were defined as CD3, CD15, CD16, CD19 and CD56 positive (Figure 1). Thresholds to determine percentage of cells expressing CCR2, CX_3CR1, TLR-2 and TLR-4 were calculated using an FMO with isotype control or negative staining population where appropriate. The frequency of mono-cyte and DC subsets is presented as per μl of whole blood (calculated using CountBright absolute counting beads) as well as the percentage of CD45 expressing PBMCs. Proportions of monocyte and DC subsets were defined as the percentage of CD45 expressing PBMCs. All analyses were performed in FlowJo 7.6.4 (Treestar, OR, USA).

Intracellular cytokine staining

Intracellular cytokine staining was performed on cryopreserved PBMCs of donors randomly selected from each age group (young adults and advanced-age, frail elderly). Briefly, 10^6 cells (4×10^6/ ml) in X-VIVO 10 media (Lonza, Basel, CH) supplemented with 10% human AB serum (Lonza, Basel, CH) were treated with PBS (mock), 50 ng/ml LPS (Sigma, MO, USA), or 500 ng/ml Pam3CSK4 (Invivogen, CA, USA), and 1x Protein Transport Inhibitor (eBioscience, CA, USA) for 6 hours at 37°C/5% CO_2. Surface staining was performed for 30 min at room temperature with the conjugated antibodies CD14-Pacific Blue (Biolegend, CA, USA), CD16 PE-Cy7, HLA-DR-PerCp Cy5.5 (eBioscience, CA, USA) and CD3-AmCyan (BD Bioscience, ON,CA), and fixed with 1x Fix/lyse buffer (eBioscience, CA, USA) for 10 min. Cells were permeabilized for 30 min with 1x Permeabilization Buffer (eBioscience, CA, USA) at room temperature, and stained with the conjugated antibodies TNF-Alexa Fluor 700, IL-1β-PE, IL-8-

Table 1. Distribution of advanced-age, frail elderly with regards to disease.

	Disease positive			Disease Negative		
	n	Mean Age	M:F	n	Mean Age	M:F
Anemia	20	85.5	3:17	116	86.8	18:98
Arrhythmia	31	86.5	6:25	105	86.6	15:90
Asthma	11	85.9	0:11	125	86.7	21:104
Coronary artery disease	37	88.4	8:29	99	85.9	13:86
Congestive heart failure	16	87.6	2:14	120	86.5	19:101
Chronic obstructive pulmonary disease	13	86.7	2:11	123	86.6	19:104
Stroke	17	88.2	3:14	119	86.4	18:101
Dementia	66	87.0	11:55	70	86.2	10:60
Diabetes mellitus	32	84.7	6:26	104	87.2	15:89

M:F, Male:Female.

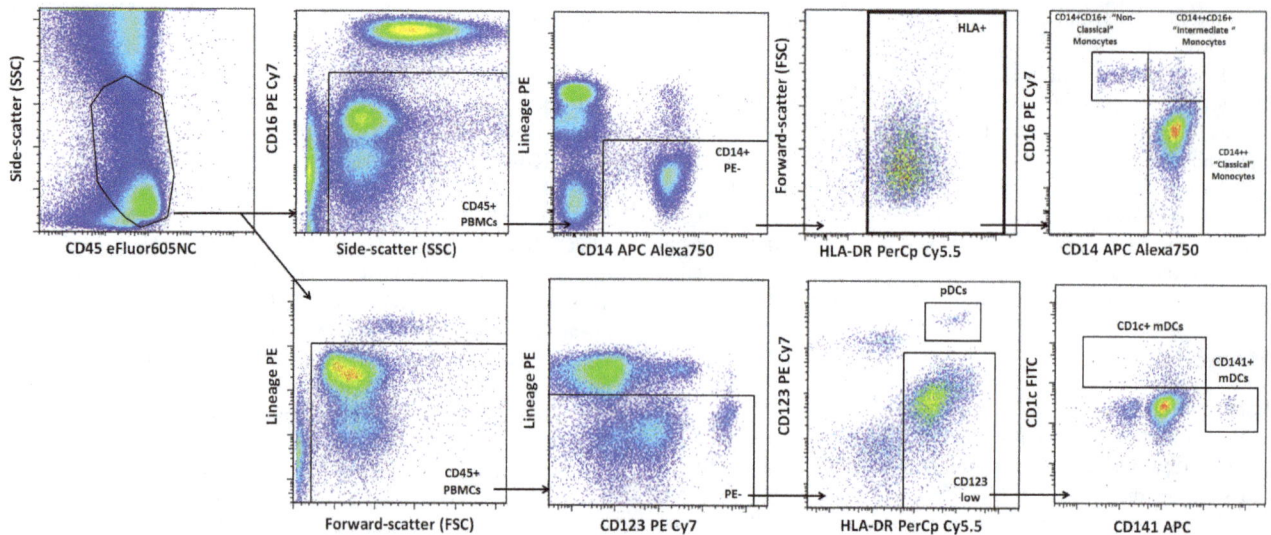

Figure 1. Summary of the gating strategy to define blood monocyte (upper panel) and dendritic cell (lower panel) subsets. Monocytes were defined as CD45 and HLA-DR expressing and lineage (CD2, CD3, CD15, CD19, CD56, NKp46) negative. Dendritic cell subsets were defined as CD45 and HLA-DR expressing, lineage (CD3, CD15, CD19, CD56) negative, and CD123 bright plasmacytoid dendritic cells (pDCs) or CD123 low, and CD1c or CD141 expressing myeloid dendritic cells (mDCs).

APC, and IL-6-FITC (eBioscience, CA, USA) for 30 min at room temperature. Cells were fixed with 2% paraformaldehyde, centrifuged and resuspended in FacsWash prior to analysis. Monocytes were defined as high front scatter (FSC)/Side scatter (SSC), and expressing CD14 and/or CD16 and HLA-DR, but not CD3. Flow cytometry and analysis was performed as described above.

Statistics

All statistical analyses were performed in R 2.11.1 (R Development Core Team, 2011) or Microsoft Excel. For immunophenotyping, differences between age groups were compared using the non-parametric Wilcoxon rank sum test. Experimental-wise significance threshold was determined using the Benjamini-Hochberg procedure for controlling false discovery rate. To determine if donor sex provided substantial bias in our comparisons between age groups, we performed an initial analysis by linear regression on log-transformed values. This indicated that sex only had a significant (experimental-wise $p < 0.05$) effect on the absolute count and proportion of classical monocytes. For associations with disease in the advanced-age, frail elderly, analysis was performed by logistic regression on log-transformed parameters, and adjusted for age. Logarithmic transformation was necessary to approximate normality, and the ratio of males to females was determined to be balanced between cases and controls (Chi-square $p > 0.05$). Comparison of intracellular cytokine production was performed by Student's t-test on log-transformed values.

Results

For our characterization of peripheral blood monocyte and DC subsets in the advanced-age, frail elderly, we included a cohort of young adults and community-dwelling seniors in order to ascertain whether the cellular frequency and receptor expression levels observed are consistent with alterations that occur over the course of aging, or if they are indeed particular to advanced-age, frail elderly individuals. The absolute frequencies of CD45+ PBMCs were found to significantly decrease with age (mean ± SEM: young adults 2,339±100, seniors 1,893±120 and advanced-age, frail elderly 1,146±107) (Table 2) whereas there was a decrease in the absolute number and percentage of classical monocytes between young adults and the aged (seniors and advanced-age, frail elderly), but no significant decrease between seniors and the advanced-age, frail elderly (Table 2). Consistent with previous studies [8,10], the ratio of classical to intermediate monocytes is reduced with age and we observe that this reduction is more dramatic in the advanced-age, frail elderly (mean ± SEM: young adults: 25.5±1.8, seniors: 20.5±2.4, advanced-age, frail elderly: 14.4±1.3). As has been previously observed [6,7,9], there was a reduction in circulating myeloid (CD1c+ and CD141+) DCs, which we found is further decreased in the advanced-age, frail elderly, while plasmacytoid DCs were significantly reduced in seniors and the advanced-age, frail elderly.

In addition to measurements of frequency, the expression of innate pattern recognition receptors TLR-2 and TLR-4 were measured on monocytes and DCs, and the expression of chemokine receptors CX_3CR1 and CCR2 on monocytes alone (Table 2). It would appear that the percentage of TLR-2 expressing myeloid DCs is increased in the advanced-age, frail elderly, while no differences were observed for monocytes. It should be noted that although the trends regarding TLR-2 expression suggest an increase from young adults, to seniors, to the advanced-age, frail elderly. However, the subtlety in these alterations and degree of variation do not allow us to conclude as such. A subtle, but significant increase in the percentage of TLR-4 expressing classical monocytes was also observed in the advanced-age, frail elderly. There is an age-related reduction in the percentage of monocytes expressing CCR2, but no significant difference between community-dwelling seniors and the advanced-age, frail elderly. For CX_3CR1 however, a reduction in the percentage of expressing monocytes appears to be limited to the advanced-age, frail elderly.

Although only subtle differences in the expression of TLR-2 and -4 were observed for monocytes from the advanced-age, frail elderly, we sought to additionally characterize the functional

Table 2. Immunophenotyping of peripheral blood mononuclear cells (PBMCs) from young adults, community-dwelling seniors, and advanced-age, frail elderly.

		Adults (19–59 yrs, n = 35)	Seniors (61–76 yrs, n = 45)	Elderly (81–100 yrs, n = 49)	Wilcoxon Rank-Sum P-value		
					AdultxSenior	AdultxElderly	SeniorxElderly
CD45+ PBMCs	Cells/µL	2,339±100	1,893±120	1,146±107	<0.001	<0.001	<0.001
CD14++ "Classical" monocytes	Cells/µL	177±11	104±9	98±10	<0.001	<0.001	-
	Rel. PBMCs (%)	8.36±0.66	5.13±0.42	7.23±0.89	<0.001	0.017	-
	CCR2+ (%)	19.3±3.1	5.1±1.2	8.7±2.3	<0.001	<0.001	0.170
	CX3CR1+ (%)	92.9±1.0	90.5±2.1	77.6±3.7	-	0.005	0.002
	TLR-2+ (%)	100.0±0.01	100.0±0.01	100.0±0.01	-	-	-
	TLR-4+ (%)	1.4±0.12	1.4±0.10	1.7±0.09	-	0.006	0.061
CD14++CD16+ "Intermediate" monocytes	Cells/µL	7.92±0.70	6.50±0.64	7.77±0.68	0.057	-	0.145
	Rel. PBMCs (%)	0.37±0.03	0.31±0.03	0.58±0.06	-	0.046	0.001
	CCR2+ (%)	10.2±1.7	2.56±0.40	4.91±1.19	<0.001	<0.001	-
	CX3CR1+ (%)	95.7±0.7	93.4±1.6	78.9±3.5	-	<0.001	<0.001
	TLR-2+ (%)	100.0±0.02	99.9±0.03	100.0±0.01	-	-	-
	TLR-4+ (%)	2.0±0.43	1.7±0.22	1.6±0.23	-	-	-
CD14+CD16+ "Non-classical" monocytes	Cells/µL	13.9±1.3	13.1±1.3	7.9±0.8	-	<0.001	<0.001
	Rel. PBMCs (%)	0.64±0.06	0.62±0.05	0.55±0.06	-	0.140	0.160
	CCR2+ (%)	1.52±0.24	1.17±0.13	1.05±0.16	-	0.069	0.222
	CX3CR1+ (%)	99.7±0.1	99.6±0.1	98.5±0.4	-	0.016	0.003
	TLR-2+ (%)	99.3±0.3	99.7±0.1	99.7±0.1	0.100	-	-
	TLR-4+ (%)	1.2±0.16	1.2±0.14	1.3±0.15	-	-	-
Classical/Intermediate ratio		25.5±1.8	20.5±2.4	14.4±1.3	0.003	<0.001	0.014
Intermediate/Non-classical ratio		0.65±0.04	0.55±0.05	1.45±0.19	0.042	<0.001	<0.001
CD141++ myeloid dendritic cells	Cells/µL	0.68±0.06	0.67±0.06	0.26±0.03	-	<0.001	<0.001
	Rel. PBMCs (%)	0.031±0.004	0.038±0.003	0.025±0.002	0.123	0.147	0.002
	TLR-2+ (%)	26.1±2.1	34.7±3.3	40.2±3.9	0.137	0.011	-
	TLR-4+ (%)	14.5±1.6	15.7±1.6	17.0±2.3	-	-	-
CD1c+ myeloid dendritic cells	Cells/µL	11.7±1.2	11.2±0.6	7.3±0.7	0.121	0.005	<0.001
	Rel. PBMCs (%)	0.52±0.06	0.64±0.04	0.68±0.04	-	-	-
	TLR-2+ (%)	90.1±0.8	91.4±0.7	92.4±1.0	-	0.005	0.040
	TLR-4+ (%)	16.6±0.8	17.6±1.1	19.3±1.2	-	-	-

Table 2. Cont.

		Adults	Seniors	Elderly	Wilcoxon Rank-Sum P-value		
		(19-59 yrs, n = 35)	(61-76 yrs, n = 45)	(81-100 yrs, n = 49)	AdultxSenior	AdultxElderly	SeniorxElderly
CD123++ plasmacytoid dendritic cells	Cells/µL	7.39±0.56	4.03±0.22	2.45±0.31	<0.001	<0.001	<0.001
	Rel. PBMCs (%)	0.32±0.02	0.23±0.01	0.22±0.02	0.004	0.002	-
	TLR-2+ (%)	11.3±1.2	13.5±1.1	10.0±1.0	0.094	-	-
	TLR-4+ (%)	5.2±0.39	5.6±0.55	6.5±0.66	-	0.017	-

Mean and standard error presented. Only values with comparison-wise (Wilcoxon rank-sum test) significance at p<0.25 shown; Bolded values indicated experimental-wise (Benjamin-Hochberg FDR) significance at p<0.05. Cells/µL, cells per microliter of blood (absolute count); Rel. PBMCs, relative to PBMCs.

capacity of monocyte subsets from this age group to respond to stimulus via these receptors. Using intracellular cytokine staining, the production of IL-1β, IL-6, IL-8 and TNF by monocytes subsets in response to Pam3CSK4 (TLR-2 agonist) and LPS (TLR-4 agonist) were quantified in PBMCs from the advanced-age, frail elderly and young adults. Consistent with previous literature [11,15,16] the relative production of cytokine by monocyte subsets are as follows: IL-1β, Classical = Intermediate > Non-classical; IL-6, Intermediate > Classical > Non-classical; IL-8, Classical = Intermediate > Non-classical; TNF, Intermediate ≥ Non-classical > Classical (Figure 2A-D). No significant differences between age-groups in the overall production of IL-1β (Figure 2A) or IL-6 (Figure 2B) were observed. Classical monocytes from the advanced-age, frail elderly produced more IL-8 in response to LPS as compared to young adults (Figure 2D), and for all subsets, with exception to intermediate monocytes stimulated with LPS, TNF production was greater in the advanced-age, frail elderly at baseline (PBS mock control) and in response to Pam3CSK4 or LPS (Figure 2D). Interestingly, while the overall production of TNF was greater in the advanced-age, frail elderly, the relative induction of TNF (versus PBS mock control) was significantly lower for all subsets compared to young adults (Figure 2E). No differences between age-groups were observed for the relative induction of IL-1β, IL-6 or IL-8 (data not shown).

To determine whether the observed alterations to monocyte and DC frequency and monocyte CCR2 and CX₃CR1 expression in the advanced-age, frail elderly are associated with chronic disease, we analyzed a larger, second cohort of 136 participants (Table 1). This cohort second cohort was deemed necessary in order to have sufficient statistical power to perform the desired association tests. Within the advanced-age, frail elderly cohort we performed logistic regression for each of the monocyte and DC markers in a univariate manner against the presence of chronic obstructive pulmonary disease, congestive heart failure, coronary artery disease, asthma, dementia, cerebral vascular accident, diabetes mellitus, arrhythmia or anemia (Table 3). Other than a positive association between pDC frequency and dementia, no significant associations were observed for the frequencies of blood DCs. Although the senior and advanced-age, frail elderly groups had fewer monocytes expressing CCR2, there was no statistically significant association between monocyte CCR2 expression and disease (data not shown). In contrast, reductions in CX₃CR1 expression only occurred in the advanced-age, frail elderly and individuals with elevated levels of CX₃CR1 had a greater likelihood of having dementia, while reduced expression was associated with an increased risk of diabetes and anemia (Figure 3A). In addition there was a significant correlation between monocyte frequency and dementia, diabetes and anemia. The likelihood of having dementia was positively associated with monocytes and the classical to intermediate monocyte ratio, whereas for diabetes and anemia, opposite trends were observed (Figure 3B).

Discussion

Our results indicate that for many, but not all myeloid cell populations, age-related alterations tend to become more pronounced with advanced-age and frailty. These changes in circulating myeloid cell populations may reflect changes in precursor generation or emigration from the bone marrow. As an example, the recent finding in mice that a reduction of circulating pDCs stimulates myelopoiesis and increases circulating myeloid-derived suppressor cells (MDSCs) [17], whose numbers increase in the advanced-age, frail elderly [14], implies that there

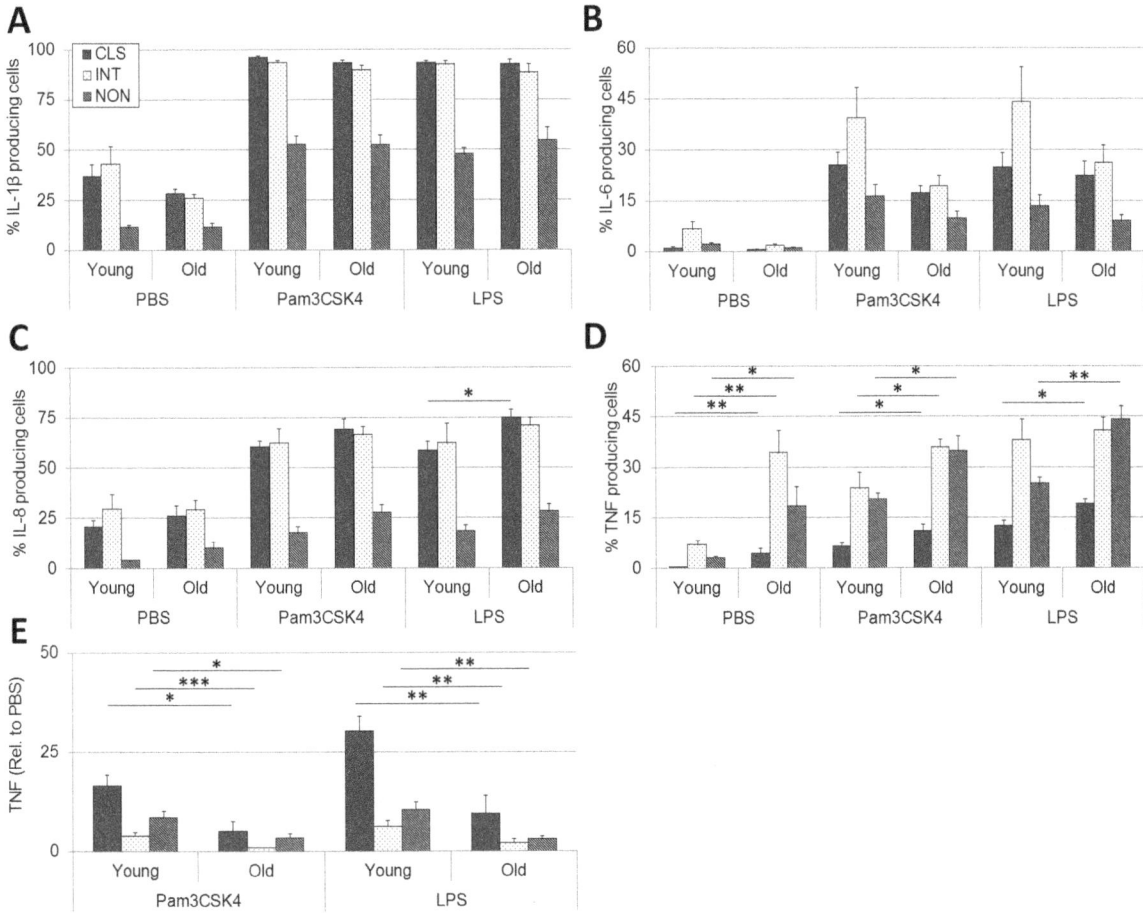

Figure 2. Cytokine production, but not induction, is elevated in monocytes from the advanced-age, frail elderly as compared to young adults. PBMCs were stimulated with mock (PBS), and TLR-2 (Pam3CSK4, Pam) and TLR-4 (LPS) agonists, and the production of A) IL-1β, B) IL-6, C) IL-8 and D) TNF in classical (CLS), intermediate (INT) and non-classical (NON) monocytes was measured by flow cytometry. Relative to mock, the induction of E) TNF was significantly lower in the advanced-age, frail elderly. n = 5–8 per group, per treatment. Comparison-wise p-value, ***p<0.001, **p<0.01, *p<0.05.

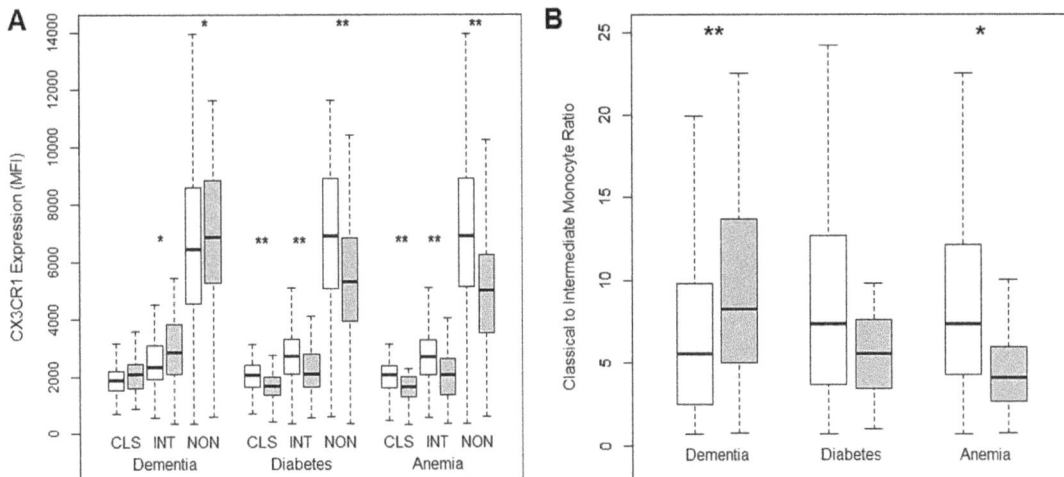

Figure 3. Representation of the differences in A) the expression of CX₃CR1 on the classical (CLS), intermediate (INT) and non-classical (NON) monocyte subsets and B) the classical to intermediate monocyte ratio, between cases (grey) and controls (white) for dementia, diabetes mellitus and anemia. Comparison-wise p-value, **p<0.01, *p<0.05.

Table 3. Associations between blood monocyte and DC markers and disease in the advanced-age, frail elderly.

		Chronic obstructive pulmonary disease	Congestive heart failure	Coronary artery disease	Asthma	Dementia	Cerebral vascular accident	Diabetes mellitus	Arrhythmia	Anemia
Monocytes	CD45%	2.47 (0.70–9.24)	-	-	-	**2.49 (1.16–5.66)** *	-	0.44 (0.17–1.12)	-	**0.33 (0.10–0.99)**
Classical	CD45%	2.13 (0.80–6.16)	-	-	-	1.66 (0.95–3.02)	-	**0.52 (0.26–1.03)**	0.60 (0.30–1.15)	**0.40 (0.18–0.88)** *
	CX_3CR1 (MFI)	-	-	1.93 (0.70–6.05)	0.24 (0.06–1.01) *	2.07 (0.83–5.62)	-	**0.22 (0.07–0.62)** **	-	**0.20 (0.06–0.64)** **
Intermediate	CD45%	-	-	1.55 (0.91–2.69)	-	0.67 (0.41–1.06)	0.52 (0.25–1.05)	-	1.89 (1.08–3.46) *	-
	CX_3CR1 (MFI)	-	-	-	0.24 (0.06–0.91) *	**2.90 (1.24–7.41)** *	-	**0.19 (0.06–0.50)** **	0.43 (0.16–1.08)	**0.18 (0.05–0.52)** **
Non-classical	CD45%	-	-	-	-	1.41 (0.84–2.40)	-	**0.35 (0.18–0.67)** **	-	0.54 (0.26–1.09)
	CX_3CR1 (MFI)	-	-	1.72 (0.82–4.15)	0.38 (0.14–1.02) *	**2.07 (1.04–4.48)** *	-	**0.32 (0.14–0.67)** **	-	**0.32 (0.13–0.72)** **
Classical:Intermediate ratio	CD45%	1.69 (0.87–3.48)	-	0.76 (0.49–1.17)	-	**1.74 (1.16–2.69)** **	1.68 (0.92–3.23)	0.72 (0.45–1.15)	**0.49 (0.30–0.79)** **	**0.55 (0.31–0.94)** *
pDC	CD45%	-	-	-	-	**0.56 (0.30–0.98)** *	-	0.51 (0.25–1.00)	-	-
CD1c+ mDC	CD45%	-	-	-	2.79 (0.71–12.07)	-	-	0.44 (0.18–1.08)	-	-
CD141+ mDC	CD45%	-	-	-	-	-	-	-	-	0.56 (0.28–1.12)

Odds ratios and 95% confidence intervals presented. Only comparison-wise (logistic regression) significance at p<0.25 shown;
*p<0.05,
**p<0.01. Bolded observations indicate experimental-wise (Benjamini-Hochberg FDR) significance at p<0.15. CD45%, percentage of cells relative to CD45+ PBMCs; MFI, mean fluorescent intensity.

may be previously unappreciated feedback mechanisms between circulating DCs and the bone marrow compartment.

In addition to changes in frequency, changes in phenotype and function have been shown to occur with age and it has been proposed that these phenotypic changes may contribute to age-associated chronic disease, especially those with inflammatory etiology. There have been conflicting reports, for example, as to whether monocytes have hypo- or hyper-inflammatory responses to TLR ligands and whether these might be due to changes in TLR expression [18,19]. While we observed only a slight increase in the percentage of TLR-4 expressing classical monocytes and no changes to the expression of monocyte TLR-2, the production of TNF, and to a lesser extent IL-8, was significantly higher in monocyte subsets from the advanced-age, frail elderly, both at baseline and in response to TLR-2 and -4 stimuli. This is similar to what has been shown in previous reports [8,11], and supports the theory that constitutive over-production of cytokines by monocyte subsets may predispose elderly individuals to a higher risk of chronic disease.

Another potential contributor to the development of chronic disease in the elderly is the ability of circulating monocytes to migrate to the tissues. Both CCR2 and CX$_3$CR1, receptors for the chemokines MCP-1 (CCL2) and fractalkine (CX$_3$CL1), are potently involved in the migration and recruitment of monocytes in the host. Monocyte recruitment via chemokine receptors has been linked to the development of inflammatory diseases such as atherosclerosis and cancer [20,21], and an increased expression of the monocyte/macrophage chemoattractant CX$_3$CL1 has been observed in cardiovascular disease and Alzheimer's disease [22,23]. Although correlations of increased CX$_3$CR1 expression and dementia have not been previously demonstrated in humans, our observations are consistent with mouse models of Alzheimer's disease in which either a loss of CX$_3$CR1 gene expression [24] or a reduction in signalling through CX$_3$CR1 [25] results in an improved outcome. Little is known regarding monocyte phenotype or CX$_3$CR1 expression and diabetes, although it has been shown

that monocytes display an activated phenotype in diabetics [26,27] and the production of CX$_3$CL1, likely by adipocytes, is found at higher levels in diabetics [28]. Whether monocytes expressing lower levels of CX$_3$CR1 contribute to insulin resistance and diabetes in the frail elderly is not known. We also observed associations of decreased monocyte numbers and CX$_3$CR1 expression with anemia. Chronic inflammation anemia is extremely common in the frail elderly [29] and is associated with elevated levels of inflammatory cytokines, especially IL-6 [30]. Since monocytes and erythrocytes share a common progenitor in the bone marrow, this association may be due to a common mechanism of suppressed myelopoeisis due to the aging or the immune status of the host.

In summary, changes in monocyte frequency, phenotype and function occur in the advanced-age, frail elderly and correlate with chronic disease. However, we do not know if these changes predispose individuals to age-related diseases or whether the overall immune status associated with many of these conditions is what ultimately impacts monocyte development and function. Future longitudinal studies will need to be performed to dissect the cause and effect of these changes as individuals approach advanced-age. Changes in circulating monocyte frequency and phenotype may be robust markers of immune risk in the aged.

Acknowledgments

The authors would like to acknowledge Amy Bartholomew for nursing assistance and Dr. Frédéric Geissmann for advice on the immunophenotyping protocol.

Author Contributions

Conceived and designed the experiments: CV DMEB. Performed the experiments: CV JM RP AL. Analyzed the data: CV. Contributed reagents/materials/analysis tools: JB. Contributed to the writing of the manuscript: CV DMEB. Organized and managed experimental cohorts: JJ ML.

References

1. Larbi A, Franceschi C, Mazzatti D, Solana R, Wikby A, et al. (2008) Aging of the immune system as a prognostic factor for human longevity. Physiology (Bethesda) 23: 64–74. 23/2/64 [pii];10.1152/physiol.00040.2007 [doi].

2. van den Biggelaar AH, Huizinga TW, de Craen AJ, Gussekloo J, Heijmans BT, et al. (2004) Impaired innate immunity predicts frailty in old age. The Leiden 85-plus study. Exp Gerontol 39: 1407–1414. S0531-5565(04)00213-X [pii];10.1016/j.exger.2004.06.009 [doi].

3. Rosenkranz D, Weyer S, Tolosa E, Gaenslen A, Berg D, et al. (2007) Higher frequency of regulatory T cells in the elderly and increased suppressive activity in neurodegeneration. J Neuroimmunol 188: 117–127. S0165-5728(07)00174-9 [pii];10.1016/j.jneuroim.2007.05.011 [doi].

4. Korkosz M, Bukowska-Strakova K, Sadis S, Grodzicki T, Siedlar M (2012) Monoclonal antibodies against macrophage colony-stimulating factor diminish the number of circulating intermediate and nonclassical (CD14(++)CD16(+)/CD14(+)CD16(++)) monocytes in rheumatoid arthritis patient. Blood 119: 5329–5330. 119/22/5329 [pii];10.1182/blood-2012-02-412551 [doi].

5. Wikby A, Maxson P, Olsson J, Johansson B, Ferguson FG (1998) Changes in CD8 and CD4 lymphocyte subsets, T cell proliferation responses and non-survival in the very old: the Swedish longitudinal OCTO-immune study. Mech Ageing Dev 102: 187–198.

6. Della BS, Bierti L, Presicce P, Arienti R, Valenti M, et al. (2007) Peripheral blood dendritic cells and monocytes are differently regulated in the elderly. Clin Immunol 122: 220–228. S1521-6616(06)00902-8 [pii];10.1016/j.clim.2006.09.012 [doi].

7. Jing Y, Shaheen E, Drake RR, Chen N, Gravenstein S, et al. (2009) Aging is associated with a numerical and functional decline in plasmacytoid dendritic cells, whereas myeloid dendritic cells are relatively unaltered in human peripheral blood. Hum Immunol 70: 777–784. S0198-8859(09)00171-2 [pii];10.1016/j.humimm.2009.07.005 [doi].

8. Nyugen J, Agrawal S, Gollapudi S, Gupta S (2010) Impaired functions of peripheral blood monocyte subpopulations in aged humans. J Clin Immunol 30: 806–813. 10.1007/s10875-010-9448-8 [doi].

9. Perez-Cabezas B, Naranjo-Gomez M, Fernandez MA, Grifols JR, Pujol-Borrell R, et al. (2007) Reduced numbers of plasmacytoid dendritic cells in aged blood donors. Exp Gerontol 42: 1033–1038. S0531-5565(07)00130-1 [pii];10.1016/j.exger.2007.05.010 [doi].

10. Seidler S, Zimmermann HW, Bartneck M, Trautwein C, Tacke F (2010) Age-dependent alterations of monocyte subsets and monocyte-related chemokine pathways in healthy adults. BMC Immunol 11: 30. 1471-2172-11-30 [pii];10.1186/1471-2172-11-30 [doi].

11. Hearps AC, Martin GE, Angelovich TA, Cheng WJ, Maisa A, et al. (2012) Aging is associated with chronic innate immune activation and dysregulation of monocyte phenotype and function. Aging Cell 11: 867–875. 10.1111/j.1474-9726.2012.00851.x [doi].

12. Ziegler-Heitbrock L, Ancuta P, Crowe S, Dalod M, Grau V, et al. (2010) Nomenclature of monocytes and dendritic cells in blood. Blood 116: e74–e80. blood-2010-02-258558 [pii];10.1182/blood-2010-02-258558 [doi].

13. Rockwood K, Abeysundera MJ, Mitnitski A (2007) How should we grade frailty in nursing home patients? J Am Med Dir Assoc 8: 595–603. S1525-8610(07)00351-9 [pii];10.1016/j.jamda.2007.07.012 [doi].

14. Verschoor CP, Johnstone J, Millar J, Dorrington MG, Habibagahi M, et al. (2013) Blood CD33(+)HLA-DR(-) myeloid-derived suppressor cells are increased with age and a history of cancer. J Leukoc Biol. jlb.0912461 [pii];10.1189/jlb.0912461 [doi].

15. Cros J, Cagnard N, Woollard K, Patey N, Zhang SY, et al. (2010) Human CD14dim monocytes patrol and sense nucleic acids and viruses via TLR7 and TLR8 receptors. Immunity 33: 375–386. S1074-7613(10)00317-1 [pii];10.1016/j.immuni.2010.08.012 [doi].

16. Sanchez-Torres C, Garcia-Romo GS, Cornejo-Cortes MA, Rivas-Carvalho A, Sanchez-Schmitz G (2001) CD16+ and CD16- human blood monocyte subsets differentiate in vitro to dendritic cells with different abilities to stimulate CD4+ T cells. Int Immunol 13: 1571–1581.

17. Ioannou M, Alissafi T, Boon L, Boumpas D, Verginis P (2013) In Vivo Ablation of Plasmacytoid Dendritic Cells Inhibits Autoimmunity through Expansion of

Myeloid-Derived Suppressor Cells. J Immunol 190: 2631–2640. jimmu-nol.1201897 [pii];10.4049/jimmunol.1201897 [doi].

18. Balistreri CR, Colonna-Romano G, Lio D, Candore G, Caruso C (2009) TLR4 polymorphisms and ageing: implications for the pathophysiology of age-related diseases. J Clin Immunol 29: 406–415. 10.1007/s10875-009-9297-5 [doi].

19. Renshaw M, Rockwell J, Engleman C, Gewirtz A, Katz J, et al. (2002) Cutting edge: impaired Toll-like receptor expression and function in aging. J Immunol 169: 4697–4701.

20. Qian BZ, Li J, Zhang H, Kitamura T, Zhang J, et al. (2011) CCL2 recruits inflammatory monocytes to facilitate breast-tumour metastasis. Nature 475: 222–225. nature10138 [pii];10.1038/nature10138 [doi].

21. Swirski FK, Nahrendorf M (2013) Leukocyte behavior in atherosclerosis, myocardial infarction, and heart failure. Science 339: 161–166. 339/6116/161 [pii];10.1126/science.1230719 [doi].

22. Kim TS, Lim HK, Lee JY, Kim DJ, Park S, et al. (2008) Changes in the levels of plasma soluble fractalkine in patients with mild cognitive impairment and Alzheimer's disease. Neurosci Lett 436: 196–200. S0304-3940(08)00319-4 [pii];10.1016/j.neulet.2008.03.019 [doi].

23. Wong BW, Wong D, McManus BM (2002) Characterization of fractalkine (CX3CL1) and CX3CR1 in human coronary arteries with native atherosclerosis, diabetes mellitus, and transplant vascular disease. Cardiovasc Pathol 11: 332–338. S1054880702001114 [pii].

24. Fuhrmann M, Bittner T, Jung CK, Burgold S, Page RM, et al. (2010) Microglial Cx3cr1 knockout prevents neuron loss in a mouse model of Alzheimer's disease. Nat Neurosci 13: 411–413. nn.2511 [pii];10.1038/nn.2511 [doi].

25. Lee S, Varvel NH, Konerth ME, Xu G, Cardona AE, et al. (2010) CX3CR1 deficiency alters microglial activation and reduces beta-amyloid deposition in two Alzheimer's disease mouse models. Am J Pathol 177: 2549–2562. S0002-9440(10)60305-7 [pii];10.2353/ajpath.2010.100265 [doi].

26. Cipolletta C, Ryan KE, Hanna EV, Trimble ER (2005) Activation of peripheral blood CD14+ monocytes occurs in diabetes. Diabetes 54: 2779–2786. 54/9/2779 [pii].

27. Min D, Brooks B, Wong J, Salomon R, Bao W, et al. (2012) Alterations in monocyte CD16 in association with diabetes complications. Mediators Inflamm 2012: 649083. 10.1155/2012/649083 [doi].

28. Shah R, Hinkle CC, Ferguson JF, Mehta NN, Li M, et al. (2011) Fractalkine is a novel human adipochemokine associated with type 2 diabetes. Diabetes 60: 1512–1518. 60/5/1512 [pii];10.2337/db10-0956 [doi].

29. Artz AS, Fergusson D, Drinka PJ, Gerald M, Bidenbender R, et al. (2004) Mechanisms of unexplained anemia in the nursing home. J Am Geriatr Soc 52: 423–427. 52116 [pii].

30. Ershler WB (2003) Biological interactions of aging and anemia: a focus on cytokines. J Am Geriatr Soc 51: S18–S21. jgs5102 [pii].

12

Interhemispheric Cerebral Blood Flow Balance during Recovery of Motor Hand Function after Ischemic Stroke—A Longitudinal MRI Study Using Arterial Spin Labeling Perfusion

Roland Wiest[1][*][◑], Eugenio Abela[1,4][◑], John Missimer[3], Gerhard Schroth[1], Christian W. Hess[4], Matthias Sturzenegger[4], Danny J. J. Wang[5], Bruno Weder[1,2,4], Andrea Federspiel[6]

1 Support Center for Advanced Neuroimaging (SCAN), Institute for Diagnostic and Interventional Neuroradiology, University Hospital Inselspital and University of Bern, Bern, Switzerland, 2 Department of Neurology, Kantonsspital St. Gallen, St. Gallen, Switzerland, 3 Paul Scherrer Institute, Laboratory of Biomolecular Research, Villigen, Switzerland, 4 Department of Neurology, University Hospital Inselspital and University of Bern, Bern, Switzerland, 5 Department of Neurology, Ahmanson-Lovelace Brain Mapping Center, University of California Los Angeles, Los Angeles, California, United States of America, 6 Department of Psychiatric Neurophysiology, University Hospital of Psychiatry and University of Bern, Bern, Switzerland

Abstract

Background: Unilateral ischemic stroke disrupts the well balanced interactions within bilateral cortical networks. Restitution of interhemispheric balance is thought to contribute to post-stroke recovery. Longitudinal measurements of cerebral blood flow (CBF) changes might act as surrogate marker for this process.

Objective: To quantify longitudinal CBF changes using arterial spin labeling MRI (ASL) and interhemispheric balance within the cortical sensorimotor network and to assess their relationship with motor hand function recovery.

Methods: Longitudinal CBF data were acquired in 23 patients at 3 and 9 months after cortical sensorimotor stroke and in 20 healthy controls using pulsed ASL. Recovery of grip force and manual dexterity was assessed with tasks requiring power and precision grips. Voxel-based analysis was performed to identify areas of significant CBF change. Region-of-interest analyses were used to quantify the interhemispheric balance across nodes of the cortical sensorimotor network.

Results: Dexterity was more affected, and recovered at a slower pace than grip force. In patients with successful recovery of dexterous hand function, CBF decreased over time in the contralesional supplementary motor area, paralimbic anterior cingulate cortex and superior precuneus, and interhemispheric balance returned to healthy control levels. In contrast, patients with poor recovery presented with sustained hypoperfusion in the sensorimotor cortices encompassing the ischemic tissue, and CBF remained lateralized to the contralesional hemisphere.

Conclusions: Sustained perfusion imbalance within the cortical sensorimotor network, as measured with task-unrelated ASL, is associated with poor recovery of dexterous hand function after stroke. CBF at rest might be used to monitor recovery and gain prognostic information.

Editor: Felix Schlachetzki, University of Regensburg, Germany

Funding: This study was granted by the Swiss National Foundation Grant (SNF 3200B0-118018) to BW and Swiss National Foundation Grant (SPUM 124114) to GS (www.snf.ch). The funders had no role in study design, data collection and analysis, decision to publish, or preparation of the manuscript.

Competing Interests: The authors have declared that no competing interests exist.

* Email: roland.wiest@insel.ch

◑ These authors contributed equally to this work.

Introduction

Widely distributed brain networks are involved in motor recovery after acute ischemic stroke. This has been evidenced by functional and effective connectivity analyses at rest and during tasks, the latter exemplified by changes in excitatory and inhibitory interactions between nodes of the somatomotor network [1]. Neuroimaging studies using blood-oxygen level dependent

(BOLD) contrast have shown modulations of task-evoked activity in extended fronto-parietal and striato-cerebellar networks within the ipsi- and contralesional hemispheres during recovery of hand motor skills [2,3,4,5,6]. Such dynamics of BOLD contrast are the result of complex interactions within specific cortico-subcortical circuits and may be evoked also after a lesion of a remote subcortical node [7]. Inman et al. found reduced spontaneous resting-state connectivity in the ipsilesional hemisphere between the superior parietal cortex and both the primary sensorimotor (SM1) and supplementary motor area (SMA) during recovery in the subacute stage of stroke [8]. Two longitudinal studies disclosed significant spatial reorganizations of motor networks both in the ipsi- and contralesional hemisphere from early to late recovery phase [7,9]. Implicated is the issue of interhemispheric balance which has been studied in the sensorimotor system of normal volunteers by Fox and Raichle [10]. They showed a bihemispheric coherence of somatomotor cortex, including medial motor areas, and secondary somatosensory association cortices in correlation maps relying on resting state BOLD. Instroke patients, disruption of functional connectivity in the somatomotor network correlated with motor impairment of upper extremity after stroke [11]. Finally, bihemispheric structural alterations were identified after stroke, reflected by increases in grey matter volume of the contralesional precuneus (PRE) and ipsilesional paralimbic anterior cingulate cortex (pACC). These structural patterns were positively correlated with recovery of motor function [12]. In sum, these studies suggest that functional and structural changes in both hemispheres are associated with motor recovery and, furthermore, the degree of interhemispheric balance may be of significance.

The most frequently employed imaging technique to map network activity is BOLD-fMRI [13]. Arterial spin labeling (ASL) offers advantages over BOLD-fMRI in applications where slowly varying changes in brain function are investigated [14]. The ASL signal is straightforward because it facilitates the direct quantification of cerebral blood flow (CBF). In comparison to the BOLD signal, it correlates well with the actual site of metabolism and neuronal involvement [15]. In cerebrovascular disease, ASL has been applied to investigate several issues such as perfusion changes, collateral flow, low-flow conditions and the effects of arterial stenosis [16,17,18,19,20].

Here, we examine the association between recovery of motor hand function relying on specific and standardized motor tasks and perfusion patterns, using serial ASL measurements in the early chronic phase after cortical ischemic stroke. We hypothesized that CBF patterns and their dynamics might allow drawing conclusions to precondition of recovery, implicated nodes of specific motor networks and interhemispheric CBF balance. We chose deliberately the time points for imaging at three and nine months in order to control for the duration of recovery processes. In addition, the three month examination should facilitate the comparison with studies dealing with CBF balance [21,22,23,24].

Materials and Methods

Participants

We prospectively recruited patients at two comprehensive stroke centers (Departments of Neurology, University Hospital Bern and Kantonsspital St. Gallen, Switzerland) from January 01th, 2008 through July 31th, 2010. The study received ethical approval from both research centers (Ethikkommission des Kantons St. Gallen (EKSG), Kantonsspital St. Gallen, 9007 St. Gallen and Kantonale Ethikkommission Bern (KEK), 3010Bern, Switzerland) and all participants gave written informed consent before enrollment. Data from this cohort have been previously employed for a lesion analysis study [25]. Inclusion criteria were: (1) first-ever stroke, (2) clinically significant contralesional hand plegia or paresis as a main symptom, and (3) involvement of the pre-and/or postcentral gyri confirmed on diffusion-weighted (DWI) and fluid attenuated inversion recovery (FLAIR) scans. Exclusion criteria were: (1) aphasia or cognitive deficits severe enough to preclude understanding of study purposes, (2) prior cerebrovascular events, (3)

significant stenosis (70–99% according to NASCET) or occlusion of the carotid and intracranial arteries on MR–angiography, (4) purely subcortical stroke, (5) other medical conditions interfering with task performance.

We studied 23 consecutive stroke patients (4 women, age range 41–78 y, mean age $\pm$ SD: 62.7$\pm$11.8 y). As a control group, we recruited 20 healthy participants from the local community (10 women, age range 55–75, mean age$\pm$SD: 63.6$\pm$6.5 y). Groups were matched for age (two-sample t-test: t (41) = 2.4,p<.23) and (premorbid) handedness according to the Edinburgh Handedness Questionnaire (patients: median 82, range 65–100; controls: median 82, range 75–90, Mann-Whitney U-test U=14.5, p< .35). For the patient group, behavioral data were recorded during the first week after stroke (baseline, days post-stroke, mean$\pm$SD: 5.6$\pm$3.6 d), at 3 months (93.2$\pm$8.3 d) and 9 months (277.3$\pm$13.2 d). All patient received neurorehabilitative treatment according to their clinical needs. In addition to the main measurement time-points, monthly control visits with assessment of motor hand function (see below) were performed to ensure appropriate intensity of neurorehabilitative treatment. Controls were tested at two visits separated by one month (29.5$\pm$1.3 d between examinations). ASL imaging was performed at 3 and 9 months post-stroke for patients, and repeated in 10 controls to assess the reliability of CBF measurements.

Behavioral Data

Clinical and motor hand function assessment. Details on measurement procedures can be found in the supplementary materials. Stroke etiologies were classified according to the TOAST criteria [26]. Clinical stroke severity was assessed using the National Institutes of Health Stroke Scale (NIHSS) [27,28]. Hand motor function was assessed with two outcome variables, grip force and dexterity. Grip force was measured by hand dynamometry (HD) with a Jamar Dynamometer [29]. Dexterous hand function was measured using the modified Jebsen-Taylor Test (JTT), a standardized quantitative assessment that consists of five timed subtests that simulate everyday activities [30,31,32]. For our current analysis, we relied on data from the JTT subtest "Picking Small Objects" (PSO), which consists of picking six common objects (2 paper clips, 2 bottle caps, 2 coins) and dropping them into an empty can as fast as possible. As previously shown by our group, PSO explains by far most of the longitudinal variance in JTT scores and allows accurate classification of patient subgroups [25]. The two motor tasks measure complementary aspects of hand motor function. Behaviorally, HD is performed with a simple power grip using the whole hand, whereas PSO necessitates successive precision grips (e.g. characterized by opposition of the thumb against one or two fingers) [33]. Neuroanatomically, each grip form is controlled by different cerebral networks: power grips are mainly controlled by the primary sensorimotor cortices, whereas precision grip control includes the premotor and posterior parietal cortices [34,35].

Imaging Data

Details on acquisition parameters and preprocessing algorithms for all image modalities can be found in supporting information S1. We summarize the main procedures below.

Acquisition. All images were acquired on a 3T Siemens Magnetom Trio (Erlangen, Germany) equipped with a 12-channel radiofrequency head coil. We measured CBF using the pulsed arterial spin labeling (PASL) technique [36,37] and obtained high-resolutionT1-weighted MR images with a 3D Modified Driven Equilibrium Fourier Transform (MDEFT) sequence [38].

Preprocessing. High-resolution anatomical images were normalized to standard Montreal Neuroimaging Institute (MNI) space using an unified normalization-segmentation algorithm, resulting in normalized anatomical image as well as normalized grey matter (GM), white matter and cerebrospinal fluid tissue maps [39]. Binary lesion masks were used to exclude voxels within the lesion from the normalization process to avoid image distortions [40,41]. Raw PASL images were first realigned to reduce movement artifacts. Quantified CBF flow time-series and average CBF maps for the entire acquisition were then calculated [42,43]. Average CBF maps were coregistered to the anatomical image and normalized using the individual normalization parameters derived from the segmentation algorithm. Next, CBF maps were constrained to the GM by masking CBF images with normalized GM partitions that were binarized at a density threshold of 0.2. This empirical value assured that GM density values of at least 68% were included in the GM images. Finally, CBF images were smoothed with a 3D Gaussian kernel of 8×8×8 mm Full-Width at Half Maximum (FWHM) to reduce inter-individual anatomical differences. Before statistical analysis, all images were flipped such that the lesioned hemisphere was on the right. For quality control, we assessed the signal-to-noise ratio and test-retest reliability of CBF measurements for patients and controls before statistical analysis (see supporting information S1).

Statistical analysis

Behavioral data. We used Fisher's exact test for count data. All behavioral variables were tested for normality using the Shapiro-Wilk test. Non-parametric tests were used where appropriate. Motor performance data were converted to z-scores using the mean and standard deviation of corresponding healthy control scores (HD: 36.0±12.0 kg, PSO: 5.9±1.2 s), such that lower z-scores represented lower motor performance. As in our previous work, patients that attained a PSO z-score of >-2.5 (p<.01, one-tailed) at Month 9 were empirically classified as successfully recovered (SR), all others as impaired recovered (IR) [25].

Imaging data. Lesion masks of patient subgroups were summed and binarized such that only voxels lesioned in ≥50% of the patients in each subgroup were retained. For voxel-wise analysis of CBF maps, we first performed a between-group comparison within the framework of the general linear model in SPM8 using a mixed-design analysis of variance (ANOVA) in order to assess the main effect of group (group factor with three levels: one for healthy controls, two for the repeated measurements of stroke patient subgroups at month 3 and month 9). Age and global mean CBF values were included as nuisance covariates. In order to account for stroke severity, all voxel-wise analyses were repeated after adjusting global mean CBF for total lesion volume using linear regression.

The resulting statistical parametric map was thresholded at p< .05, Family-Wise Error (FWE) corrected for multiple comparisons. Post-hoc unpaired t-tests were computed to compare cross-sectional between-group effects (patients at each exam against controls). Finally, paired t-test for longitudinal within-group effects, the main focus of this study, were computed (each patient subgroup separately). T-tests were calculated without equal variance assumptions. The resulting statistical parametric maps were explored using a threshold of p<.001(uncorrected), constrained to a cluster size of ≥ 50voxels. To assess the neuroanatomical distribution of lesions and significant CBF clusters, we used a cytoarchitectonic probabilistic atlas in MNI space (see supporting information S2).

To analyze changes of interhemispheric balance within the sensorimotor network in each subject, we extracted CBF values

from functionally defined cortical regions of interest (ROI) as derived from our previous fMRI studies in healthy volunteers during tactile object manipulation [44,45]. The rationale for doing so was that this task required fine-tuned sensory-guided finger movements, very similar to the PSO test used here to assess dexterous recovery and classify patient subgroups. These ROI included the dorsal premotor cortex (dPMC), supplementary motor area (SMA), paralimbic anterior cingulate cortex (pACC), primary motor cortex (M1), primary somatosensory cortex (S1), intraparietal sulcus (IPS), and superior precuneus (sPRE). Additionally, and ROI of the dorsolateral prefrontal cortex (dlPFC), which also participates in motor execution, was derived from an atlas of resting-state fMRI networks (http://findlab.stanford.edu/functional_ROIs.html). For details on ROI see table S1, supporting information S1. Laterality indices (LI) between hemispheres were calculated according to the standard formula [46]:

$$LI = \frac{(CBF_c - CBF_i)}{(CBF_c + CBF_i)}$$

where c and i denote the contra- and ipsilesional hemisphere, respectively [36]. LI were calculated for each ROI individually, as well as across the whole network (by summing all individual ROI-LI), defined as "sensorimotor LI" throughout the paper.

Results

Behavioral data

According to our classification criterion, 17 patients were classified as SR and 6 as IR. Subgroup characteristics and motor examination results are summarized in Table 1. Proportions of male versus female patients (Fisher's exact test, p = .27, odds ratio [95%CI]: 3.5 [0.2–63.6]), and left versus right sided paresis (Fisher's exact test, p = .62, 0.3 [.01–4.7]) as well as mean age (Welch's t-test, t (41) = 1.4, p = .36) were not statistically different between subgroups. The IR group showed a trend for higher NIHSS scores at Baseline (Wilcoxon rank sum test, W = 21.5, p = .07) and significantly higher scores at month 9 (W = 14, p< .02).

Concerning motor hand function, grip force (as measured by HD) and dexterity (as assessed with PSO) showed markedly different recovery time courses (Figure 1). Grip force between month 3 and month 9 was statistically different for both subgroups (Wilcoxon signed rank test for SR: W = 17, p < 0.01, for IR: W = 0, p<.05), but these changes occurred within the range of healthy control performance (Figure 1, right panel). Dexterity (PSO performance) showed no statistically significant change between examinations (SR: W = 42, p=.19, IR: W = 6, p=.43). SR patients performed at 3 months already within healthy control performance (p = .12), and IR patients remained impaired throughout examinations (both p<.001 versus healthy control performance) (Figure 1, left panel). At month 9 PSO and NIHSS had a significant negative correlation (Spearman's rank correlation, ρ = −0.45, p<0.05), in contrast to HD and NIHSS (ρ = −0.26, p = .22).

Lesion data

Lesion distribution maps of both subgroups are shown in supporting information S2 and quantified using cytoarchitectonic maps in Table 2. Overall, patients in the IR group had a significantly higher lesion volume (Welch's t-test t = 4.1, p<0.02) than SR patients. Moreover, although in both groups the lesion core covered the primary sensorimotor cortices, the IR lesion map affected these areas more extensively, and included a large portion

Table 1. Clinical characteristics of recovery subgroups.

	Successful Recovery(n = 17)			Impaired Recovery(n = 6)		
Gender(M/F)	15/2			4/2		
Affected Hand(L/R)	11/6			5/1		
Etiology (n)*	LA (5), CE (7), OC(1), UN(4)			LA (2), CE (3), OC (1)		
Age(y)	64.2±12.3(41–78)			59.0±10.3 (49–78)		
Lesion volume(cm³)	16.0±21.0 (5.3–23.5)			68.6±37.8 (35.8–121.2)		
	Baseline	*Month 3*	*Month 9*	*Baseline*	*Month 3*	*Month 9*
NIHSS	3.8±1.3	1.6±0.8	0.6±0.8	6.8±3.1	5.0±3.3	3.3±2.7
HD (kg)	21.2±14.1	36.5±11.9	41.9±10.5	2.0±12.5	23.0±17.0	33.2±17.2
HD (z-scores)	−1.2±1.2	0.0±1.0	0.5±0.9	−1.3±1.1	−1.1±1.4	−0.2±1.4
PSO (s)	10.2±9.2	7.4±3.5	6.5±2.0	27.4±14.6	17.1±13.5	10.9±3.3
PSO (z-scores)	−2.9±5.6	−1.2±2.9	−0.5±1.7	−18.3±11.7	−9.3±11.3	−4.1±2.8

Abbreviations: HD, hand dynamometry; NIHSS, National Institutes of Health Stroke scale; PSO, picking small objects. All values are mean ± SD (range), except for gender and affected hand (absolute numbers). *Etiology according to the TOAST criteria: LA, large artery arteriosclerosis; CE, cardioembolism; SO, small-vessel occlusion; OC, other determined cause; UN, undetermined cause.

of the posterior parietal cortex, covering areas of IPS, supramarginal gyrus and parietal operculum. Higher lesion load in IR patients corresponds to our previous observations [25]. Additionally, we quantified lesion load on the cortico-spinal tract (CST) and superior longitudinal fascicle (SLF). Adjusting for total lesion volume, none of them showed a statistically significant difference across groups (both p>.1).

Cross-sectional CBF differences between patients and healthy controls

In the ANOVA model, we identified overall between-group differences almost exclusively in the ipsilesional hemisphere, i.e. in

SMA (Area 6), the lower M1 and S1 (Area 4p and 3b), the secondary somatosensory cortex (SII) and subregions of the inferior parietal cortex. ROI analyses on raw CBF values revealed that the overall differences corresponded to hypoperfusion relative to healthy controls. T-tests between patients and healthy controls at each time point revealed that most differences apparent at month 3 were reversible at month 9. As the results were expected with respect to the lesion topography, this analysis provided a quality control for the evaluation of the longitudinal analysis between IR and SR subgroups (see Fig. S1 and Table S2 in supporting information S2).

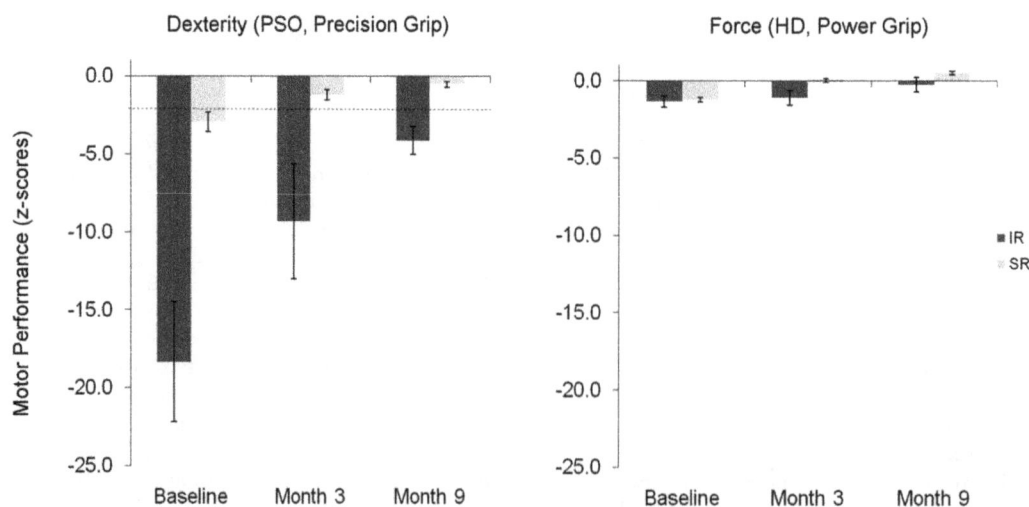

Figure 1. Time course of motor hand function in impaired (IR) and successful recovery (SR) subgroups. Left panel shows the recovery of dexterity, as measured with the picking small objects (PSO) task. The right panel shows the recovery of grip force, as measured with hand dynamometry (HD). Motor performance (y-axis) is given in z-scores task compared to healthy controls (lower scores indicate worse motor performance). Dashed line indicate thresholds for z = −2.5 (p<.01).

Table 2. Affected neuroanatomical areas in the lesion core of patient subgroups.

Anatomical Region	Cytoarchitectonic Area	SR				IR			
		Vol%	x	y	z	Vol%	x	y	z
Lesion core center of gravity			33	−17	44		46	−16	30
Affected areas									
Precentral gyrus	Area 4p	33.9	33	−31	45	80.6	37	−20	44
Postcentral gyrus	Area 3a	19.9	30	−32	48	72.4	32	−30	40
	Area 3b	8.9	41	−21	48	7.0	42	−17	40
	Area 1	0.9	48	−21	55	72.4	50	−19	51
	Area 2	0.1	46	−24	49	56.4	45	−10	43
Intraparietal sulcus	hIP2	0.0	-	-	-	73.9	46	−38	45
Inferior parietal lobule	IPC (PF)	0.0	-	-	-	63.6	51	−17	28
	IPC (PFcm)	0.0	-	-	-	70.8	53	−23	35
	IPC (PFop)	0.0	-	-	-	100	56	−24	30
	IPC (PFt)	0.0	-	-	-	99.7	54	−30	44
Parietal operculum	OP 1	0.0	-	-	-	100.0	53	−26	24
	OP 2	6.9	37	−22	28	100.0	38	−24	21
	OP 3	9.7	39	−19	27	100.0	44	−16	21
	OP 4	0.0	-	-	-	99.9	58	−13	19
Cortico-spinal tract	CST	48.8	33	−16	43	56.5	45	−20	34
Superior longitudinal fascicle	SLF	35.1	30	−21	28	86.2	31	−40	38

Abbreviations: hIP, human intraparietal sulcus; IPC (inferior parietal cortex), OP, operculum. Vol% indicates volume percent of each area covered by the lesion core map of each subgroup. Only areas damaged above 50% of their volume in any of the two groups are shown. Coordinates indicate the center of gravity of the lesion core in MNI space (x/y/z, in mm).

Longitudinal CBF differences in patients with successful and impaired recovery

Voxel-wise comparisons revealed spatially distinct patterns of CBF change between exams and recovery subgroups (Figure 2). SR patients showed significant changes within two extended *contralesional* clusters involving midline motor nodes, i.e. the midline portion of the SMA, pACC and sPRE. Results were not qualitatively different when adjusting for total lesion volume (Fig. S2 in supporting information S3). In contrast, IR patients showed *ipsilesional* clusters of significant CBF change in the caudal portion of the postcentral gyrus, reaching into the inferior parietal lobule. In the SR group, CBF values in contralesional SMA/pACC and sPRE showed a reduction during recovery, whereas CBF values within the ipsilesional postcentral gyrus were unchanged. Conversely, CBF in the IR group remained extremely low in the ipsilesional postcentral gyrus and low in the contralesional midline motor nodes (Table 3). Again in contrast to the SR group, adjustment for total lesion volume lead to a disappearance of these effects, indicating a strong dependence of local CBF on stroke severity in IR patients (Fig. S2 in supporting information S3).

Interhemispheric CBF balance in the sensorimotor network

The time-course of the sensorimotor LI in the patient subgroups and its reproducibility in ten healthy volunteers with repeated ASL is shown in Figure 3. The detailed LIs according to regions and patient subgroups are specified in Fig. S3 in supporting information S3. The sensorimotor LI showed a trend level difference between all subgroups (both patient subgroups and healthy controls) at month 3 (Kruskal-Wallis test, K = 5.6, p = .06), but became significantly different at month 9 (K = 73, p<.05). Closer examination indicated that this occurred due to a significant reversal in laterality in the SR subgroup between time points (Wilcoxon rank sum test, W = 109.5, p<.05), whereas the IR group remained unchanged (W = 15.3, n.s.). The lower panel

of Fig. 3 shows that balance returned to levels comparable to healthy controls in SR patients, whereas persisting imbalance is evident in the IR subgroup. Given the strong relationship between CBF and total lesion volume in this subgroup (see above), we further tested for a correlation between sensorimotor LI at 3 and 9 months and lesion volume. Rank correlation indeed revealed a significant dependence of the sensorimotor LI on stroke size in the IR subgroup (at 3 months: ρ = .78, p<.04, at 9 months: ρ = .81, p<.04), which was absent in SR patients (at 3 months: ρ = −.11, p<.45 at 9 months: ρ = −.29, p<.25). This indicates that above a given level of ischemic damage the capacity to re-balance interhemispheric CBF within the sensorimotor network was abolished in our cohort, impeding successful recovery.

Discussion

This is a longitudinal study of a selected cohort of first-ever stroke patients with ischemic lesions involving the primary sensorimotor cortices, without connected upstream artery stenosis. All patients were examined at precisely defined time points post-stroke after 3 and 9 months. At this stage we observed a clinically dichotomized recovery, i.e.: i.) subjects who recovered mainly motor hand skill requiring precision grip in comparison with healthy volunteers (SR) and ii.) subjects retaining a significant chronic deficit in this regard (IR). Group differences were characterized exclusively by deficient precision grip, but not by power grip. Between groups, we verified simultaneously discordant courses of longitudinal CBF.

Apart from the primary sensorimotor cortex as a common denominator, the structural lesions in the IR-subgroup were more extended and involved the posterior parietal cortex, preferentially intraparietal sulcus, inferior parietal lobule and parietal operculum. Hypoperfused areas were located in this subgroup around the core lesion in the postcentral and supramarginal gyrus and persisted during the observation period. Similar reductions of

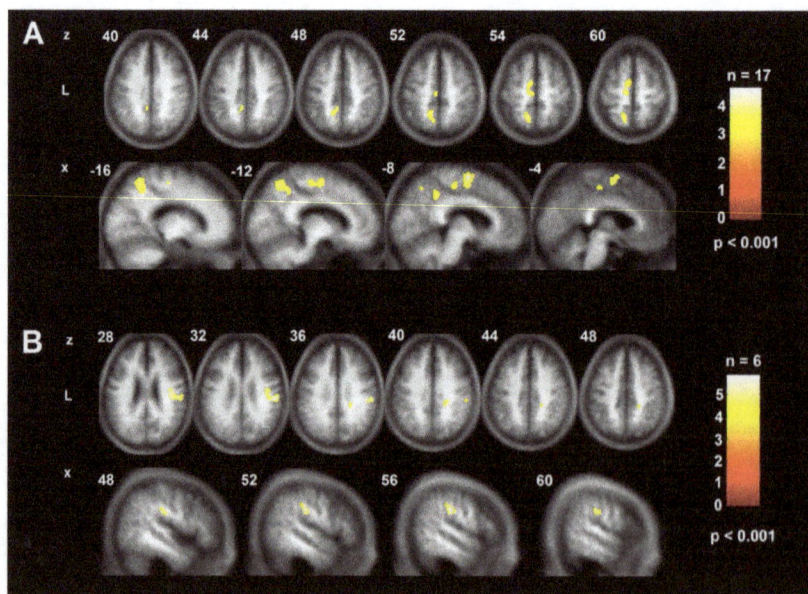

Figure 2. Longitudinal CBF differences between three and nine months for patients with successful and impaired recovery. A longitudinal decrease in supplementary motor area, paralimbic anterior cingulate cortex and superior precuneus is apparent in the SR group (panel A); whereas chronic sustained hypoperfusion in postcentral and supramarginal gyrus is found in the IR group (panel B). Maps are projected onto axial (z) and sagittal (x) slices of an average anatomical image of the complete patient cohort in neurological convention (L, left). The affected hemisphere is on the right side. Coordinates are given in MNI space (mm).

Table 3. Longitudinal changes of CBF in patient subgroups between 3 and 9 months.

Anatomical region	Cytoarchitectonic area (Vol%)*	x	y	z	Size	SR CBF Month 3	SR CBF Month 9	IR CBF Month 3	IR CBF Month 9	HC CBF
Contralesional Clusters										
Supplementary Motor Area Paralimbic Anterior Cingulate Cortex	Area6(87.1) n. a.	-9 -2	0 61	46	589	61.5±12.1	48.7±11.2	37.7±13.2	36.4±8.7	64.6±22.1
Superior Precuneus	SPL7A(67.8)	-13	-57	54	237	47.6±12.5	34.8±17.8	36.81±11.1	39.91±10.6	50.1±18.6
Ipsilesional Cluster										
Inferior parietal lobule Postcentral gyrus	IPC(PFt)(21.4) Area3b(12.5)	54	-37	30	688	43.96±12.07	40.35±10.76	25.8±23.6	25.4±20.2	48.3±13.6

Abbreviations: CBF, cerebral blood flow (values are mean ± SD in ml/100 mg/min.); HC, healthy controls; n.a., not available. *Percent of cluster on each area.

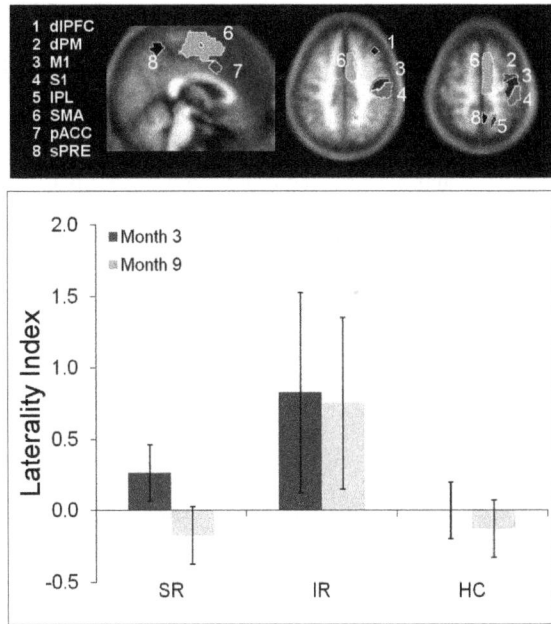

Figure 3. Longitudinal changes in sensorimotor laterality index in patient subgroups and healthy controls. Upper panel shows the set of regions-of-interest that defines the motor network. Only right hemispheric regions are shown for clarity. Lower panel shows sensorimotor laterality indices (LI) according to the defined network for patient subgroups and healthy controls at both examinations (for patients, Exam 1 denotes measurement at three months, Exam 2 nine months. For healthy controls, both examinations were one month apart). Positive values indicate contralesional lateralization. Note reversion of sensorimotor LI to lesioned hemisphere between examinations at 3 and 9 months for the successful recovered (SR) patients, whereas a persistent lateralization to the contralesional hemisphere is evident in impaired recovered (IR) patients. Healthy controls (HC) remain balanced. Bars indicate mean ±95% confidence intervals.

perilesional CBF levels that are correlated with infarct size have already been reported in chronic stroke patients using ASL, indicating sustained hypoperfusion in the affected sensorimotor cortex [47]. In contrast, lesions in the SR subgroup were rather localized to the primary sensorimotor cortex and hypoperfusion had resolved in the stroke-affected hemisphere. However, significant reductions of CBF in the contralesional hemisphere along the evaluated time period could be identified within medially located nodes of the specific sensorimotor network: i.e. in the SMA, pACC and sPRE. Considering longitudinal CBF changes according to these subgroups, the preconditions of a double dissociation are fulfilled [51]: The IR-subgroup differed by an unchanged severe reduction of CBF between month 3 and 9 in the perilesional cortex, whereas SR-subgroup showed a significant reduction of CBF at month 9 confined to medial motor areas of the contralesional hemisphere. Overall, our data confirm the importance of restoring CBF in critical cortical network nodes for successful recovery of specific functions, as recently shown using ROI-analysis of MR-perfusion data in patients with cortical and subcortical stroke-associated aphasia [48,49] and hemispatial neglect [50].

Laterality indices within the sensorimotor network

There are few systematic studies on the subject of contrasting CBF-changes in both hemispheres after stroke, i.e. by the analysis of laterality indices, LIs [21,22,23,24,51]. Calautti et al. refined the computation of Cramer at al. by calculating a weighted LI of fMRI BOLD-response reflecting the changed bilateral distribution of activation fields evoked after motor stimulation of the recovered hand in the early chronic stage after a subcortical ischemic stroke. There were statistically significant correlations between maximum finger tapping and the LI for M1 and S1 after recovery. Marshall and coworkers computed LIs using fMRI and BOLD-response in subcortical ischemic stroke lesions during the immediate post-stroke and at early chronic stage, 3 to 6 months after stroke. They observed an evolution of activation in the sensorimotor cortex from early contralesional activity to late ipsilesional activity during movement of the paretic hand following regained function. Both studies admit only indirect inferences for CBF analysis, since they were possibly confounded by the influence of complex interhemi-spheric neuronal interactions of mutual interhemispheric inhibi-tion, by disinhibition and the relativity of the BOLD signal [1]. BOLD responses are dependent on the severity of motor impairment as well as on CBF decreases at rest. Thus, task-related increases of the BOLD signal fMRI studies during recovery, as well as their reductions to physiological levels after 6–12 months may be partially addressed to CBF changes. Overall, longitudinal normalization of the BOLD signal is associated with good outcome [4,52,53,54].

We complemented these studies in several regards: i.) evaluation in cortical strokes with a common, overlapping lesion site in the primary motor and sensory cortices, ii.) examination at rest, iii.) unbiased quantification of CBF by ASL instead of relative BOLD signal changes and iv.) analysis in cortical nodes of specific sensorimotor networks as previously identified by a sensorimotor fMRI activation study [44]. In healthy controls there was reproducible, stable balance within narrow margins over time within the nodes of sensorimotor circuits. Patients revealed a considerable variance of laterality indices across the time span. In the IR-subgroup the sensorimotor LI remained unchanged and shifted to the contralesional hemisphere. In the SR-subgroup the sensorimotor LI indicated a significant reversion to the lesioned hemisphere while the mean CBF decreased in the contralesional medial motor nodes. The crucial observation of an augmentative CBF dynamic is thus recognizable only in the SR-group: Changes of CBF and associated LIs may reflect ongoing neuronal reorganization associated with recovery. These findings support the significance of the image analysis as the areas of decreased CBF in both subgroups have been shown to be part of the constituents of sensorimotor networks distributed over both hemispheres. In contrast, the more extensive lesions with sustained poor perfusion, as exemplified by the IR-subgroup, seem to hinder the restitution of favorable interhemispheric balance. Indeed, the strong positive correlations between contralesional CBF shift (positive LI) and lesion volume in the IR subgroup indicate that above a certain threshold of ischemic damage longitudinal CBF adjustments cannot occur any longer. Interestingly, loss of interhemispheric CBF dynamics within the sensorimotor network does not preclude substantial gains in motor performance during recovery in the IR group (see Figure 1), but rather seems to provide an upper bound to motor performance. One explanation for this apparent paradox might be the recruitment of additional neural circuits that might provide compensatory, but coarse and ineffective behavioral output. Indeed, we have recently shown that extensive grey matter remodeling occurs in subcortical and cortical nodes of a basal ganglia-dorsolateral prefrontal network in IR-type patients, i. e. outside the "canonical" cortical motor loop, and the relationship between this phenomenon and CBF lateralization remains to be explored [55].

Functional implications

Dynamic changes of CBF in the contralesional medial motor nodes of SR patients might represent a set point adjustment to reinstate interhemispheric balance with homologous motor nodes of the primarily lesioned hemisphere. This might be paralleled by diminished recruitment of these structures in the contralesional hemisphere, which in part subserve focused attention and motor execution [2,11]. In this respect the pACC, a structure connected also to the dorsolateral prefrontal cortex, plays an important role in monitoring motor control, sensory perception, cognitive function and attention [56,57]. The superior precuneus cluster identified in our study lies ventral to the superior parietal sulcus just above the subparietal sulcus. It has bilateral and reciprocal cortico-cortical connections with the adjacent posteromedial cortex, providing an anatomical basis for their functional coupling [58]. Beyond the parietal lobe, extensive connections exist between the superior precuneus and the dorsal premotor area, the supplementary motor area (SMA) and the anterior cingulate cortex [59,60]. The posteromedial parietal cortex acts with the lateral parietal areas in elaborating information about egocentric spatial relations for body movement control (motor imagery), voluntary attention shift and mental imagery tasks. The lateral aspect of the posterior parietal cortex, the posterior parietal lobe and inferior posterior lobule are involved in controlling spatial aspects of motor behavior, e.g. during sensory guided finger movements [61]. By virtue of its connectivity, the superior precuneus is involved into the execution or preparation of spatially guided motor behavior, such as pointing and reaching, and in particular in coordination of both upper limbs during task execution [62]. Interestingly, a study by Marshall et al. has recently shown that early BOLD activity in precuneus and posterior parietal cortex during hand movements might be predictive for later recovery [46].

Limitations

A few limitations must be kept in mind when interpreting our results. Sample sizes are small, especially for the IR subgroup, and thus generalization is difficult based on our results. However, this subgroup represents in our view an interesting and generally underrepresented subset in CBF studies, exhibiting hypoperfusion in the absence of (significant) arterial stenosis. The clarification of its underlying pathophysiological mechanisms remains a challenge for future studies of this peculiar association [47]. One methodical limitation to consider is that CBF quantification was done under the assumption that T1 relaxation of blood be constant over the whole brain. This is clearly an oversimplification which might cause biased CBF estimates in lesioned brain areas. We therefore included explicit lesion masks during CBF reconstruction to mitigate this bias. Also, the ASL sequence we used does not cover the cerebellum, and thus, we could not evaluate the well-known diaschisis effects and its role for recovery [63]. Furthermore, conclusions from ASL studies allow no direct comparison with activation studies performed with BOLD fMRI [47].

Conclusions

ASL measurements during rest are capable to delineate subtle CBF-changes within nodes of specific large scale networks during the early chronic phase after a sensorimotor stroke. Such changes related to hand motor skill as shown by voxel-based analysis may exhibit an asymmetric pattern due to interhemispheric imbalance. Reversion of the laterality indices underlying this pattern in favor of the lesioned hemisphere goes along with recovery. Of note, the time course of recovery processes, clearly outlasts the first three months post stroke, indicating that not only acute [64,65], but also early and late chronic measurements of cerebral hemodynamics are important to understand stroke recovery. The data provide us with a method to monitor recovery of specific motor hand functions and to evaluate the interrelation between chronic sustained hypoperfusion, infarct size and BOLD response.

Supporting Information

Supporting Information S1 Contains supplementary methods. These include a description of the behavioral testing procedures, the MR data acquisition and processing and magnetic resonance image acquisition parameters.

Acknowledgments

We thank our patients and their caregivers for participating in our study.

Author Contributions

Conceived and designed the experiments: RW EA AF BW. Performed the experiments: EA. Analyzed the data: RW EA JM BW AF. Contributed reagents/materials/analysis tools: CH GS MS DJJW. Contributed to the writing of the manuscript: RW EA JM BW AF DJJW.

References

1. Rehme AK, Grefkes C (2013) Cerebral network disorders after stroke: evidence from imaging-based connectivity analyses of active and resting brain states in humans. J Physiol 591: 17–31.
2. Grefkes C, Nowak DA, Eickhoff SB, Dafotakis M, Kust J, et al. (2008) Cortical connectivity after subcortical stroke assessed with functional magnetic resonance imaging. Ann Neurol 63: 236–246.
3. Mosier K, Lau C, Wang Y, Venkadesan M, Valero-Cuevas FJ (2011) Controlling instabilities in manipulation requires specific cortical-striatal-cerebellar networks. J Neurophysiol 105: 1295–1305.
4. Rehme AK, Fink GR, von Cramon DY, Grefkes C (2011) The role of the contralesional motor cortex for motor recovery in the early days after stroke assessed with longitudinal FMRI. Cereb Cortex 21: 756–768.
5. Ward NS, Brown MM, Thompson AJ, Frackowiak RS (2003) Neural correlates of motor recovery after stroke: a longitudinal fMRI study. Brain 126: 2476–2496.
6. Ward NS, Brown MM, Thompson AJ, Frackowiak RS (2003) Neural correlates of outcome after stroke: a cross-sectional fMRI study. Brain 126: 1430–1448.
7. Wang L, Yu C, Chen H, Qin W, He Y, et al. (2010) Dynamic functional reorganization of the motor execution network after stroke. Brain 133: 1224–1238.
8. Inman CS, James GA, Hamann S, Rajendra JK, Pagnoni G, et al. (2012) Altered resting-state effective connectivity of fronto-parietal motor control systems on the primary motor network following stroke. Neuroimage 59: 227–237.
9. Park CH, Chang WH, Ohn SH, Kim ST, Bang OY, et al. (2011) Longitudinal changes of resting-state functional connectivity during motor recovery after stroke. Stroke 42: 1357–1362.
10. Fox MD, Raichle ME (2007) Spontaneous fluctuations in brain activity observed with functional magnetic resonance imaging. Nat Rev Neurosci 8: 700–711.
11. Carter AR, Astafiev SV, Lang CE, Connor LT, Rengachary J, et al. (2010) Resting interhemispheric functional magnetic resonance imaging connectivity predicts performance after stroke. Ann Neurol 67: 365–375.
12. Fan F, Zhu C, Chen H, Qin W, Ji X, et al. (2013) Dynamic brain structural changes after left hemisphere subcortical stroke. Hum Brain Mapp 34: 1872–1881.
13. Lee MH, Smyser CD, Shimony JS (2013) Resting-state fMRI: a review of methods and clinical applications. AJNR Am J Neuroradiol 34: 1866–1872.
14. Wang J, Aguirre GK, Kimberg DY, Roc AC, Li L, et al. (2003) Arterial spin labeling perfusion fMRI with very low task frequency. Magn Reson Med 49: 796–802.
15. Wang J, Alsop DC, Li L, Listerud J, Gonzalez-At JB, et al. (2002) Comparison of quantitative perfusion imaging using arterial spin labeling at 1.5 and 4.0 Tesla. Magn Reson Med 48: 242–254.
16. Detre JA, Wang J, Wang Z, Rao H (2009) Arterial spin-labeled perfusion MRI in basic and clinical neuroscience. Curr Opin Neurol 22: 348–355.
17. Hendrikse J, Petersen ET, Golay X (2012) Vascular disorders: insights from arterial spin labeling. Neuroimaging Clin N Am 22: 259–269, x-xi.
18. Alsop DC, Detre JA, Golay X, Gunther M, Hendrikse J, et al. (2014) Recommended implementation of arterial spin-labeled perfusion MRI for clinical applications: A consensus of the ISMRM perfusion study group and the European consortium for ASL in dementia. Magn Reson Med.
19. Donahue MJ, Hussey E, Rane S, Wilson T, van Osch M, et al. (2014) Vessel-encoded arterial spin labeling (VE-ASL) reveals elevated flow territory asymmetry in older adults with substandard verbal memory performance. J Magn Reson Imaging 39: 377–386.

20. Bokkers RP, Hernandez DA, Merino JG, Mirasol RV, van Osch MJ, et al. (2012) Whole-brain arterial spin labeling perfusion MRI in patients with acute stroke. Stroke 43: 1290–1294.
21. Calautti C, Naccarato M, Jones PS, Sharma N, Day DD, et al. (2007) The relationship between motor deficit and hemisphere activation balance after stroke: A 3T fMRI study. Neuroimage 34: 322–331.
22. Marshall RS, Perera GM, Lazar RM, Krakauer JW, Constantine RC, et al. (2000) Evolution of cortical activation during recovery from corticospinal tract infarction. Stroke 31: 656–661.
23. Nhan H, Barquist K, Bell K, Esselman P, Odderson IR, et al. (2004) Brain function early after stroke in relation to subsequent recovery. J Cereb Blood Flow Metab 24: 756–763.
24. Ward NS, Brown MM, Thompson AJ, Frackowiak RS (2004) The influence of time after stroke on brain activations during a motor task. Ann Neurol 55: 829–834.
25. Abela E, Missimer J, Wiest R, Federspiel A, Hess C, et al. (2012) Lesions to primary sensory and posterior parietal cortices impair recovery from hand paresis after stroke. PLoS One 7: e31275.
26. Adams HP Jr, Bendixen BH, Kappelle LJ, Biller J, Love BB, et al. (1993) Classification of subtype of acute ischemic stroke. Definitions for use in a multicenter clinical trial. TOAST. Trial of Org 10172 in Acute Stroke Treatment. Stroke 24: 35–41.
27. Lyden P, Lu M, Jackson C, Marler J, Kothari R, et al. (1999) Underlying structure of the National Institutes of Health Stroke Scale: results of a factor analysis. NINDS tPA Stroke Trial Investigators. Stroke 30: 2347–2354.
28. Lyden PD, Hantson L (1998) Assessment scales for the evaluation of stroke patients. J Stroke Cerebrovasc Dis 7: 113–127.
29. Mathiowetz V, Weber K, Volland G, Kashman N (1984) Reliability and validity of grip and pinch strength evaluations. J Hand Surg Am 9: 222–226.
30. Jebsen RH, Griffith ER, Long EW, Fowler R (1971) Function of "normal" hand in stroke patients. Arch Phys Med Rehabil 52: 170–174 passim.
31. Jebsen RH, Taylor N, Trieschmann RB, Trotter MJ, Howard LA (1969) An objective and standardized test of hand function. Arch Phys Med Rehabil 50: 311–319.
32. Stern EB (1992) Stability of the Jebsen-Taylor Hand Function Test across three test sessions. Am J Occup Ther 46: 647–649.
33. Castiello U (2005) The neuroscience of grasping. Nat Rev Neurosci 6: 726–736.
34. Binkofski F, Buccino G (2004) Motor functions of the Broca's region. Brain Lang 89: 362–369.
35. Ehrsson HH, Fagergren E, Forssberg H (2001) Differential fronto-parietal activation depending on force used in a precision grip task: an fMRI study. J Neurophysiol 85: 2613–2623.
36. Wu WC, Fernandez-Seara M, Detre JA, Wehrli FW, Wang J (2007) A theoretical and experimental investigation of the tagging efficiency of pseudocontinuous arterial spin labeling. Magn Reson Med 58: 1020–1027.
37. Dai W, Garcia D, de Bazelaire C, Alsop DC (2008) Continuous flow-driven inversion for arterial spin labeling using pulsed radio frequency and gradient fields. Magn Reson Med 60: 1488–1497.
38. Deichmann R, Schwarzbauer C, Turner R (2004) Optimisation of the 3D MDEFT sequence for anatomical brain imaging: technical implications at 1.5 and 3 T. Neuroimage 21: 757–767.
39. Ashburner J, Friston KJ (2005) Unified segmentation. Neuroimage 26: 839–851.
40. Andersen SM, Rapcsak SZ, Beeson PM (2010) Cost function masking during normalization of brains with focal lesions: still a necessity? Neuroimage 53: 78–84.
41. Brett M, Leff AP, Rorden C, Ashburner J (2001) Spatial normalization of brain images with focal lesions using cost function masking. Neuroimage 14: 486–500.

42. Wang J, Alsop DC, Song HK, Maldjian JA, Tang K, et al. (2003) Arterial transit time imaging with flow encoding arterial spin tagging (FEAST). Magn Reson Med 50: 599–607.

43. Federspiel A, Muller TJ, Horn H, Kiefer C, Strik WK (2006) Comparison of spatial and temporal pattern for fMRI obtained with BOLD and arterial spin labeling. J Neural Transm 113: 1403–1415.

44. Kagi G, Missimer JH, Abela E, Seitz RJ, Weder BJ (2010) Neural networks engaged in tactile object manipulation: patterns of expression among healthy individuals. Behav Brain Funct 6: 71.

45. Hartmann S, Missimer JH, Stoeckel C, Abela E, Shah J, et al. (2008) Functional connectivity in tactile object discrimination: a principal component analysis of an event related fMRI-Study. PLoS One 3: e3831.

46. Marshall RS, Zarahn E, Alon L, Minzer B, Lazar RM, et al. (2009) Early imaging correlates of subsequent motor recovery after stroke. Ann Neurol 65: 596–602.

47. Richardson JD, Baker JM, Morgan PS, Rorden C, Bonilha L, et al. (2011) Cerebral perfusion in chronic stroke: implications for lesion-symptom mapping and functional MRI. Behav Neurol 24: 117–122.

48. Hillis AE, Kleinman JT, Newhart M, Heidler-Gary J, Gottesman R, et al. (2006) Restoring cerebral blood flow reveals neural regions critical for naming. J Neurosci 26: 8069–8073.

49. Hillis AE, Barker PB, Wityk RJ, Aldrich EM, Restrepo L, et al. (2004) Variability in subcortical aphasia is due to variable sites of cortical hypoperfusion. Brain Lang 89: 524–530.

50. Khurshid S, Trupe LA, Newhart M, Davis C, Molitoris JJ, et al. (2012) Reperfusion of specific cortical areas is associated with improvement in distinct forms of hemispatial neglect. Cortex 48: 530–539.

51. Cramer SC, Nelles G, Benson RR, Kaplan JD, Parker RA, et al. (1997) A functional MRI study of subjects recovered from hemiparetic stroke. Stroke 28: 2518–2527.

52. Calautti C, Leroy F, Guincestre JY, Marie RM, Baron JC (2001) Sequential activation brain mapping after subcortical stroke: changes in hemispheric balance and recovery. Neuroreport 12: 3883–3886.

53. Seifritz E, Bilecen D, Hanggi D, Haselhorst R, Radu EW, et al. (2000) Effect of ethanol on BOLD response to acoustic stimulation: implications for neuropharmacological fMRI. Psychiatry Res 99: 1–13.

54. Enzinger C, Johansen-Berg H, Dawes H, Bogdanovic M, Collett J, et al. (2008) Functional MRI correlates of lower limb function in stroke victims with gait impairment. Stroke 39: 1507–1513.

55. Abela E, Seiler A, Missimer JH, Federspiel A, Hess CW, et al. (2014) Grey matter volumetric changes related to recovery from hand paresis after cortical sensorimotor stroke. Brain Struct Funct.

56. Paus T, Castro-Alamancos MA, Petrides M (2001) Cortico-cortical connectivity of the human mid-dorsolateral frontal cortex and its modulation by repetitive transcranial magnetic stimulation. Eur J Neurosci 14: 1405–1411.

57. Seitz RJ, Roland E, Bohm C, Greitz T, Stone-Elander S (1990) Motor learning in man: a positron emission tomographic study. Neuroreport 1: 57–60.

58. Cavanna AE, Trimble MR (2006) The precuneus: a review of its functional anatomy and behavioural correlates. Brain 129: 564–583.

59. Goldman-Rakic PS (1988) Topography of cognition: parallel distributed networks in primate association cortex. Annu Rev Neurosci 11: 137–156.

60. Leichnetz GR (2001) Connections of the medial posterior parietal cortex (area 7m) in the monkey. Anat Rec 263: 215–236.

61. Seitz RJ, Binkofski F (2003) Modular organization of parietal lobe functions as revealed by functional activation studies. Adv Neurol 93: 281–292.

62. Wenderoth N, Debaere F, Sunaert S, Swinnen SP (2005) The role of anterior cingulate cortex and precuneus in the coordination of motor behaviour. Eur J Neurosci 22: 235–246.

63. Infeld B, Davis SM, Lichtenstein M, Mitchell PJ, Hopper JL (1995) Crossed cerebellar diaschisis and brain recovery after stroke. Stroke 26: 90–95.

64. Matteis M, Vernieri F, Troisi E, Pasqualetti P, Tibuzzi F, et al. (2003) Early cerebral hemodynamic changes during passive movements and motor recovery after stroke. J Neurol 250: 810–817.

65. Silvestrini M, Troisi E, Matteis M, Razzano C, Caltagirone C (1998) Correlations of flow velocity changes during mental activity and recovery from aphasia in ischemic stroke. Neurology 50: 191–195.

13

The Influence of Very Low Illumination on the Postural Sway of Young and Elderly Adults

Darja Rugelj[1]*, **Gregor Gomišček**[1,2], **France Sevšek**[1]

1 Biomechanical Laboratory, Faculty of Health Sciences, University of Ljubljana, Ljubljana, Slovenia, **2** Institute for Biophysics, Medical Faculty, University of Ljubljana, Ljubljana, Slovenia

Abstract

The purpose of the present study was to evaluate the influence of very low ambient illumination and complete darkness on the postural sway of young and elderly adults. Eighteen healthy young participants aged 23.8±1.5 years and 26 community-dwelling elderly aged 69.8±5.6 years were studied. Each participant performed four tests while standing on a force platform in the following conditions: in normal light (215 lx) with open eyes and with closed eyes, in very low illumination (0.25 lx) with open eyes, and in complete darkness with open eyes. The sequences of the tests in the altered visual conditions were determined by random blocs. Postural sway was assessed by means of the force platform measurements. The centre of pressure variables: the medio-lateral and antero-posterior path lengths, mean velocities, sway areas, and fractal dimensions were analysed. Very low illumination resulted in a statistically significant increase in postural sway in both the young and elderly groups compared to normal light, although the increase was significantly smaller than those observed in the eyes closed and complete darkness condition, and no significant effects of illumination on fractal dimensions were detected. The gains of the sways in the very low or no illumination conditions relative to the normal light condition were significantly larger in the group of young participants than in the group of elderly participants (up to 50% and 25%, respectively). However, the response patterns to changes in illumination were similar in the young and elderly participants, with the exception of the short-range fractal dimension of the medio-lateral sway. In conclusion, very low illumination resulted in increased postural sway compared to normal illumination; however, in the closed eye and complete darkness conditions, postural sway was significantly higher than in the very low illumination condition regardless of the age of the participants.

Editor: Ramesh Balasubramaniam, University of California, Merced, United States of America

Funding: No external sources of funding were received. The trial was supported by the existing resources of the Faculty of Health Sciences at University of Ljubljana. The funders had no role in study design, data collection and analysis, decision to publish, or preparation of the manuscript.

Competing Interests: The authors have declared that no competing interests exist.

* Email: darja.rugelj@zf.uni-lj.si

Introduction

The human balance control system depends on important resources, such as cognitive processing, biomechanical constrains, age, and movement strategies [1], and is based on feedback from the somatosensory, vestibular and visual systems. The effect of the absence of visual information on balance can be assessed by the time for which a person is able to stand with their eyes closed [2] and can be measured as changes in postural steadiness via stabilometry [3,4]. It has often been reported that, without visual information, postural steadiness significantly decreases [3,4,5,6,7]. This phenomenon has been documented in both young and older persons [7,8], and postural sway is typically larger in elderly persons than in middle-aged and young persons [9,10,11,8]. Dark environments thus affect adults in all age groups, although the effect is smaller in young adults than in middle-aged adults [12], and elderly persons are the most destabilised in conditions with no vision [12,13,11,8].

However, different functional situations are present in environments with low and very low illumination. Such environments are commonly met indoors, for example, in corridors or in bedrooms and bathrooms at night [14]. These areas are considered to present the highest risk of falls for elderly people; it is estimated that approximately 20 to 55 per cent of all falls occur at home at night among the population that is 65 years or older [7,15]. One of the possible reasons for this estimate is the fact that older people tend to rely more on the visual information for the postural stabilisation, and this effect increases with age [10]. Additionally, changes in the sensory context require a person to re-weight sensory flow to maintain stability [1]. Very low illumination is an example of such an environmental context in which sensory re-weighting is required. Subliminal pathologies and age-related changes in the somatosensory systems, including vision [11], contribute to decreased postural steadiness in the elderly. Individuals with specific sensory loss are therefore limited in their abilities to re-weight postural sensory dependence and are thus at higher risks of falling in particular sensory context [1]. It has been shown that the postural response of the elderly to low illumination can increase the risk for instability and falls [16]. Low levels of illumination and the optical patterns associated with specific surface layouts (e.g., escalators) have been identified as environmental factors that have detrimental effects on older people's postural controls [6]. The rate of falls in elderly adults with poor vision is markedly higher than that among the elderly with normal vision [17].

There is no agreement between the studies that have investigated the influence of reduced levels of the ambient illumination on postural steadiness. Low illumination (between 1 and 3 lx) has been determined to have no influence on postural sway in a group of 9–10 year-old school children [18,19]. However, for elderly populations, the reported results regarding the influence of very low ambient illumination are conflicting. Some authors have reported increases in postural sway in environments with very low illumination compared to those with normal illumination [3,6,13], while others were unable to find any significant increase in postural sway [20].

A review of the current and past literature did not identify any study that compared the responses to closed eyes, very low illumination and complete darkness between young and elderly persons. The early studies of the influences of various illumination conditions, including complete darkness, that were performed by Edwards [3] revealed, for example, a strong dependency on visual information input and the amount of illumination. However, this author did not allow the participants time to adapt to the transitions between different illumination conditions. Therefore, the results of this author might partially be attributable to the adaptation process, which has been found to last up to 30 seconds and to affect postural stability [7].

Thus, the main purpose of the present study was to investigate the effects of different levels of illumination on postural steadiness. Furthermore, we studied and compared these effects between a group of young and a group of elderly participants. To address these effects, we measured postural sway in four different experimental conditions: normal light with eyes open, normal light with closed eyes, very low illumination (dim light), and complete darkness with eyes open. We hypothesised that very low levels of illumination would affect postural stability and increase postural sway. We also hypothesised that younger participants would be less affected by changes in illumination (i.e., very low illumination) than would the older participants.

Methods

1 Participants

The forty-four adults that participated in this study included 18 young healthy participants (12 female and 6 male) and 26 elderly community-dwelling participants (20 female and 6 male). The details of the participants are presented in Table 1. The exclusion criteria were the use of any medication known to compromise balance, diabetes, impaired vision and injuries to the lower extremities or spine. The participants were also required to express no fear of darkness or of small spaces (e.g., elevators). The study was approved by Slovenian National Medical Ethic Committee. Prior to any measurements, all participants read information about the test protocol, received additional verbal explanations when required and provided written informed consent.

2 Experimental procedure

Each participant underwent five consecutive measurements, each of which lasted 70 seconds. During each measurement, the participant was instructed to stand as still as possible while barefoot and with their feet close together on the force platform, while their hands were hanging relaxed, and their gaze was focused on a dot that was pasted to the wall. During the first trial (1) in the normal lighting conditions (215 lx), the participant's eyes were open. The following three trials were characterised as follows: (2) normal lighting conditions with closed eyes (215 lx), (3) a very low level of illumination (dim light) (0.25 lx) with open eyes, and (4) complete darkness with open eyes. The sequences of the trials with the altered visual conditions (trials 2, 3 and 4) were randomised by using random blocks.

In the trials in the normal lighting conditions with closed eyes, the participants were told to keep their eyes closed, and this requirement was additionally enforced by covering the eyes with opaque night glasses. In the very low level of illumination trials, the assistant turned off the main light, turned on the dimmed light, and let the participant adapt to the new lightening conditions for 30 seconds. The same procedure was followed for the complete darkness with open eye trials with the exception of turning the dim light on.

3 Illumination

The room was illuminated either by a regular ceiling lamp or by a desk lamp. The illumination of the desk lamp was adjustable via voltage regulation with a transformer (ISKRA TRN, Slovenia). The illuminance was determined with a luxmeter (Luxmeter Testo 545 Lux, Fc Germany) that was placed at the gaze fixation point on the wall. Because the lowest illuminance levels at the gaze fixation point were close or below the detection level of the luxmeter, these levels were determined based on illuminance measurements taken from a selected position in close proximity to the desk lamp. To determine the illuminance values in this experimental condition, the correlation between the two luminance values was determined at higher levels of illuminance and extrapolated to the experimental conditions. Thus, illuminance below the detection limit of the luxmeter and more precise determinations at levels close to the detection limit at the gaze fixation point of the participant were possible.

3.1 Illumination characteristics. The characteristics of illumination of the room, i.e., increases, stability and magnitude, were determined by measuring the illuminance in close proximity to the desk lamp during the first 5 minutes after the lamp was turned on. These measurements were performed at 5-second intervals during the first 100 seconds and at 30-second intervals thereafter. The variability in the room illumination measurements was below 1%. Thus, the room illumination was determined to have good temporal stability, and no significant time dependency was noticeable over the time interval of 70 seconds. The final illuminance value had already been reached in the first 5 seconds.

4 Instrumentation and data processing

Stabilometry was used to assess the amount of postural sway during upright quiet standing. The centre of pressure (CoP) movement position data were collected at a 50 Hz sampling rate using a portable force platform (Kistler 9286 AA, Winthertur, Switzerland). The raw data were stored on the disk of a PC-type computer using Kistler's BioWare program. The data were later uploaded to a server running the Linux (Fedora 18) operating system. Data analysis was performed with a web-based software that was specially developed for the stabilometric measurements in our laboratory [21]. After smoothing the acquired CoP positions with Gaussian averaging over 3 adjacent points, the first 10 seconds of each data series were excluded, and the remaining 60 seconds of the data series were used for the analysis. We excluded the first 10 seconds from the analysis to eliminate the possible consequences of the transitions between different illumination conditions and to avoid the transition between stepping on the force plate and steady standing [22,13,23]. From the resulting data, the time domain and fractal measures were calculated. A number of measures in both domains have been used to investigate postural steadiness in response to changing illuminance levels. In the time domain these measures are the mean values and standard deviations of the CoP displacements and velocities and the total path length, and the lengths of the medio-lateral and antero-posterior CoP movements. Additionally, the area and the outline

Table 1. Descriptive data for the participants in the study.

	Number of participants	Mean ± SD	Minimum	Maximum
Age (years)				
Young	18	23.8±1.5	22	26
Elderly	26	69.8±5.6	60	82
Body mass (kg)				
Young	18	66.3±11.6	45	88
Elderly	26	72.3±13.5	49	105
Body height (cm)				
Young	18	169.9±0.1	155	181
Elderly	26	163.9±0.1	155	180

shape of the measured stabilogram were determined, and the fractal dimensions were calculated from the time series of the CoP movements.

The procedures to determine the spatiotemporal parameters of the stabilogram and the outline and sway area have been described elsewhere [24]. Briefly, the antero-posterior (AP) and medio-lateral (ML) path lengths were calculated from the measured time series of the COP positions Y_i and X_i as follows:

$$PathAP = \sum_{i=1}^{N-1} |(Y_{i+1} - Y_i)| \text{ and } PathML = \sum_{i=1}^{N-1} |(X_{i+1} - X_i)|,$$

where the summation of the absolute values occurred over all N points. Similarly, the total CoP path length was determined as follows:

$$Path = \sum_{i=1}^{N-1} \sqrt{(X_{i+1} - X_i)^2 + (Y_{i+1} - Y_i)^2}$$

The mean velocity was obtained simply as Path/T, where T stands for the total measurement time of the N points.

To determine the sway area shape, the experimental data points were converted into polar coordinates relative to the data centre, and the points that were the furthest from the centre were determined in consecutive angular intervals. An analytic expression was fitted to these outline points [25] that determined the distance $(R(\varphi))$ from a chosen centre at a given angle φ via a Fourier series of N_{max} coefficients a_m and b_m:

$$R(\varphi) = R_0 + \sum_{m=1}^{Nmax} (a_m \cos m\varphi + b_m \sin m\varphi)$$

The origin of the coordinate system was then shifted to the centre of the calculated contour, and the procedure was repeated. Consequently, the shape of the smooth outline of the postural sway region is given by

$$U_m = \sqrt{a_m^2 + b_m^2}$$

from which the surface area can be approximated as [26]:

$$\text{Area} = \pi R_0^2 + \pi \sum_{m=1}^{Nmax} U_m^2.$$

In addition to this area, the area of the elliptical region was calculated by principal component analysis (PCA) of the covariant matrix [27]. Here, the eigenvalues (σ_0^2) were calculated from the covariant matrix σ_{xy}^2

$$\sigma_{xy}^2 = \frac{1}{N} \sum_{i=1}^{N} (X_i - \overline{X}).(Y_i - \overline{Y}),$$

where $\overline{X}$ and $\overline{Y}$ are the mean values, and the summation was performed over all N measured points.

The two eigenvalues are thus

$$\sigma_0^2 = \frac{1}{2} (\sigma_{xx}^2 + \sigma_{yy}^2 \pm \sqrt{(\sigma_{xx}^2 - \sigma_{yy}^2)^2 + 4(\sigma_{xy}^2)^2}).$$

The sway area (Area_{PCA}) may then by reproduced by an ellipse with the two principal axes $1.96 \sigma_0$. If the distribution is a bivariate Gaussian, such an ellipse includes 95% of the data points along each axis; consequently, 85.35% of all points lie within its perimeter [27].

The fractal dimensions of the ML and AP CoP positions time series were determined by the Higutchi method [28]. For a chosen time interval k, the length of the curve starting at m in the interval from 1 to k is determined as follows:

$$L_m(k) = \frac{1}{k} \cdot \frac{N-1}{\text{Int}((N-m)/k).k} \sum_{i=1}^{\text{Int}((N-m)/k)} |X_{m+ik} - X_{m+(i-1)k}|.$$

The length of the curve L(k) is then calculated by averaging over k values of m. If the curve in the given interval of k values is fractal, its length L(k) is proportional to k^{-D}. The exponent D is the fractal dimension of the curve and can be easily determined by linear regression as the slope of the function $\ln(L(k))$ versus $\ln(k)$. This procedure was tested by applying it to a time series that was

Table 2. Mean values for the time domain postural sway variables in the different illumination conditions for the groups of 18 young and 26 elderly participants (the bold figures indicate significant differences compared to the initial normal light eyes open condition).

	Mean velocity ± SD (cm/s)	ML path ± SD (cm)	AP path ± SD (cm)	Sway area ± SD (cm^2)
Normal light - open eyes				
Young	1.11±0.23	46.38±8.82	38.25±10.1	3.34±1.16
Elderly	1.51±0.33	66.08±15.85	48.95±12.21	5.29±2.35
Normal light - closed eyes				
Young	**1.54±0.46**	**67.29±20.28**	**50.07±16.56**	4.84±2.12
Elderly	**1.86±0.44***	**80.76±18.89***	**57.75±14.38****	5.57±1.91
Very low illumination				
Young	**1.31±0.36**	**56.22±13.95**	**43.02±14.98**	3.99±1.77
Elderly	**1.68±0.42****	**72.89±18.34****	**55.28±14.92****	**5.66±2.06****
Complete darkness - open eyes				
Young	**1.51±0.39**	**65.23±18.25**	**49.11±14.03**	4.69±1.96
Elderly	**1.82±0.42***	**78.23±18.52***	**58.24±13.7***	5.08±2.59

ML - medio-lateral, AP - antero-posterior, SD - standard deviation, **p<0.01, ***p<0.001.

generated as the sum of Gaussian noise in which the dimension was known to be 1.5 [28].

The following four sway parameters in the time domain were chosen for our analysis: (1) the mean CoP velocity during the 60 s measurement interval, (2) the medio-lateral and (3) antero-posterior path lengths, and (4) the sway area. The latter was calculated as the best area outline represented by the first $N_{max} = 25$ Fourier coefficients calculated from 100 angular intervals. In the fractal domain, the dimensions were calculated from the unfiltered ML and AP time series of the CoP positions for the two time intervals from 0 to 0.3 s and from 0.8 to 12 s. These short and long time intervals were chosen to exclude the transition region and to assure two predominantly linear relations of ln(L(k)) versus ln(k).

The calculation of the Romberg's quotient was extended to encompass all of the illumination conditions. Thus, the gain for a variable in any particular condition was calculated as the quotient between that variable and the one obtained under the normal illumination with open eyes condition. The gains for time domain were calculated for both groups and for all variables.

5 Statistical analyses

The Statistical Package for Social Sciences (SPSS 20, SPSS Inc., Chicago, IL USA) was used for the statistical analyses. One-way repeated measures analyses of variance (ANOVAs) were performed to identify the effects of illumination and age on each of the dependent variables. Significant ANOVA findings were followed by LSD post hoc tests. To evaluate the differences between the age groups in the gains, t-tests for independent samples were used. The significance level was set at $p<0.05$.

Results

1 Time domain variables

One-way repeated measures ANOVAs for the illumination conditions and age were calculated to compare the postural sway variables between the two groups of participants of different ages in each of the four different experimental conditions. Significant main effects of illumination condition were found for all four time domain variables. The calculated values for the mean CoP velocity

was $F_{3,126} = 25.852$ ($p<0.001$), for the medio-lateral path length, $F_{3,126} = 25.150$ ($p = 0.001$), for the antero-posterior path length, $F_{3,126} = 22.694$ ($p = 0.001$), and for the sway area, $F_{3,126} = 4.174$ ($p = 0.007$). These findings indicate that there were effects of the amount of light on the postural sway variables. Significant main effects of age were also found for all of the analysed postural sway variables as follows: mean CoP velocity ($F_{1,42} = 12.072$, $p<0.001$), medio-lateral path length ($F_{1,42} = 14.012$, $p<0.001$), antero-posterior path length ($F_{1,42} = 8.64$, $p = 0.007$), and sway area ($F_{1,42} = 7.484$, $p = 0.009$). These findings indicate that age had effects on the postural sway variables. However, the interactions were not significant for any of the analysed postural sway variables: mean CoP velocity ($F_{3,126} = 0.246$, $p = 0.864$), medio-lateral path length ($F_{3,126} = 0.591$, $p = 0.622$), antero-posterior path length ($F_{3,126} = 0.303$, $p = 0.823$), and sway area ($F_{3,126} = 0.551$, $p = 0.648$). These results indicate that there were not effects of group on postural sway in response to illumination.

The detailed results for all reported time domain CoP variables, which were separately determined from the experimental data recorded from 18 young and 26 elderly participants, are given in Table 2. From this table, it can be seen that the values for all four of the sway variables in the time domain were significantly higher during the initial experimental conditions (i.e., normal illumination with open eyes) in the elderly group than in the younger group. The same was true for all of the other experimental conditions (normal lighting conditions with closed eyes, very low level of illumination, and complete darkness with open eyes).

After finding no interaction of postural sway in response to illumination, we collapsed the groups and analysed the effects of different light conditions. LSD post hoc tests were performed to assess the differences between the four illumination conditions. We compared the normal illumination with open eyes to each of the following conditions: (1) closed eyes, (2) very low level of illumination, and (3) complete darkness with open eyes.

The **mean CoP velocity**: An LSD post hoc test revealed a significant increase in the mean velocity for all of the altered light conditions compared to the normal light condition ($p<0.001$). When compared to the very low level of illumination, the increases in the mean CoP velocities in both no vision conditions were significantly elevated ($p<0.001$). The **medio-lateral and**

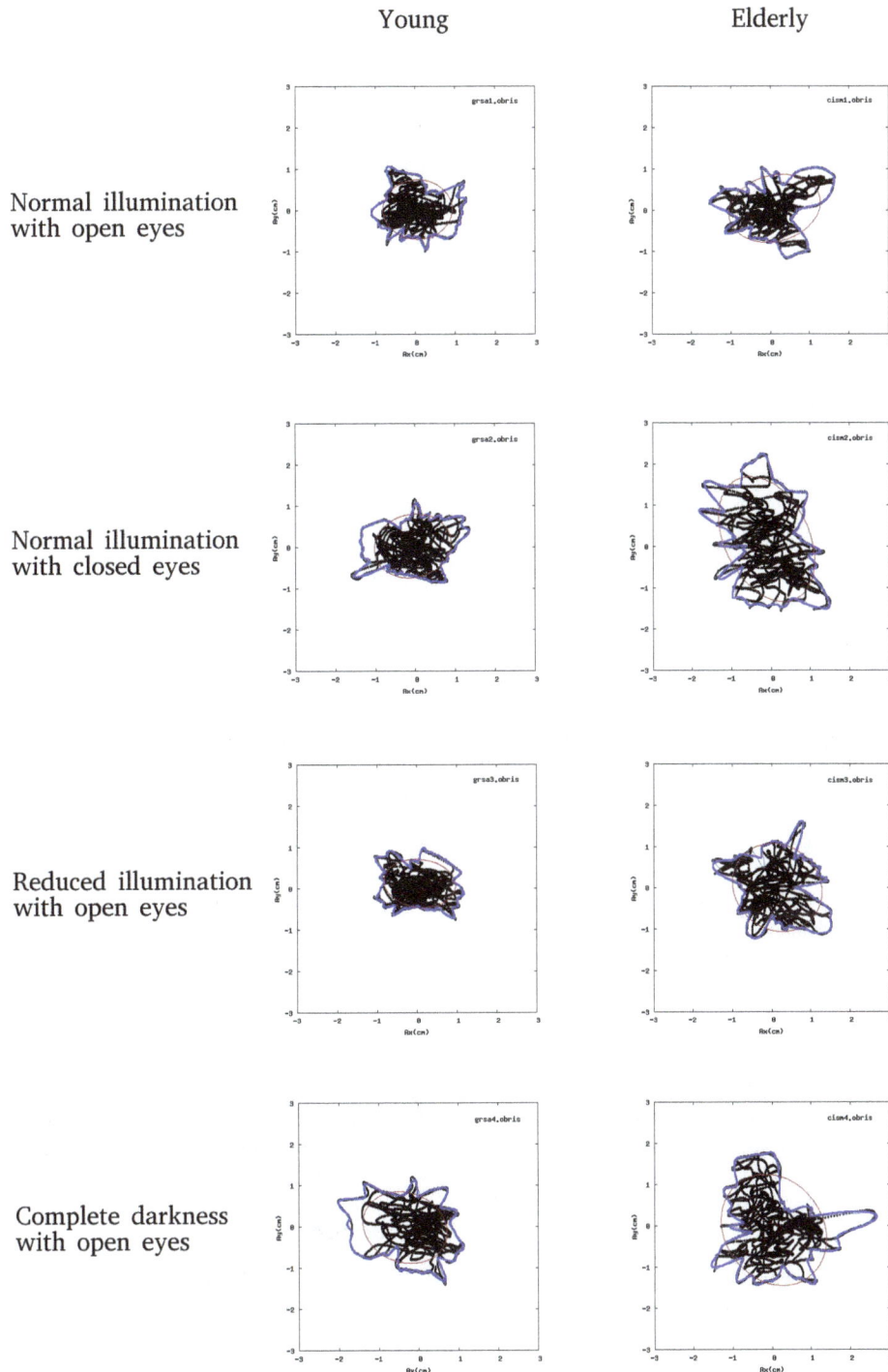

Figure 1. Typical CoP movement recordings. Typical CoP movement recordings from a young and an elderly participant under the four experimental conditions. The CoP path is indicated by the black dotted line, the CoP outline is indicated in blue, and the elliptic PCA region with 95% points along each axis is delineated by the red line.

antero-posterior path lengths increased in all of the altered light conditions relative to the normal light condition. LSD post hoc tests revealed that all of these differences were significant with p value that ranged from <0.001 to <0.003. Compared to the very low level of illumination, the increases in the medio-lateral and antero-posterior path lengths were both significantly higher in the no vision conditions (p<0.001). **Sway area:** LSD post hoc test

revealed a significant increase of sway area for closed eyes and complete darkness compared to the normal light condition, $p = 0.006$ and $p = 0.015$, respectively. When compared to the very low level of illumination, the increases did not vary significantly between the very low level of illumination and any of the other light conditions; the LSD post hoc test results were $p = 0.164$, $p = 0.088$ and $p = 0.087$ for open eyes, closed eyes and

Table 3. Fractal dimensions of the medio-lateral (D_{ML}) and antero-posterior (D_{AP}) CoP time series over short (0 s to 0.3 s) and long (0.8 s to 12 s) time intervals for the 18 young and 26 elderly participants.

	$D_{ML} \pm$ SD		$D_{AP} \pm$ SD	
	short	long	short	long
Normal light - open eyes				
Young	1.09±0.03	1.86±0.11	1.15±0.05	1.77±0.11
Elderly	1.09±0.02	1.89±0.11	1.13±0.04	1.85±0.09
Normal light - closed eyes				
Young	1.10±0.03	1.89±0.08	1.15±0.06	1.86±0.10
Elderly	1.10±0.04	1.91±0.10	1.14±0.05	1.86±0.12
Very low illumination				
Young	**1.09±0.03**	1.88±0.07	1.14±0.04	1.85±0.11
Elderly	**1.10±0.04***	1.91±0.09	1.13±0.04	1.86±0.10
Complete darkness - open eyes				
Young	1.10±0.03	1.93±0.07	1.13±0.05	1.85±0.10
Elderly	1.10±0.03	1.91±0.10	1.13±0.04	1.87±0.10

*$p<0.05$.

complete darkness, respectively. The mean values and SDs of all of the described variables are given in the last two lines of Table 2. Typical movement recordings of the CoPs in the four experimental conditions for the young and elderly participants are shown in Figure 1.

2 Fractal domain variables

One-way repeated measures ANOVAs of illumination conditions and age were calculated to compare the postural sway variables in the fractal domain between the two groups of participants. The main effect of illumination condition was only significant for D_{ML}(short) ($F_{3,126} = 5.215$ and p = 0.002), and the remaining fractal domain variables were not significant. The calculated value for D_{ML}(long) was $F_{3,126} = 2.332$ ($p = 0.077$), for D_{AP}(short) $F_{3,126} = 2.710$ ($p = 0.048$) and for D_{AP}(long) $F_{3,126} = 3.251$ ($p = 0.024$). These results indicate that there were weak effects of the amount of light on the fractal domain variables. The main effects of the age were also non-significant for all of the analysed fractal domain variables: for D_{ML}(short), $F_{1,42} = 0.242$, $p = 0.625$; for D_{ML}(long), $F_{1,42} = 0.419$, $p = 0.521$; for D_{AP}(short), $F_{1,42} = 0.563$, $p = 0.457$; and for D_{AP}(long), $F_{1,42} = 1.411$, $p = 0.241$. These findings indicate that there were no effects of age on the fractal domain variables of postural sway. The interactions were also not significant for any of the analysed fractal domain variables: for D_{ML}(short), $F_{3,126} = 1.805$, $p = 0.15$; for D_{ML}(long), $F_{3,126} = 1.507$, $p = 0.216$; for D_{AP}(short), $F_{3,126} = 1.579$, $p = 0.198$; and for D_{AP}(long), $F_{3,126} = 1.996$, $p = 0.118$. These findings indicate that there was no effect of age on postural sway in response to ambient illumination. The detailed results for all reported CoP variables in the fractal domain, which were separately determined from the experimental data recorded from the 18 young and 26 elderly participants, are given in Table 3.

3 Gain of the time domain variables

The relative gains of the CoP variables were analysed to investigate the magnitudes of the differences between the conditions and between the groups. The gains were calculated separately for each age group and for all variables as the quotients

relative to the value of the particular variable obtained under normal illumination with open eyes. Interestingly, in all of the evaluated conditions, the gains in the CoP fluctuations in the time domain were higher among the group of young participants compared to the elderly group. The gains of the elderly subjects were significantly smaller in the closed eyes condition in terms of the medio-lateral path length and sway area ($t_{42} = 2.551$, $p = 0.015$; $t_{42} = 2.393$, $p = 0.021$, respectively). The gain of the mean velocity was also smaller in the group of elderly participants; however, this difference was marginally significant ($t_{42} = 1.827$, $p = 0.075$). The same was also true for the complete darkness condition (medio-lateral path length $t_{42} = 2.547$, $p = 0.015$; sway area $t_{42} = 2.292$, $p = 0.027$, and mean velocity $t_{42} = 1.820$, $p = 0.076$). The highest relative difference was 1.50 and was observed in the increase in the sway area among the group of young participants when they were standing in normal light conditions with their eyes closed; the next largest difference (1.41) occurred in this group in the total darkness with open eyes condition (Figure 2).

Discussion

The purpose of this study was to evaluate the influence of different environmental illumination conditions on the sways of groups of healthy young and elderly adults. The results revealed that both the young and elderly participants responded in a similar manner to changes in environmental illumination. Postural sway increased (i.e., postural steadiness decreased) the most in the closed eyes conditions, followed by the complete darkness with open eyes conditions. Postural sway was least affected by the very low level of environmental illumination. The responses to the very low level of environmental illumination were sways that were significantly larger than those in the normal light and significantly smaller than those in the no light conditions among both the young and elderly adults.

Compared to the eyes open normal illumination condition, the eyes open very low level of illumination condition yielded similar responses in both age groups. The illuminance in the dark room at the gaze fixation point was estimated to be 0.25 lx. This is the

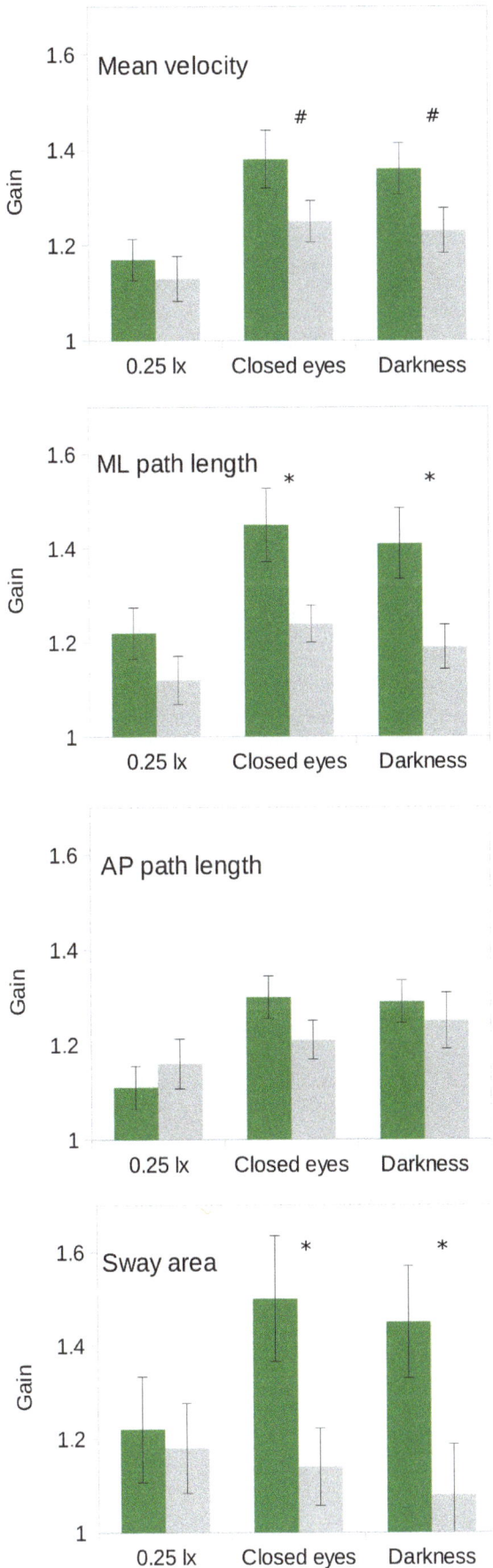

Figure 2. Gains in postural sway. Gains in postural sway expressed as the quotients between the normal light eyes opened conditions to the (1) very low illumination, (2) eyes closed and (3) total darkness conditions for the young participants (dark green) and the elderly participants (light grey). * indicates a significant difference between the two age groups at $p < 0.05$, and # indicates marginal significance at $0.05 < p < 0.08$.

lowest level of illumination that has been reported (3 lx: [3], [13] and [20], 1 lx: [6]). It seems that the amount of light provided in this condition was not sufficient for accurate visual referencing and resulted in increases in postural sway. Therefore, we conclude that very low level of ambient illumination altered postural steadiness but significantly less so than did both of the no vision conditions. These results agree with those of Simoneau et al. [20] who reported a minimal effect of dim light on postural sway (from 2.6 to 11 per cent for different time domain variables) and the results of Brooke-Wavel et al. [6] who reported increased sway in dim light. The visual referencing differed between our study and that of Brooke-Wavel et al. [6] in terms of the spatial referencing markers; in our study, a single reference point was placed in front of the participants, while Brooke-Wavel et al. [6] used vertical lines to structure the environment. However, these authors did not report whether an adaptation period was allowed prior to the beginning of the measurements. Between these two studies, the ages of both groups were similar (present study: 69.8 years and Brooke-Wavel et al. [6]: 69.7 years). Our results indicate that in very low illumination, even when sufficient time is allowed for adaptation and an anchor point is provided, young and elderly adults exhibit increased postural sway, but these increases are less than those observed in both of the no vision conditions.

In the both the closed eyes and complete darkness no vision conditions, significant increases in postural sway were observed compared to the normal condition and the very low level of illumination condition in both age groups. These results agree with previous results regarding the absence of visual inflow in young [29] and elderly adults [30]. When the results between the two no vision conditions (i.e., normal light with closed eyes and complete darkness with open eyes) were compared within each group, no significant differences were found. Therefore, the hypothesis proposed by Rougier [31] that nearly all postural sway parameters are systematically higher in no light conditions with closed eyes compared to no light conditions with open eyes might indicate that the eyelid opening-closing mechanism can interfere with postural control. Rougier [31] reported a difference in stabilogram properties between conditions of standing with eyes closed in normal light and with eyes open in darkness. However, preliminary results from our laboratory [32] have shown that participants sway in complete darkness to similar extent regardless of whether their eyes are open or closed. Additionally, the results from both of the darkness conditions did not differ from those observed in the eyes closed in normal light condition. An advantage of our experimental arrangement over that of Rougier [31] might be the use of the night goggles that allowed the research assistant to continuously ensure the closure of the eyes in the dark room.

Age had no effect on the responses to the level of environmental illumination; the same patterns were observed in the young and the old groups. A similar finding was reported by Kinsella-Shaw et al. [13]. However, the absolute values were significantly higher for the older group, which agrees with previous results of studies investigating the postural sways of young and elderly adults [6,30,33]. It is also interesting to note that neither age nor illumination condition resulted in any significant changes in the fractal dimensions as determined from the medio-lateral and antero-posterior CoP time series over short (0 s to 0.3 s) and long (0.8 s to 12 s) time intervals with the exception of the effect of illumination on D_{ML}(short). The insensitivity of the fractal dimensions to different illumination conditions agrees with the results of Stambolieva [34], who did not find any differences between open and closed eye conditions using nonlinear techniques; however, Doyle et al. [35] reported changes in antero-posterior fractal dimensions between open and closed eye conditions among elderly people using the same method reported here. This discrepancy might be because these authors used different time intervals for their dimension calculations and did not treat the short and long time intervals separately. The latter difference might also explain the generally smaller values for the calculated dimensions reported by these authors.

When the gains of the postural sway variables relative to the normal conditions (i.e., the normal illumination with open eyes condition) were compared between the two studied groups, considerably higher gains in all of the postural sway variables were observed in the young participants. Our results from the young participants revealed medio-lateral path length gains of 22 per cent gain in low illumination and 41 per cent in complete darkness. In contrast, the relative gains of the elderly participants were substantially smaller; 12 per cent was observed in very low illumination, and 19 per cent was observed in total darkness. These detected gains are significantly lower than those reported in the study by Edwards [3] who described a 32 per cent gain in postural sway in dim light and a 93.7 per cent gain in total darkness among a group of young participants. These differences might be explained by the lack of adaptation time to changes in changed illumination. Hence, a portion of the increase in postural sway might have been due to the initial phase of adaptation to changes in illumination during which higher postural sway variables could be expected. Specifically, Sozzi et al. [36] reported significant shifts in CoP position due to changes in visual input. The adaptation to darkness and decreased light requires considerable time [37], and during adulthood, the adaptation process slows with increasing age [38]. In our study, sufficient time was allowed between trials for the participants to adapt to the changes in illumination. Our results support the results and the conclusion of Johnson et al. [7] that sufficient time is needed to stabilise posture when sitting up in bed in dimly lit environments before any given action can be safely performed. However, some caution is needed when comparing these results because the participants in Johnson's study had to address changes in two conditions; changing body position (from lying to a sitting position) in which orthostatic function plays an important role, and adaptation to low levels of environmental illumination. Moreover, in more dynamic conditions, such as gait, the transition between normal and dim light rather than the low level of light itself is the most destabilising effect regardless of gait speed [39].

Smaller gains in postural sway among elderly adults as expressed as Romberg quotients were reported by Prieto et al. [11] for the time domain variables, sway area and fractal dimensions. The Romberg quotients for the elderly adults reported in this study are even smaller. The only variable that

increased more among the elderly adults than among the younger adults was the Romberg quotient for the mean velocity [11]. Why would young participants respond with higher relative gains in postural sway compared to the elderly participants when their eyes were closed or they were in complete darkness? We hypothesise that the sway of the young participants is, in normal conditions, well within the limits of stability, and although their sway increases more with decreased visual flow, it remains well within those limits. As reported by Sozzi et al. [36], in eyes closed conditions, young adults use 3% of their supporting surface, while elderly adults already use a larger support area for swaying. The perceptions of the slow velocity shifts in CoP or CoG are based on information coming from the visual and proprioceptive systems, while the vestibular system responds to higher velocity movements [40]. Therefore, it seems to be reasonable to assume that elderly persons adopt a strategy to avoid the high CoP velocities that results in increased postural sway. Thus, to prevent this increase in sway, older adults adapt to no-vision conditions with increased stiffness. This response of the elderly participants likely results from their previous experiences that are an important component for the selection of a strategy for a specific postural response [1] and on the reference of their own perceived stability borders that are a function of their egocentric reference frame [41]. This reference frame is based on information coming from the visual, proprioceptive and vestibular systems [42]. Additionally, increased activity of the ankle muscles in the no-vision conditions has been reported for young adults [36], and a similar phenomenon likely occurs in the elderly.

Thus, the main limitation of this study regarding its practical implications seems to be that the results are valid only for static situations, whereas in functional situations, the gaze moves within the visual field, which requires additional mental processing.

Conclusion

Based on the analyses of the results of experiment, we accept our first working hypothesis and reject the second hypothesis. Very low illumination increased postural sway regardless of the age of the participants. Moreover, the gains exhibited in the postural sway measures by the young participants in altered illumination conditions were higher than those of the elderly participants across all of the time domain variables; however, the patterns of responses to the illumination changes were similar in both age groups. The higher gains among the young group might be interpreted as a hallmark of normal balance performance [43].

Acknowledgments

Many thanks to Petra Pohleven for organizing the participants and help with measurements.

Author Contributions

Conceived and designed the experiments: DR GG FS. Performed the experiments: DR GG. Analyzed the data: DR GG FS. Contributed reagents/materials/analysis tools: FS. Wrote the paper: DR GG FS.

References

1. Horak FB (2006) Postural orientation and equilibrium: what do we need to know about neural control of balance to prevent falls? Age Ageing 35 (Supplement 2): ii7–ii11.

2. Springer BA, Martin R, Cyhan T, Roberts HG, Gill NW (2007) Normative values for the unipedal stance test with eyes open and closed. J Geriatric Phys Ther 30: 8–14.

3. Edwards AS (1946) Body sway and vision. J Exp Physiol 36: 526–535.

4. Paulus WM, Straube A, Brandt T (1984) Visual stabilization of posture - physiological stimulus characteristics and clinical aspects. Brain 107: 1143–1163.

5. Lanska DJ (2002) Romberg sign and early instruments for measuring postural sway. Semin Neurol 22: 409–418.

6. Broke-Wavell K, Perrett LK, Howerth PA, Haslam RA (2001) Influence of visual environment on the postural stability in healthy older. Gerontol 48: 293–297.

7. Johnson EG, Meltzer JD (2012) Effect of sitting pause times on postural stability after supine-to-standing transfer in dimly lit environments. J Ger Phys Ther 35: 15–19.

8. Kim J, Kwon Y, Eom GM, Jun JH, Lee JW, et al. (2012) Effects of vision, age and gender on structural and global posturographic features during quiet standing. Int J Precision Eng Manuf 13: 969–975.

9. Kolleger H, Baumgartner C, Wober C, Oder W, Deecke L (1992) Spontaneous body sway as a function of sex, age and visio: Posturographic study of 30 healthy adults. Eur Neurol 32: 253–259.

10. Lord SR, Ward JA (1994) Age-associated differences in sensiomotor function and balance in community dwelling women. Age Ageing, 23: 452–460.

11. Prieto TE, Myklebust JB, Hoffmann RG, Lovett EG, Myklebust BM (1996) Measures of postural steadiness: Differences between healthy young and elderly adults. IEEE Trans Biomed Eng 43: 956–966.

12. Poulain I, Giraudet G (2008) Age-related changes of visual contribution in posture control. Gait Posture 27: 1–7.

13. Kinsella-Shaw JM, Harrison SJ, Colon-Semenza C, Turvey MT (2006) Effects of visual environment on quiet standing by young and old adults. J Motor Beh 38: 251–264.

14. Tinetti ME (2003) Clinical practice. Preventing falls in elderly persons. New Eng J Med 348: 42–49.

15. Lord SR, Menz HB (2000) Visual contributions to postural stability in older adults Gerontol 46: 306–310.

16. Figuerio MG, Gras L, Qi R, Rizzo P, Rea M (2008) A novel night light system for postural control and stability in seniors. Lighting Res Tehnol 40: 111–126.

17. Lord SR, Dayhew J (2001) Visual risk factors for falls in older people. JAGS 49: 508–515.

18. Blanchard Y, McVeigh R, Graham M, Cadet M, Mwilambwe K, et al. (2007) The influence of ambient lighting levels on postural sway in healthy children ages 9 to 11. Gait Posture 26: 442–445.

19. Marucchi C, Gagey PM (1987) Postural blindness. Agressologie 28: 947–948.

20. Simoneau GG, Leibowitz HW, Ulbrecht JS, Tyrell RA, Cavanagh PR (1992) The effect of visual factors and head orientation on postural steadiness in women 55 to 70 years of age. J Gerontol 47: M151–M158.

21. Sevšek F. Stabilometrija V 1.0. Ljubljana: Visoka šola za zdravstvo, 2009. Available at: http://manus.zf.uni-lj.si/~meritev.

22. Kim S, Nusbaum MA, Madigan ML (2008) Direct parametrization of postural stability during quiet upright stance: Effects of age and altered sensory conditions. J Biomech 41: 406–411.

23. Wang Z, Newell KM (2012) Asymmetry of foot position and weight distribution channnels the inter-leg coordination dynamics of standing. Exp Brain Res 222: 333–344.

24. Rugelj D, Sevšek F (2011) The effect of load mass and its placement on postural sway. Appl Ergon 42: 860–866.

25. Sevšek F, Gomišček G (2004) Shape determination of attached fluctuating phospholipid vesicles, Comput Meth Prog Bio 73: 189–194.

26. Rugelj D, Sevšek F (2007) Postural sway area of elderly subjects. WSEAS Trans Signal Process, 3: 213–219.

27. Oliveira LF, Simpson DM, Nadal J (1996) Calculation of area of stabilometric signals using principal component analysis, Physiol Meas 17: 305–312.

28. Higuchi T (1988) Approach to an irregular time series of the basis of the fractal theory. Phys D 31: 277–283.

29. Santos BR, Delisle A, Larivière C, Plamondon A, Imbeau D (2008) Reliability of centre of pressure summary measures of postural steadiness in healthy young adults. Gait Posture 27: 408–15.

30. Raymakers JA, Samson MM, Verhaar HJJ (2005) The assessment of body sway and the choice of the stability parameter(s). Gait Posture 21: 48–58.

31. Rougier P (2003) The influence of having the eyelids open or closed on undisturbed postural control. Neuroscie Res 47: 73–83.

32. Sevšek F, Bijol L, Rugelj D (20011) Postural sway in darkness. In: XXIIIrd Congress of the International Society of Biomechanics, Brussels, July 3–7, 2011. ISB 2011: conference book: program & abstracts. Brussels: Vrije Universiteit, 2011, 174.

33. Lin D, Seol H, Nussbaum AM, Madigan LM (2008) Reliability of CoP-based postural sway measures and age-related differences. Gait Posture 28: 337–42.

34. Stambolieva K (2001) Fractal properties of postural sway during quiet stance with changed visual and proprioceptive inputs. J Physiol Sci 61: 123–130.

35. Doyle TLA. Dugan EL, Humphries B, Nweton RU (2004) Discriminating between eledrly and young using fractal dimension analysis of centre of pressure. Int J Med Sci 1: 11–20.

36. Sozzi S, Monti A, De Nunzio AM, Do MC, Schieppati M (2011) Sensori-motor integration during stance: Time adaptation of control mechanisms on adding or removing vision. Hum Mov Sci 30: 172–189.

37. Tipton DA (1984) A review of vision physiology. Aviat Space Environ Med 55: 145–149.

38. Jackson GR, Owsley C, McGwin G (1999) Aging and dark adaptation. Vision Res 39: 3975–3982.

39. Moe-Nilssen R, Helbostad JL, Akra T, Birkedal T, Nygaard HA (2006) Modulation of gait during visual adaptation to dark. J Motor Beh 38: 118–125.

40. Fitzpatrick R, McClockey DI (1994) Proprioceptive, visual and vestibular thresholds for the perception of sway during standing in humans. J Physiol MS2415: 173–186.

41. Massion J, Alexandrov A, Frolov A (2004) Why and how are posture and movement coordinated? Progress Brain Res 143: 13–27.

42. Peterka RJ (2002) Sensomotor integration in human postural control. J Neurophysiol 88: 1097–1118.

43. Brower B, Culham EG, Liston RAL, Grant T (1998) Normal variability of postural measures: Implications for the reliability of the relative balance performance outcomes. Scand J Rehabil Med 30: 131–137.

14

Systemic Adverse Events after Intravitreal Bevacizumab versus Ranibizumab for Age-Related Macular Degeneration

Wei Wang, Xiulan Zhang*

Zhongshan Ophthalmic Center, State Key Laboratory of Ophthalmology, Sun Yat-Sen University, Guangzhou, People's Republic of China

Abstract

Objective: To assess whether the incidence of systemic adverse events differs between those who used bevacizumab and those who used ranibizumab in the treatment of age-related macular degeneration (AMD).

Methods: A systematic literature search was conducted to identify randomised controlled trials (RCTs) comparing the use of intravitreal bevacizumab with the use of ranibizumab in AMD patients. Results were expressed as risk ratios (RRs) with accompanying 95% confidence intervals (CIs). The data were pooled using the fixed-effect or random-effect model according to the heterogeneity present.

Results: Four RCTs were included in the final meta-analysis. Overall, the quality of the evidence was high. There were 2,613 treated patients: 1,291 treated with bevacizumab and 1,322 treated with ranibicizumab. No significant differences between bevacizumab use and ranizumab use were found in terms of the incidence of death from all causes, arteriothrombotic events, stroke, nonfatal myocardial infarction, vascular death, venous thrombotic events, and hypertension, with the pooled RRs being 1.11 (0.77, 1.61), 1.03 (0.69,1.55), 0.84 (0.39,1.80), 0.97 (0.48, 1.96), 1.24 (0.63, 2.44), 2.38 (0.94, 6.04), and 1.02 (0.29, 3.62), respectively.

Conclusions: The meta-analysis shows that both treatments are comparably safe. However, the findings from our study must be confirmed in future research via well-designed cohort or intervention studies because of the limited number of studies.

Editor: Andreas Wedrich, Medical University Graz, Austria

Funding: This research was supported by the National Natural Science Foundation of China (81371008). No additional external funding was received. The funders had no role in study design, data collection and analysis, decision to publish, or preparation of the manuscript.

Competing Interests: The authors have declared that no competing interests exist.

* Email: zhangxl2@mail.sysu.edu.cn

Introduction

Age-related macular degeneration (AMD) is the most common cause of blindness in individuals over 50 years of age [1–3]. Although an estimated 80% of patients with AMD have the non-neovascular (dry) form, the neovascular (wet) form is responsible for almost 90% of severe visual losses resulting from AMD [4–6]. Vascular endothelial growth factor-A (VEGF-A) has been proven to play a major role in the pathogenesis of wet AMD [7,8]. Since the mid-2000s, antivascular endothelial growth factor (anti-VEGF) therapy has become the mainstay of treatment for wet AMD [9].

Ranibizumab (Lucentis, Genentech, Inc., South San Francisco, CA, USA) is a recombinant humanized immunoglobulin G1κ isotype monoclonal antibody fragment directed toward all isoforms of VEGF-A [7]. It has been approved for the treatment of wet AMD by the food and drug administration (FDA) in the US (2006), Europe (2007), Japan (2009), and many other countries. However, the cost of ranibizumab is immense: monthly injections at a dose of 0.5 mg result in an annual cost greater than US $23,000 per patient [10].

Similar to ranibizumab, bevacizumab (Avastin, Genentech, Inc., South San Francisco, CA, USA) is a recombinant humanized full-length antibody that can inhibit all isoforms of VEGF-A [11]. In 2004, it was approved for the treatment of metastatic cancer of the colon or rectum, but it has not gained FDA approval for intravitreal use. Therefore, it can be utilized only in an off-label setting. For the past several years, it has been used off-label to treat wet AMD with very encouraging results. Bevacizumab has attracted more and more interest because of its low cost, which is especially important considering the number of injections that are necessary at 4- to 6-week intervals. A report suggested that the US medicare system could save more than US$1 billion within 2 years if bevacizumab replaced ranibizumab [7,10].

Although anti-VEGF agents are injected in small quantities into the eye, concerns about systemic safety have been raised, especially for the off-label use of bevacizumab. Research has shown that the systemic administration of bevacizumab, along with chemotherapeutic agents, can increase the risk of thromboembolic events two-fold over chemotherapy alone [12]. Many recently published randomized clinical trials (RCTs) have evaluated intravitreal bevacizumab and ranibizumab for the treatment of wet AMD. The results of the comparison of the AMD Treatments Trial (CATT) and the Age-related Choroidal Neovascularization Trial (IVAN) demonstrated that bevacizumab was not inferior to ranibizumab in the treatment of wet AMD [13,14]. However, these studies were not sufficiently powerful to detect drug-specific differences in the rates of systemic adverse events. Hence, the crucial question of whether adverse effects differ between off-label bevacizumab and licensed ranibizumab has not yet been answered [15].

To determine whether the intravitreal injection of bevacizumab creates a higher risk of systemic adverse events than ranibizumab injection does, we undertook a systematic review and meta-analysis of all relevant head-to-head RCTs.

Methods

This study was reported in accordance with the Preferred Reporting Items for Systematic Reviews and Meta-Analyses (PRISMA) statement (Checklist S1) [16]. All stages of study selection, data extraction, and quality assessment were performed independently by two reviewers (W.W. and X.Z.). Any disagreement was resolved via discussion and consensus.

1. Literature Search

Studies were identified through a systematic search of Pubmed, Embase, the Chinese Biomedicine Database, and the Cochrane library from inception up to December 2013. The initial search terms were (Ranibizumab or Lucentis) AND (Bevacizumab or Avastin) AND ("Macular degeneration" or AMD), which were filtered by "Humans" and "Randomized Controlled Trial." In addition, the reference lists of identified studies were manually checked to include other potentially eligible trials. This process was performed iteratively until no additional articles could be identified.

2. Study Selection

Studies were considered acceptable for inclusion in the meta-analysis if they met the following criteria: (1) the study design included randomized clinical trials; (2) the population was patients with wet AMD; (3) the interventions were intravitreal bevacizumab and intravitreal ranibizumab, which were directly compared in head-to-head design; (4) the incidence of systemic adverse events was reported; (5) there was a follow-up time of at least 1 year; and (6) there were at least ten patients in each arm. If there were multiple reports for a particular study, the most recent publication was included. Trials were excluded if they (1) were abstracts, letters, or meeting proceedings; (2) had repeated data or did not report outcomes of interest; or (3) included patients with other indications than wet AMD, patients previously treated with VEGF inhibitors, or patients receiving systemic anti-VEGF therapy.

3. Data Extraction

The following information was extracted from each study: first author; year of publication; study design; inclusion and exclusion criteria; number of patients in each group; characteristics of the study population; adverse events; the period, and number of injections preceding an adverse event. A Thromboembolic Event (TEE) was defined as any arteriothrombotic or venous thrombotic event [17].

4. Quality Assessment

The methodological quality of each trial was evaluated using the Jadad scale [18]. The scale consists of three items describing randomization (0–2 points), blinding (0–2 points), and dropouts and withdrawals (0–1 points) in the reporting of a randomized controlled trial. A score of 1 is given for each of the points described. A further point is awarded when the method of randomization and/or blinding is given and is appropriate, whereas when it is inappropriate, a point is deducted. The quality scale ranges from 0 to 5 points. Higher scores indicate better reporting. The studies are said to be of low quality if the Jadad score is ≤ 2 and of high quality if the score is ≥ 3.

5. Statistical Analysis

All outcomes were expressed as risk ratios (RRs) with accompanying 95% confidence intervals (CIs). Outcome measure was assessed on an intent-to-treat (ITT) basis, the ITT population being comprised of all randomized patients who received the study medication and provided a valid baseline measurement. The cochrane Q test was used to detect the heterogeneity of the effects. Significant heterogeneity was defined as a P value of <0.05. A fixed-effects model or random-effects model was used, depending on the presence or absence of heterogeneity. The I^2 value was used to demonstrate the percentage of the variability attributable to heterogeneity rather than to sampling error. Studies with an I^2 statistic of <25% are considered to have no heterogeneity, those with an I^2 statistic of 25% to 50% are considered to have low heterogeneity, those with an I^2 statistic of 50% to 75% are considered to have moderate heterogeneity, and those with an I^2 statistic of >75% are considered to have high heterogeneity [19]. Sensitivity analyses were performed by investigating the influence of a single study on the overall pooled estimate via omitting one study at a time. Potential publication bias was assessed by using Begg's and Egger's tests [20,21]. A P value <0.05 was judged to be statistically significant, except when otherwise specified. All statistical analyses were performed using Stata version 12.0 (Stata Corp, College Station, TX).

Results

1. Literature Search

The selection process and reasons for exclusion are detailed in Figure 1. The initial search identified 125 potentially relevant articles, of which 71 were excluded based on the titles and abstracts. The remaining 54 were retrieved for a full-text review, and 40 of them were excluded because 38 included unqualified patients, two involved unqualified interventions, eight contained duplicated data [22–29], one did not report outcomes of interest [30], and one contained only one patients (<10) in the ranibizumab arm [31]. Thus, four RCTs [13,14,32,33] were included in the final meta-analysis.

2. Study Characteristics and Quality

The main characteristics of the four RCTs included in the meta-analysis are presented in Table 1, and the outcome data of each included trial are described in Table 2. These studies were published between 2012 and 2013. The sizes of the RCTs ranged from 317 to 1,185 patients (a total of 2,613; 1,291 with bevacizumab and 1,322 with ranibicizumab). Of the four trials, one was done in the USA [14], one in the UK [13], one in France [33], and one in Australia [32]. The trials included in this

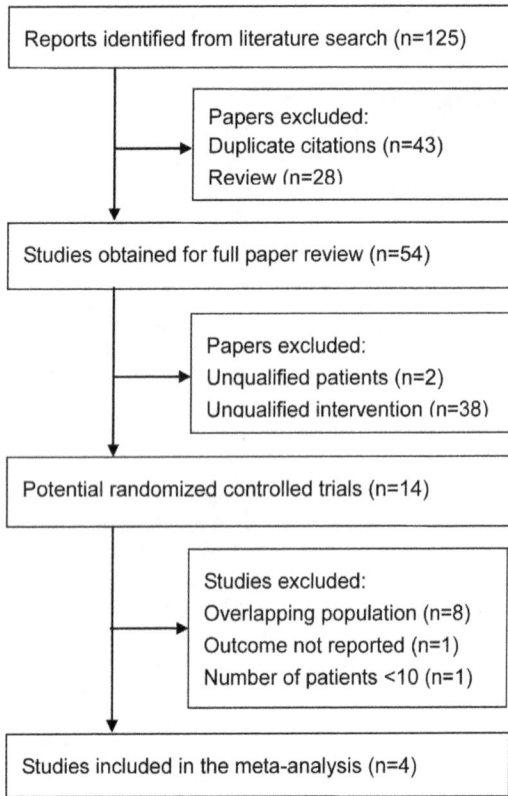

Figure 1. Flowchart of studies included in meta-analysis. RCT, randomized controlled trial.

meta-analysis appeared to have been reasonably designed and conducted. All studies had a statement regarding randomization and double-blindness. Four trials described the methods of randomization. Four trials reported withdrawals and dropouts. All trials described the main outcome, and no missing data seemed to influence the results. The Jadad score of the studies included was 5.

3. Risk of Systemic Adverse Events

The risk estimates for systemic adverse events associated with intravitreal bevacizumab, as compared with ranibizumab, were summarized in Table 3. No significant differences between bevacizumab and ranizumab were found in terms of the incidence of death from all causes, arteriothrombotic events, stroke, nonfatal myocardial infarction, vascular death, venous thrombotic events, and hypertension, with the pooled RRs being 1.11 (0.77, 1.61), 1.03 (0.69,1.55), 0.84 (0.39,1.80), 0.97 (0.48, 1.96), 1.24 (0.63, 2.44), 2.38 (0.94, 6.04), and 1.02 (0.29, 3.62), respectively. When any arteriothrombotic or venous thrombotic events, such as TEE, were combined, no significant difference was detected (RR, 1.22; 95% CI: 0.85 to 1.75; P = 0.292) (Figure 2). Furthermore, when adverse events were divided by MedDRA system organ class, there was also no significant difference between bevacizumab and ranibizumab injections. The tests for heterogeneity were all non-significant (all P>0.1). We tested the robustness of our analyses by performing sensitivity analyses excluding the CATT study (largest trial). Excluding this study did not change our final results.

Table 1. Baseline characteristics of the head-to-head studies comparing ranibizumab with bevacizumab.

Study	Location	Center	Blind	Duration	Intervention	No. of eyes	Age (years)	Male (%)	Visual acuity (letters)	Foveal thickness (mm)
CATT	USA	44	double	2 years	Ranibizumab Monthly	301	79.2±7.4	39.2%	60.1±14.3	458±184
					Bevacizumab Monthly	286	80.1±7.3	37.1%	60.2±13.1	463±196
					Ranibizumab as Needed	298	78.4±7.8	37.9%	61.5±13.2	458±193
					Bevacizumab as Needed	300	79.3±7.6	38.7%	60.4±13.4	461±175
IVAN	UK	23	double	2 years	Ranibizumab	314	77.8±7.6	41%	67.8±17.0	471.6±192.5
					Bevacizumab	296	77.7±7.3	39%	66.1±18.4	465.6±183.1
GEFAL	France	38	double	1 year	Ranibizumab	129	78.68±7.27	31.21%	55.78±13.99	354.75±109.90
					Bevacizumab	119	79.62±6.90	35.82%	54.62±14.07	359.21±120.72
MANTA	Austria	10	double	1 year	Ranibizumab	163	77.6±8.1	36.20%	56.4±13.5	365.0±8.1
					Bevacizumab	154	76.7±7.8	36.36%	57.0±13.0	374.6±8.4

CATT = The Comparison of Age-related macular degeneration Treatments Trials; IVAN = The Alternative treatments to Inhibit VEGF in Age-related choroidal Neovascularization study; MANTA = The Multicenter Anti-VEGF Trial; GEFAL = The Groupe d'Etude Français Avastin versus Lucentis dans la DMLA néovasculaire (The French Study Group Avastin versus Lucentis for neovascular AMD).

Table 2. Outcome data of randomized controlled trials included in the meta-analysis.

Adverse events	CAAT		IVAN		GEFAL		MANTA	
	Ranibizumab (N = 599)	Bevacizumab (N = 586)	Ranibizumab (N = 314)	Bevacizumab (N = 296)	Ranibizumab (N = 246)	Bevacizumab (N = 255)	Ranibizumab (N = 163)	Bevacizumab (N = 154)
Systemic adverse event								
Death-all causes	32	36	15	15	3	2	2	3
Arteriothrombotic events	28*	29	13	10	1	1	3	5
Stroke	8	8	6	3	0	0	1	1
Nonfatal myocardial infarction	9	7	4	4	1	1	2	3
Vascular death	12	14	3	4	0	0	0	0
Venous thrombotic events	3	10	3	4	0	1	0	0
Hypertension	3	4	0	0	2	1	0	0
MedDRA system organ class								
Cardiac disorders	47	62	20	19	5	2	1	1
Infections	41	54	9	12	2	4	3	3
Nervous system disorders	34	36	9	8	0	3	1	2
Injury and procedural complications	23	35	12	10	2	4	3	2
Neoplasms benign and malignant	27	22	11	14	1	1	2	1
Surgical and medical procedures	0	0	16	14	0	5	0	1
Gastrointestinal disorders	11	28	3	9	5	3	0	0
Any other system organ class	81	104	25	27	11	10	2	3

Table 3. Risk ratio of systemic adverse events associated with intravitreal bevacizumab compared with ranibizumab.

Avastin vs Lucentis	Study(n)	RR (95%CI)			Heterogeneity		Overall Effect	
		Estimate	Lower	Up	P	I^2(%)	Z	P
Death-all causes	4	1.11	0.77	1.61	0.907	0.00%	0.56	0.572
Arteriothrombotic events	4	1.03	0.69	1.55	0.828	0.00%	0.15	0.879
Stroke	3	0.84	0.39	1.80	0.737	0.00%	0.46	0.649
Nonfatal myocardial infarction	4	0.97	0.48	1.96	0.925	0.00%	0.09	0.928
Vascular death	2	1.24	0.63	2.44	0.842	0.00%	0.61	0.541
Venous thrombotic events	3	2.38	0.94	6.04	0.676	0.00%	1.83	0.067
Hypertension	2	1.02	0.29	3.62	0.471	0.00%	0.03	0.977
MedDRA system organ class								
Cardiac disorders	4	1.20	0.88	1.62	0.460	0.00%	1.16	0.245
Infections	4	1.36	0.97	1.91	0.965	0.00%	1.79	0.074
Nervous system disorders	4	1.11	0.75	1.66	0.606	0.00%	0.52	0.602
Injury and procedural complications	4	1.31	0.87	1.98	0.578	0.00%	1.30	0.194
Neoplasms benign and malignant	4	0.96	0.62	1.48	0.743	0.00%	0.18	0.854
Surgical and medical procedures	3	1.75	0.43	7.16	0.222	33.60%	0.78	0.434
Gastrointestinal disorders	3	1.90	0.78	4.62	0.141	49.00%	1.41	0.158
Any other system organ class	4	1.25	0.99	1.56	0.803	0.00%	1.90	0.058

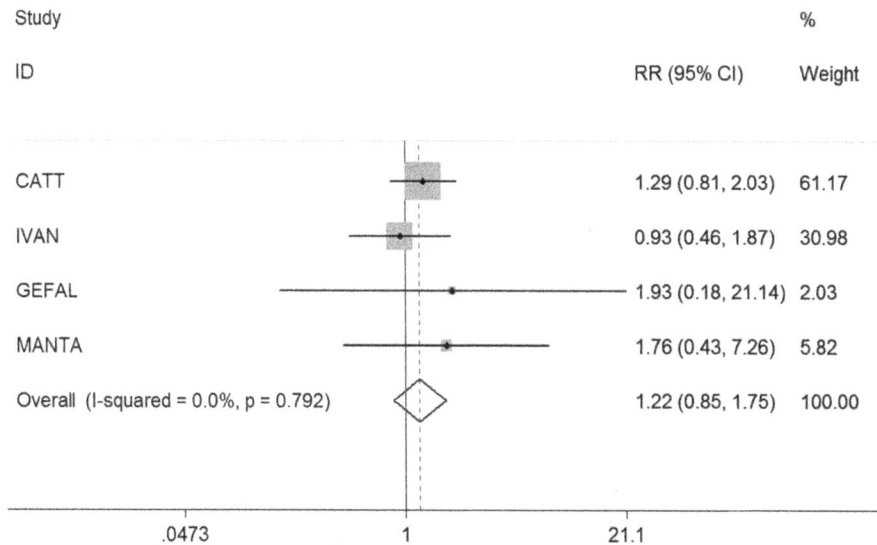

Figure 2. Risk ratio of thromboembolic events associated with intravitreal bevacizumab compared with ranibizumab. Each study is shown by the point estimate of relative risk "risk ratio" (RR) - the size of the square is proportional to the weight of the study - and 95%confidence interval for the RR (lines extending from the squares); the pooled RR and 95%confidence interval are shown as a diamond.

4. Publication Bias

Due to the limited number (<10) of studies included in each analysis, publication bias was not assessed.

Discussion

The development of VEGF inhibitors has revolutionized the treatment of AMD. Bevacizumab and ranibizumab are the two most common VEGF inhibitors in ophthalmic practice [34]. Although anti-VEGF agents are injected into the eye in small quantities, concerns about systemic safety have been raised [35]. Until relatively recently, high-quality data comparing the efficacy and safety of ranibizumab and bevacizumab in AMD were lacking. Because many adverse events are relatively uncommon, clinical trials often lack the power to detect small but clinically important risk differences. Hence, meta-analyses pooling data from multiple studies provide important insights [15,36]. The main aim of this study is to provide an evidence-based analysis of the safety profile for bevacizumab versus that of intravitreal ranibizumab injections in patients with AMD. In the present meta-analysis, we have reviewed the literature regarding the safety of intravitreal bevacizumab as compared with that of ranibizumab. The pooled results suggest that the incidence of specific systemic complications did not differ significant between bevacizumab and ranibizumab. Also, no heterogeneity was observed across the studies.

Several high-quality non-randomized studies [37–40] focusing on adverse effects for bevacizumab versus ranibizumab are summarized in Table 4. All of them reported that the rates of specific systemic adverse events, such as all-cause mortality, stroke, acute myocardial infarction, and venous thromboembolism during the bevacizumab and ranibizumab periods were not different. However, the limitation of these studies was that a non-randomized study design was used (case control or cohort study). The principal finding of our meta-analysis is consistent with the aforementioned studies on the topic.

Thus far, ranibizumab and bevacizumab have been evaluated in several systematic reviews [11,17,34,41]. However, the published reviews focused on the beneficial effects and clinical effectiveness of VEGF inhibitors, without adequately addressing their adverse effects. Furthermore, they are mainly based on indirect comparative studies; this may lower the evidence level. In Schmucker and colleagues' report [41], only one multiple-center, head-to-head RCT (CATT) was included; it had relatively modest sample sizes. In another meta-analysis by Chakravarthy et al. [13], no difference in the frequency of death, arterial thrombotic events, or hospital admission for heart failure was recorded between the drugs. Their study is limited by the fact that only 1-year CATT data were included. In our study, we incorporated the 2-year CATT data and two other well-designed RCTs. We found a similar risk of specific adverse events between the bevacizumab and ranibizumab groups. From a theoretical viewpoint, the risk of the development of systemic adverse events may be higher with bevacizumab than with ranibizumab [10]. Bevacizumab is more likely to induce immunologic activation and will remain in systemic circulation than ranibizumab. Thus, bevacizumab administration may create a higher risk of systemic adverse events. These highlight the need for ongoing surveillance and large population-based studies to investigate these outcomes [15].

The results of this meta-analysis must be interpreted cautiously in light of the strengths and limitations of the included trials. A key strength of this study is the fact that all the studies included in this meta-analysis were published by established centers of excellence using a randomized controlled design and all of them were well-performed and of high quality. In addition, with the enlarged sample size, we have enhanced statistical power to provide more precise and reliable effect estimates. Despite our rigorous methodology, some limitations of the current study should not be ignored. First, we cannot fully exclude publication bias. The number of included studies is insufficient to carry out further statistical testing to detect publication bias through an asymmetry plot. In addition, we did not attempt to gain access to unpublished results. More RCTs are warranted to confirm or refute our finding in the future update meta-analysis. Second, all studies have come from western populations with predominately Caucasian participants. The relatively good distribution of the study population makes findings from this meta-analysis a fair representation of the general population. The safety of these drugs for other ethnicities,

Table 4. Summary of high-quality non-randomized studies comparing ranibizumab with bevacizumab.

Author, country	Design	Population	Method	Results
Campbell et al., 2012, Canada	Population based nested case-control study	Older adults with a history of physician diagnosed retinal disease identified between 1 April 2006 and 31 March 2011.	Cases were patients admitted to hospital for ischaemic stroke, acute myocardial infarction, venous thromboembolism, for congestive heart failure. Event-free controls were matched to cases on the basis of year of birth, sex, history of the outcome in the previous 5 years, and diabetes	Adjusted odds ratios for bevacizumab relative to ranibizumab were 1.03 (0.67 to 1.60) for ischaemic stroke, 1.23 (0.85 to 1.77) for acute myocardial infarction, 0.92 (0.51 to 1.69) for venous thromboembolism, and 1.35 (0.93 to 1.95) for congestive heart failure. Results showed these risks did not differ significantly between bevacizumab and ranibizumab injections.
Campbell et al., 2012, Canada	Population-based, time series analysis	All patients aged 66 years or older with physician-diagnosed retinal disease between 2002 and 2010 (N = 116 388).	Segmented regression analysis was used to evaluate changes in the rate of hospitalization for ischemic stroke associated with the introduction of bevacizumab and ranibizumab.	Bevacizumab trend change coefficient: -0.0026 stroke hospitalizations/1000 subjects/month (P = 0.20); Ranibizumab trend change coefficient: -0.0011 stroke hospitalizations/1000 subjects/month (P = 0.78). Results showed that stroke rates in the bevacizumab and ranibizumab periods were not different.
French et al., 2011, USA	Cohort study	Beneficiaries of the Veterans Health Administration aged ≥55 years with AMD in fiscal years 2007-2009 were included.	Anti-vascular endothelial growth factor exposure was identified through pharmacy records. Cox proportional hazard model was adjusted for age, gender, number of injections, and ocular and medical comorbidities.	The adjusted HR for all-cause mortality were 0.94 (95%CI: 0.72 to 1.22) for bevacizumab and 0.85 (95%CI: 0.67 to1.08) for ranibizumab. Results showed lack an association between the use of either ranibizumab or bevacizumab and mortality.
Curtis et al., 2010, USA	Cohort study	Medicare beneficiaries 65 years or older with a claim for AMD in fiscal years 2005-2006 were included.	When the patients received a therapy different from the initial therapy, the data were censored. The associations between anti-VEGF therapies and the risks of all-cause mortality, incident myocardial infarction, bleeding, and incident stroke were calculated.	Adjusted HRs for ranibizumab relative to bevacizumab were 0.90 (0.79-1.02) for all-cause mortality, 0.84 (0.66-1.06) for myocardial infarction, 1.03 (0.93-1.15) for bleeding, 0.81 (0.68-0.98) for stroke. Results showed these risks did not differ significantly between bevacizumab and ranibizumab injections.

such as Asians, must be tested. Furthermore, patients enrolled in RCTs meet strict eligibility criteria, which may exclude many patients at a higher risk for systemic adverse events. These limitations likely resulted in an underestimation of the incidence of systemic adverse events. However, the determination of the risk of systemic adverse events associated with bevacizumab versus ranibizumab was not likely affected, because this underestimation should have had similar impacts on both arms. Finally, given that the treatment of wet AMD is not limited to 2 years, more data from studies of longer durations are needed to determine the relative safety of each anti-VEGF agent over the long term.

In conclusion, there is no difference between bevacizumab and ranibizumab in terms of the risk of specific systemic adverse events. However, the results should be interpreted cautiously because the relevant evidence remains limited, and the findings must be confirmed through future research involving well-designed cohort studies or RCTs.

Author Contributions

Conceived and designed the experiments: WW XZ. Performed the experiments: WW XZ. Analyzed the data: WW XZ. Contributed reagents/materials/analysis tools: WW XZ. Wrote the paper: WW XZ.

References

1. Owen CG, Jarrar Z, Wormald R, Cook DG, Fletcher AE, et al. (2012) The estimated prevalence and incidence of late stage age related macular degeneration in the UK. Br J Ophthalmol 96: 752–756.
2. Rudnicka AR, Jarrar Z, Wormald R, Cook DG, Fletcher A, et al. (2012) Age and gender variations in age-related macular degeneration prevalence in populations of European ancestry: a meta-analysis. Ophthalmology 119: 571–580.
3. Kawasaki R, Yasuda M, Song SJ, Chen SJ, Jonas JB, et al. (2010) The prevalence of age-related macular degeneration in Asians: a systematic review and meta-analysis. Ophthalmology 117: 921–927.
4. Schmier JK, Jones ML, Halpern MT (2006) The burden of age-related macular degeneration. Pharmacoeconomics 24: 319–334.
5. Brown MM, Brown GC, Sharma S, Stein JD, Roth Z, et al. (2006) The burden of age-related macular degeneration: a value-based analysis. Curr Opin Ophthalmol 17: 257–266.
6. Ferris FR, Wilkinson CP, Bird A, Chakravarthy U, Chew E, et al. (2013) Clinical classification of age-related macular degeneration. Ophthalmology 120: 844–851.
7. Frampton JE (2013) Ranibizumab: a review of its use in the treatment of neovascular age-related macular degeneration. Drugs Aging 30: 331–358.
8. Ambati J, Fowler BJ (2012) Mechanisms of age-related macular degeneration. Neuron 75: 26–39.
9. Lally DR, Gerstenblith AT, Regillo CD (2012) Preferred therapies for neovascular age-related macular degeneration. Curr Opin Ophthalmol 23: 182–188.
10. Campbell RJ, Bell CM, Campbell EL, Gill SS (2013) Systemic effects of intravitreal vascular endothelial growth factor inhibitors. Curr Opin Ophthalmol 24: 197–204.
11. Schmucker C, Ehlken C, Hansen LL, Antes G, Agostini HT, et al. (2010) Intravitreal bevacizumab (Avastin) vs. ranibizumab (Lucentis) for the treatment of age-related macular degeneration: a systematic review. Curr Opin Ophthalmol 21: 218–226.
12. Hurwitz HI, Tebbutt NC, Kabbinavar F, Giantonio BJ, Guan ZZ, et al. (2013) Efficacy and safety of bevacizumab in metastatic colorectal cancer: pooled analysis from seven randomized controlled trials. Oncologist 18: 1004–1012.
13. Chakravarthy U, Harding SP, Rogers CA, Downes SM, Lotery AJ, et al. (2013) Alternative treatments to inhibit VEGF in age-related choroidal neovascularisation: 2-year findings of the IVAN randomised controlled trial. Lancet 382: 1258–1267.

14. Martin DF, Maguire MG, Fine SL, Ying GS, Jaffe GJ, et al. (2012) Ranibizumab and bevacizumab for treatment of neovascular age-related macular degeneration: two-year results. Ophthalmology 119: 1388–1398.

15. Cheung CM, Wong TY (2013) Treatment of age-related macular degeneration. Lancet 382: 1230–1232.

16. Moher D, Liberati A, Tetzlaff J, Altman DG (2009) Preferred reporting items for systematic reviews and meta-analyses: the PRISMA statement. J Clin Epidemiol 62: 1006–1012.

17. Abouammoh MA (2013) Ranibizumab injection for diabetic macular edema: meta-analysis of systemic safety and systematic review. Can J Ophthalmol 48: 317–323.

18. Jadad AR, Moore RA, Carroll D, Jenkinson C, Reynolds DJ, et al. (1996) Assessing the quality of reports of randomized clinical trials: is blinding necessary? Control Clin Trials 17: 1–12.

19. Higgins JP, Thompson SG, Deeks JJ, Altman DG (2003) Measuring inconsistency in meta-analyses. BMJ 327: 557–560.

20. Egger M, Davey SG, Schneider M, Minder C (1997) Bias in meta-analysis detected by a simple, graphical test. BMJ 315: 629–634.

21. Begg CB, Mazumdar M (1994) Operating characteristics of a rank correlation test for publication bias. Biometrics 50: 1088–1101.

22. Ying GS, Huang J, Maguire MG, Jaffe GJ, Grunwald JE, et al. (2013) Baseline predictors for one-year visual outcomes with ranibizumab or bevacizumab for neovascular age-related macular degeneration. Ophthalmology 120: 122–129.

23. Jaffe GJ, Martin DF, Toth CA, Daniel E, Maguire MG, et al. (2013) Macular morphology and visual acuity in the comparison of age-related macular degeneration treatments trials. Ophthalmology 120: 1860–1870.

24. DeCroos FC, Toth CA, Stinnett SS, Heydary CS, Burns R, et al. (2012) Optical coherence tomography grading reproducibility during the Comparison of Age-related Macular Degeneration Treatments Trials. Ophthalmology 119: 2549–2557.

25. Chakravarthy U, Harding SP, Rogers CA, Downes SM, Lotery AJ, et al. (2012) Ranibizumab versus bevacizumab to treat neovascular age-related macular degeneration: one-year findings from the IVAN randomized trial. Ophthalmology 119: 1399–1411.

26. Grunwald JE, Daniel E, Ying GS, Pistilli M, Maguire MG, et al. (2012) Photographic assessment of baseline fundus morphologic features in the Comparison of Age-Related Macular Degeneration Treatments Trials. Ophthalmology 119: 1634–1641.

27. Martin DF, Maguire MG, Ying GS, Grunwald JE, Fine SL, et al. (2011) Ranibizumab and bevacizumab for neovascular age-related macular degeneration. N Engl J Med 364: 1897–1908.

28. Donahue SP, Recchia F, Sternberg PJ (2010) Bevacizumab vs ranibizumab for age-related macular degeneration: early results of a prospective double-masked, randomized clinical trial. Am J Ophthalmol 150: 287, 287.

29. Subramanian ML, Ness S, Abedi G, Ahmed E, Daly M, et al. (2009) Bevacizumab vs ranibizumab for age-related macular degeneration: early results of a prospective double-masked, randomized clinical trial. Am J Ophthalmol 148: 875–882.

30. Biswas P, Sengupta S, Choudhary R, Home S, Paul A, et al. (2011) Comparative role of intravitreal ranibizumab versus bevacizumab in choroidal neovascular membrane in age-related macular degeneration. Indian J Ophthalmol 59: 191–196.

31. Subramanian ML, Abedi G, Ness S, Ahmed E, Fenberg M, et al. (2010) Bevacizumab vs ranibizumab for age-related macular degeneration: 1-year outcomes of a prospective, double-masked randomised clinical trial. Eye (Lond) 24: 1708–1715.

32. Krebs I, Schmetterer L, Boltz A, Told R, Vecsei-Marlovits V, et al. (2013) A randomised double-masked trial comparing the visual outcome after treatment with ranibizumab or bevacizumab in patients with neovascular age-related macular degeneration. Br J Ophthalmol 97: 266–271.

33. Kodjikian L, Souied EH, Mimoun G, Mauget-Faysse M, Behar-Cohen F, et al. (2013) Ranibizumab versus Bevacizumab for Neovascular Age-related Macular Degeneration: Results from the GEFAL Noninferiority Randomized Trial. Ophthalmology.

34. Mitchell P (2011) A systematic review of the efficacy and safety outcomes of anti-VEGF agents used for treating neovascular age-related macular degeneration: comparison of ranibizumab and bevacizumab. Curr Med Res Opin 27: 1465–1475.

35. Aujla JS (2012) Replacing ranibizumab with bevacizumab on the Pharmaceutical Benefits Scheme: where does the current evidence leave us? Clin Exp Optom 95: 538–540.

36. Torjesen I (2013) Avastin is as effective as Lucentis in treating wet age related macular degeneration, study finds. BMJ 347: f4678.

37. Campbell RJ, Gill SS, Bronskill SE, Paterson JM, Whitehead M, et al. (2012) Adverse events with intravitreal injection of vascular endothelial growth factor inhibitors: nested case-control study. BMJ 345: e4203.

38. Campbell RJ, Bell CM, Paterson JM, Bronskill SE, Moineddin R, et al. (2012) Stroke rates after introduction of vascular endothelial growth factor inhibitors for macular degeneration: a time series analysis. Ophthalmology 119: 1604–1608.

39. French DD, Margo CE (2011) Age-related macular degeneration, anti-vascular endothelial growth factor agents, and short-term mortality: a postmarketing medication safety and surveillance study. Retina 31: 1036–1042.

40. Curtis LH, Hammill BG, Schulman KA, Cousins SW (2010) Risks of mortality, myocardial infarction, bleeding, and stroke associated with therapies for age-related macular degeneration. Arch Ophthalmol 128: 1273–1279.

41. Schmucker C, Ehlken C, Agostini HT, Antes G, Ruecker G, et al. (2012) A safety review and meta-analyses of bevacizumab and ranibizumab: off-label versus goldstandard. PLoS One 7: e42701.

15

Blood Pressure Associates with Standing Balance in Elderly Outpatients

Jantsje H. Pasma[1], Astrid Y. Bijlsma[2,3], Janneke M. Klip[2], Marjon Stijntjes[2,3], Gerard Jan Blauw[2,4], Majon Muller[2], Carel G. M. Meskers[5], Andrea B. Maier[3]*

1 Department of Rehabilitation Medicine, Leiden University Medical Center, Leiden, The Netherlands, 2 Department of Gerontology and Geriatrics, Leiden University Medical Center, Leiden, The Netherlands, 3 Department of Internal Medicine, Section of Gerontology and Geriatrics, VU University Medical Center, Amsterdam, The Netherlands, 4 Department of Geriatrics, Bronovo Hospital, The Hague, The Netherlands, 5 Department of Rehabilitation Medicine, VU University Medical Center, Amsterdam, The Netherlands

Abstract

Objectives: Assessment of the association of blood pressure measurements in supine and standing position after a postural change, as a proxy for blood pressure regulation, with standing balance in a clinically relevant cohort of elderly, is of special interest as blood pressure may be important to identify patients at risk of having impaired standing balance in routine geriatric assessment.

Materials and Methods: In a cross-sectional cohort study, 197 community-dwelling elderly referred to a geriatric outpatient clinic of a middle-sized teaching hospital were included. Blood pressure was measured intermittently (n = 197) and continuously (subsample, n = 58) before and after a controlled postural change from supine to standing position. The ability to maintain standing balance was assessed during ten seconds of side-by-side, semi-tandem and tandem stance, with both eyes open and eyes closed. Self-reported impaired standing balance and history of falls were recorded by questionnaires. Logistic regression analyses were used to examine the association between blood pressure and 1) the ability to maintain standing balance; 2) self-reported impaired standing balance; and 3) history of falls, adjusted for age and sex.

Results: Blood pressure decrease after postural change, measured continuously, was associated with reduced ability to maintain standing balance in semi-tandem stance with eyes closed and with increased self-reported impaired standing balance and falls. Presence of orthostatic hypotension was associated with reduced ability to maintain standing balance in semi-tandem stance with eyes closed for both intermittent and continuous measurements and with increased self-reported impaired standing balance for continuous measurements.

Conclusion: Continuous blood pressure measurements are of additional value to identify patients at risk of having impaired standing balance and may therefore be useful in routine geriatric care.

Editor: Nandu Goswami, Medical University of Graz, Austria

Funding: This study was supported by the Dutch Technology Foundation STW, which is part of the Netherlands Organisation for Scientific Research (NWO) and which is partly funded by the Ministry of Economic Affairs. Furthermore, this study was supported by the seventh framework program MYOAGE (HEALTH-2007-2.4.5-10) and 050-060-810 Netherlands Consortium for Healthy Aging (NCHA). The funders had no role in study design, data collection and analysis, decision to publish, or preparation of the manuscript.

Competing Interests: The authors have declared no competing interests exist.

* Email: a.maier@vumc.nl

Introduction

Five to 30 percent and 53 to 78 percent of elderly aged above 65 years suffer from orthostatic hypotension (OH) [1] and hypertension [2], respectively. Both OH and hypertension are signs of impaired blood pressure regulation [3,4], which is associated with increased risk of cardiovascular events [5–7], falls [8–14], and mortality [15–18]. Another important risk factor of falls is impaired standing balance [13,19,20] resulting from the deterioration of underlying systems, i.e. the sensory systems (proprioception, vision and vestibular), muscles and neural control [21].

Few studies investigated the relation between blood pressure regulation and standing balance [22–25]. In healthy elderly aged above 65 years, hypertension was found to be unrelated to quality of standing balance measured by Center of Pressure (CoP) movement [24], but was related to the score on a dynamic pull test investigating postural stability [25]. Furthermore, in healthy elderly and patients with Parkinson's disease, OH was found to be associated with higher Center of Mass (CoM) movement during standing [22,23].

In clinical practice, comparison of blood pressure measurements before and after a postural change from supine to standing position is used as a proxy for blood pressure regulation. In this study, we assessed the association of both intermittent and continuous blood pressure measurements before and after a postural change with three measures of standing balance: 1) the ability to maintain standing balance, 2) self-reported impaired standing balance and 3) history of falls, in community-dwelling elderly referred to a geriatric outpatient clinic. Results are relevant for design of routine geriatric assessment and therapeutic strategies.

Materials and Methods

Setting and study population

This cross-sectional study included 207 community-dwelling elderly who were referred to a geriatric outpatient clinic in a middle-sized teaching hospital (Bronovo Hospital, The Hague, Netherlands) for a comprehensive geriatric assessment (CGA) between March 2011 and January 2012. CGA was performed during a two hour visit including questionnaires and physical and cognitive measurements. All tests were performed by trained nurses or medical staff. The study was reviewed and approved by the institutional review board of the Leiden University Medical Center (Committee Medical Ethics (CME), Leiden, the Netherlands). The need for individual informed consent was waived, as this research was based on patient care. Ten elderly patients (4.8%) were excluded due to missing data on standing balance, leaving 197 patients for analyses. Continuous blood pressure measurements were added to the CGA in June 2012 and were subsequently available in 62 patients. Data of four patients were excluded because of technical problems, leaving 58 patients for analysis. Of two patients who visited the outpatient clinic twice, data were used from the second visit that included the continuous blood pressure measurements.

Blood pressure measurements

Blood pressure was measured in supine position and during 3 minutes in standing position after postural change. Patients were in supine position for at least 5 minutes. An automatic lift chair (Vario 570, Fitform B.V., Best, The Netherlands) was used to provide automated support from a supine to a raised position. Subsequently patients were asked to stand up and stand unsupported for 3 minutes.

Intermittent blood pressure measurements. Systolic and diastolic blood pressure measurements were determined intermittently using an automated sphygmomanometer on the left arm (Welch Allyn, Skaneateles, USA). Blood pressure was measured after at least 5 minutes in supine position before postural change and after 1 and 3 minutes in standing position. Three blood pressure measures were determined: 1) supine blood pressure was defined as the blood pressure measured in supine position before postural change; 2) blood pressure decrease was calculated for two time points by subtracting the blood pressure taken at 1 or 3 minutes in standing position from the supine blood pressure; 3) $OH_{intermittent}$ was defined as a decrease of at least 20 mmHg systolic blood pressure or 10 mmHg diastolic blood pressure at 1 or 3 minutes in standing position compared to supine blood pressure [26].

Continuous blood pressure measurements. At the same time, systolic and diastolic blood pressure measurements were determined continuously and non-invasively using a digital photoplethysmograph with a cuff placed on the right middle finger (Finometer PRO, Finapres Medical Systems BV, Amsterdam, The Netherlands) [27]. Data were analyzed using BeatScope 1.1 software (Finapres Medical systems BV, Amsterdam, The Netherlands) resulting in beat-to-beat blood pressure data. Beat-

to-beat blood pressure data were exported to Matlab (The Mathworks, Natick, MA) and averaged over 5 seconds intervals [28]. Three blood pressure measures were determined: 1) supine blood pressure was defined as the mean blood pressure in supine position during the last 60 seconds before postural change; 2) blood pressure decrease was calculated for three consecutive time periods, i.e. 0 to 15 seconds, 15 to 60 seconds and 60 to 180 seconds after postural change by subtracting the lowest averaged blood pressure measured during the time period from the supine blood pressure; 3) $OH_{continuous}$ was defined as a decrease of at least 20 mmHg systolic blood pressure or 10 mmHg diastolic blood pressure after 15 to 180 seconds in standing position compared to supine blood pressure. In addition, initial OH (iOH) was included in the definition of $OH_{continuous}$ defined as a decrease of at least 40 mmHg systolic blood pressure or 20 mmHg diastolic blood pressure during the first 15 seconds compared to supine blood pressure [29,30].

Standing balance

The ability to maintain standing balance was assessed in three standing positions characterized by a progressive narrowing of the base of support performed both with eyes open and eyes closed. Patients, wearing non-slip socks, were instructed to maintain balance for 10 seconds in each standing condition. During side-by-side stance, patients were instructed to stand with the medial malleoli as close together as possible; during semi-tandem stance, with the medial side of the heel of one foot touching the big toe of the other foot; and during tandem stance, with both feet in line while the heel of one foot touched the toes of the other. Standing positions with eyes open were first assessed as part of the Short Physical Performance Battery (SPPB) [31]. Subsequently, all standing positions were repeated with eyes closed. Patients were allowed three trials if standing balance was lost prematurely. When the patients could not complete a standing position, consecutive positions were omitted. Six patients did not attempt the standing positions with eyes closed due to lack of time or lack of motivation, leaving 191 patients for analyses of standing balance positions with eyes closed. Impaired standing balance was self-reported by answering the question whether and how often the patient experienced problems with standing balance. A positive answer was registered when the answer option 'regularly' or 'always' was given. History of falls was self-reported by answering the question whether falls in the past 12 months were experienced.

Characteristics of patients

Aforementioned items were part of a larger questionnaire obtaining information on marital status, living arrangements, smoking, alcohol use and use of walking aid. Body mass index was calculated by measuring body weight and height. Information on diseases and use of medication was extracted from medical charts. Multimorbidity was rated as the presence of two or more diseases including chronic obstructive pulmonary disease, heart failure, diabetes mellitus, hypertension, malignancy, myocardial infarction, Parkinson's disease, (osteo)arthritis, transient ischemic attack and stroke. The Hospital Anxiety Depression Scale (HADS) was used to detect depressive symptoms [32]; a score higher than 8 out of 21 points indicated depressive symptoms. Global cognitive functioning was assessed using the Mini Mental State Examination (MMSE) [33]. Handgrip strength was measured in standing position using a hand dynamometer (Jamar, Sammons Preston, Inc., Bolingbrook, IL, USA). The best performance of three trials alternately for each hand was used for analyses. Physical functioning was measured with a 10 meter walking test at usual pace in steady state, and with the SPPB. The SPPB comprises the

Table 1. Characteristics of all elderly patients and of subgroup of elderly patients who underwent additional continuous blood pressure measurements.

	All (n = 197)	Subgroup (n = 58)
Socio-demographics		
Age, years	81.9 (7.1)	80.6 (7.0)
Men, n (%)	78 (39.6)	25 (43.1)
Widowed, n (%)	80 (41.5)	17 (29.8)
Independent living, n (%)	154 (79.4)	46 (79.3)
Current smoking, n (%)[a]	22 (16.2)	9 (15.5)
Excessive alcohol use, n (%)[e]	8 (4.1)	6 (10.3)
Health characteristics		
BMI, kg/m^2[b]	25.8 (4.5)	26.4 (4.9)
Multimorbidity, n (%)[b, f]	95 (50.3)	26 (46.4)
Number of medication, median (IQR)[b]	5 (3–7)	5 (3–7)
HADS, depression > 8; n (%)[c]	28 (23.1)	10 (20.4)
MMSE, points; median (IQR)	27 (24–29)	28 (25–29)
Physical functioning		
Handgrip strength, kg	26.1 (8.2)	27.2 (7.9)
Gait speed, m/s	0.87 (0.29)	0.87 (0.29)
SPPB, points; median (IQR)	7 (5–10)	8 (6–10)
Self-reported, n (%)		
Fall incident previous 12 months	127 (64.5)	34 (58.6)
Impaired standing balance[g]	88 (45.1)	20 (35.1)
Use of walking aid	108 (55.1)	29 (50.0)
Supine blood pressure[h, b]		
Systolic blood pressure, mmHg	142 (24)	141 (25)
Diastolic blood pressure, mmHg	74.6 (10.1)	74.4 (11.0)
Blood pressure decrease after postural change		
Orthostatic hypotension, n (%)[i]	29 (15.4)	7 (12.5)
Systolic blood pressure decrease, mmHg[j, d]		
1 minute	3.15 (15.94)	−0.62 (18.24)
3 minutes	−0.80 (15.55)	−4.37 (16.03)
Diastolic blood pressure decrease, mmHg[j, d]		
1 minute	−2.90 (7.18)	−4.53 (7.10)
3 minutes	−4.17 (8.27)	−5.76 (9.54)

All parameters are presented as mean with standard deviation unless indicated otherwise. Data available in [a] n = 136, [b] n = 190, [c] n = 121, [d] n = 181. [e] Defined as > 14 units per week for females and > 21 units per week for males. [f] Present in case of two or more diseases, including chronic obstructive pulmonary diseases, heart failure, diabetes mellitus, hypertension, malignancy, myocardial infarction, Parkinson's disease, (osteo)arthritis, transient ischemic attack and stroke. [g] Defined as regularly or always self-reported impaired standing balance. [h] Measured after at least 5 minutes in supine position. [i] Orthostatic hypotension defined as decrease in systolic blood pressure of ≥ 20 mmHg or decrease in diastolic blood pressure of ≥ 10 mmHg at 1 or at 3 minutes after postural change, intermittently measured. [j] Supine blood pressure minus blood pressure at 1 or 3 minutes after postural change. IQR: inter quartile range. BMI: Body Mass Index. HADS: Hospital Anxiety and Depression Scale. MMSE: Mini Mental State Examination. SPPB: Short Physical Performance Battery.

ability to maintain balance in three standing positions with eyes open, a timed four meter walk and a timed sit-to-stand test.

Statistical analyses

Continuous variables with Gaussian distribution are presented as mean and standard deviation; otherwise as number and percentage or median and interquartile range. The association between blood pressure measures and 1) the ability to maintain standing balance; 2) impaired standing balance; and 3) history of falls were analyzed using logistic regression models including adjustment for demographics, i.e. age and sex. P values less than 0.05 were considered statistically significant. Statistical analyses

were performed using SPSS for Windows (SPSS Inc, Chicago, USA), version 20. For visualization purposes, tertiles of blood pressure decrease were calculated. Graphs were made with GraphPad Prism 5 (GraphPad Software, Inc., La Jolla, USA).

Results

Characteristics of patients

Characteristics of patients, including intermittent blood pressure measures, are presented in Table 1. Continuous blood pressure measures for the subgroup of patients are shown in Table S1. The mean age of all patients was 81.9 years. OH$_{intermittent}$ was present

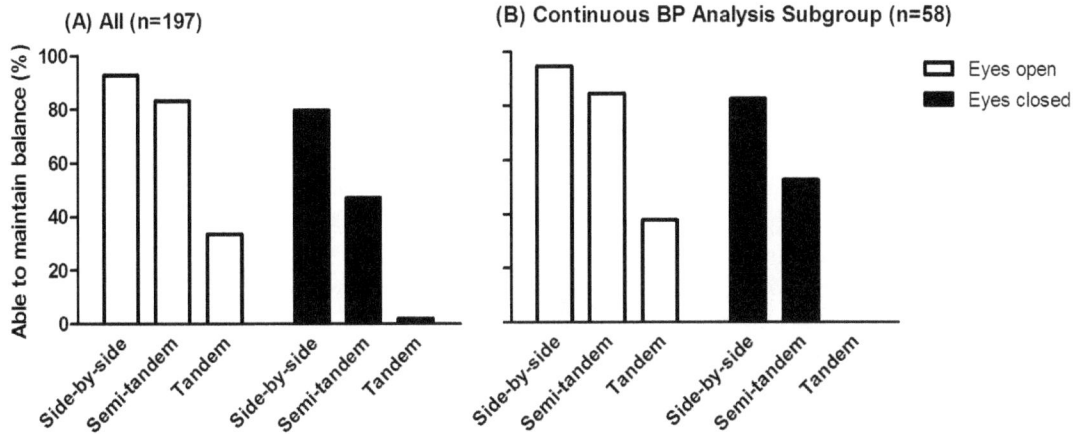

Figure 1. Ability to maintain balance in several standing positions with eyes open and eyes closed. A) all elderly patients (n = 197) and for B) subgroup who underwent additional continuous blood pressure measurements (n = 58).

in 29 out of 197 patients (15%). $OH_{continuous}$ was present in 33 out of 58 patients (57%); in 19 patients (58%) also initial OH was present and in 5 patients (15%) only iOH was present. In 26 of 33 patients (79%) in which OH was present using continuous measurements, no OH was present using intermittent measurements.

Standing balance

Ability to maintain standing balance is shown in Figure 1. The number of patients able to maintain standing balance was lower with increasing difficulty of the standing positions, both for eyes open and eyes closed conditions. In tandem stance with eyes closed 4 (2%) patients were able to maintain balance. Comparable percentages were found for the subgroup who underwent additional continuous blood pressure measurements as shown in Figure 1B. Table 1 shows that 45% of the patients reported impaired standing balance and 65% of the patients reported at least one fall incident in the 12 months prior to the visit to the outpatient clinic.

Blood pressure measures and standing balance

Intermittent blood pressure measurements. The associations between intermittent blood pressure measures and the ability to maintain standing balance adjusted for age and sex are presented in Table 2. In standing positions with eyes open, intermittent blood pressure measures were not associated with the ability to maintain balance. In standing positions with eyes closed, intermittent blood pressure measures, except $OH_{intermittent}$, were not associated with the ability to maintain standing balance. Patients with $OH_{intermittent}$ were significantly less likely to be able to maintain balance in semi-tandem stance with eyes closed. All intermittent blood pressure measures were not associated with self-reported impaired standing balance and history of falls as presented in Table S2. Additional adjustments for BMI, gait speed, MMSE score and handgrip strength did not influence the results.

Continuous blood pressure measurements. The associations between continuous blood pressure measures and the ability to maintain standing balance adjusted for age and sex are displayed in Table S3. The main findings are visualized in Figure 2. In standing positions with eyes open, blood pressure measures were not associated with the ability to maintain balance. In standing positions with eyes closed, patients with a higher

decrease in systolic blood pressure in each time period after postural change and patients with a higher decrease in diastolic blood pressure during the first 15 seconds or during 15 to 60 seconds after postural change were significantly less likely to be able to maintain balance in semi-tandem stance with eyes closed. Patients with $OH_{continuous}$ were significantly less likely to be able to maintain balance in semi-tandem stance with eyes closed. Additional adjustments for BMI, gait speed, MMSE score and handgrip strength did not influence the results.

The associations between continuous blood pressure measures and self-reported impaired standing balance and history of falls adjusted for age and sex are displayed in Figure 3 using a forest plot. This plot shows the odds ratio and 95% confidence interval per association, in which no overlap with 1.0 indicates a significant difference. Patients with a higher decrease in systolic or diastolic blood pressure during the first 15 seconds or during 15 to 60 seconds after postural change were significantly more likely to report impaired standing balance. Patients with a higher decrease in systolic or diastolic blood pressure during 15 to 60 seconds after postural change were significantly more likely to experience falls in the last 12 months. In addition, patients with a higher decrease in diastolic blood pressure in the first 15 seconds after postural change were significantly more likely to have a history of falls. Patients with $OH_{continuous}$ were significantly more likely to report impaired standing balance, but not to experience falls in the last 12 months. Additional adjustments for BMI, gait speed, MMSE score and handgrip strength did not influence the results.

Discussion

Significant associations between continuously measured blood pressure decrease after postural change and the ability to maintain standing balance in conditions with eyes closed, self-reported impaired standing balance and history of falls were found in community-dwelling elderly referred to a geriatric outpatient clinic. Furthermore, OH determined with continuous measurements was associated with reduced ability to maintain standing balance and with increased self-reported impaired standing balance, but not with falls.

This is the first study that investigated the association of blood pressure measures with ability to maintain standing balance and self-reported impaired standing balance in elderly outpatients. In previous studies, no association was found between hypertension

Table 2. Association between intermittent blood pressure measures and the ability to maintain standing balance in all elderly patients (n = 197).

	Eyes open conditions						Eyes closed conditions					
	Side-by-side		Semi-tandem		Tandem		Side-by-side		Semi-tandem		Tandem	
	OR (95% CI)	p	OR (95% CI)	p	OR (95% CI)	p	OR (95% CI)	p	OR (95% CI)	p	OR (95% CI)	p
Supine blood pressure[a]												
Systolic BP	1.01 (0.99–1.04)	.33	1.00 (0.98–1.01)	.65	1.00 (0.99–1.02)	.79	1.00 (0.98–1.01)	.79	1.00 (0.98–1.01)	.91		.42
Diastolic BP	1.04 (0.99–1.10)	.15	1.01 (0.97–1.04)	.76	1.00 (0.90–1.03)	.93	1.03 (0.99–1.07)	.93	1.01 (0.98–1.04)	.13		.59
Blood pressure decrease after postural change												
Orthostatic hypotension[b]	1.32 (0.25–7.01)	.75	1.10 (0.37–3.29)	.75	0.82 (0.31–2.17)	.87	0.66 (0.25–1.72)	.69	0.33 (0.12–0.89)	**.03**	n.a.	
Systolic BP decrease[c]												
1 minute	1.04 (1.00–1.08)	.07	1.01 (0.98–1.03)	.51	1.01 (0.98–1.03)	.51	1.01 (0.99–1.03)	.60	1.00 (0.98–1.02)	.48		.73
3 minutes	1.02 (0.98–1.07)	.34	1.00 (0.98–1.03)	.86	1.01 (0.98–1.03)	.86	1.00 (0.98–1.03)	.64	0.99 (0.97–1.02)	.84		.60
Diastolic BP decrease[c]												
1 minute	1.05 (0.96–1.14)	.32	1.05 (0.99–1.11)	.09	1.00 (0.96–1.05)	.09	1.03 (0.98–1.08)	.88	0.99 (0.95–1.04)	.32		.75
3 minutes	1.02 (0.93–1.12)	.63	1.01 (0.96–1.07)	.63	1.01 (0.96–1.05)	.63	0.99 (0.94–1.04)	.82	0.99 (0.95–1.03)	.57		.63

All data are from logistic regression analysis with adjustments for age and sex. Ability to maintain standing balance: 0 = unable, 1 = able. [a] Measured after at least 5 minutes in supine position. [b] Orthostatic hypotension: 0 = absent, 1 = present; defined as decrease in systolic blood pressure of ≥ 20 mmHg or decrease in diastolic blood pressure of ≥ 10 mmHg during 3 minutes after postural change. [c] Supine blood pressure minus blood pressure at 1 or 3 minutes after postural change. n.a. = not applicable, number of elderly patients able to maintain this balance condition is less than 5.

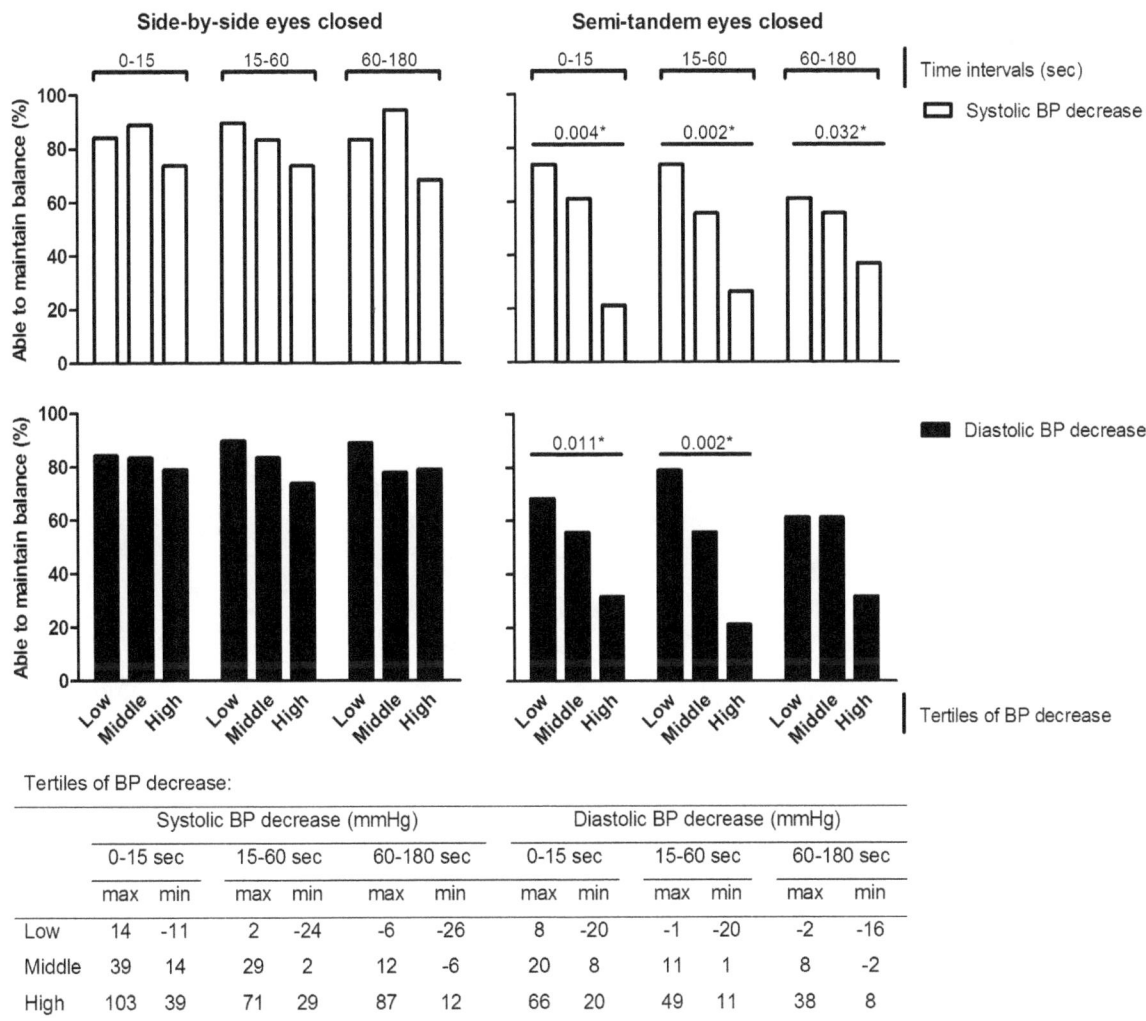

Figure 2. Percentage of elderly patients able to maintain balance during side-by-side and semi-tandem stance with eyes closed. Data is given for tertiles of systolic and diastolic blood pressure (BP) decrease, continuously measured, during the time period in seconds after postural change. *P values derived from logistic regression analyses with adjustments for age and sex.

Tertiles of BP decrease:

	Systolic BP decrease (mmHg)						Diastolic BP decrease (mmHg)					
	0-15 sec		15-60 sec		60-180 sec		0-15 sec		15-60 sec		60-180 sec	
	max	min	max	min	max	min	max	min	max	min	max	min
Low	14	-11	2	-24	-6	-26	8	-20	-1	-20	-2	-16
Middle	39	14	29	2	12	-6	20	8	11	1	8	-2
High	103	39	71	29	87	12	66	20	49	11	38	8

and quality of standing balance, measured by CoP movement, in healthy elderly [24]. However, hypertension has been associated with standing balance during a dynamic test, in which the patient was pulled backward and the response was quantified [25]. In this study, no association was found between blood pressure in supine position and measures of standing balance. Previous studies in healthy elderly and Parkinson patients found an association between OH, determined using blood pressure measurements at rest, after standing up and after one, two and three minutes of standing, and quality of standing balance, measured by CoM movement; elderly with OH were found to have an increased CoM movement during stance compared to elderly without OH [22,23]. In accordance with those studies, we found an association of presence of OH and blood pressure decrease with subjective (i.e. self-reported impaired standing balance) and objective (i.e. ability to maintain standing balance) measures of standing balance.

Previous studies investigated the association between blood pressure measures and falls. In this study continuous blood pressure measures did associate with falls, which is conflicting with other studies [9,12,28]. In accordance with other studies, no association was found between intermittent blood pressure

measures and falls [8,11,28]. Conflicting results could be due to variance in assessment and the lack of an uniform definition of OH. Furthermore, falls were assessed in different ways, i.e. retrospective, self-reported versus prospective assessment during a follow up period or use of self-administrated fall risk profiles.

The association between blood pressure decrease and reduced ability to maintain standing balance may be explained by cerebral hypoperfusion. Cerebral autoregulation modulates cerebral blood flow and cerebral perfusion in order to maintain sufficient oxygenation of the brain regions with fluctuations in blood pressure [34] and is affected by impaired blood pressure regulation [35,36]. As a result, rapid or large decreases in blood pressure may lead to a decrease in cerebral blood flow [37–39], which increases the risk of repetitive transient hypoperfusion of the brain resulting in ischemic brain damage and impaired neural control [40–43]. As neural control is involved in standing balance, this can result in impaired standing balance. This hypothesis is supported by previous findings of a negative association between ischemic brain damage quantified by white matter hyperintensities on magnetic resonance imaging (MRI) and the ability to maintain balance during specific conditions [42,44–46]. Furthermore, white matter

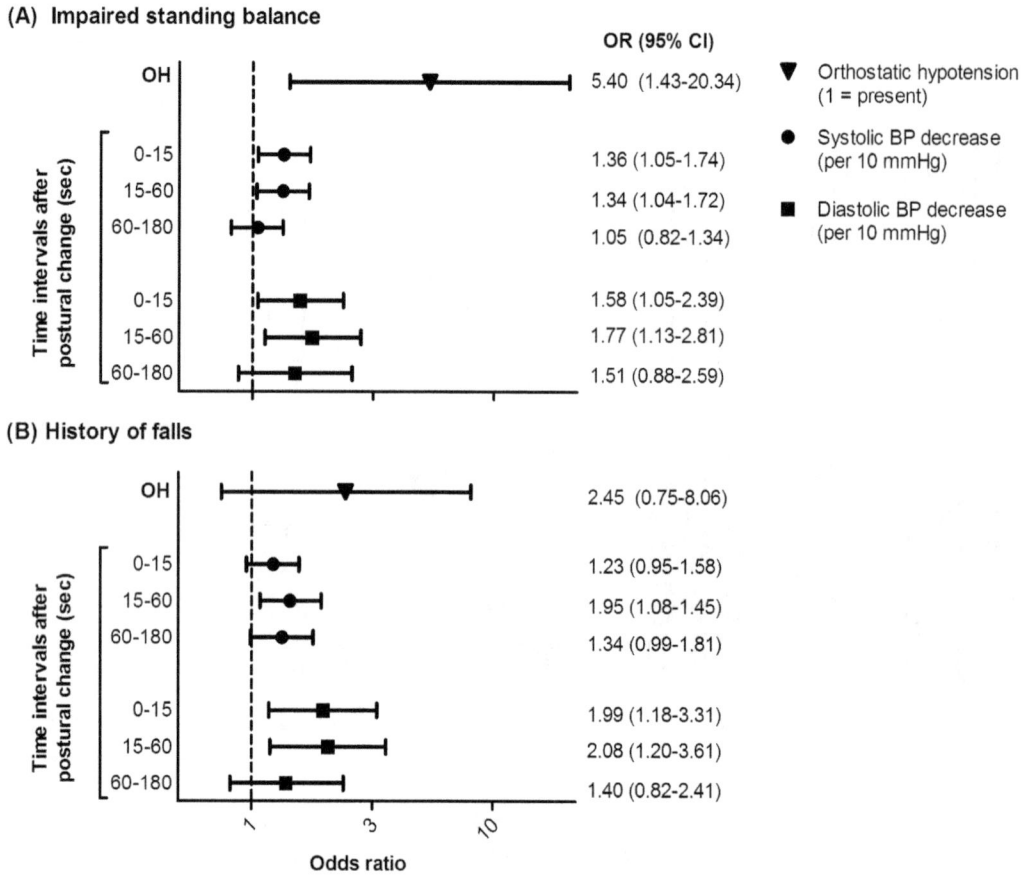

Figure 3. Forest plots of the association between blood pressure and A) reported impaired standing balance and B) history of falls. Blood pressure measures were determined with continuous measurements in subgroup who underwent additional continuous blood pressure measurements (n = 58). Orthostatic hypotension: 0 = absent, 1 = present; defined as a decrease in systolic blood pressure of ≥ 40 mmHg or in diastolic blood pressure of ≥ 20 mmHg during 15 seconds after postural change or a decrease in systolic blood pressure of ≥ 20 mmHg or diastolic blood pressure of ≥ 10 mmHg between 15 and 180 seconds after postural change. Reported impaired balance: 0 = never or sometimes, 1 = regularly or always. History of falls: 0 = no falls, 1 = falls. Results are presented in odds ratios per 10 mmHg blood pressure decrease and 95% confidence intervals with adjustments for age and sex. No overlap with 1.0 indicates a significant difference.

hyperintensities were associated with higher CoP movement which is assumed to reflect poor quality of standing balance [47]. An alternative explanation may be a common-cause, i.e. impaired blood pressure regulation and impaired standing balance both are the result of the same factor, e.g. comorbidities, neurodegeneration or cerebrovascular lesions without a direct causal relation. Further research is needed to get better insight in the causal underlying mechanisms between blood pressure and standing balance.

The association between blood pressure decrease and the ability to maintain standing balance became apparent in standing positions with eyes closed. During this specific standing condition, the nervous system has to compensate for the elimination of visual information by use of sensory reweighting [48]. The sensory systems deteriorates with increasing age [49] and elderly have to rely on less accurate and reliable sensory information in case of elimination of the visual information, which makes standing with eyes closed more difficult. Besides the sensory systems involved in standing balance, sensory systems involved in blood pressure regulation, e.g. baroreceptors, deteriorate with age and age related diseases [50,51]. This is a possible explanation for the fact that the association between blood pressure decrease and the ability to maintain standing balance was only present in standing positions with eyes closed.

The association between blood pressure decrease and standing balance was detected using objective (i.e. the ability to maintain standing balance) as well as subjective measures of standing balance (i.e. self-reported impaired standing balance and history of falls). Comparable results for the ability to maintain balance and falls were found, as impaired standing balance is a risk factor for falls[13,19,20]. Comparable results between the ability to maintain balance and self-reported impaired balance confirm the relation between the subjective and objective measures of standing balance and strengthen the clinical value of the outcome.

No association was observed between supine blood pressure and the ability to maintain standing balance, self-reported impaired standing balance or history of falls. However, previous research showed that hypertension, measured in sitting position, was associated with an increase in brain damage and concurrent impairments in mobility, cognition and mood in elderly with a mean age of 75 years [40,42]. These conflicting results might be explained by age differences. In the very old (aged above 85 years) high blood pressure is associated with better survival, mediated by poor health status and frailty in the subject with lower blood pressure. In contrast, high blood pressure in a younger population (mean age 74 years) is associated with poor survival[18]. It is unknown if there is a certain age or state of cardiovascular disease in which a high blood pressure becomes of benefit due to better perfusion. A next step would be to focus on different age groups, which will be of clinical added value. This requires large study sample sizes.

In this study, the largest decrease in blood pressure was found during the first 60 seconds after postural change by use of continuous blood pressure measurements, which is in accordance with previous research [12]. Using intermittent blood pressure measurements only one time point is recorded, which has as consequence that peak blood pressure decreases may be missed. In this study, OH determined with intermittent measurements was present in 15 percent of the patients compared to 57 percent of the patients when OH was established with continuous measurements, which is in accordance with previous findings [52]. Seventy-nine percent of these elderly were established as OH patients only with continuous measurements. The use of intermittent measurements may therefore underestimate the number of OH patients.

Strength of this study was the unique study population of elderly patients. No exclusion criteria were applied. The population is representative for the community-dwelling elderly visiting the geriatric outpatient clinic. Furthermore, the use of continuous blood pressure measurements provided additional information about the blood pressure during the first 60 seconds after postural change and made it possible to include iOH in the analyses. As blood pressure was measured during 3 minutes after postural change, delayed OH, which occurs ten minutes or more after postural change [53], could not be measured. Limitation of this study is the cross-sectional design, which makes it impossible to draw conclusions about a causal relation between blood pressure regulation and standing balance. Furthermore, history of falls was measured using questionnaires which could result in recall bias. Despite the lower number of patients with continuous blood pressure measurements, we were able to find valuable associations of blood pressure decrease with standing balance.

impaired standing balance and history of falls were found. The fact that previous associations could not be detected with intermittent blood pressure measurements, demonstrates the additional value of continuous over intermittent blood pressure measurements in routine geriatric assessment.

Conclusions

In conclusion, only by using continuous blood pressure measurements as a proxy for blood pressure regulation, associations with the ability to maintain standing balance, self-reported

Author Contributions

Conceived and designed the experiments: ABM CGMM GJB JHP MS. Performed the experiments: JHP MS JMK. Analyzed the data: JHP JMK AYB ABM MM. Contributed reagents/materials/analysis tools: ABM CGMM GJB. Contributed to the writing of the manuscript: JHP JMK AYB. Obtained funding: ABM CGMM GJB. Critical revision: MS ABM CGMM GJB MM. Study supervision: ABM CGMM.

References

1. Low PA (2008) Prevalence of orthostatic hypotension. Clin Auton Res 18 Suppl 1: 8–13. 10.1007/s10286-007-1001-3.
2. Wolf-Maier K, Cooper RS, Banegas JR, Giampaoli S, Hense HW, et al. (2003) Hypertension prevalence and blood pressure levels in 6 European countries, Canada, and the United States. JAMA 289: 2363–2369. 10.1001/jama.289.18.2363.
3. Lipsitz LA (1989) Orthostatic hypotension in the elderly. N Engl J Med 321: 952–957. 10.1056/NEJM198910053211407.
4. James MA, Potter JF (1999) Orthostatic blood pressure changes and arterial baroreflex sensitivity in elderly subjects. Age Ageing 28: 522–530.
5. Masley SC, Phillips SE, Schocken DD (2006) Blood pressure as a predictor of cardiovascular events in the elderly: the William Hale Research Program. J Hum Hypertens 20: 392–397. 10.1038/sj.jhh.1002002.
6. Dart AM, Gatzka CD, Kingwell BA, Willson K, Cameron JD, et al. (2006) Brachial blood pressure but not carotid arterial waveforms predict cardiovascular events in elderly female hypertensives. Hypertension 47: 785–790. 10.1161/01.HYP.0000209340.33592.50.
7. Benvenuto LJ, Krakoff LR (2011) Morbidity and mortality of orthostatic hypotension: implications for management of cardiovascular disease. Am J Hypertens 24: 135–144. 10.1038/ajh.2010.146.
8. Liu BA, Topper AK, Reeves RA, Gryfe C, Maki BE (1995) Falls among older people: relationship to medication use and orthostatic hypotension. J Am Geriatr Soc 43: 1141–1145.
9. Heitterachi E, Lord SR, Meyerkort P, McCloskey I, Fitzpatrick R (2002) Blood pressure changes on upright tilting predict falls in older people. Age Ageing 31: 181–186.
10. Gangavati A, Hajjar I, Quach L, Jones RN, Kiely DK, et al. (2011) Hypertension, orthostatic hypotension, and the risk of falls in a community-dwelling elderly population: the maintenance of balance, independent living, intellect, and zest in the elderly of Boston study. J Am Geriatr Soc 59: 383–389. 10.1111/j.1532-5415.2011.03317.x.
11. van Hateren KJ, Kleefstra N, Blanker MH, Ubink-Veltmaat LJ, Groenier KH, et al. (2012) Orthostatic hypotension, diabetes, and falling in older patients: a cross-sectional study. Br J Gen Pract 62: e696–e702. 10.3399/bjgp12X656838.
12. Maurer MS, Cohen S, Cheng H (2004) The degree and timing of orthostatic blood pressure changes in relation to falls in nursing home residents. J Am Med Dir Assoc 5: 233–238. 10.1097/01.JAM.0000129837.51514.93.
13. Tinetti ME, Speechley M, Ginter SF (1988) Risk factors for falls among elderly persons living in the community. N Engl J Med 319: 1701–1707. 10.1056/NEJM198812293192604.
14. Romero-Ortuno R, Cogan L, Foran T, Kenny RA, Fan CW (2011) Continuous noninvasive orthostatic blood pressure measurements and their relationship with orthostatic intolerance, falls, and frailty in older people. J Am Geriatr Soc 59: 655–665. 10.1111/j.1532-5415.2011.03352.x.
15. Rockwood MR, Howlett SE, Rockwood K (2012) Orthostatic hypotension (OH) and mortality in relation to age, blood pressure and frailty. Arch Gerontol Geriatr 54: e255–e260. 10.1016/j.archger.2011.12.009.
16. Verwoert GC, Mattace-Raso FU, Hofman A, Heeringa J, Stricker BH, et al. (2008) Orthostatic hypotension and risk of cardiovascular disease in elderly people: the Rotterdam study. J Am Geriatr Soc 56: 1816–1820. 10.1111/j.1532-5415.2008.01946.x.
17. Lagro J, Laurenssen NC, Schalk BW, Schoon Y, Claassen JA, et al. (2012) Diastolic blood pressure drop after standing as a clinical sign for increased mortality in older falls clinic patients. J Hypertens 30: 1195–1202. 10.1097/HJH.0b013e328352b9fd.

18. Odden MC, Peralta CA, Haan MN, Covinsky KE (2012) Rethinking the association of high blood pressure with mortality in elderly adults: the impact of frailty. Arch Intern Med 172: 1162–1168. 10.1001/archinternmed.2012.2555.

19. Muir SW, Berg K, Chesworth B, Klar N, Speechley M (2010) Quantifying the magnitude of risk for balance impairment on falls in community-dwelling older adults: a systematic review and meta-analysis. J Clin Epidemiol 63: 389–406. 10.1016/j.jclinepi.2009.06.010.

20. Rubenstein LZ (2006) Falls in older people: epidemiology, risk factors and strategies for prevention. Age Ageing 35 Suppl 2: ii37–ii41. 10.1093/ageing/afl084.

21. Horak FB, Shupert CL, Mirka A (1989) Components of postural dyscontrol in the elderly: a review. Neurobiol Aging 10: 727–738.

22. Overstall PW, Exton-Smith AN, Imms FJ, Johnson AL (1977) Falls in the elderly related to postural imbalance. Br Med J 1: 261–264.

23. Matinolli M, Korpelainen JT, Korpelainen R, Sotaniemi KA, Myllyla VV (2009) Orthostatic hypotension, balance and falls in Parkinson's disease. Mov Disord 24: 745–751. 10.1002/mds.22457.

24. Abate M1, Di Iorio A, Pini B, Battaglini C, Di Nicola I, et al. (2009) Effects of hypertension on balance assessed by computerized posturography in the elderly. Arch Gerontol Geriatr 49: 113–117. 10.1016/j.archger.2008.05.008.

25. Hausdorff JM, Herman T, Baltadjieva R, Gurevich T, Giladi N (2003) Balance and gait in older adults with systemic hypertension. Am J Cardiol 91: 643–645.

26. The Consensus Committee of the American Autonomic Society and the American Academy of Neurology (1996) Consensus statement on the definition of orthostatic hypotension, pure autonomic failure, and multiple system atrophy. Neurology 46: 1470.

27. Imholz BP, Wieling W, van Montfrans GA, Wesseling KH (1998) Fifteen years experience with finger arterial pressure monitoring: assessment of the technology. Cardiovasc Res 38: 605–616.

28. van der Velde N, van den Meiracker AH, Stricker BH, van der Cammen TJ (2007) Measuring orthostatic hypotension with the Finometer device: is a blood pressure drop of one heartbeat clinically relevant? Blood Press Monit 12: 167–171. 10.1097/MBP.0b013e3280b083bd.

29. Wieling W, Krediet CT, van Dijk N, Linzer M, Tschakovsky ME (2007) Initial orthostatic hypotension: review of a forgotten condition. Clin Sci (Lond) 112: 157–165. 10.1042/CS20060091.

30. Wieling W, Schatz IJ (2009) The consensus statement on the definition of orthostatic hypotension: a revisit after 13 years. J Hypertens 27: 935–938. 10.1097/HJH.0b013e32832b1145.

31. Guralnik JM, Simonsick EM, Ferrucci L, Glynn RJ, Berkman LF, et al. (1994) A short physical performance battery assessing lower extremity function: association with self-reported disability and prediction of mortality and nursing home admission. J Gerontol 49: M85–M94.

32. Zigmond AS, Snaith RP (1983) The hospital anxiety and depression scale. Acta Psychiatr Scand 67: 361–370.

33. Folstein MF, Folstein SE, McHugh PR (1975) "Mini-mental state". A practical method for grading the cognitive state of patients for the clinician. J Psychiatr Res 12: 189–198.

34. Lucas SJ, Tzeng YC, Galvin SD, Thomas KN, Ogoh S, et al. (2010) Influence of changes in blood pressure on cerebral perfusion and oxygenation. Hypertension 55: 698–705. 10.1161/HYPERTENSIONAHA.109.146290.

35. Strandgaard S, Paulson OB (1995) Cerebral blood flow in untreated and treated hypertension. Neth J Med 47: 180–184.

36. Novak V, Novak P, Spies JM, Low PA (1998) Autoregulation of cerebral blood flow in orthostatic hypotension. Stroke 29: 104–111.

37. Rickards CA, Cohen KD, Bergeron LL, Burton BL, Khatri PJ, et al. (2007) Cerebral blood flow response and its association with symptoms during orthostatic hypotension. Aviat Space Environ Med 78: 653–658.

38. Lipsitz LA, Mukai S, Hamner J, Gagnon M, Babikian V (2000) Dynamic regulation of middle cerebral artery blood flow velocity in aging and hypertension. Stroke 31: 1897–1903.

39. Mehagnoul-Schipper DJ, Vloet LC, Colier WN, Hoefnagels WH, Jansen RW (2000) Cerebral oxygenation declines in healthy elderly subjects in response to assuming the upright position. Stroke 31: 1615–1620.

40. Hajjar I, Quach L, Yang F, Chaves PH, Newman AB, et al. (2011) Hypertension, white matter hyperintensities, and concurrent impairments in mobility, cognition, and mood: the Cardiovascular Health Study. Circulation 123: 858–865. 10.1161/CIRCULATIONAHA.110.978114.

41. Pantoni L, Garcia JH (1997) Pathogenesis of leukoaraiosis: a review. Stroke 28: 652–659.

42. Whitman GT, Tang Y, Lin A, Baloh RW (2001) A prospective study of cerebral white matter abnormalities in older people with gait dysfunction. Neurology 57: 990–994.

43. Vernooij MW, van der Lugt A, Ikram MA, Wielopolski PA, Vrooman HA, et al. (2008) Total cerebral blood flow and total brain perfusion in the general population: the Rotterdam Scan Study. J Cereb Blood Flow Metab 28: 412–419. 10.1038/sj.jcbfm.9600526.

44. Baloh RW, Yue Q, Socotch TM, Jacobson KM (1995) White matter lesions and disequilibrium in older people. I. Case-control comparison. Arch Neurol 52: 970–974.

45. Tell GS, Lefkowitz DS, Diehr P, Elster AD (1998) Relationship between balance and abnormalities in cerebral magnetic resonance imaging in older adults. Arch Neurol 55: 73–79.

46. Starr JM, Leaper SA, Murray AD, Lemmon HA, Staff RT, et al. (2003) Brain white matter lesions detected by magnetic resonance [correction of resosnance] imaging are associated with balance and gait speed. J Neurol Neurosurg Psychiatry 74: 94–98.

47. Novak V, Haertle M, Zhao P, Hu K, Munshi M, et al. (2009) White matter hyperintensities and dynamics of postural control. Magn Reson Imaging 27: 752–759. 10.1016/j.mri.2009.01.010.

48. Peterka RJ (2002) Sensorimotor integration in human postural control. J Neurophysiol 88: 1097–1118.

49. Horak FB, Shupert CL, Mirka A (1989) Components of postural dyscontrol in the elderly: a review. Neurobiol Aging 10: 727–738.

50. Mancia G, Ferrari A, Gregorini L, Parati G, Pomidossi G, et al. (1983) Blood pressure and heart rate variabilities in normotensive and hypertensive human beings. Circ Res 53: 96–104.

51. Duschek S, Werner NS, Reyes Del Paso GA (2013) The behavioral impact of baroreflex function: A review. Psychophysiology. 10.1111/psyp.12136.

52. Cooke J, Carew S, Quinn C, O'Connor M, Curtin J, et al. (2013) The prevalence and pathological correlates of orthostatic hypotension and its subtypes when measured using beat-to-beat technology in a sample of older adults living in the community. Age Ageing. 10.1093/ageing/aft112.

53. Gibbons CH, Freeman R (2006) Delayed orthostatic hypotension: a frequent cause of orthostatic intolerance. Neurology 67: 28–32. 10.1212/01.wnl.0000223828.28215.0b.

16

Relationship between Neural Rhythm Generation Disorders and Physical Disabilities in Parkinson's Disease Patients' Walking

Leo Ota[1]*, **Hirotaka Uchitomi**[1], **Ken-ichiro Ogawa**[1], **Satoshi Orimo**[2], **Yoshihiro Miyake**[1]

1 Department of Computational Intelligence and Systems Science, Tokyo Institute of Technology, Yokohama, Kanagawa, Japan, 2 Department of Neurology, Kanto Central Hospital, Setagaya, Tokyo, Japan

Abstract

Walking is generated by the interaction between neural rhythmic and physical activities. In fact, Parkinson's disease (PD), which is an example of disease, causes not only neural rhythm generation disorders but also physical disabilities. However, the relationship between neural rhythm generation disorders and physical disabilities has not been determined. The aim of this study was to identify the mechanism of gait rhythm generation. In former research, neural rhythm generation disorders in PD patients' walking were characterized by stride intervals, which are more variable and fluctuate randomly. The variability and fluctuation property were quantified using the coefficient of variation (CV) and scaling exponent α. Conversely, because walking is a dynamic process, postural reflex disorder (PRD) is considered the best way to estimate physical disabilities in walking. Therefore, we classified the severity of PRD using CV and α. Specifically, PD patients and healthy elderly were classified into three groups: no-PRD, mild-PRD, and obvious-PRD. We compared the contributions of CV and α to the accuracy of this classification. In this study, 45 PD patients and 17 healthy elderly people walked 200 m. The severity of PRD was determined using the modified Hoehn–Yahr scale (mH-Y). People with mH-Y scores of 2.5 and 3 had mild-PRD and obvious-PRD, respectively. As a result, CV differentiated no-PRD from PRD, indicating the correlation between CV and PRD. Considering that PRD is independent of neural rhythm generation, this result suggests the existence of feedback process from physical activities to neural rhythmic activities. Moreover, α differentiated obvious-PRD from mild-PRD. Considering α reflects the intensity of interaction between factors, this result suggests the change of the interaction. Therefore, the interaction between neural rhythmic and physical activities is thought to plays an important role for gait rhythm generation. These characteristics have potential to evaluate the symptoms of PD.

Editor: Oscar Arias-Carrion, Hospital General Dr. Manuel Gea González, Mexico

Funding: This work was supported by the Ministry of Education, Culture, Sports, Science and Technology (MEXT) Grant-in-Aid for Scientific Research (B) to Dr. Miyake (MEXT KAKENHI Grant Number 23300209, URL: http://www.mext.go.jp/english/). The funders had no role in study design, data collection and analysis, decision to publish, or preparation of the manuscript.

Competing Interests: The authors have declared that no competing interests exist.

* Email: ohta@myk.dis.titech.ac.jp

Introduction

Walking is one of the most fundamental factors in our daily behaviors. The gait dynamics is thought to be generated by the interaction between neural rhythmic activity and physical activity [1,2]. However, because this interaction is difficult to estimate in healthy gait dynamics, we focused on the patients with Parkinson's disease (PD) (as a typical example of neurodegenerative disease) [3], which causes not only neural rhythm generation disorders, but also physical disabilities. To identify the mechanism of gait rhythm generation, we attempted to examine the relationship between neural rhythmic activity and physical activity in PD patients.

In previous studies, two symptoms were reported as neural rhythm generation disorders in PD patients' walking. One symptom was the increase in the variability of gait rhythm [4,5], and the other symptom was a change in the fluctuation property of gait rhythm from the normal $1/f$-like fluctuation property [6–8]. In healthy young people, gait rhythm is not constant; rather, it changes subtly. This change can be described by a pair of physical measures. One is the coefficient of variation (CV), which

represents the variability of gait rhythm. The other is the scaling exponent α, which represents the fluctuation property of gait rhythm and can be calculated by detrended fluctuation analysis (DFA). In particular, the fluctuation in gait rhythm is an important feature of walking. In healthy young people, the gait rhythm exhibits small variation and $1/f$-like fluctuation properties [9].

For each of these symptoms, two types of gait rehabilitation methods using sensory cues have been proposed. One is gait training with rhythmic stimuli, which is based on forced entrainment for human, including rhythmic auditory stimulation (RAS) gait training [10] and treadmill training [11]. The other is gait training with rhythmic stimuli, which is based on mutual entrainment with human, such as WalkMate gait training [12]. In RAS gait training, fixed-tempo rhythmic auditory stimuli are input to PD patients [10]. This type of rehabilitation improves mainly the variability of gait rhythm. In other words, RAS gait training decreases CV but does not change α much [8,13]. We have been developing the WalkMate system [12]. In WalkMate gait training, rhythmic auditory stimuli mutually entrained with the gait rhythm of PD patients [14]. This type of rehabilitation improves mainly the fluctuation property of gait rhythm [14]. In one study, α improved substantially, but CV did not change much after four consecutive days of WalkMate gait training [15]. These findings suggest that RAS gait training and WalkMate gait training improve different features of neural rhythm generation disorders in PD patients' walking.

Conversely, PD patients often also show physical disabilities. Postural instability is one of the main motor symptoms of physical disability in PD, and its clinical manifestations are a festinant and shuffling gait, poor postural alignment, and defective postural reflexes. There are many tests for assessing the postural instability and balance control related to the risk of falling [16]. Regarding gait dynamics, the pull test [17], which is a test of postural reflex disorder (PRD), is the most suitable to evaluate physical disabilities during a dynamic state, such as walking.

However, it is not clear whether CV and α, which evaluates the different features of neural rhythm generation disorders, are related to PRD, which evaluate physical disabilities. The purpose of this study was to examine the relationship between the set of CV and α, and PRD on a platform aimed at evaluating the gait rhythm in PD patients, to identify the mechanism of gait rhythm generation. To construct this evaluation platform, we focused on a combination of CV and α, because it can be considered as a feature amount that represents neural rhythm generation disorders. Subsequently, we classified the subjects according to the presence or absence of PRD using the platform for gait rhythm. Furthermore, the severity of PRD in a group of PD patients was classified using the platform for gait rhythm. The modified Hoehn–Yahr (mH-Y) scale [18,19] was used as the method of evaluation of the clinical signs of PRD.

In the Methods section, we describe the demographic information of participants, gait task, and the method of measurement of stride interval. Then, we explain the calculation of two dynamic indicators: the variability of the stride interval (CV) and the fluctuation property of the stride interval (α). We mention a linear discriminant analysis using a combination of CV and α, and the classification of PRD using mH-Y. In the Results section, the results of the two classifications are shown, and the accuracy and contribution of CV or α to the classifications are reported. In the Discussion section, we discuss the mechanism underlying neural rhythm generation disorders in PD patients' walking and a potential application of this platform to evaluate the motor symptoms of PD.

Methods

Participants

Forty-five patients (21 men, 24 women; mean age $\pm$ SD, 69.8 ± 8.2 years) with PD and 17 age-matched healthy people (10 men, seven women; mean age, 70.2 ± 2.8 years) participated in this study (Table 1). The mean disease duration ($\pm$ SD) was 4.7 ± 3.9 years. The mH-Y classifications and number of subjects were mH-Y 1–2 ($n = 19$), mH-Y 2.5 ($n = 11$), and mH-Y 3 ($n = 15$). All patients were taking at least one of antiparkinsonian medications during the experiment. The antiparkinsonian medications included levodopa/carbidopa, dopamine receptor agonist, selegiline, amantadine, and anticholinergics. Those were taken at maximum two hours before the start time of measurement. All participants could walk without a cane or walker. These experimental procedures were approved by the Kanto Central Hospital Ethics Committee. Before the experiment, we obtained written informed consent from the participants.

Gait tasks and measurement of stride interval

Participants walked at their preferred pace along a 200 m round course. We measured gait rhythm once for each participant and calculated the stride interval time series. Stride interval is defined as the time duration between two consecutive foot contacts on the same side. Foot switches (OT-21BP-G, Ojiden, Japan) were attached under the shoes and were used to detect the gait rhythm. The mean number ($\pm$ SD) of stride intervals was 154 ± 23 strides for the 200 m. Data for foot contact timing were sent to a laptop PC (CF-W5AWDBJR, Panasonic, Japan) via a wireless transmitter (S-1019M1F, Smart Sensor Technology, Japan). The sampling frequency was 100 Hz. We used only the data obtained for the left side because no significant differences between stride interval were observed between the left and right sides (left side: mean $= 1.06 \pm 0.09$ s, CV $= 2.73\% \pm 1.09\%$, $\alpha = 0.80 \pm 0.21$; right side: mean $= 1.06 \pm 0.09$ s, CV $= 2.78\% \pm 1.62\%$, $\alpha = 0.81 \pm 0.22$; P-values based on Welch's two-sample t test: $P = 0.97$ for mean, $P = 0.82$ for CV, $P = 0.92$ for α). We analyzed the data obtained for the right side in only one patient because a high noise level was observed in the data for the left side. To assess only the stable stride interval phase, the first 10 strides and last five strides (i.e., the transient stride interval phase) were not analyzed.

CV

We focused on the CV as a dynamic indicator to evaluate the variability of stride interval in the participants. CV represents the variability of time-series data, and is calculated as the standard deviation normalized to the mean value: CV $=$ SD/Mean$\times 100$ [%]. The CV of healthy people is 1%–2.5%, and the CV of PD patients is 2.5%–4% [6].

DFA

We focused on the scaling exponent α as the other dynamic indicator to evaluate the fluctuation property. The scaling exponent α can be quantified by DFA as a long-range correlation in time series data [20,21]. We selected this method because it can also be applied to relatively short intervals [22].

If the α is nearly equal to 0.5, the time series is characterized by white noise. On the other hand, if α is near 1.0, the series is characterized by $1/f$ fluctuation and is suggested to be generated by chaos dynamics or limit cycle dynamics coupled with noise [23–26]. The α of the stride interval at the preferred pace has been reported as 0.50–0.85 in PD patients [6,8] and as 0.8–1.2 in healthy young people [27,28]. In healthy elderly people, the α of the stride interval is decreased to 0.7–0.9, although the CV remains unchanged [7,28,29].

Linear discriminant analysis

Fisher's linear discriminant analysis was used with a combination of CV and α to obtain a function for dividing the measured data into two groups [30].

The leave-one-out cross-validation method was used to estimate the classification rate, and the following were calculated: (1) accuracy, the rate of truly classified data among all data; (2) sensitivity, the accuracy rate for identifying positive data (participants with more severe symptoms); and (3) specificity, the accuracy rate for identifying negative data (participants with mild symptoms). To compare the individual contribution to the classification of CV and α, these two variables were normalized using a Z score, and the angle between the normalized CV axis and the boundary line was calculated by a linear discriminant function.

Table 1. Characteristics of the participants.

Classification	Difference between PRD and no-PRD			Difference between obvious-PRD and mild-PRD		
Positive/Negative	Positive (PRD, $n=26$)	Negative (no-PRD, $n=36$)	P	Positive (obvious-PRD, $n=15$)	Negative (mild-PRD, $n=11$)	P
Age (years, mean ± SD)	72.7±7.0	68.1±6.9	0.01	72.5±6.7	72.4±7.5	0.83
Sex (male:female)	15:11	16:20	0.31	8:7	7:4	0.61
Disease duration (years, mean ± SD)	4.9±4.6	2.3±3.1	0.01	6.2±5.5	4.0±2.8	0.35
mH-Y score in "on" state (median, range)	3, 2.5–3	1.25, 0–2	–	3, 3	2.5, 2.5	–

P values were calculated using Welch's two-sample t test.
PRD, postural reflex disorder; mH-Y, modified Hoehn–Yahr scale.

Classification of PRD

Walking is controlled in parallel with posture and muscle-tone control [31–34]. Postural instability, which is one of the physical disabilities, can be often evaluated by the Berg Balance Test [16]. However, when considering gait dynamics, the pull test (30th item in the Unified Parkinson's Disease Rating Scale) is the most suitable for estimating the ability of physical activities in walking [17]. Therefore, we focused on the pull test to identify the presence or absence of PRD and its severity. In the pull test, the shoulder of a PD patient is pulled backward and forward while the patient remains standing. An overview of the classification is shown in Figure 1. Performance on the pull test is associated with mH-Y, which is one of the clinical indicators used for the assessment of motor symptoms of PD [19].

The scores in the original H-Y range from 1 to 5, in increments of 1. The mH-Y includes added stages 1.5, and 2.5 [19]. We separated participants into three groups based on their mH-Y score and performance on the pull test: mH-Y score of 2 or less

with no problems on the pull test (no-PRD), mH-Y = 2.5 with signs of mild disorder on the pull test (mild-PRD), and mH-Y = 3 with obvious signs of disorder on the pull test (obvious-PRD). No-PRD was determined by a normal postural reflex in the pull test. Mild-PRD was defined by very mild postural impairment (suggestive, but not diagnostic; usually one or two steps before recovery from a postural threat) [19]. Obvious-PRD was determined by the presence of retropulsion, which is defined by (1) the appearance of more than three backward steps during the pull test, followed by unaided recovery, (2) the absence of postural reflex, or (3) the indication of falling if the examinee is not supported [17]. Although the examiner's decision regarding need of support in the pull test is subjective, we paid careful attention to the classification of PRD. All participants were examined by the same doctor in the same environment. Furthermore, the doctor is a PD expert who is authorized by the Japanese Society of Neurology. Therefore, the results of the mH-Y staging were reproducible.

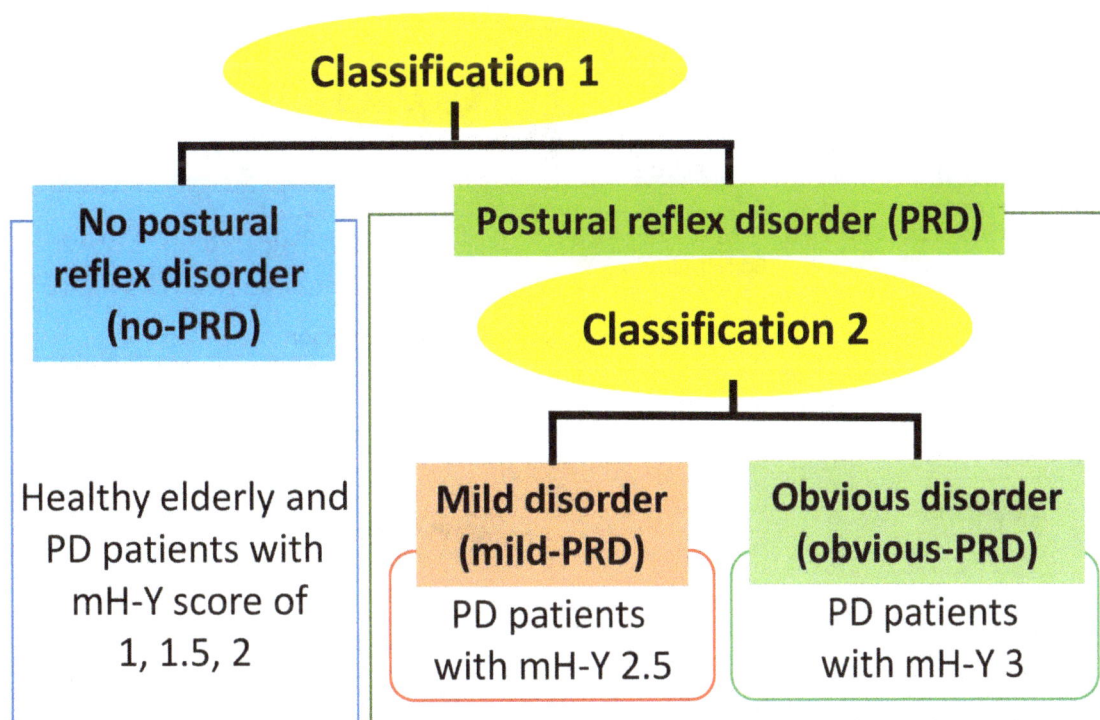

Figure 1. Classification of the severity of postural reflex disorder (PRD).

We first classified participants according to the presence and absence of PRD (Classification 1 in Figure 1, see Table 1). This classification segregated the no-PRD group (17 healthy elderly people and two PD patients, one with an mH-Y score of 1 and one with a score of 1.5) from the PRD group. We then divided the PRD group of patients into the mild-PRD and obvious-PRD groups (Classification 2 in Figure 1, see Table 1).

Results

Figure 2 shows a sample result of the gait analysis, including the stride interval time series and the result of DFA. The CV of the stride interval was larger in PD patients with PRD (Figure 2A, B) than in healthy people (Figure 2C). The α of the stride interval (Figure 2A) was lower in PD patients with obvious-PRD than in PD patients with mild-PRD (Figure 2B), in PD patients with no-PRD (Figure 2C), or in healthy elderly people (Figure 2D).

Classification 1: The presence or absence of PRD

First, we classified the PD patients and healthy elderly people into two groups according to the presence or absence of PRD. The no-PRD group comprised healthy elderly participants and PD patients with an mH-Y score of 1–2, and the PRD group comprised PD patients with an mH-Y score of 2.5–3. Figure 3A shows the distribution of all participants' data for the feature space configured by CV and α of the stride interval; namely, (CV, α) plane. The x-axis represents CV, and the y-axis represents α. The blue points represent the data for the no-PRD group, and the green points represent the data for the PRD group. On the y-axis of α in Figure 3A, the data for each group overlapped between 0.5 and 1.0. In contrast, the no-PRD group data were distributed in a

scattered pattern in the low-CV area, and the data for the PRD group were scattered in the high-CV area.

Figure 3B shows the distribution of normalized data, to indicate which axis contributes to the classification of the two groups regardless of the variation in each axis. The solid line represents the boundary line between the two groups. When we defined the no-PRD group as negative and the PRD group as positive, the accuracy was 74%, the sensitivity was 50%, and the specificity was 92%. The angle between the normalized CV axis and the boundary line shown in Figure 3B was 91°. The large angle observed between the normalized CV axis and the boundary line suggests that the CV can be used to differentiate between the presence and absence of PRD.

Classification 2: Obvious-PRD or mild-PRD

Next, we focused on the two PRD groups: obvious-PRD and mild-PRD. The mild-PRD group comprised PD patients with an mH-Y score of 2.5, and the obvious-PRD group comprised PD patients with an mH-Y score of 3. Figure 4A shows the distribution of data of the PRD group in CV, α) plane. The red points represent the data for the mild-PRD group, and the light-green points represent the data for the obvious-PRD group. On the x-axis of CV in Figure 4A, the data for both groups overlap between 2.5 and 6.0. By contrast, the α for the mild-PRD group tended to scatter near 1.0 (i.e., the $1/f$-like fluctuation property was observed), and the α for the obvious-PRD group tended to scatter around 0.6 (i.e., the $1/f$-like fluctuation property was detected less often).

When we defined the mild-PRD group as negative and the obvious-PRD group as positive, the accuracy was 69%, the

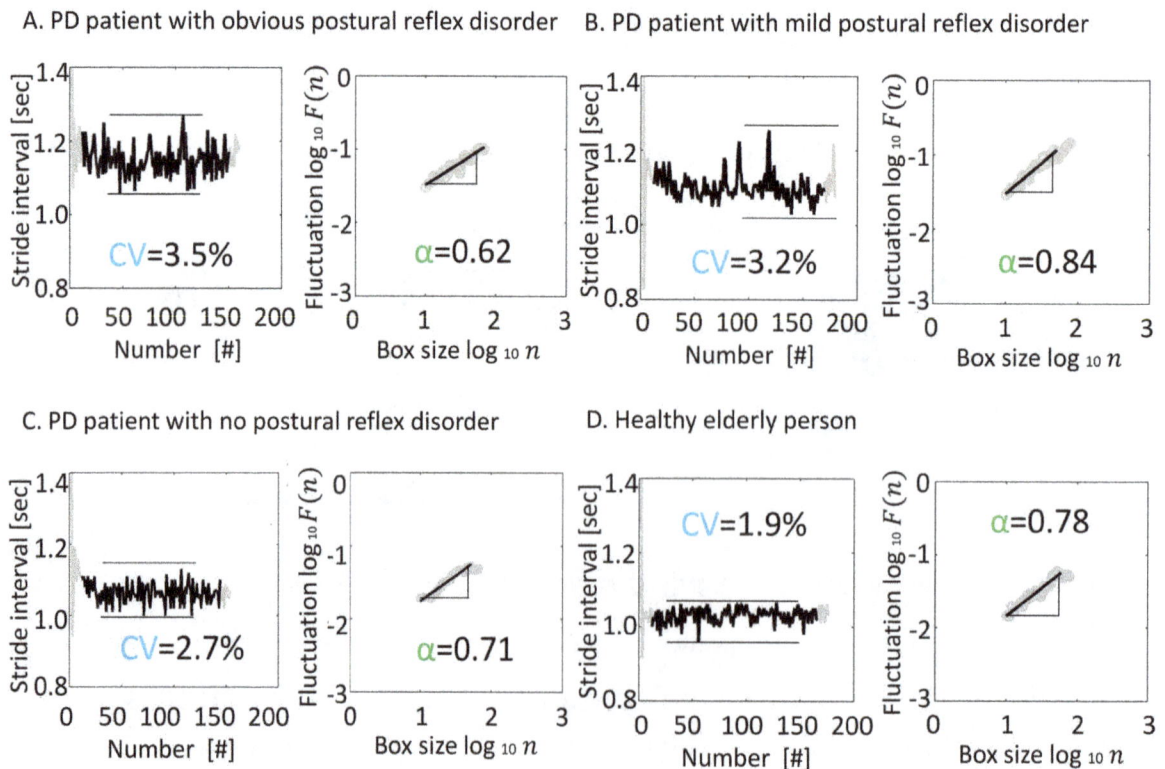

A. PD patient with obvious postural reflex disorder   B. PD patient with mild postural reflex disorder

C. PD patient with no postural reflex disorder   D. Healthy elderly person

Figure 2. A sample of the stride interval and the fluctuation relative to box size. (A) PD patient with obvious postural reflex disorder (mH-Y score, 3; age 76 years; male). (B) PD patient with mild postural reflex disorder (mH-Y score, 2.5; age, 70 years; male). (C) PD patient with no postural reflex disorder (mH-Y score, 2; age, 76 years; male). (D) Healthy elderly person (age. 71 years; male).

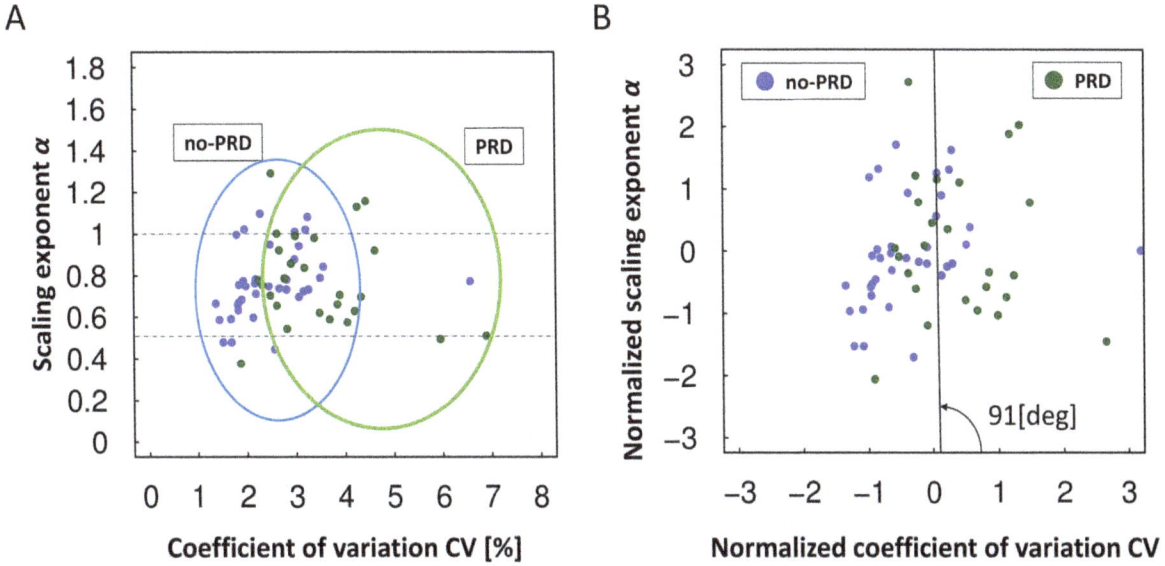

Figure 3. Classification according to the presence or absence of postural reflex disorder. The no postural reflex disorder group (no-PRD) is indicated by blue points, and the postural reflex disorder group (PRD) is indicated by green points. The x-axis represents the CV, and the y-axis represents α. The data for the no-PRD group are distributed in a small CV region around 2%, whereas those for the PRD group are distributed in a large CV region roughly from 2.5% to 5%. The two groups have a wide and overlapping distribution of α. (A) Distribution of the original data. (B) Distribution of the normalized data. The solid line represents the boundary between the no-PRD group and the PRD group.

sensitivity was 80%, and the specificity was 55%. The solid line represents the boundary line between the two groups, and the dashed line represents a horizontal line that corresponds to the average level of the original value of α. The angle between the normalized CV axis and the boundary line shown in Figure 4B was 5.7°. The small angle observed between the normalized CV axis and the boundary line suggests that α can be used to differentiate obvious-PRD from mild-PRD.

Discussion

In this study, we used CV to evaluate the variability of gait rhythm, and the scaling exponent α to evaluate the fluctuation property of gait rhythm. These are two important indicators of neural rhythm generation disorders in PD patients. We performed a linear discriminant analysis based on a combination of CV and α to differentiate between the presence and absence of PRD, and between obvious-PRD and mild-PRD. As a result, CV differentiated between the presence and absence of PRD, indicating the

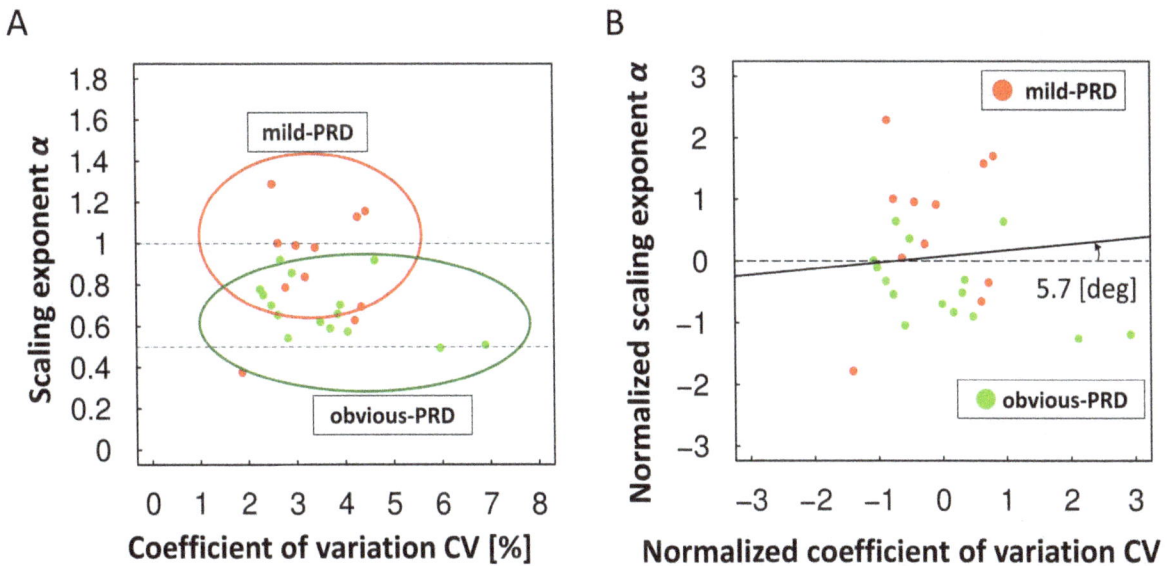

Figure 4. Classification of obvious and mild postural reflex disorder. The mild postural reflex disorder group (mild-PRD) is indicated by red points, and the obvious postural reflex disorder group (obvious-PRD) is indicated by light-green points. The x-axis represents the CV, and the y-axis represents α. (A) Distribution of the original data. (B) Distribution of the normalized data. The solid line represents the boundary between the mild-PRD and obvious-PRD groups.

strong correlation between the change of CV and symptoms of PRD. Considering that the mechanism of PRD is independent of the neural rhythmic activities, this result suggests the existence of feedback process from physical activities to neural rhythmic activities. Furthermore, α differentiated between mild-PRD and obvious-PRD. Considering α reflects the strength of interaction or relationship between factors, this result suggests the existence of interaction between physical activities and neural rhythmic activities. Therefore, the interaction between neural rhythmic activities and physical activities is thought to play an important role for gait disabilities in PD.

We now discuss the relationship between neural rhythm generation disorders and physical disabilities based on the results obtained in this study. Figure 5 summarizes the results of the classification used in this study. CV and α are dynamic indicators of neural rhythm generation disorders, and PRD is a clinical indicator of the severity of a physical disability. Area A in Figure 5 represents a low CV: i.e., the variability of the gait rhythm of the participants was small. Moreover, the participants who appeared in this area had no symptoms of PRD. Area B represents a large CV and a high α: i.e., the variability was large but the $1/f$-like fluctuation property was observed. In addition, these patients had mild symptoms of PRD. Area C represents a large CV and a low α: i.e., the variability of the gait rhythm of the patients was large, and the $1/f$-like fluctuation property was not observed. In addition, these patients showed obvious symptoms of PRD.

When considering the manner in which neural rhythm generation disorders progress during the transition from the healthy state to obvious-PRD, we find an important factor in walking. At first, the patient's gait rhythm tends to transfer from the area A to area B in (CV, α) plane during the transition from no-PRD to mild-PRD. This result shows that there are strong correlation between the occurrence of PRD and the increase of CV. It might be natural to be considered that the change of neural rhythm generation give rise to the disabilities for physical activity. However the mechanism of PRD is independent of development of neural rhythmic generation, because the enhancement and suppression function of the muscle tone, which is related to the occurrence of PRD, is considered to work in parallel with the function of gait rhythm generation [31–34]. Therefore, this means that physical activity is fed back to neural rhythm activity in walking. Considering the fact that neural rhythmic activity always affects the physical activity, our result suggests the existence of interaction between neural rhythmic activity and physical activity. Next, the gait rhythm tends to transfer from area B to area C during the transition from mild-PRD to PRD. This shows that there are strong correlation between progression of the severity of PRD and the decrease of α. In other words, this transition is observed as the weakening process of the $1/f$ fluctuation from the state we can observe the $1/f$ fluctuation. The $1/f$ fluctuation property is defined by the frequency spectrum whose power is proportional to the inverse of frequency. In general, $1/f$-like

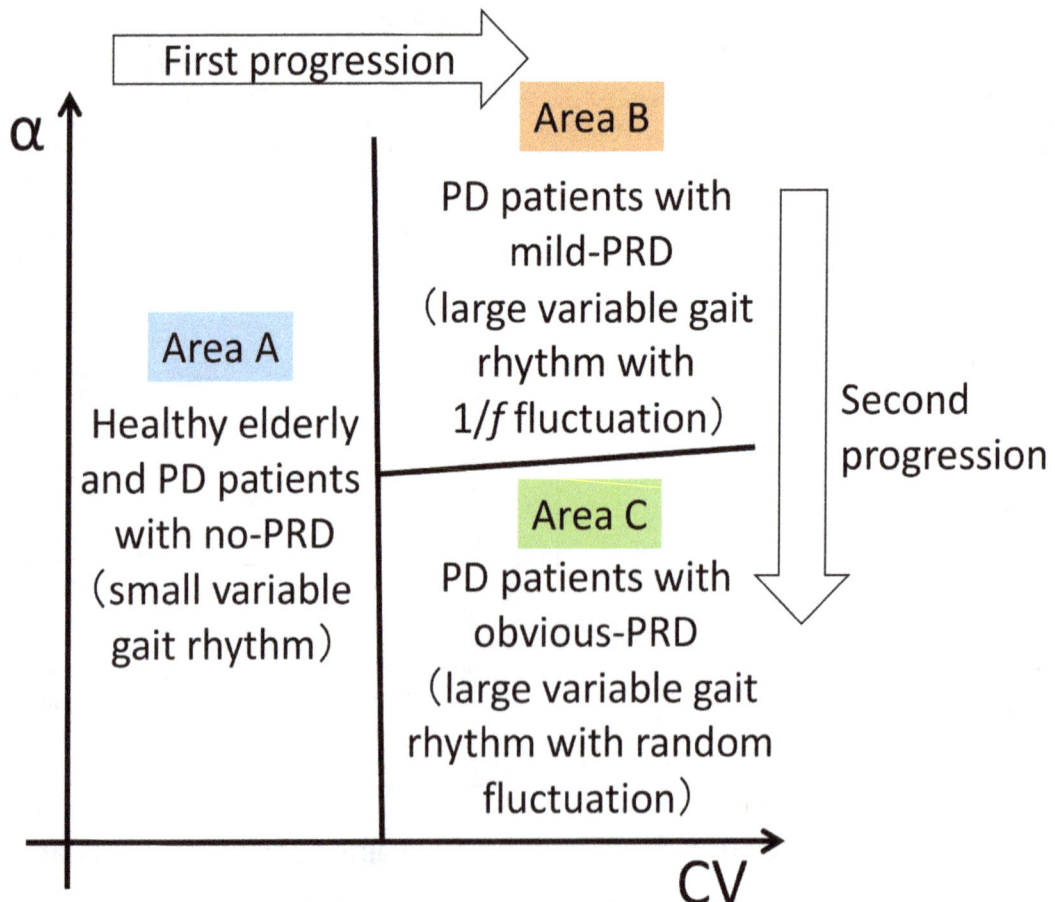

Figure 5. Concept of the evaluation platform. The x-axis is related to the CV of the stride interval, and the y-axis is related to the α of the stride interval. PRD, postural reflex disorder.

fluctuation is mainly generated by the interaction between multiple factors [9,23–28]. Therefore, the change of time series structure of the gait rhythm can be regarded as the intensity change of interaction. This result suggests that the intensity of interaction on the mechanism of gait rhythm generation is weakened by the progression of severity of PRD. This complement the fact that the interaction between neural rhythmic activity and physical activity plays an important role in gait rhythm generation.

When considering all these points, we summarize the development mechanism of gait rhythm generation disorders. The gait rhythm of the patients in area A (small CV) in Figure 5 represented the state without physical disabilities. The gait rhythm of the patients in area B (large CV, high α) represented the state that is controlled mainly by the interaction between neural rhythmic and physical activities against the physical disabilities. The gait rhythm of the patients in area C (large CV, low α) represented the destabilized state in response to weakening of the interaction between neural rhythmic and physical activities. These findings suggest that it is possible to construct an evaluation platform for neural rhythm generation disorders by combining the CV and α parameters, and to use this system to evaluate the progression of physical disabilities.

This information on Figure 5 may provide clues for evaluating the progress of PD patients during rehabilitation using RAS gait training or WalkMate gait training. RAS gait training decreases CV [8,13]. This type of gait training may improve the first progression involving variability of gait rhythm: i.e., transition from the right half-plane (area B or area C) to the left half-plane (area A) in (CV, α) plane. On the other hand, the WalkMate gait training increases the $1/f$-like fluctuation property [14,15]. This type of gait training may improve the second progression involving the fluctuation property: i.e., the transition from area C to area B. Therefore, based on this platform, we were able to extract information not only on the presence or absence of PRD, but also on the severity of PRD using (CV, α) plane for evaluating neural rhythm generation disorders. Using this system to evaluate neural rhythm generation disorders may help physical therapists to choose a rehabilitation method that fits the severity of the patients' physical disabilities.

Acknowledgments

We would like to thank all participants at the Kanto Central Hospital for their cooperation with this study. We are also grateful to the researchers who gave us useful information and to our colleagues, particularly Michael J. Hove at Harvard University and Kazuki Suzuki, Toshitaka Nomura, and Shou Itou at the Tokyo Institute of Technology for their support and for instructive comments about gait measurement and analysis.

Author Contributions

Conceived and designed the experiments: LO HU KO SO YM. Performed the experiments: LO HU SO YM. Analyzed the data: LO HU KO YM. Contributed reagents/materials/analysis tools: LO HU YM. Wrote the paper: LO HU KO SO YM. Subject recruitment: SO.

References

1. Pearson KG (2000) Neural adaptation in the generation of rhythmic behavior. Annu Rev Physiol 62: 723–753.
2. Taga G, Yamaguchi Y, Shimizu H (1991) Self-organized control of bipedal locomotion by neural oscillators in unpredictable environment. Biol Cybern 65: 147–159.
3. Jankovic J (2008) Parkinson's disease: clinical features and diagnosis. J Neurol Neurosurg Psychiatry 79: 368–376.
4. Hausdorff JM, Cudkowicz ME, Firtion R, Wei JY, Goldberger AL (1998) Gait variability and basal ganglia disorders: stride-to-stride variations of gait cycle timing in Parkinson's disease and Huntington's disease. Mov Disord 13: 428–437.
5. Schaafsma JD, Giladi N, Balash Y, Bartels AL, Gurevich T, et al. (2003) Gait dynamics in Parkinson's disease: relationship to Parkinsonian features, falls and response to levodopa. J Neurol Sci 212: 47–53.
6. Hausdorff JM, Lertratanakul A, Cudkowicz ME, Peterson AL, Kaliton D, et al. (2000) Dynamic markers of altered gait rhythm in amyotrophic lateral sclerosis. J Appl Physiol 88: 2045–2053.
7. Hausdorff JM (2007) Gait dynamics, fractals and falls: finding meaning in the stride-to-stride fluctuations of human walking. Hum Mov Sci 26: 555–589.
8. Hausdorff JM (2009) Gait dynamics in Parkinson's disease: common and distinct behavior among stride length, gait variability, and fractal-like scaling. Chaos 19: 026113. doi:10.1063/1.3147408.
9. Hausdorff JM, Peng CK, Ladin Z, Wei JY, Goldberger AL (1995) Is walking a random walk? Evidence for long-range correlations in stride interval of human gait. J Appl Physiol 78: 349–358.
10. Thaut MH, Abiru M (2010) Rhythmic auditory stimulation in rehabilitation of movement disorders: a review of the current research. Music Percept 27: 263–269.
11. Rubinstein TC, Giladi N, Haausdorff JM (2002) The power of cueing to circumvent dopamine deficits: a review of physical therapy treatment of gait disturbances in Parkinson's disease. Mov Disord 17: 1148–1160.
12. Miyake Y (2009) Interpersonal synchronization of body motion and the Walk-Mate walking support robot. Robot IEEE Trans 25: 638–644.
13. Hausdorff JM, Lowenthal J, Herman T, Gruendlinger L, Peretz C, et al. (2007) Rhythmic auditory stimulation modulates gait variability in Parkinson's disease. Eur J Neurosci 26: 2369–2375.
14. Hove MJ, Suzuki K, Uchitomi H, Orimo S, Miyake Y (2012) Interactive rhythmic auditory stimulation reinstates natural $1/f$ timing in gait of Parkinson's patients. PLoS ONE 7: e32600.
15. Uchitomi H, Ota L, Ogawa K-i, Orimo S, Miyake Y (2013) Interactive rhythmic cue facilitates gait relearning in patients with Parkinson's disease. PLoS ONE 8: e72176.
16. Thorbahn LDB, Newton RA (1996) Use of the Berg Balance Test to predict falls in elderly persons. Phys Ther 76: 576–583.
17. Bloem BR, Beckley DJ, Van Hilten BJ, Roos RAC (1998) Clinimetrics of postural instability in Parkinson's disease. J Neurol 245: 669–673.
18. Hoehn MM, Yahr MD (1967) Parkinsonism: onset, progression, and mortality. Neurology 17: 427–442.
19. Goetz CG, Poewe W, Rascol O, Sampaio C, Stebbins GT, et al. (2004) Movement Disorder Society Task Force report on the Hoehn and Yahr staging scale: status and recommendations. Mov Disord 19: 1020–1028.
20. Peng C-K, Buldyrev SV, Havlin S, Simons M, Stanley HE, et al. (1994) Mosaic organization of DNA nucleotides. Phys Rev E Stat Phys Plasmas Fluids Relat Interdiscip Topics 49: 1685–1689.
21. Peng C-K, Havlin S, Stanley HE, Goldberger AL (1995) Quantification of scaling exponents and crossover phenomena in nonstationary heartbeat time series. Chaos 5: 82–87.
22. Delignieres D, Ramdani S, Lemoine L, Torre K, Fortes M, et al. (2006) Fractal analyses for 'short' time series: a re-assessment of classical methods. J Math Psychol 50: 525–544.
23. Goldberger AL, Amaral LA, Hausdorff JM, Ivanov PC, Peng CK, et al. (2002) Fractal dynamics in physiology: alterations with disease and aging. Proc Natl Acad Sci U S A 99: 2466–2472.
24. Gates DH, Su JL, Dingwell JB (2007) Possible biomechanical origins of the long-range correlations in stride intervals of walking. Physica A 380: 259–270.
25. Ivanov PCh, Ma QDY, Bartsch RP, Hausdorff JM, Amaral LAN, et al. (2009) Levels of complexity in scale-invariant neural signals. Phys Rev E Stat Nonlin Soft Matter Phys 79: 041920.
26. Ahn J, Hogan N (2013) Long-range correlations in stride intervals may emerge from non-chaotic walking dynamics. PLoS ONE 8: e73239.
27. Hausdorff JM, Purdon PL, Peng CK, Ladin Z, Wei JY, et al. (1996) Fractal dynamics of human gait: stability of long-range correlations in stride interval fluctuation. J Appl Physiol 80: 1448–1457.
28. Hausdorff JM, Ashkenazy Y, Peng C-K, Ivanov PC, Stanley HE, et al. (2001) When human walking becomes random walking: fractal analysis and modeling of gait rhythm fluctuations. Physica 302: 138–147.
29. Hausdorff JM, Mitchell SL, Firtion R, Peng CK, Cudkowicz ME, et al. (1997) Altered fractal dynamics of gait: reduced stride-interval correlations with aging and Huntington's disease. J Appl Physiol 82: 262–269.
30. Duda RO, Hart PE, Stork DG (2001) Pattern classification. 2nd ed. New York: Wiley. 654 p.
31. Takakusaki K, Hanaguchi T, Ohtinata-Sugimoto J, Saitoh K, Sakamoto T (2003) Basal ganglia efferents to the brainstem centers controlling postural muscle tone and locomotion: a new concept for understanding motor disorders in basal ganglia dysfunction. Neuroscience 119: 293–308.
32. Takakusaki K, Saitoh K, Harada H, Kashiwayanagi M (2004) Role of basal ganglia-brainstem pathways in the control of motor behaviors. Neurosci Res 50: 137–151.

33. Tomita N, Yano M (2007) Bipedal robot controlled by the basal ganglia and brainstem systems adjusting to indefinite environment. Proc 2007 IEEE/ICME International Conference on Complex Medical Engineering: 116–121.

34. Takakusaki K, Tomita N, Yano M (2008) Substrates for normal gait and pathophysiology of gait disturbances with respect to the basal ganglia dysfunction. J Neurol 255[Suppl 4]: 19–29.

17

Human *NR5A1*/SF-1 Mutations Show Decreased Activity on BDNF (Brain-Derived Neurotrophic Factor), an Important Regulator of Energy Balance: Testing Impact of Novel SF-1 Mutations Beyond Steroidogenesis

Jana Malikova[1,2¶], Núria Camats[2¶], Mónica Fernández-Cancio[3], Karen Heath[4], Isabel González[5], María Caimarí[6], Miguel del Campo[7], Marian Albisu[3], Stanislava Kolouskova[1], Laura Audí[3], Christa E. Flück[2]*

1 Department of Pediatrics, 2nd Faculty of Medicine, Charles University in Prague and University Hospital Motol, Prague, Czech Republic, 2 Pediatric Endocrinology, Department of Pediatrics and Department of Clinical Research, University Children's Hospital Bern, Bern, Switzerland, 3 Pediatric Endocrinology, Vall d'Hebron Research Institute VHIR, CIBERER, Autonomous University, Barcelona, Spain, 4 Institute of Medical and Molecular Genetics INGEMM, Hospital Universitario La Paz, Universidad Autónoma de Madrid, IdiPAZ, Madrid, Spain, 5 Pediatric Endocrinology Service, Hospital Universitario La Paz, Universidad Autónoma de Madrid, IdiPAZ, Madrid, Spain, 6 Pediatric Endocrinology, Son Espases University Hospital, Palma de Mallorca, Spain, 7 Genetic Service, Hospital Vall d'Hebron, Barcelona, Spain

Abstract

Context: Human *NR5A1*/SF-1 mutations cause 46,XY disorder of sex development (DSD) with broad phenotypic variability, and rarely cause adrenal insufficiency although SF-1 is an important transcription factor for many genes involved in steroidogenesis. In addition, the Sf-1 knockout mouse develops obesity with age. Obesity might be mediated through Sf-1 regulating activity of brain-derived neurotrophic factor (BDNF), an important regulator of energy balance in the ventromedial hypothalamus.

Objective: To characterize novel SF-1 gene variants in 4 families, clinical, genetic and functional studies were performed with respect to steroidogenesis and energy balance.

Patients: 5 patients with 46,XY DSD were found to harbor *NR5A1*/SF-1 mutations including 2 novel variations. One patient harboring a novel mutation also suffered from adrenal insufficiency.

Methods: SF-1 mutations were studied in cell systems (HEK293, JEG3) for impact on transcription of genes involved in steroidogenesis (*CYP11A1*, *CYP17A1*, *HSD3B2*) and in energy balance (*BDNF*). BDNF regulation by SF-1 was studied by promoter assays (JEG3).

Results: Two novel *NR5A1*/SF-1 mutations (Glu7Stop, His408Profs*159) were confirmed. Glu7Stop is the 4th reported SF-1 mutation causing DSD and adrenal insufficiency. *In vitro* studies revealed that transcription of the *BDNF* gene is regulated by SF-1, and that mutant SF-1 decreased *BDNF* promoter activation (similar to steroid enzyme promoters). However, clinical data from 16 subjects carrying SF-1 mutations showed normal birth weight and BMI.

Conclusions: Glu7Stop and His408Profs*159 are novel SF-1 mutations identified in patients with 46,XY DSD and adrenal insufficiency (Glu7Stop). *In vitro*, SF-1 mutations affect not only steroidogenesis but also transcription of BDNF which is involved in energy balance. However, in contrast to mice, consequences on weight were not found in humans with SF-1 mutations.

Editor: Michal Hetman, University of Louisville, United States of America

Funding: This work was supported by grants of the Swiss National Science Foundation (320030-146127) to CEF, the Instituto de Salud Carlos III, Madrid, Spain CIBERER U-712 to MFC and the AGAUR (University and Research Management and Evaluation Agency), Barcelona, Spain (2009SGR31) to LA, and by ESPE (European Society of Pediatric Endocrinology) Research Fellowship grants to JM and NC (sponsored by Novo Nordisk A/S). The funders had no role in study design, data collection and analysis, decision to publish, or preparation of the manuscript.

Competing Interests: The authors declare that Novo Nordisk A/S partly funded this study. There are no patents, products in development or marketed products to declare.

* Email: christa.flueck@dkf.unibe.ch

¶ JM and NC are joint first authors on this work.

Introduction

The nuclear receptor steroidogenic factor 1 (SF-1/*NR5A1*) is a master regulator of adrenal and gonadal development, including sexual determination and differentiation, as well as steroidogenesis and reproduction [1,2]. SF-1 also plays a pivotal role in the development of the ventromedial hypothalamic nucleus (VMH) and for functions of the pituitary gland [3,4]. In addition, expression of SF-1 has been identified in the spleen, skin and in small amounts in the placenta [5,6,7]. SF-1 was first identified in 1992 for its function as a transcriptional regulator of steroidogenic genes and was named accordingly [8]. Later, the Sf-1 KO mice were reported with a severe phenotype including lack of adrenal glands and a complete sex reversal of 46,XY animals [9]. Finally in 1999, the first human being with adrenal insufficiency and 46,XY disorder of sexual development (DSD) harboring a heterozygote SF-1 mutation was described [10]. Meanwhile, numerous SF-1 mutations have been identified [2], yet the exact function of SF-1 explaining the broad phenotype associated with SF-1 mutations remains elusive [11,12].

SF-1 is encoded by the *NR5A1* gene which is located on the long arm of chromosome 9 (9q33). The gene consists of 7 exons but only 6 exons are coding. SF-1 has 461 amino acids and comprises a DNA binding domain with two zinc fingers, an accessory DNA binding domain, a hinge region and a ligand binding domain [1]. The structure of SF-1 is greatly conserved among animal species [13]. To date more than 70 human *NR5A1* mutations have been described (Human Gene Mutations Database, www.hgmd.cf.ac.uk). Most of these mutations are found in a heterozygote state [11,14] and only a few in a homozygote [15], or compound heterozygote state [16]. So far, no correlation between phenotype and genotype, and also no clear pattern of heredity has been seen as both sporadic and familiar presentations exist [11]. Furthermore, possibility of dominant negative effect of heterozygote *NR5A1* mutations has been debated without convincing results [11].

The clinical presentation of SF-1 deficiency is very variable. The first human individual with a heterozygote Gly35Glu SF-1 mutation had 46,XY DSD and adrenal insufficiency [10]. So far, only two additional SF-1 mutations causing adrenal insufficiency have been reported [15,17]. The heterozygote Arg255Leu mutation was found in a girl with symptoms of adrenal insufficiency and normal ovarian differentiation and function [17], and the homozygote Arg92Gln mutation was present in a boy with adrenal failure and 46,XY DSD [15]. By contrast, *NR5A1* mutations are frequently found in patients with 46,XY DSD with apparently normal function of the adrenal cortex [11,14,18]. Similarly, some *NR5A1* mutations were found in 46,XX females with premature ovarian failure or ovarian insufficiency with normal adrenal function [11,19].

SF-1 deficiency also affects the central regulation of reproduction and energy balance [20]. The pituitary Sf-1 KO mouse model showed that SF-1 is an essential regulator of gonadotropin (LH, FSH) expression [4,21,22]. These mice present with hypogonadotropic hypogonadism reflected by sexual immaturity, low weight of gonads and sterility [4]. Apart from the pituitary gland, SF-1 is also required for the development, organization and function of the ventromedial hypothalamus (VMH) [3,23]. Mouse models have shown that a loss of SF-1 stimulation leads to disorganization of the VMH, thereby impairing its function related to anxiety, thermoregulation, sexual behavior and energy balance [24]. Selective deletion of Sf-1 in the VMH in mice prenatally resulted in late onset obesity [25], while the same deletion postnatally led to

diet induced obesity and deregulated thermogenesis [25]. However, these possible effects of SF-1 deficiency have not yet been studied in humans harboring SF-1 mutations.

In this context, the brain-derived neurotrophic factor (BDNF) is an important regulator of energy balance [26]. It is a highly conserved neurotrophin which is thought to be a SF-1 target gene [27]. BDNF is expressed in several appetite-regulating centers in the hypothalamus and the hindbrain in both mouse and human [28]. Depletion of *Bdnf* or its receptor (TrkB) in mice results in excessive feeding, weight gain and features accompanied by the metabolic syndrome [26,29]. Abnormal locomotor activity and late-onset obesity was also observed in a *Bdnf* heterozygote knockout mouse model or when *Bdnf* was inactivated in the central nervous system [29,30]. In addition, reduced expression of BDNF was described in association with obesity in the leptin receptor deficient mouse [31], the Alzheimer disease mouse [32] and the Sf-1 KO mouse [3]. In humans, two reports show a relationship between BDNF (locus 11p14) and obesity [33,34]. Patients with WAGR syndrome (Wilm's tumor, aniridia, genito-urinary anomalies and mental retardation, OMIM 194072) with a heterozygous 11p14 deletion including the *BDNF* gene suffer all from childhood onset obesity, while WAGR syndrome patients without genetic anomalies including the *BDNF* gene have normal prevalence of obesity [33]. Additionally, a girl with obesity and impaired cognitive function who has only one functional copy of the *BDNF* gene has been described [34].

We hypothesize that human SF-1 mutations may affect metabolism and that this effect could be mediated in part through BDNF. Therefore, in this study we characterize novel *NR5A1* mutations, one being associated with the rare phenotype of adrenal insufficiency and 46,XY DSD. We describe the effect of these SF-1 mutations *in vitro* on transcription of genes involved in steroidogenesis and on the *BDNF* gene which is important for central regulation of food intake. Finally, we describe some weight related parameters in our small cohort of *NR5A1* patients.

Patients and Methods

Patients and ethical approval

Five patients of Czech Republic and Spanish origin with unsolved 46,XY DSD were studied. Main characteristics of patients and families are shown in Table 1, family trees are depicted in Figure 1A and biochemical data are available as Table S1. All studied subjects and/or their legal guardians gave written informed consent for the hormonal and molecular studies, which were approved by the respective ethical committees of the involved centers: Ethics commissions of Vall d'Hebron Research Institute and CIBERER, Barcelona, Spain, and University Hospital Bern, Switzerland.

Case reports (Table 1 and 2, Figure 1, Table S1)

Patient 1 from Czech Republic, was delivered at 31 weeks gestation because of HELLP (hemolysis, elevated liver enzymes, low platelets) syndrome of the mother. Birth weight was 1430 g (5–10th percentile) and length was 38 cm (5–10th percentile). Physical exam revealed perineal hypospadias but no other anomalies. Karyotype was 46,XY. Neonatal period was unremarkable. However, at the age of three months, he was admitted for adrenal failure (hyponatremia, hyperkalemia, episode of hypoglycemia, dehydration) in the course of an acute, viral respiratory infection. Baseline levels of ACTH and plasma renin activity were elevated. Cortisol response to ACTH stimulation was low confirming adrenal insufficiency.

Table 1. Clinical and genetic characteristics of 5 patients harboring mutations in the *NR5A1* gene.

Patient	Origin, YOB	Karyotype	Assigned sex	Genital anatomy at birth	Gonadal function (age)	Adrenal function (age)	NR5A1 gene mutation	Family history
1	Czech, 2010	46,XY	Male	Perineal hypospadia. Palpable testicles.	At 12 months: Baseline T low, FSH slightly elevated.	Adrenal insufficiency (high ACTH, low cortisol, high PRA, normal aldosterone).	Compound heterozygote: c.19G>T, p.Glu7Stop; c.887C>T, p.Thr296Met	F = c.887C>T, p.Thr296Met M = WT
2	Spanish, 2013	46,XY	Male to female at 4 months	Clitoris with redundant skin. Palpable glans but no corpora cavernosa. Posterior labial fusion. Gonads palpable in genital folds (<1 ml). No Müllerian ducts.	Abnormal at 3.5 months: Baseline T low, FSH high; Very low T response to hCG stimulation.	Normal at baseline aged 3.5 months.	Heterozygote: c.1222_1223insC, p.His408Profs*159	M = WT F = "carrier" (hypospadias) ICSI product from both parents' gametes.
3	Spanish, 2011	46,XY	Male	Scrotal hypospadias. Penis length 2 cm. Bilateral scrotal gonads. No Müllerian ducts.	Abnormal: T slightly decreased, but normal precursor response to hCG stimulation. AMH low at age 17–20 days.	Normal at baseline aged 17 days.	Heterozygote: c.937C>T, p.Arg313Cys	F = WT M = WT
4	Spanish, 2010 1st twin	46,XY	Male	Scrotal hypospadias. Penis length 1.5 cm. Bilateral scrotal gonads (1 ml). No Müllerian ducts.	T high at birth. AMH low at 2 months.	ND	Heterozygote: c.937C>T, p.Arg313Cys	Bichorial twin of patient 5. F = carrier (operated hypospadias; testis volume L 6 ml/R 12 ml). M = unknown ICSI product from donor ova and father's sperm.
5	Spanish, 2010 2nd twin	46,XY	Male	Scrotal hypospadias. Penis length 1.5 cm. Unilateral cryptorchidism, scrotal testis 0.5 ml.	T high at birth. AMH low at 2 months.	ND	Heterozygote: c.937C>T, p.Arg313Cys	Bichorial twin of patient 4.

YOB: year of birth; F: father; M: mother; WT: wild type; L: left; R: right; ND – not determined.

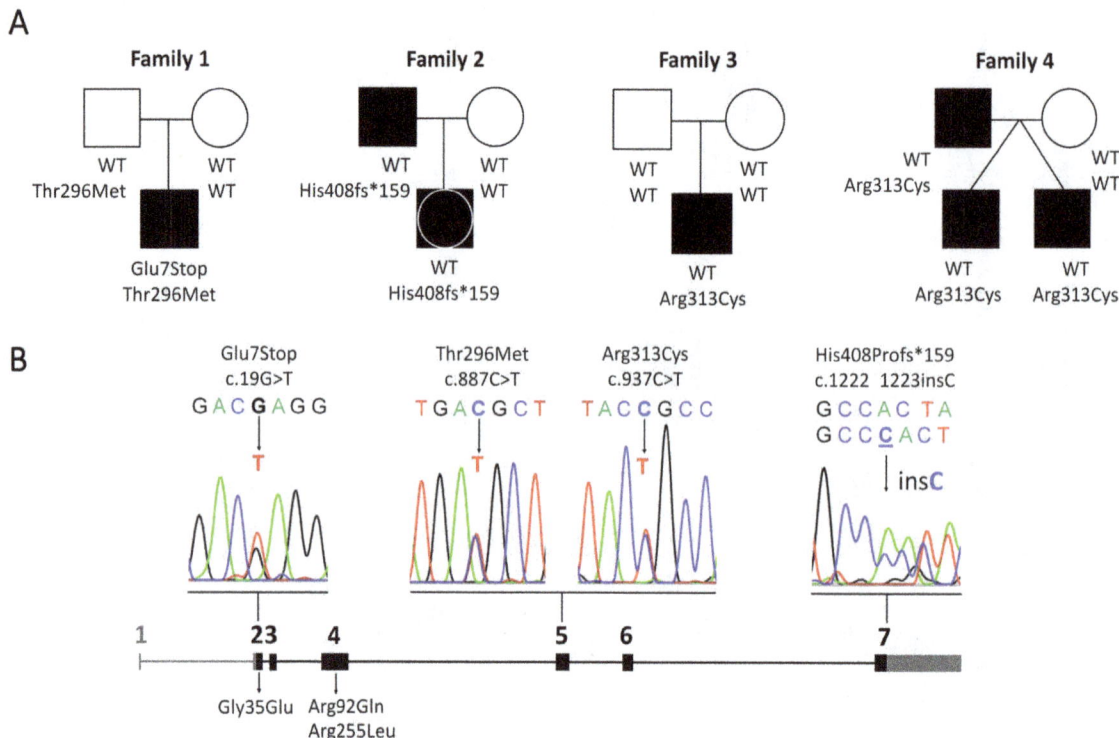

Figure 1. Genetic information on 5 subjects carrying *NR5A1* mutations. A. Family trees of 4 families and 7 affected individuals (5 patients and 2 parents) are shown. Scheme of the *NR5A1* gene showing the mutations identified in the reported patients (above the scheme) and all reported SF-1 mutations causing adrenal insufficiency (below the scheme). Electropherograms of novel mutations are also depicted. The *NR5A1* gene is composed of coding (*black*) and non-coding sequences (*gray*). Exons are indicated by *numbers*.

Patient 2 from Spain (with parents from Argentina of European descents) was investigated during fetal development because of a discordant genital sex by ultrasound (female) compared to the genetic sex (46,XY). He was conceived by ICSI from both parents gametes. Owing to the father's history of hypospadias, the *NR5A1* gene was analysed in the father showing an heterozygous mutation. The same mutation was detected in fetal material. Although there was no consanguinity, the mother was also analysed to predict possible compound heterozygocity or homozygocity. The patient was delivered at 40 weeks gestation with a normal weight and length. External genitalia showed a clitoris-like genital tubercle, posterior labial fusion, no visible urethral meatus nor vaginal opening. Small (<1 ml) gonads were palpable in the genital folds. Male sex was assigned. The neonatal period was uneventful and endocrine evaluation was not performed until the age of 3.5 months when baseline ACTH, cortisol and 17-hydroxy-progesterone (17OHP) were normal, while baseline testosterone (T) was low and FSH high for age; T response to hCG stimulation was low. Therefore, at 4 months of age, gender was reassigned to female due to the severely feminized external genitalia.

Patient 3 from Spain was delivered at 38 weeks gestation with normal weight and length; he was evaluated at 14 days due to ambiguous genitalia (scrotal hypospadias, penis length 2 cm and gonads palpable in the scrotal folds). Karyotype was 46,XY. Baseline cortisol and aldosterone were normal as were the measured steroid precursors. Baseline FSH was slightly elevated, AMH and inhibin B were low. T response to hCG stimulation was low while the T/DHT ratio was normal.

Patients 4 and 5 from Spain were delivered as bichorionic twins at 36 weeks gestation with the 1st twin showing normal weight and lenght while the 2nd was small for gestational age (SGA). They

were obtained by ICSI from the father's sperm and a donated ova to avoid the mother's genetic disease (epidermiolysis bullosa). Both babies presented with ambiguous genitalia: scrotal hypospadias with a penis length of 1.5 cm, both gonads palpable (1 ml) in the scrotal folds (1st twin) and unilateral cryptorchidism and one palpable gonad (0.5 ml in the 2nd twin). The father had been operated for hypospadias during childhood. His testes biopsies at 9 years of age revealed diminished seminiferous tubule diameter and fertility index in the left testis while these parameters were normal in the right testis). Neonatal period was uneventful in both twins. At birth (2 days), baseline T, precursors and gonadotropins were normal for age and AMH was low at 2 months.

Genetic analyses

Genomic DNA was isolated from peripheral blood leukocytes. All exons and part of adjacent introns of the *NR5A1* gene were amplified and sequenced as previously described [11]. Obtained sequences were analysed against the *NR5A1*/SF-1 GenBank entries NT_008470.19 (genomic DNA), NM_004959.4 (mRNA) and NP_004950.2 (protein).

In vitro functional studies

Human embryonic kidney cells (HEK293) and human placental choriocarcinoma cells (JEG3) were used for functional studies. HEK293 cells were cultured in DMEM supplemented with 10% fetal calf serum, 1% penicillin/streptomycin and 1% sodium pyruvate (Gibco, Paisley, UK). JEG3 cells were cultured in MEM supplemented with 10% fetal calf serum, 1% penicillin/strepto-mycin and 1% L-glutamine (Gibco).

Table 2. Weight related parameters of subjects carrying (heterozygote) *NR5A1* mutations.

Subject	Karyotype	NR5A1 mutation(s)	Gestational age at birth (weeks)	Birth weight (g)	(SD)	Current age (y, m)	Actual weight (kg)	(SD)	BMI (kg/m²)	(SD)
Present study (Figure 1)										
F1, II.1	46,XY	Glu7Stop; Thr296Met	31	1430	−0.83	3 y 1 m	16.30	0.59	17.80	1.39
F2, II.1	46,XY	His408Profs*159	40	3200	−0.76	-	-	-	-	-
F3, II.1	46,XY	Arg313Cys	38	2630	−1.77	-	-	-	-	-
F4, II.1	46,XY	Arg313Cys	36	2470	−0.75	1 y 10 m	12.70	0.30	15.30	−0.26
F4, II.2	46,XY	Arg313Cys	36	1390	−4.87	1 y 10 m	13.00	0.57	15.40	−0.47
F2, I.1_Fa	46,XY	His408Profs*159	-	-	-	32 y	80.00	-	27.00	0.50
F4, I.1_Fa	46,XY	Arg313Cys	-	-	-	30 y	90.00	-	26.60	0.40
Patients from Camats et al. (Table 1, Ref. 11)										
1	46,XY	Val20Leu	41	2970	−1.90	5 y	21.80	0.80	15.30	0
2	46,XY	His24Tyr	40	3600	0	17 y	85.00	-	25.70	1.33
5	46,XY	Gly90Arg	40	3100	−1.28	14 y 6 m	51.40	0	19.70	0.04
6	46,XY	Pro130ArgfsX165	-	-	-	1 y	8.90	−1.15	15.90	−0.69
7	46,XY	Gln206ThrfsX20	41	3820	1.21	5 y	26.30	2.90	21.70	2.81
8	46,XY	Leu231_Leu233dup	40	3280	−0.67	5.5 y	28.00	2.85	21.40	2.45
9	46,XX	Pro235Leu	-	-	-	19 y	58.00	-	24.00	0.60
1_Fa	46,XY	Val20Leu	-	-	-	32 y	71.00	-	24.00	0.84
5_Mo	46,XX	Gly90Arg	-	-	-	35 y	63.00	-	23.40	0.76

F: family; Fa: father; Mo: mother.

Promoter luciferase reporter vectors for steroidogenic enzymes HSD3B2, CYP11A1, CYP17A1 (-227CYP17A1_Δluc, -152CYP11A1_pGL3, -301HSD3B2_pGL3) and corresponding empty control vectors (Δ_luc, pGL3), as well as cDNA for wild-type (WT) SF-1/NR5A1 were available from previous work [35,36]. Luciferase reporter vectors for human promoters I, IV, V and VII of the BDNF gene (pGL4.15_hBDNFpI, pGL4.15_hBDNFpIV, pGL4.15_hBDNFpV, pGL4.15_hBDNFpVII) were kindly provided by Dr. P. Pruunsild and Prof. T. Timmusk (Tallinn University of Technology, Tallinn, Estonia). Mutant NR5A1 expression vectors (c.19T, c.887T, c.937T, c.1222_1223insC) and SF-1 cis element mutant pGL4.15_hBDNFpI (c.-876_873CTTT) were generated by PCR-based site-directed mutagenesis using specific primers (available upon request) following the QuickChange protocol by Stratagene (Agilent Technologies Inc., Santa Clara, CA, USA).

For promoter activity studies, cells were cultured in 24-well plates and transiently transfected with WT or mutant NR5A1 and WT or mutant promoter luciferase reporter constructs using Lipofectamine 2000 (Invitrogen, AG, Basel, Switzerland) for 48 hours, and the Dual-Luciferase Reporter (DLR) Assay System (Promega AG, Wallisellen, Switzerland) was used for readout as previously described [11]. Specific Firefly luciferase readings were normalized against Renilla control readings and expressed as relative light units (RLU). Experiments were repeated at least 3 times in duplicates.

Statistical analysis

Data are shown as mean±SEM of at least three independent experiments. Statistical analysis was examined by t-test with Microsoft Office Excel (Windows 2003, Microsoft Inc.). Significance was set at *$p<0.05$, **$p<0.01$.

Results

Genetic analysis

We identified 2 novel and 2 known NR5A1 sequence variations in 5 patients newly diagnosed with SF-1 deficiency (Figure 1). Patient 1 (family 1), a boy with adrenal insufficiency and 46,XY DSD harbored compound heterozygote novel c.19G>T and c.887C>T variations in the NR5A1 gene coding for Glu7Stop in the DNA binding domain and Thr296Met in the ligand binding domain. Glu7Stop was not found in either parents, thus qualifying as a de novo mutation. By contrast, heterozygocity for Thr296Met was detected in the healthy father (Figure 1). Patient 2 (family 2) was heterozygote for a novel insertion c.1222_1223insC which is predicted to result in a frameshift elongating the SF-1 protein by 159 amino acids (His408Profs*159). The mutation was inherited from an affected carrier father (Figure 1). In patients 3 to 5 from two families (3 and 4), a heterozygote c.937C>T mutation in exon 5 was found changing Arg313Cys in the ligand-binding domain (Table 1, Figure 1). In family 3, the mutation was de novo (patient 3), whereas in family 4 (patients 4 and 5), the mutation was inherited in two dizygotic twins from an affected carrier father (Table 1, Figure 1). This mutation was recently reported in a patient manifesting with distal hypospadias and a bifid scrotum containing testes [37].

In vitro studies of the impact of SF-1 variants on steroidogenesis and energy balance

Impact of identified SF-1 mutations on steroidogenesis was studied in non-steroidogenic HEK293 cells by assessing their transcriptional activity on the promoters of the HSD3B2, CYP11A1 and CYP17A1 genes (Figure 2). The Glu7Stop mutation revealed a complete lack of transcriptional activation for all promoter constructs. The Thr296Met variant showed similar transactivation activity as WT SF-1 indicating that it is not a disease-causing variant but rather a polymorphism (SNP). Interestingly, the His408Profs*159 and Arg313Cys mutations showed normal activity when tested on the HSD3B2 promoter construct, but their transactivation activity was significantly decreased when tested on the CYP11A1 and CYP17A1 promoters.

To study potential involvement of SF-1 on central energy balance, the transcriptional regulation of SF-1 on the promoters of the BDNF gene was assessed in JEG3 cells. According to literature, there are many alternative BDNF variants (17 BDNF and 12 antisense BDNF variants) in human due to use of different promoters [28]. For initial experiments, we used four different human BDNF promoter constructs, namely hBDNF I, IV, V and VII. Promoter constructs I and IV were chosen as mouse Bdnf transcripts I and IV are primarily expressed in the brain (area of VMH) and their promoters are reported to be regulated by Sf-1 [27]. Similarly, promoters V and VII were assessed for reported expression in the human brain [28]. In our JEG3 cell system, among those promoters, we were only able to transactivate the hBDNF promoter I by WT SF-1 (data not shown). Thus, further studies involving SF-1 and human BDNF were performed with this hBDNF promoter I (Figure 3). In this promoter, we found a putative SF-1 cis-element at c.-874 to -867 (CAAGGACA). To confirm that this cis-element in the hBDNF promoter is regulated by SF-1, we constructed a promoter with a mutant SF-1 site and assessed its activity by co-transfection with WT SF-1. Upon co-transfection with WT SF-1, the mutant BDNF promoter lost activity when compared with the WT promoter (Figure 3A). In this system, SF-1 mutants Glu7Stop, Arg313Cys and His408Profs*159 showed only weak transactivation activity compared to WT SF-1 confirming a possible effect of SF-1 on BDNF and thus energy balance. By contrast, the Thr296Met sequence variation had similar transactivation power on the hBNDF promoter I as seen with WT SF-1 (Figure 3B).

Weight related parameters of patients harboring SF-1 mutations

To address the question whether SF-1 deficiency may have metabolic consequences, we collected clinical data from our cohort of patients with SF-1 mutations. We were able to obtain data from 16 subjects with heterozygote SF-1 mutations including patients and their (affected) relatives (Table 2). Birth weight in singletons was normal (n = 8; median −0.83 SD, range −1.9 to 1.21). BMI of subjects currently being 1–17 years of age was also normal (n = 9; median 0.04 SD, range −0.69 to 2.81), as was BMI of 5 adults (median 0.6 SD, range 0.4 to 0.84). Thus in our small cohort of rather young patients with heterozygote SF-1 mutations overweight or obesity seems not an issue.

Discussion

In this study, two novel SF-1 mutations (Glu7Stop, His408Profs*159) were identified in 5 patients with SF-1 deficiency, all manifesting with 46,XY DSD and one (Glu7Stop) presenting with adrenal insufficiency that is rarely associated with SF-1 mutations. The disease causing impact of the identified mutations was confirmed by functional studies in cell models assessing transcriptional activity of wild-type and mutant SF-1 on genes involved in steroidogenesis (CYP11A1, CYP17A1, HSD3B2) and central energy balance (BDNF).

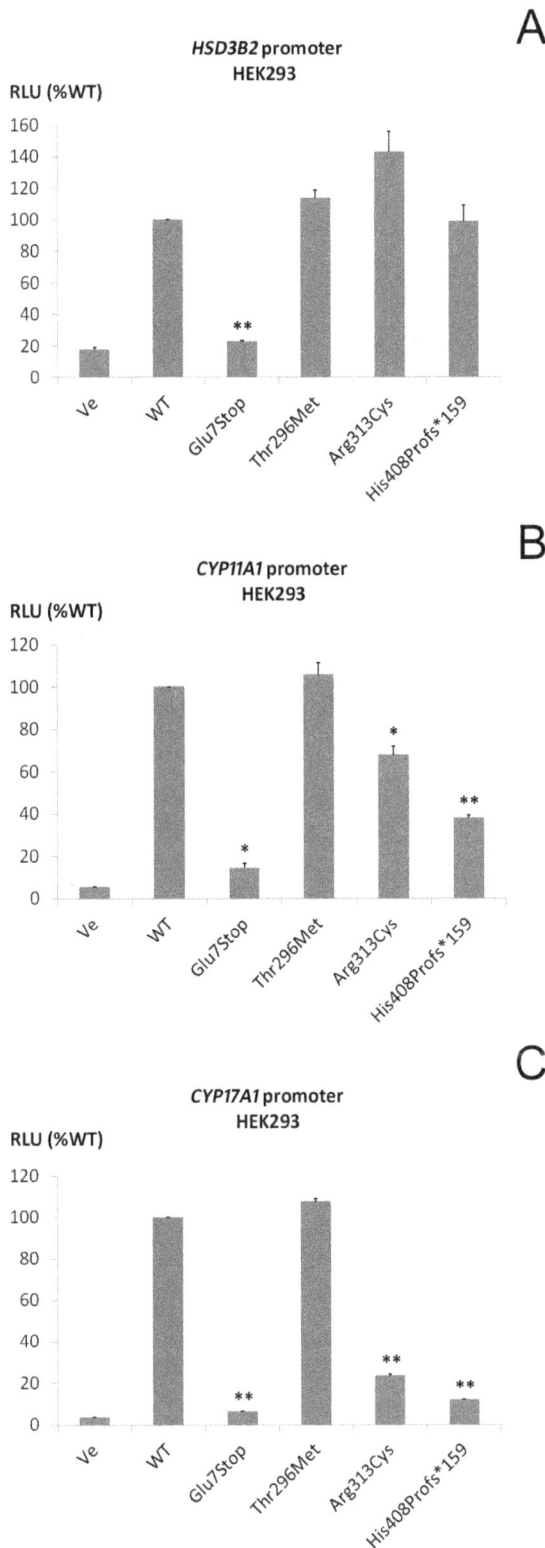

Figure 2. Promoter reporter studies for reported *NR5A1* mutations. Human embryonic kidney HEK293 cells were transiently transfected with wild-type (WT) or mutant SF-1 and promoter luciferase reporter constructs of the genes for steroidogenic enzymes *HSD3B2* (A), *CYP11A1* (B), *CYP17A1* (C). Luciferase activity was measured with the Promega Dual Luciferase assay system. Results are expressed as percentage of WT SF-1 activity. Independent experiments were performed in duplicate at least 3 times. Error bars represent the mean and SEM. *$p<0.05$; **$p<0.01$.

To date, only three SF-1 mutations have been implicated with adrenal insufficiency (heterozygote Gly35Glu and Arg255Leu, homozygote Arg92Gln) [10,15,17]. With patient 1, we add a novel SF-1 mutation (Glu7Stop) to this series. Our *in vitro* studies suggest that Glu7Stop is a loss of function SF-1 mutation. By contrast, the second SF-1 sequence variation (Thr296Met) identified in patient 1 is rather a simple polymorphism. First, it does not differ in functional assays when compared to WT SF-1. Second, this variant (rs201151141) has also been detected at an allelic frequency of 0.001 in a cohort of 662 normal subjects studied for a large-scale genome sequencing project (dbSNP database, http://www.ncbi.nlm.nih.gov/projects/SNP/snp).

The novel His408Profs*159 mutation identified in the SF-1 gene in patient 2 codes for a longer protein of 567 amino acids compared to WT SF-1 (461 aa). This mutant had an impact on both the steroidogenic promoters and the *BDNF* promoter (Figure 2). Interestingly, this heterozygous mutation was first detected in the father when investigated because of his history of childhood hypospadias and infertility. He nevertheless fathered a child through ICSI but the fetus's genetic and phenotypic sex was discordant. At birth the 46,XY child's genital phenotype was almost completely feminized and hormonal work-up at 4 months of age revealed low androgens prompting female sex assignment although the mutation was the same as in the father. This illustrates again for a novel *NR5A1* mutation the wide phenotypic spectrum within the same family.

The Arg313Cys mutation found in patients 3–5 in our study was recently reported in a patient with hypospadias [37]. Similar to our functional assays, Arg313Cys showed reduced transactivation on the promoters of the *AMH* and *CYP11A1* genes [37]. Although Arg313 is located in the highly conserved helix 5 of the ligand-binding domain, this same position has also been described for an Arg313His change (c.838G>A) in males with hypospadias [38,39]. Thus, position Arg313 of SF-1 may be a hot spot for mutations. Interestingly, this mutation appeared *de novo* in our family 4, while in family 5, the mutation was transmitted by an affected father.

In theory, SF-1 mutations could also have metabolic consequences for affected patients. But so far, no clinical data existed on this topic. Observations from the Sf-1 KO mice models suggest that loss of SF-1 is associated with impaired energy balance and low temperature expenditure leading to late-onset type of obesity [25]. Deletion of *BDNF* gene was described in obese patients with WAGR syndrome [33]. Among many other factors regulating appetite, SF-1 together with BDNF are expressed in the VMH of mice. Tran *et al.* described a significantly decreased expression of the *Bdnf* gene in Sf-1 +/− KO mice [27]. They also identified two promoter variants of the murine *Bdnf* gene which were specifically used in the VMH and their activity was related to SF-1 dosage [27]. In the presented study, we tried to establish the role of SF-1 in the regulation of human BDNF, an important player for central energy balance and thus obesity [40]. In fact, our experiments now show that the human *BDNF* promoter I is regulated by SF-1, and that SF-1 mutations have impaired transactivation activity on this promoter similar to impaired effect on promoters regulating genes of steroidogenesis. These results indicate that SF-1 might be a co-regulator of energy balance and that mutations in SF-1 may therefore also lead to metabolic consequences (e.g. obesity) in humans.

In addition to the *in vitro* studies, we were also able to collect some clinical data related to energy balance in 16 patients with heterozygote SF-1 mutations (Table 2). However, in our small cohort of 9 patients aged 1–17 years and 5 adults, we did not find weights and BMIs consistent with overweight or obesity.

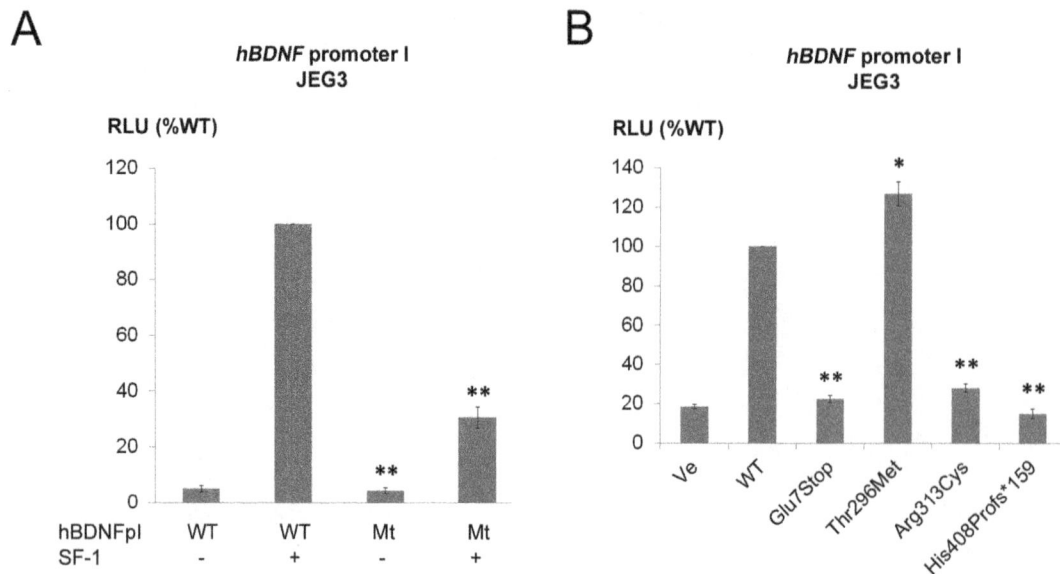

Figure 3. Promoter reporter studies for SF-1 regulating the human *BDNF* promoter I and comparative studies of specific *NR5A1* mutations on *BDNF* promoter activity. A consensus SF-1 transcription binding site was identified in the wild-type (WT) human BDNF promoter I. This *cis*-element was mutated to assess the role of SF-1 on BDNF transcription. Human placental JEG3 cells were transiently transfected with the WT or the SF-1 element mutant (Mt) BDNF promoter reporter with or without SF-1, and promoter activity was assessed by the Promega Dual Luciferase assay (A). After showing that SF-1 regulates the WT BDNF promoter I specifically (A), the ability of specific SF-1 mutations to *trans*-activate the *BDNF* promoter I was investigated (B). Results are expressed as percentage of WT SF-1 activity. Independent experiments were performed in duplicate 3 times. Error bars represent the mean and SEM. *$p < 0.05$; **$p < 0.01$.

Therefore, presented clinical data in humans are not in line with data found in mice [25,26], although *in vitro* data in human and mouse are similar [25,27]. These negative results might be 'true' negative results or may be explained by the following shortcomings of our presented study. First, small number of studied patients, which are in addition too young to observe metabolic consequences. Second, all patients are heterozygote for their SF-1 mutation and carry one wild-type SF-1 allele while most studied mice were Sf-1 complete KO. Further collaborative studies are therefore needed to gather clinical data of more patients and follow-up on a bigger cohort longitudinally.

Supporting Information

Table S1 Biochemical data of patients included in this study. Values outside the age- and sex-specific reference range

are given in **bold**. [1]PRA: plasma renin activity; [2]AMH: anti-Müllerian hormone; [3]Synacthen (250 µg/1.73 m^2 BSA); [4]hCG: 600 IU/48 h×6; [5]hCG: 1000 IU/24 h×3.

Author Contributions

Conceived and designed the experiments: JM NC MFC LA CEF. Performed the experiments: JM NC MFC KH IG MC MdC MA SK LA CEF. Analyzed the data: JM NC MFC LA CEF. Contributed reagents/materials/analysis tools: KH IG MC MdC MA SK. Contributed to the writing of the manuscript: JM NC LA CEF. Clinical evaluations: KH IG MC MdC MA SK.

References

1. Hoivik EA, Lewis AE, Aumo L, Bakke M (2010) Molecular aspects of steroidogenic factor 1 (SF-1). Mol Cell Endocrinol 315: 27–39.
2. Ferraz-de-Souza B, Lin L, Achermann JC (2011) Steroidogenic factor-1 (SF-1, NR5A1) and human disease. Mol Cell Endocrinol 336: 198–205.
3. Tran PV, Lee MB, Marin O, Xu B, Jones KR, et al. (2003) Requirement of the orphan nuclear receptor SF-1 in terminal differentiation of ventromedial hypothalamic neurons. Mol Cell Neurosci 22: 441–453.
4. Zhao L, Bakke M, Krimkevich Y, Cushman LJ, Parlow AF, et al. (2001) Steroidogenic factor 1 (SF1) is essential for pituitary gonadotrope function. Development 128: 147–154.
5. Morohashi K, Tsuboi-Asai H, Matsushita S, Suda M, Nakashima M, et al. (1999) Structural and functional abnormalities in the spleen of an mFtz-F1 gene-disrupted mouse. Blood 93: 1586–1594.
6. Patel MV, McKay IA, Burrin JM (2001) Transcriptional regulators of steroidogenesis, DAX-1 and SF-1, are expressed in human skin. J Invest Dermatol 117: 1559–1565.
7. Ramayya MS, Zhou J, Kino T, Segars JH, Bondy CA, et al. (1997) Steroidogenic factor 1 messenger ribonucleic acid expression in steroidogenic and nonsteroidogenic human tissues: Northern blot and in situ hybridization studies. J Clin Endocrinol Metab 82: 1799–1806.

8. Lala DS, Rice DA, Parker KL (1992) Steroidogenic factor I, a key regulator of steroidogenic enzyme expression, is the mouse homolog of fushi tarazu-factor I. Mol Endocrinol 6: 1249–1258.
9. Sadovsky Y, Crawford PA, Woodson KG, Polish JA, Clements MA, et al. (1995) Mice deficient in the orphan receptor steroidogenic factor 1 lack adrenal glands and gonads but express P450 side-chain-cleavage enzyme in the placenta and have normal embryonic serum levels of corticosteroids. Proc Natl Acad Sci U S A 92: 10939–10943.
10. Achermann JC, Ito M, Hindmarsh PC, Jameson JL (1999) A mutation in the gene encoding steroidogenic factor-1 causes XY sex reversal and adrenal failure in humans. Nat Genet 22: 125–126.
11. Camats N, Pandey AV, Fernandez-Cancio M, Andaluz P, Janner M, et al. (2012) Ten novel mutations in the NR5A1 gene cause disordered sex development in 46,XY and ovarian insufficiency in 46,XX individuals. J Clin Endocrinol Metab 97: E1294–1306.
12. Sarafoglou K, Ahmed SF (2012) Disorders of sex development: challenges for the future. J Clin Endocrinol Metab 97: 2292–2294.
13. Taketo M, Parker KL, Howard TA, Tsukiyama T, Wong M, et al. (1995) Homologs of Drosophila Fushi-Tarazu factor 1 map to mouse chromosome 2 and human chromosome 9q33. Genomics 25: 565–567.

14. Kohler B, Lin L, Ferraz-de-Souza B, Wieacker P, Heidemann P, et al. (2008) Five novel mutations in steroidogenic factor 1 (SF1, NR5A1) in 46,XY patients with severe underandrogenization but without adrenal insufficiency. Hum Mutat 29: 59–64.

15. Achermann JC, Ozisik G, Ito M, Orun UA, Harmanci K, et al. (2002) Gonadal determination and adrenal development are regulated by the orphan nuclear receptor steroidogenic factor-1, in a dose-dependent manner. J Clin Endocrinol Metab 87: 1829–1833.

16. Bashamboo A, Ferraz-de-Souza B, Lourenco D, Lin L, Sebire NJ, et al. (2010) Human male infertility associated with mutations in NR5A1 encoding steroidogenic factor 1. Am J Hum Genet 87: 505–512.

17. Biason-Lauber A, Schoenle EJ (2000) Apparently normal ovarian differentiation in a prepubertal girl with transcriptionally inactive steroidogenic factor 1 (NR5A1/SF-1) and adrenocortical insufficiency. Am J Hum Genet 67: 1563–1568.

18. Lin L, Achermann JC (2008) Steroidogenic factor-1 (SF-1, Ad4BP, NR5A1) and disorders of testis development. Sex Dev 2: 200–209.

19. Lourenco D, Brauner R, Lin L, De Perdigo A, Weryha G, et al. (2009) Mutations in NR5A1 associated with ovarian insufficiency. N Engl J Med 360: 1200–1210.

20. Majdic G, Young M, Gomez-Sanchez E, Anderson P, Szczepaniak LS, et al. (2002) Knockout mice lacking steroidogenic factor 1 are a novel genetic model of hypothalamic obesity. Endocrinology 143: 607–614.

21. Jacobs SB, Coss D, McGillivray SM, Mellon PL (2003) Nuclear factor Y and steroidogenic factor 1 physically and functionally interact to contribute to cell-specific expression of the mouse Follicle-stimulating hormone-beta gene. Mol Endocrinol 17: 1470–1483.

22. Halvorson LM, Kaiser UB, Chin WW (1996) Stimulation of luteinizing hormone beta gene promoter activity by the orphan nuclear receptor, steroidogenic factor-1. J Biol Chem 271: 6645–6650.

23. Ikeda Y, Luo X, Abbud R, Nilson JH, Parker KL (1995) The nuclear receptor steroidogenic factor 1 is essential for the formation of the ventromedial hypothalamic nucleus. Mol Endocrinol 9: 478–486.

24. Schimmer BP, White PC (2010) Minireview: steroidogenic factor 1: its roles in differentiation, development, and disease. Mol Endocrinol 24: 1322–1337.

25. Kim KW, Zhao L, Donato J, Jr., Kohno D, Xu Y, et al. (2011) Steroidogenic factor 1 directs programs regulating diet-induced thermogenesis and leptin action in the ventral medial hypothalamic nucleus. Proc Natl Acad Sci U S A 108: 10673–10678.

26. Unger TJ, Calderon GA, Bradley LC, Sena-Esteves M, Rios M (2007) Selective deletion of Bdnf in the ventromedial and dorsomedial hypothalamus of adult mice results in hyperphagic behavior and obesity. J Neurosci 27: 14265–14274.

27. Tran PV, Akana SF, Malkovska I, Dallman MF, Parada LF, et al. (2006) Diminished hypothalamic bdnf expression and impaired VMH function are associated with reduced SF-1 gene dosage. J Comp Neurol 498: 637–648.

28. Pruunsild P, Kazantseva A, Aid T, Palm K, Timmusk T (2007) Dissecting the human BDNF locus: bidirectional transcription, complex splicing, and multiple promoters. Genomics 90: 397–406.

29. Kernie SG, Liebl DJ, Parada LF (2000) BDNF regulates eating behavior and locomotor activity in mice. EMBO J 19: 1290–1300.

30. Rios M, Fan G, Fekete C, Kelly J, Bates B, et al. (2001) Conditional deletion of brain-derived neurotrophic factor in the postnatal brain leads to obesity and hyperactivity. Mol Endocrinol 15: 1748–1757.

31. Stranahan AM, Arumugam TV, Mattson MP (2011) Lowering corticosterone levels reinstates hippocampal brain-derived neurotropic factor and Trkb expression without influencing deficits in hypothalamic brain-derived neurotropic factor expression in leptin receptor-deficient mice. Neuroendocrinology 93: 58–64.

32. Kohjima M, Sun Y, Chan L (2010) Increased food intake leads to obesity and insulin resistance in the tg2576 Alzheimer's disease mouse model. Endocrinology 151: 1532–1540.

33. Han JC, Liu QR, Jones M, Levinn RL, Menzie CM, et al. (2008) Brain-derived neurotrophic factor and obesity in the WAGR syndrome. N Engl J Med 359: 918–927.

34. Gray J, Yeo GS, Cox JJ, Morton J, Adlam AL, et al. (2006) Hyperphagia, severe obesity, impaired cognitive function, and hyperactivity associated with functional loss of one copy of the brain-derived neurotrophic factor (BDNF) gene. Diabetes 55: 3366–3371.

35. Huang N, Miller WL (2000) Cloning of factors related to HIV-inducible LBP proteins that regulate steroidogenic factor-1-independent human placental transcription of the cholesterol side-chain cleavage enzyme, P450scc. J Biol Chem 275: 2852–2858.

36. Fluck CE, Miller WL (2004) GATA-4 and GATA-6 modulate tissue-specific transcription of the human gene for P450c17 by direct interaction with Sp1. Mol Endocrinol 18: 1144–1157.

37. Allali S, Muller JB, Brauner R, Lourenco D, Boudjenah R, et al. (2011) Mutation analysis of NR5A1 encoding steroidogenic factor 1 in 77 patients with 46, XY disorders of sex development (DSD) including hypospadias. PLoS One 6: e24117.

38. Ciaccio M, Costanzo M, Guercio G, De Dona V, Marino R, et al. (2012) Preserved fertility in a patient with a 46,XY disorder of sex development due to a new heterozygous mutation in the NR5A1/SF-1 gene: evidence of 46,XY and 46,XX gonadal dysgenesis phenotype variability in multiple members of an affected kindred. Horm Res Paediatr 78: 119–126.

39. Adamovic T, Chen Y, Thai HT, Zhang X, Markljung E, et al. (2012) The p.G146A and p.P125P polymorphisms in the steroidogenic factor-1 (SF-1) gene do not affect the risk for hypospadias in Caucasians. Sex Dev 6: 292–297.

40. Rios M (2013) BDNF and the central control of feeding: accidental bystander or essential player? Trends Neurosci 36: 83–90.

18

The Concordance of Care for Age Related Macular Degeneration with the Chronic Care Model: A Multi-Centered Cross-Sectional Study

Stefan Markun[1]*, Elisabeth Brändle[1], Avraham Dishy[2], Thomas Rosemann[1], Anja Frei[1,3]

1 Institute of General Practice and Health Service Research, University of Zurich, University Hospital of Zurich, Zurich, Switzerland, **2** Department of Ophthalmology, Cantonal Hospital Aarau, Aarau, Switzerland, **3** Institute of Social and Preventive Medicine, University of Zurich, Zurich, Switzerland

Abstract

Aims: The aim of the study was to assess the concordance of care for age related macular degeneration with the evidence-based framework for care for chronic medical conditions known as the chronic care model. Furthermore we aimed to identify factors associated with the concordance of care with the chronic care model.

Methods: Multi-centered cross-sectional study. 169 patients beginning medical treatment for age related macular degeneration were recruited and analyzed. Patients completed the Patient Assessment of Chronic Illness Care (PACIC) questionnaire, reflecting accordance to the chronic care model from a patient's perspective, the National Eye Institute Visual Functioning Questionnaire-25 (NEI-VFQ-25) and Patient Health Questionnaire (PHQ-9). Visual acuity and chronic medical conditions were assessed. Nonparametric tests and correlation analyses were performed, also multivariable regression analysis.

Results: The median PACIC summary score was 2.4 (interquartile range 1.75 to 3.25), the lowest PACIC subscale score was "follow-up/coordination" with a median of 1.8 (interquartile range 1.00 to 2.60). In multivariable regression analysis the presence of diabetes type 2 was strongly associated with low PACIC scores (coefficient = −0.85, p = 0.007).

Conclusion: Generally, care for patients with age related macular degeneration by ophthalmologists is in moderate concordance with the chronic care model. Concerning follow-up and coordination of health service, large improvements are possible. Future research should answer the question how healthcare delivery can be improved effecting relevant benefits to patients with AMD.

Editor: Tammy Clifford, Canadian Agency for Drugs and Technologies in Health, Canada

Funding: This trial was supported by the non-commercial foundation "Zukunft Hausarzt, Zürcher Stiftung zur Förderung der Hausarztmedizin", Zürich (www.zukunfthausarzt.ch). The funders had no role in study design, data collection and analysis, decision to publish, or preparation of the manuscript.

Competing Interests: The authors have declared that no competing interests exist.

* Email: stefan.markun@usz.ch

Introduction

Health care in general is being challenged by the unprecedented increase in chronic conditions. [1,2] The need to react to this epidemiological transition has led to initiatives, targeting to improve care for chronic conditions. [3] The chronic care model (CCM) developed by Wagner and colleagues is an evidence-based multifaceted recommendation package, targeting to improve care in different categories that are regarded as determinants for adequate care of chronic conditions. [4–6] These categories are organization of healthcare, clinical information systems, delivery-system design, decision support, self-management support and community resources. The CCM is supported by the WHO and has gained widespread acceptance because interventions enhancing the concordance with the CCM effectively improved relevant outcomes in chronic diseases such as diabetes, osteoarthritis or depression. [7–9] A validated tool to measure the concordance of care with the CCM from the patient's perspective has been developed [10].

Age related macular degeneration (AMD) is a chronic condition with severe potential impact on diseased patients. In AMD, visual loss is for the greatest part triggered by the growth of abnormal blood vessels in proximity of the retina. These abnormal blood vessels cause leakage of blood constituents with consecutive anatomic disruption, cell death and ultimately loss of central vision. The growth of new blood vessels including the consequences on visual function, however, can be effectively antagonized by therapies targeting the vascular endothelial growth factor

A (VEGF-A). [11] These therapies are applied by periodic intravitreal injections. Current treatment strategies aim to administer injections in phases of disease activity notable by sudden deteriorations of visual function. [12,13] This individualized and patient-centered approach potentially reduces unnecessary injections, however, it requires health services to provide a thorough follow-up management. Furthermore patients need to be adequately informed and empowered as they take great responsibility by self-monitoring their disease. This is especially important in stages of presumed disease inactivity, when re-occurrence of neovascularizations should prompt immediate re-uptake of an anti-VEGF-A therapy capable of slowing down or even avert permanent visual loss. Such features of healthcare delivery are represented in the CCM, which is therefore relevant in AMD on both the caregivers' and the patients' levels. Whether care for AMD is in concordance with the CCM, however, is currently unknown.

The aim of this study was to assess if and to what extent care for patients with AMD is in concordance with the CCM in Swiss ophthalmology clinics (1). Furthermore we aimed to identify factors that determine the concordance of care with the CCM (2).

Materials and Methods

Study design

This is a cross-sectional study, based on the baseline data gathered for the randomized trial "The chronic care for age-related macular degeneration study" (CHARMED). The study has been registered at Current Controlled Trials (ISRCTN32507927), the study protocol is publically available. [14] In brief about 20 ophthalmologists from 20 leading ophthalmology clinics in Switzerland providing therapy for patients with AMD were invited to participate in the study by a formal letter. Participating ophthalmologists where trained to gather outcome measures in a standardized format. Also in every participating clinic chronic care coaches where trained to deliver chronic care and conduct structured interviews for outcome measurements. According to the trial's power calculation 352 patients where intended to be recruited, however, recruiting was stopped after 20 months when the number of newly recruited patients per month reached zero.

Ethics statement

Ethics committee approval was obtained (ethics committee of the Canton Zurich, KEK-ZH-NR: 2010-04391/1). The study was performed adhering to the tenets of the Declaration of Helsinki and according to Good Clinical Practice Guidelines.

Patients

Patients were recruited consecutively from April 1 2011 until January 28 2013 by the participating ophthalmologists during clinical visits.

To be eligible for inclusion, patients were required to meet the following inclusion criteria: Diagnosis of wet AMD, age above 50 years, eligible for antiangiogenic drug therapy and visual acuity of at least 20 letters in the assessment with the Early Treatment Diabetic Retinopathy Study (ETDRS) chart. Written informed consent in the study participation was obtained before any study related procedures were taken. Exclusion criteria were former invasive medical treatment for AMD, severe general illness (i.e. advanced malignant tumors or dementia), severe psychological illness and insufficient German or French language skills.

Measures and data collection

Data collection was performed directly after written informed consent was obtained. A questionnaire was filled in by the ophthalmologists containing the following measures retrieved at the recruitment visit: Visual acuity (using ETDRS charts, standardized measurements were assured by conducting a visit with a teaching session at each ophthalmology clinic); central retinal thickness by optical coherence tomography; specific comorbidities such as hypertension, diabetes type 2, diabetic retinopathy, coronary artery disease, congestive heart failure, stroke or transient ischemic attack, asthma or chronic obstructive lung disease and neoplasms; family anamnesis of wet AMD; smoking status; current medication; estimation of the patients compliance on a four-point scale (range from 1 = very good to 4 = very bad).

A second questionnaire was given to the patients at the recruiting visit to fill in and return directly to the University of Zurich using a readily stamped and accordingly addressed envelope. The questionnaire was self-administered and contained the Patient Assessment of Chronic Illness Care (PACIC) as a measure for concordance of care with the CCM, [10] the PHQ-9 questionnaire as a measure for depression [15] and questions about socio-demographic data and health service utilization.

The PACIC is a validated self-administered instrument that measures the concordance of care with the CCM from the patient's perspective. According to the key-elements of the CCM the PACIC is organized containing five essential categories of chronic care asked in 20 individual items. In specific these categories are patient activation, delivery system design/decision support, goal setting/tailoring, problem solving/contextual counselling and follow-up/coordination. Each of the individual items are scored on a five point Likert-scale ranging from "almost never" (= 1, corresponding to poorest concordance with the CCM) to "almost always" (= 5, corresponding to highest concordance with the CCM). The PACIC summary score is the mean score of the 20 individual items and gives an overall rating of the concordance with the CCM. Five subscales are defined that allow estimations of the CCM concordance with the respective essential categories of chronic care. Such as the CCM, the PACIC itself has shown to be associated with favorable outcomes in chronic conditions. [16] The PACIC summary score was our predefined primary outcome.

The Patient Health Questionnaire (PHQ-9) is a self-administered tool that allows rapid screening for depression and rating severity that recently has showed consistency in patients with visual impairment. [17,18] The PHQ-9 was introduced in the measurements as a confounder control, because depression is known to be highly prevalent among patients with AMD and might influence outcomes of the CHARMED randomized trial (not discussed in this article) [19].

In a face-to-face or telephone interview with the patients the trained chronic care coaches operated the National Eye Institute Visual Functioning Questionnaire-25 (NEI-VFQ-25) in the interviewer administered format. [20] The NEI-VFQ-25 is a validated measure of the visual disability specific quality of life and functioning, it consists of 25 vision-targeted questions that generate 11 subscales of vision related health and functioning [21,22].

Patients and ophthalmologists' answers remained concealed from each other; the University of Zurich had no access to the patients' personal informations ensuring anonymity.

Statistical analysis

Continuous variables are presented as means and standard deviations or medians and interquartile ranges if not otherwise

Table 1. Demographical and social characteristics of study patients, smoking status and patient compliance from the ophthalmologist's perspective; table n = 169.

Variable	Category	n	percent
Gender	Male	62	36.7
	Female	107	63.3
	Missing information	0	0.0
Age	<60 years old	3	1.8
	60–69 years old	33	19.5
	70–79 years old	69	40.8
	80–89 years old	58	34.3
	≥90 years old	6	3.6
	Missing information	0	0.0
Living situation	Living with partner or family	103	60.9
	Living alone	53	31.4
	Missing information	13	7.7
Working situation	Still working	12	7.1
	Retired	144	85.2
	Missing information	13	7.7
Education years completed	≤6 years	2	1.2
	7 to 9 years	41	24.3
	10 to 12 years	56	33.1
	≥13 years	56	33.1
	Missing information	14	8.3
Smoking status	Current smoker	26	15.4
	Former smoker	49	29.0
	Never smoker	94	55.6
	Missing information	0	0.0
Compliance	Very good	96	56.8
	Rather good	69	40.8
	Rather bad	3	1.8
	Very bad	1	0.6
	Missing information	0	0

declared; categorical data is presented as frequencies and percentages. Bivariate association between the PACIC summary score and continuous variables were conducted using Spearman correlations, between PACIC summary score and categorical variables using Mann-Whitney-U Test and Kruskal-Wallis Test (more than two groups). Potential determinants of the PACIC summary score were investigated by multivariable regression model. We included all variables in the model that showed both a significant bivariate relationship with the PACIC summary score on a 5% level and could be interpreted in terms of content as potential determinants. We further controlled for the cluster-effect of clinics, thus taking into account that patient observations are not independent, i.e. observations in one cluster tend to be more similar to each other than to individuals in the rest of the sample. A two-sided alpha of 0.05 was set as level of significance for all comparisons. Missing data were left as missing, for the construction of the PACIC summary score one missing item (out of 20) was allowed. Analyses were calculated using the software SPSS version 21.0 and STATA version 12.

Results

Ophthalmologist characteristics

Twelve different ophthalmologists from twelve different clinics could be recruited for the study. Amongst the clinics, three different categories of organization type were found: Three clinics were single handed practices (median number of patients recruited = 7, range 2–12), five clinics were group practices (median number of patients recruited = 5, range 1–18), four were clinics run within hospitals (median number of patients recruited = 25, range 11–54).

Patient characteristics and clinical measures

In total, 169 patients were enrolled in the study. 21 (12.4%) patients were recruited in single handed practices, 32 (18.9%) in group practices and 116 (68.6%) in clinics run within hospitals. 107 (63.3%) of the patients were female, the mean age was 76.7 (±8.0) years. The average of total education years absolved was 12.0 (±3.4). In all patients, treatment with ranibizumab was started. Further characteristics are shown in Table 1.

Table 2. Vision-specific variables of study patients: visual acuity was assessed with the Early Treatment Diabetic Retinopathy Study (ETDRS) Chart; disability was assessed with the National Eye Institute Visual Functioning Questionnaire-25 (NEI-VFQ-25), range 0 to 100 (0 represents worst, 100 represents best possible visual functioning); table n = 169.

Variable	Category	Mean	Standard deviation	n	Percent
ETDRS Visual acuity better eye	Total ETDRS letters correct	74.1	14.9		
	<31 ETRDS letters correct			4	2.4
	31–50 ETRDS letters correct			9	5.3
	51–70 ETRDS letters correct			30	17.8
	>70 ETRDS letters correct			118	69.8
	Missing information			8	4.7
ETDRS Visual acuity worse eye	Total ETDRS letters correct	52.6	18.9		
	<31 ETRDS letters correct			18	10.7
	31–50 ETRDS letters correct			48	28.4
	51–70 ETRDS letters correct			68	40.2
	>70 ETRDS letters correct			27	16.0
	Missing information			8	4.7
NEI-VFQ-25 subscales*	General health	54.6	19.5		
	General vision	67.0	13.6		
	Ocular pain	90.0	15.8		
	Near activities	76.4	20.6		
	Distant activities	79.9	19.9		
	Social functioning	94.0	14.2		
	Mental health	78.7	18.7		
	Role difficulties	82.1	24.6		
	Dependency	93.8	17.0		
	Driving	68.8	33.9		
	Color vision	96.2	13.8		
	Peripheral vision	88.7	18.9		

*) Missing information for all items ranged from 6 to 8, except for "Driving" which was unanswered in 83 cases.

The mean number (± standard deviation) of correctly identified ETDRS letters was 74.1 (±14.9) with the better eye and 52.6 (±18.9) with the worse eye. The mean (± standard deviation) NEI-VFQ-25 composite score was 83.8 (±12.4). The mean general health rating (not component of the composite score) was 54.6 (±19.5). Detailed vision-specific information is given in Table 2.

In 111 (65.7%) of the patients at least one co-occurring chronic medical condition was present. 99 (58.6%) of the patients had cardiovascular comorbidities. The median number of ophthalmologist consultations within one year was 2 (interquartile range 1 to 3), the median number of GP consultations was 3 (interquartile range 1 to 6). 37 (21.9%) patients had at least one hospitalization during the last year, 27 (16.0%) had emergency hospitalizations. Data about comorbidities and healthcare utilization is displayed in Table 3.

PACIC scores

The median PACIC summary score was 2.4 (interquartile range 1.75 to 3.25). There were substantial differences between the different PACIC subscale scores. The subscale score "follow-up/coordination" resulted lowest with a median subscale score of 1.8 (interquartile range 1.00 to 2.60), corresponding with an average rating of the items in the PACIC questionnaire somewhat lower than "generally not". The highest subscale score was "delivery

system design/decision support" with a median subscale score of 3.7 (interquartile range 2.33 to 4.67), corresponding with an average rating of the items in the PACIC questionnaire between "sometimes" and "most of the time". Details about the distribution of the PACIC summary score and subscale results are displayed in Table 4 and Figure 1.

Bivariate associations with PACIC summary score

The PACIC summary score was not significantly associated with the practice organization type (single handed, group practices and ambulatory clinics in hospitals: independent sample Kruskal-Wallis Test p = 0.187). No significant associations with the PACIC summary score were found for patients' socio-demographic characteristics, smoking status or physician-reported compliance. Also no significant association with the PACIC summary score was found for the number of comorbidities and for the PHQ-9. The presence of diabetes type 2 was significantly associated with lower PACIC scores (median [interquartile range] PACIC summary score of group with diabetes type 2=1.5 [1.11 to 2.13]), group without diabetes type 2=2.7 [1.83 to 3.28]; Mann Whitney U Test p = 0.002). Also the presence of coronary artery disease was significantly associated with lower PACIC scores (median [interquartile range] PACIC summary score of group with coronary artery disease = 2.0 [1.37 to 2.89], group without coronary artery disease = 2.7 [1.80 to 3.30]; Mann Whitney U Test p = 0.037). No

Table 3. Comorbidity and Health Service Utilization; table n = 169.

Variable	Category	n	percent
Number of comorbidities	0 comorbidities	58	34.3
	1 comorbidity	60	35.5
	2 comorbidities	34	20.1
	3 comorbidities	10	5.9
	≥4 comorbidities	6	3.6
	Missing information	1	0.6
Specific comorbidities	Hypertension	92	54.4
	Diabetes type 2	14	8.3
	Diabetic retinopathy	0	0.0
	Coronary artery disease	29	17.2
	Congestive heart failure	8	4.7
	Stroke/TIA[1]	14	8.3
	Asthma/COPD[2]	16	9.5
	Neoplasm	11	6.5
Depression according to PHQ-9[3]	No depression	116	68.6
	Mild depression	32	18.9
	Moderate major depression	3	1.8
	Severe major depression	2	1.2
	Missing information	16	9.5
Number of ophthalmologist consultations last year	1–2 consultations	87	51.5
	3–4 consultations	38	22.5
	5–6 consultations	14	8.3
	≥7 consultations	8	4.7
	Missing information	22	13.0
Number of GP[4] consultations last year	0–2 consultations	65	38.5
	3–4 consultations	36	21.3
	5–6 consultations	23	13.6
	≥7 consultations	31	18.3
	Missing information	14	8.3
Number of days in hospital last year	0 days	117	69.2
	1–3 days	8	4.7
	4–10 days	18	10.7
	≥11 days	11	6.5
	Missing information	15	8.9

[1]TIA = Transient ischemic attack;
[2]COPD = Chronic obstructive pulmonary disease;
[3]PHQ-9 = Patient Health Questionnaire-9;
[4]GP = General practitioner.

vision-specific variable showed association with the PACIC summary score.

Multivariate associations with PACIC summary score

For the multivariable regression model we considered the comorbidity diabetes type 2 and coronary artery disease (both significant in bivariate analysis), gender and age (potential confounders) and visual acuity of the better eye (as an indicator for the severity of visual loss). The model was controlled for the cluster-effect originating from the different study clinics.

After application of the model, the only significant determinant of the PACIC summary score was diabetes type 2 (coefficient = −0.85, p = 0.007). Coronary artery disease closely missed signif-

icance (coefficient = −0.44, p = 0.059), the other variables showed no association (Table 5).

Discussion

The CCM is an evidence-based template for the care for patients with chronic illnesses. We aimed to measure the concordance of care with the CCM in patients treated for AMD. We found that patients perceived moderate overall concordance with the CCM, especially low concordance was found in the "follow-up/coordination" subscale score.

A broad spectrum of different types of ophthalmology clinics participated in the study. Interestingly the PACIC summary score

Table 4. Patient Assessment of Chronic Illness Care (PACIC) scores; range 1 to 5, 1 corresponds to poorest concordance with the Chronic Care Model (CCM), 5 corresponds to highest concordance with the CCM; for the construction of the PACIC summary score one missing item was allowed.

PACIC Scores	Valid n	Median	Interquartile range
Summary score[1]	131	2.4	1.75 to 3.25
Subscale "Patient activation"	141	3.0	1.67 to 4.67
Subscale "Delivery system design/decision support"	133	3.7	2.33 to 4.67
Subscale "Goal setting/tailoring"	138	2.2	1.30 to 3.40
Subscale "Problem solving/contextual counselling"	138	2.0	1.19 to 3.81
Subscale "Follow-up/coordination"	139	1.8	1.00 to 2.60

[1]For calculation of PACIC summary score one missing item (out of twenty) in the questionnaire was allowed.

showed no significant association with the organization type of the clinics. Although relevant structural differences between hospital-run ophthalmology clinics and single handed ophthalmology practices must be assumed, those differences did not affect the concordance with the CCM from the patients perspective.

According to the inclusion and exclusion criteria, patients that just newly qualified for antiangiogenic therapy were recruited in this study. The sample is thus representative for AMD patients at the beginning of their chronic care situation. The relatively intact ETDRS visual acuity and the high NEI-VFQ-25 scores showed that these patients are mostly in early stages of the disease and have therefore the highest potential to benefit from preventive interventions enabled by successful healthcare delivery.

PACIC scores we identified, however, were modest. The subscale score "follow-up/coordination" was particularly low also in comparison to PACIC scores from research done in other chronic conditions such as diabetes, osteoarthritis or inflammatory bowel disease. [23–25] In AMD, however, a low concordance of follow-up organization with the CCM is especially undesirable because successful follow-up is regarded to be critical for outcomes. [26] It remains, however, debatable whether the PACIC subscales truly represent the different domains of the CCM, because of the high internal consistency of the total PACIC score itself [10,27].

Furthermore, we found specific comorbidities to be associated with low PACIC scores in ophthalmological care. In the case of

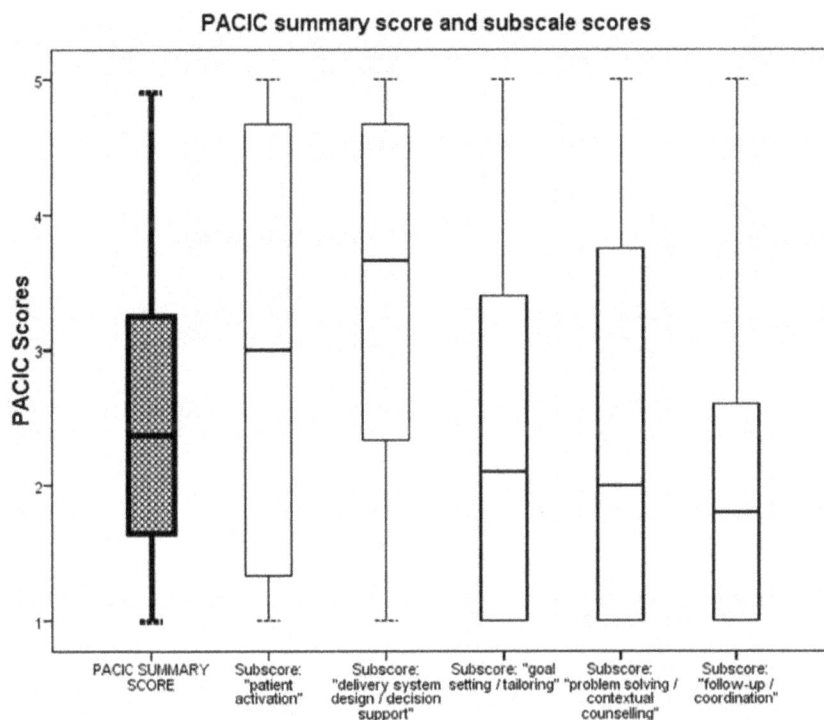

Figure 1. Distribution of PACIC summary score and subscale scores. PACIC scores are represented in boxplots. The PACIC summary score is displayed on the left, other boxplots are the respective PACIC subscale scores. The lower and the upper margin of the box indicate the 25th and 75th percentile respectively. The bar inside the box indicates the median. Whiskers extend to the most extreme data point within 1.5 times the interquartile range.

Table 5. Adjusted Regression Coefficients (95%CI) for the Patient Assessment of Chronic Illness Care (PACIC) summary score (n = 126)[1].

Variable	Category	Adjusted Regression Coefficient (95%CI)
Gender	Male	Ref
	Female	−0.06 (−0.41 to 0.29)
Age	Years	0.01 (−0.02 to 0.03)
Visual acuity of better eye	ETDRS	0.008 (−0.004 to 0.02)
Diabetes Type 2	Absent	Ref
	Present	−0.85 (−1.47 to −0.24)*
Coronary artery disease	Absent	Ref
	Present	−0.44 (−0.91; 0.02)†

[1]Multivariable regression model adjusted for all determinants in column and additionally controlled for the cluster-effect originating from the different study clinics (n = 126 patients with complete determinant and PACIC data); there was a significant cluster-effect resulting in an intra-class correlation coefficient (ICC) of 9.1% (p = 0.027).
*p = 0.007.
†p = 0.059.

diabetes type 2 this is troublesome because patients with both AMD and diabetes are in the highest need for successful chronic care as their visual acuity is endangered by two treatable chronic conditions simultaneously. With our data we cannot explain this finding of co-occurring conditions being associated with decreased PACIC scores. A possible explanation for this finding could be that ophthalmologists feel less responsible for care for multimorbid patients since they assume that the GP coordinates the care for them.

Limitations

Undoubtedly, the implementation of the different important elements of chronic care is a dynamic process requiring several contacts of healthcare professionals with the individual patient. Patients in our sample, however, were newly entering a chronic care situation for AMD. The PACIC results we obtained might therefore be representative for patients in an early stage of chronic care implementation, thus showing the gaps that still need to be filled. This might especially apply to our results in the "follow-up/ coordination" subscale. Only 131 of 169 patients provided enough data to allow calculation of the PACIC summary score. A greater number of cases would have provided more power to detect significant results. Also, we cannot exclude bias from selective answering; we assume, however, that patients dissatisfied with their healthcare would be less motivated to answer the questionnaire, thus causing bias towards false high PACIC scores. PACIC scores in our study would thus tend to be overestimated, the potential for enhancements even greater. Finally, the PACIC score

reflects the patient perspective of chronic illness care only, leaving the healthcare provider's perspective unclear.

Conclusion

Generally, care for patients with age related macular degeneration by ophthalmologists is in moderate concordance with the chronic care model. Concerning follow-up and coordination of health service, large improvements are possible, for example with follow-up calls by health service professionals (in order to prevent loss of follow-up during inactive stage of the disease) or with coordination of health service between primary care and specialized ophthalmologic care (in order to allocate responsibilities and avoid under- or overtreatment especially if additional chronic diseases as diabetes exist). Future research should answer the question how healthcare delivery can be improved effecting relevant benefits to patients with AMD.

Acknowledgments

The authors thank Oliver Senn, PhD for statistical assistance.

Author Contributions

Conceived and designed the experiments: TR AF. Performed the experiments: SM AF. Analyzed the data: SM EB AF. Contributed reagents/materials/analysis tools: AF. Contributed to the writing of the manuscript: SM EB AD TR AF. Interpretation of data: SM EB AD TR AF.

References

1. Lochner KA, Cox CS (2013) Prevalence of multiple chronic conditions among Medicare beneficiaries, United States, 2010. Prev Chronic Dis 10: E61.
2. Thorpe KE, Ogden LL, Galactionova K (2010) Chronic conditions account for rise in Medicare spending from 1987 to 2006. Health Aff (Millwood) 29: 718–724.
3. Tsai AC, Morton SC, Mangione CM, Keeler EB (2005) A meta-analysis of interventions to improve care for chronic illnesses. Am J Manag Care 11: 478–488.
4. Wagner EH (1998) Chronic disease management: what will it take to improve care for chronic illness? Eff Clin Pract 1: 2–4.
5. Wagner EH, Austin BT, Davis C, Hindmarsh M, Schaefer J, et al. (2001) Improving chronic illness care: translating evidence into action. Health Aff (Millwood) 20: 64–78.
6. Epping-Jordan JE, Pruitt SD, Bengoa R, Wagner EH (2004) Improving the quality of health care for chronic conditions. Qual Saf Health Care 13: 299–305.
7. Stellefson M, Dipnarine K, Stopka C (2013) The chronic care model and diabetes management in US primary care settings: a systematic review. Prev Chronic Dis 10: E26.
8. Rosemann T, Joos S, Laux G, Gensichen J, Szecsenyi J (2007) Case management of arthritis patients in primary care: a cluster-randomized controlled trial. Arthritis Rheum 57: 1390–1397.
9. Gensichen J, von Korff M, Peitz M, Muth C, Beyer M, et al. (2009) Case management for depression by health care assistants in small primary care practices: a cluster randomized trial. Ann Intern Med 151: 369–378.

10. Glasgow RE, Wagner EH, Schaefer J, Mahoney LD, Reid RJ, et al. (2005) Development and validation of the Patient Assessment of Chronic Illness Care (PACIC). Med Care 43: 436–444.

11. Vedula SS, Krzystolik MG (2008) Antiangiogenic therapy with anti-vascular endothelial growth factor modalities for neovascular age-related macular degeneration. Cochrane Database Syst Rev: CD005139.

12. Chakravarthy U, Williams M, Group AG (2013) The Royal College of Ophthalmologists Guidelines on AMD: Executive Summary. Eye (Lond) 27: 1429–1431.

13. Brand CS (2012) Management of retinal vascular diseases: a patient-centric approach. Eye (Lond) 26 Suppl 2: S1–16.

14. Frei A, Woitzek K, Wang M, Held U, Rosemann T (2011) The chronic care for age-related macular degeneration study (CHARMED): study protocol for a randomized controlled trial. Trials 12: 221.

15. Lowe B, Kroenke K, Herzog W, Grafe K (2004) Measuring depression outcome with a brief self-report instrument: sensitivity to change of the Patient Health Questionnaire (PHQ-9). J Affect Disord 81: 61–66.

16. Schmittdiel J, Mosen DM, Glasgow RE, Hibbard J, Remmers C, et al. (2008) Patient Assessment of Chronic Illness Care (PACIC) and improved patient-centered outcomes for chronic conditions. J Gen Intern Med 23: 77–80.

17. Lamoureux EL, Tee HW, Pesudovs K, Pallant JF, Keeffe JE, et al. (2009) Can clinicians use the PHQ-9 to assess depression in people with vision loss? Optom Vis Sci 86: 139–145.

18. Kroenke K, Spitzer RL, Williams JB (2001) The PHQ-9: validity of a brief depression severity measure. J Gen Intern Med 16: 606–613.

19. Brody BL, Gamst AC, Williams RA, Smith AR, Lau PW, et al. (2001) Depression, visual acuity, comorbidity, and disability associated with age-related macular degeneration. Ophthalmology 108: 1893–1900; discussion 1900–1891.

20. Mangione CM, Lee PP, Gutierrez PR, Spritzer K, Berry S, et al. (2001) Development of the 25-item National Eye Institute Visual Function Questionnaire. Arch Ophthalmol 119: 1050–1058.

21. Revicki DA, Rentz AM, Harnam N, Thomas VS, Lanzetta P (2010) Reliability and validity of the National Eye Institute Visual Function Questionnaire-25 in patients with age-related macular degeneration. Invest Ophthalmol Vis Sci 51: 712–717.

22. Mangione CM (2000) The National Eye Institute 25-Item Visual Function Questionnaire (VFQ-25) - Version 2000. Available: http://www.nei.nih.gov/resources/visionfunction/manual_cm2000.pdf. Accessed 2013 Nov 6.

23. Rosemann T, Laux G, Droesemeyer S, Gensichen J, Szecsenyi J (2007) Evaluation of a culturally adapted German version of the Patient Assessment of Chronic Illness Care (PACIC 5A) questionnaire in a sample of osteoarthritis patients. J Eval Clin Pract 13: 806–813.

24. Frei A, Herzog S, Woitzek K, Held U, Senn O, et al. (2012) Characteristics of poorly controlled Type 2 diabetes patients in Swiss primary care. Cardiovasc Diabetol 11: 70.

25. Randell RL, Long MD, Martin CF, Sandler RS, Chen W, et al. (2013) Patient perception of chronic illness care in a large inflammatory bowel disease cohort. Inflammatory bowel diseases 19: 1428–1433.

26. Rasmussen A, Bloch SB, Fuchs J, Hansen LH, Larsen M, et al. (2013) A 4-Year Longitudinal Study of 555 Patients Treated with Ranibizumab for Neovascular Age-related Macular Degeneration. Ophthalmology 120: 2630–2636.

27. Gugiu C, Coryn CL, Applegate B (2010) Structure and measurement properties of the Patient Assessment of Chronic Illness Care instrument. J Eval Clin Pract 16: 509–516.

19

Development of Two Barthel Index-Based Supplementary Scales for Patients with Stroke

Ya-Chen Lee[1], Sheng-Shiung Chen[2], Chia-Lin Koh[1], I-Ping Hsueh[3,4]*, Kai-Ping Yao[5], Ching-Lin Hsieh[3,4]

1 School of Occupational Therapy, College of Medicine, National Taiwan University, Taipei, Taiwan, 2 Department of Physical Medicine and Rehabilitation, E-Da Hospital/I-Shou University, Kaohsiung, Taiwan, 3 School of Occupational Therapy, College of Medicine, National Taiwan University, Taipei, Taiwan, 4 Department of Physical Medicine and Rehabilitation, National Taiwan University Hospital, Zhongzheng District, Taipei, Taiwan, 5 Department of Psychology, College of Science, National Taiwan University, Taipei, Taiwan

Abstract

Background: The Barthel Index (BI) assesses actual performance of activities of daily living (ADL). However, comprehensive assessment of ADL functions should include two other constructs: self-perceived difficulty and ability.

Objective: The aims of this study were to develop two BI-based Supplementary Scales (BI-SS), namely, the Self-perceived Difficulty Scale and the Ability Scale, and to examine the construct validity of the BI-SS in patients with stroke.

Method: The BI-SS was first developed by consultation with experts and then tested on patients to confirm the clarity and feasibility of administration. A total of 306 participants participated in the construct validity study. Construct validity was investigated using Mokken scale analysis and analyzing associations between scales. The agreement between each pair of the scales' scores was further examined.

Results: The Self-perceived Difficulty Scale consisted of 10 items, and the Ability Scale included 8 items (excluding both bladder and bowel control items). Items in each individual scale were unidimensional ($H \geq 0.5$). The scores of the Self-perceived Difficulty and Ability Scales were highly correlated with those of the BI (rho = 0.78 and 0.90, respectively). The scores of the two BI-SS scales and BI were significantly different from each other (p<.001). These results indicate that both BI-SS scales assessed unique constructs.

Conclusions: The BI-SS had overall good construct validity in patients with stroke. The BI-SS can be used as supplementary scales for the BI to comprehensively assess patients' ADL functions in order to identify patients' difficulties in performing ADL tasks, plan intervention strategies, and assess outcomes.

Editor: Yiru Fang, Shanghai Mental Health Center, Shanghai Jiao Tong University School of Medicine, China

Funding: This study was supported by a research grant from the E-Da Hospital (EDAHT 101016), http://www.edah.org.tw/index.asp. The funders had no role in study design, data collection and analysis, decision to publish, or preparation of the manuscript.

Competing Interests: The authors have declared that no competing interests exist.

* Email: iping@ntu.edu.tw

Introduction

Stroke is the leading cause of disability or dependence in activities of daily living (ADL) among the elderly [1–3]. Increasing independence in ADL is often a central aim of stroke management. Assessing a patient's ADL functions enable clinicians to set reasonable treatment goals, to make appropriate discharge arrangements, and to anticipate the need for community support [2,4].Thus, ADL measures have been widely used for clinical decision making, treatment planning, and outcome measurement.

There are at least three different constructs for ADL measures: actual performance, self-perceived difficulty, and ability [5–9]. Each construct has unique characteristics and provides unique information for users. Actual performance refers to what a person actually does in his/her daily environment and is similar in concept to the qualifier of "performance" in the International Classification of Functioning, Disability and Health (ICF) [8,10–14]. Assessing actual performance can assist users in identifying an individual's level of dependence in ADL in real life situations [5,15]. Ability describes a person's ability to execute an ADL task in a standardized, controlled context and is similar in concept to the qualifier of "capacity" in the ICF [5,6,10,14]. Assessing ADL ability provides concrete/objective information about each ADL task that an individual is physically capable (or incapable) of doing [16]. Self-perceived difficulty defines the difficulty level that a person subjectively perceives when performing ADL without assistance in daily life [5,9,17]. Assessing self-perceived difficulty in performing ADL is useful in identifying an individual's need for assistance and is in line with a patient-centered approach, which recently has been strongly advocated [5,18].

Because the three ADL constructs differ in concept and clinical utility, assessing all three constructs simultaneously helps users comprehensively understand an individual's ADL functions. For example, a patient may be capable of going to the toilet by him/herself in a standardized context, but he/she might need assistance in his/her daily life because of the inaccessible condition (e.g., a narrow door to the bathroom) in his/her living environment. On the other hand, although the patient may not be able to do an ADL task in a standardized context, he/she may accomplish it at home through home modification or the use of assistive devices. In addition, patients might report difficulty in performing ADL in spite of being fully able and actually independent in real life. Thus, assessing the three ADL constructs simultaneously will improve the efficacy of stroke management and related research.

To our knowledge, no existing ADL measures assess all three ADL constructs simultaneously. Among the ADL measures, the Barthel Index (BI) has been widely used to assess stroke patients' actual performance on ADL functions in both clinical and research settings due to its ease of administration and sound psychometric properties [5,19–21]. Thus, the BI has been adopted by the British Geriatric Society and the Royal College of General Practitioners as the recommended scale for assessment of ADL [22]. However, the BI does not assess the other two constructs (i.e., self-perceived difficulty and ability). Thus, the purposes of this study were (1) to develop two supplementary scales (Self-perceived Difficulty Scale and Ability Scale) for the BI, the BI-based Supplementary Scales (BI-SS), in order to comprehensively assess ADL functions; and (2) to examine the construct validity of the BI-SS, which is critical for differentiating the three ADL constructs, in patients with stroke.

Methods

Phase 1: Development of the BI-SS

The development process had two stages:

Stage one: Consultation with experts to determine the response categories, modes of administration, and administrative instructions of the BI-SS. Two meetings of the expert panel were held in stage one. The panels consisted of 2 senior occupational therapists, 2 psychometricians, and 3 researchers in the field of occupational therapy. The main purpose of the first meeting was to decide response categories and modes of administration (e.g., face-to-face interview or performance observation) for the Self-perceived Difficulty Scale and the Ability Scale, respectively. The definitions of ADL constructs were explained and the 10 items of the BI were provided to the panel members to act as reference items for the Self-perceived Difficulty Scale and the Ability Scale. In the second meeting, the expert panel developed the standardized administrative instructions for each item of the BI-SS based on the modes of administration determined from the first meeting. In addition, the panel members determined whether any tools or materials would be needed for assessment. All 7 of the panel members attended and participated in these two meetings. It was considered that consensus was achieved when at least 80% of the panel members indicated agreement with a proposal.

Stage 2: A pilot test of the BI-SS in patients with stroke. A pilot test was conducted with the patients to examine the clarity of the administrative instructions and the feasibility of administration of the BI-SS. We tried to recruit participants having characteristics similar to those of the target patients. All procedures were carried out by the first author in an assessment room. Participants were individually tested and encouraged to identify any administrative instructions or response categories that seemed difficult to understand or ambiguous to them. The comments were reviewed and changes were made after 4 participants were tested. This process (testing and revisions) was repeated until no more substantial comments were made.

Phase 2: Examination of the construct validity of the BI-SS

Subjects. Patients undergoing outpatient or inpatient rehabilitation were recruited from 7 rehabilitation departments in Taiwan (including northern (4 hospitals), central (2 hospitals), and southern (1 hospital) parts of Taiwan) between January 2011 and August 2012.

Participants were included in the study if they met the following criteria: (1) diagnosis (*International Classification of Disease, Ninth Revision, Clinical Modification codes*) of cerebral hemorrhage (431), cerebral infarction (434), or other (430, 432, 433, 436, 437); and (2) ability to follow instructions. In addition, we excluded patients with any co-morbidity (e.g., dementia, Parkinsonism, limb amputation, or spinal cord injury) that might otherwise affect the patient's performance on ADL. All participants gave informed consent prior to their inclusion in the study. Demographic characteristics and information on co-morbidities were collected from their medical records.

Ethics statement. This study was approved by the Research Ethics Committee Office of E-DA Hospital and the Institutional Review Board of Kaohsiung Medical University Chung-Ho Memorial Hospital.

Procedure. Each participant was assessed with the BI-SS and BI once by one of the two trained raters in an assessment room. The BI was administered to the participants via face-to-face interview with the original scoring criteria [23].

Prior to the study, the raters (independent of the expert panel) familiarized themselves with the BI-SS and BI. Both raters studied the user manual of the BI-SS and BI and received 2 hours of training on the administration of the BI-SS and BI. At the end of the training, both raters individually administered the BI-SS and BI to two patients while the first author observed and scored the patients at the same time. The raters' scoring results were checked by the first author. Any discrepancies in score results were discussed to ensure that the raters were thoroughly familiar with the standardized process of administration and scoring criteria.

Data analysis. We validated the construct validity of the BI-SS by examining the unidimensionality and convergent validity of the BI-SS.

Unidimensionality. We examined the unidimensionality of each scale of the BI-SS individually using Mokken scale analysis with the MSP5.0 computer program [3]. Mokken scale analysis is a nonparametric item response theory (IRT). The model of monotone homogeneity (MH) of Mokken scale analysis examines the accuracy of ordering of between persons' raw sum scores on a measure to determine undimensionality [3,22]. The MH model of the Mokken scale was used because it is believed to exemplify the simplest form of unidimensionality [24,25]. Other parametric IRT models, such as the Rasch model, further require a parametric functional form of the item response function (IRF) [25,26]. However, with rigorous assumptions, the Rasch model tends to exclude items that do fit the unidimensionality assumption (e.g., the Mokken model's expectations) but not the parametric IRF form assumption. Thus, the Mokken model is likely to include more items from a pool of items in a scale while still holding the essential of unidimensionality [24].

The MH model has three assumptions: (1) items form a unidimensional scale (measuring the same construct; e.g., ADL ability); (2) item scores are locally independent (e.g., the scores on a given set of items are stochastically independent of each other within a group of persons with the same level of ADL ability); and (3) the item response function for each item is a steadily increasing function of the latent trait which means that patients with a higher level of ADL function would have a higher probability of scoring higher for an item that fits MH [24,27]. Given a set of items (e.g., 8 items of the Ability Scale) that satisfies the assumptions of the MH model, then unidimensionality will hold, and it is justified to sum the score of each items to create a total score to represent the construct of interest (e.g., ADL ability) [25,28].

The fit of the MH model was evaluated by calculating the scalability coefficient H for each of the individual items i (Hi) and for the entire measure (H). The Hi value was evaluated to determine whether an item was coherent enough to be included in a unidimensional scale. In general, all Hi in a unidimensional scale should be ≥ 0.3 [27]. Thus, we removed items from the BI-SS that had a Hi below 0.3. The H value is a global indicator of the degree to which participants can be accurately ordered on the underlying construct by means of their sum scores. Higher values of H indicate fewer violations of the assumption and a better scale [3,24,25]. Therefore, unidimensionality was considered to be strongly supported if $H \geq 0.5$ [3].

Convergent validity. Spearman's rho correlation coefficient was used to examine the association between the BI-SS and the BI to determine the convergent validity of the BI-SS. A rho value ≥ 0.75 was considered high, 0.40–0.74 moderate, and ≤ 0.39 low [29]. We expected that the three scales would have moderate to high associations with each other.

We further examined the agreement between each pair of scores of the three scales (i.e., BI and BI-SS) to confirm that they were distinguished scales. First, the Wilcoxon signed rank test was used to examine whether the scores of the three scales were significantly differently from each other. The Wilcoxon signed rank test is a nonparametric statistical hypothesis test used to investigate the difference between the magnitudes of paired (dependent) observations (i.e., the BI and BI-SS in this study) [30]. Second, the minimal important difference (MID; also known as the minimal clinically importance difference [31,32]) of the BI (i.e., 1.85 points) [33] was used as a threshold to present a meaningful difference in the responses of each participant between the scales. The proportions of the patients whose response differences between each pair of scales exceeded 1.85 points were calculated. To visualize the magnitude of response differences and the degree of agreement between scales, Bland-Altman plots with 95% limits of agreement (LOA) [34] were also plotted. The LOA provided insight into the amount of variation between scales. The agreement and variation of each patient's responses to each pair of the three scales could also be seen on the plot. The range of difference was largely defined by interval between the upper bound and the lower bound of the 95% LOA ($d \pm 1.96 \times SD$), where d represents the mean differences of the each pair of scores and SD represents the standard deviation of differences [34]. If a pair of scale assesses the same construct, then the pair of scores will agree very closely and the ranges of differences between both scales will be small. Third, we compared the numbers of patients with the lowest and highest scores in the BI against the two BI-SS scales.

Results

Phase 1: Development of the BI-SS

Stage one: Consultation with experts to determine the response categories, modes of administration, and administrative instructions of the BI-SS. Based on the results of expert panel discussions, each of the 10 items of the Self-perceived Difficulty Scale used 3 response categories ranging from 0 (with much difficulty), 1 (with some difficulty), and 2

(without any difficulty), with a total score of 20 (Appendix S1 in File S1). The higher the score, the lower the patient's self-perceived difficulty in performing ADL.

Regarding the mode of administration, the face-to-face interviews method was decided for the Self-perceived Difficulty Scale. Thus, the Self-perceived Difficulty Scale was administered by asking patients to respond to questions such as "How much difficulty do you have in performing grooming?" Because self-perceived difficulty is based on a patient's own perception, it will be valid only if the responses are from the patient him/herself.

Two items (bowel and bladder control) were removed from the Ability Scale due to their infeasibility and non-practicality to be assessed in clinical settings, leaving only eight items. The items of the Ability Scale had 3 or 4 response categories. For example, 'grooming' could be rated 0 (unable to perform), 1 (able to complete partially), or 2 (able to complete), while 'transferring' could be rated 0 (unable to perform), 1 (barely able to complete), 2 (almost able to complete), or 3 (able to complete) (Appendix S1 in File S1). The total score ranged from 0 to 18, with higher scores implying a higher level of ability to carry out the ADL. Further detailed instructions for scoring the Ability Scale can be found in Appendix S1 in File S1.

Regarding the mode of administration, observation-based testing was used for the Ability Scale. In addition, the panel members recommended that the Ability Scale be assessed in a standardized context (e.g., an assessment room without distractors such as physical obstacles or other people) to eliminate the varying impacts of different contexts on the performance of a patient. Furthermore, panel members decided on the tools/materials to be used for assessing the items of feeding, grooming, dressing, and bathing in the Ability Scale: chopsticks, spoons, a bowl, a brush, toothpaste, clothes, and towels. Thus, the Ability Scale was assessed by observing patients as they carried out a specific ADL task, such as "put the jacket on and zip it up". Then the rater rated the patient's level of ability in doing this task.

Stage two: A pilot test of the BI-SS in patients with stroke. A total of 12 patients participated in the stage two of pilot testing to confirm the administrative instructions and feasibility of the BI-SS. Three rounds of testing were carried out. In the first and second rounds of testing, patients gave comments on the ambiguous wordings of instructions for, e.g., the eating task with chopsticks and the dressing task. Thus, the revisions were made accordingly. In the third round of testing, no substantial changes were suggested. The final version of standardized administrative instructions for each item of the BI-SS was clear, and the modes of administration and response categories were understandable to the patients. Thus, no further testing was conducted. In addition, on the basis of the third round of testing, the time required to complete the BI-SS was about 15 minutes.

Phase 2: Examination of the construct validity of the BI-SS

A total of 306 participants participated in this study. Their mean age was about 61 (SD = 13.8) years, and 64.1% of the patients were male. Of these participants, 62.1% of stroke was caused by cerebral infarction. The scores of the BI ranged from 0 to 20 (i.e., the full possible score range), indicating that the participants had a wide range of ADL function. Further characteristics of the participants are shown in Table 1.

Table 2 summarizes the results of the evaluation of the Mokken scale analysis for the BI-SS. The scalability coefficients Hi for the items in relation to each individual scale were all above 0.3 (ranging from 0.49 to 0.82). In addition, scalability coefficients H of the 10 items of the Self-perceived Difficulty Scale and 8 items of

Table 1. Characteristics of the participants (n = 306).

Characteristic	
Gender (male/female) (%)	196/110 (64.1%/35.9%)
Age, mean (SD)	61.82 (13.8)
Days after onset, median (1st quartile – 3rd quartile)	77.5 (28–416)
Diagnosis, n	
Cerebral hemorrhage (%)	116 (37.9%)
Cerebral infarction (%)	190 (62.1%)
Side of hemiplegia, n	
Right	176
Left	120
Bilateral	10
BI score, median (1st quartile – 3rd quartile)	13.0 (8–17)
Self-perceived Scale score, median (1st quartile – 3rd quartile)	12.0 (7–17)
Ability Scale score, median (1st quartile – 3rd quartile)	12.5 (8–16)

the Ability Scale were greater than 0.5 ($H \geq 0.63$), strongly supporting the unidimensionality of the items of each scale.

Figures 1, 2, and 3 show association and agreement between scores of the three scales. The BI was highly correlated with the Self-perceived Difficulty Scale (rho = 0.78) and the Ability Scale (rho = 0.90), respectively. The Self-perceived Difficulty Scale was highly correlated with the Ability Scale (rho = 0.75).

In order to further compare the three scales, the scores of the Ability Scale were linearly transformed into the same score ranges as those of the other two scales (0–20). First, the Wilcoxon signed rank test showed that the scores of the three scales were significantly different from each other (p<.001) (Table 3). Second, the proportion of the patients whose difference between two scales was beyond 1.85 points (MID) were 60.1% for the BI and Self-perceived Difficulty Scale, 41.8% for the BI and Ability Scale, and 61.4% for the Self-perceived Difficulty Scale and Ability Scale. The ranges of differences between each pair of the three scales are shown in the Bland-Altman plots (Figs. 1, 2, 3). The width of LOA was 15.1 for the BI and Self-perceived Difficulty Scale (75.5% of

the maximal score range, 20), 9.7 for the BI and Ability Scale (48.5% of the maximal score range, 20), and 15.9 for the Self-perceived Difficulty Scale and Ability Scale (79.5% of the maximal score range, 20).

Third, to further present the differences in the patients' scores on the three scales, we compared the numbers of patients who obtained extreme scores on these scales. A total of 17 patients scored 0 (with much difficulty) on the Self-perceived Difficulty Scale, but more than half (n = 9) of these 17 patients obtained total scores >0 on the BI. Twenty-one patients scored 20 (without any difficulty) on the Self-perceived Difficulty Scale, but nearly half (n = 10) of these 21 patients obtained total scores <20 on the BI. A total of 32 patients scored the highest possible score on the Ability Scale, but about 60% (n = 19) of these 32 patients did not obtain the highest possible score on the BI. A total of 4 patients scored the lowest possible score on the Ability Scale, but 75% (n = 3) of these patients did not obtain the lowest possible score on the Self-perceived Difficulty Scale.

Table 2. Results of Mokken scale analysis on the items of the BI-SS (n = 306).

Item		Self-perceived Difficulty Scale	Ability Scale
		Hi	Hi
1	Feeding	0.49	0.59
2	Grooming	0.55	0.61
3	Dressing	0.67	0.69
4	Bathing	0.64	0.71
5	Bowels	0.68	-
6	Bladder	0.62	-
7	Toilet use	0.71	0.82
8	Transfer	0.66	0.80
9	Mobility	0.63	0.76
10	Stairs	0.62	0.79
Scale H		0.63	0.75

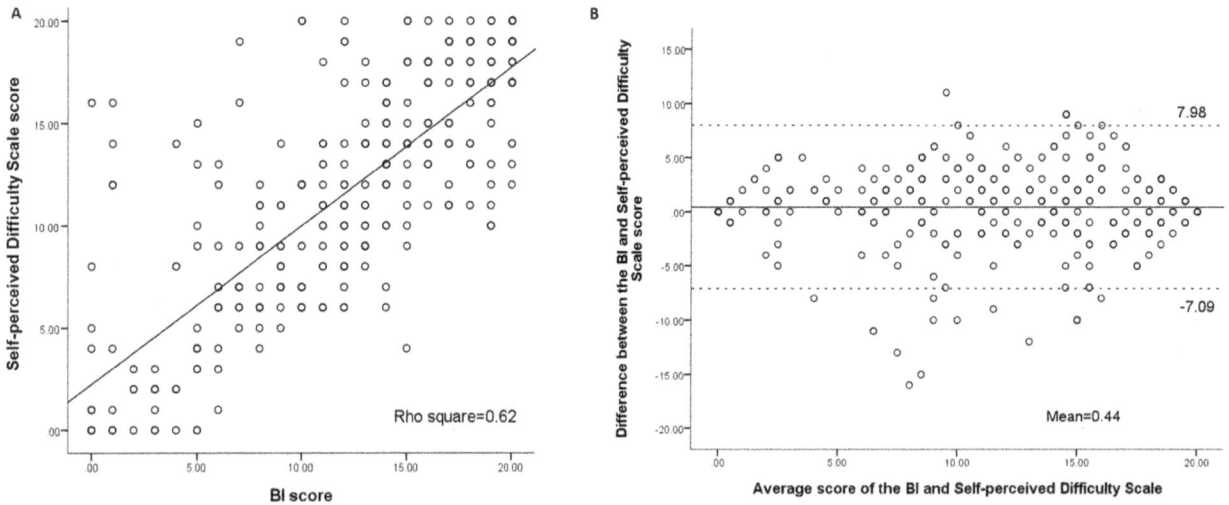

Figure 1. Correlation (A) and Bland-Altman plot (B) for the BI and Self-perceived Difficulty Scale. Bland-Altman method for plotting the scores of the difference between the BI and Self-perceived Difficulty Scale. The 2 dashed lines define the limits of agreement (mean of difference ±1.96 SD).

Discussion

The aim of this study was to develop a supplementary measure based on the original BI, the BI-SS, in order to comprehensively assess ADL functions. Analyzed with the MH model of Mokken scale analysis, our results showed that the unidimensionality of the two ADL construct scales were strong ($H \geq 0.63$). The results indicated that the 10 items of the Self-perceived Difficulty Scale assessed a single dimension, as did the 8 items of the Ability Scale. Because the items of each scale of BI-SS assessed the same dimension, the results supported summating the raw score of each item in each individual scale to create a total score for their respective scales to represent patients' level of function on self-perceived difficulty and ability.

We used the original BI as a criterion to examine the convergent validity of both the Self-perceived Difficulty Scale and the Ability Scale. Our results showed a high degree of correlation between the original BI and the two scales (rho = 0.78 and 0.90, respectively),

indicating that both constructs measured by the BI-SS, self-perceived difficulty and ability, were highly related to the actual performance construct in patients with stroke. The results confirm our hypotheses and support the convergent validity of the BI-SS in patients with stroke. Combining the results of sufficient unidimensionality and convergent validity of the BI-SS, the construct validity of the BI-SS is highly supported.

Although the associations between any pairs of the three scales were high, the other results showed that the three scales were different from each other. First, the unexplained variance between the scales was substantial (i.e., 19.1% unexplained variance existing between the BI and Ability Scale, 38% between the BI and Self-perceived Difficulty Scale, and 43.8% between the Self-perceived Difficulty Scale and Ability Scale). Second, the range of disagreement between scales was widely distributed. The LOAs revealed large variations between scales. Particularly, about half (41.861.4%) of the patients had important differences (>1.85) between scales. Third, about half to three quarters (47.675.0%) of

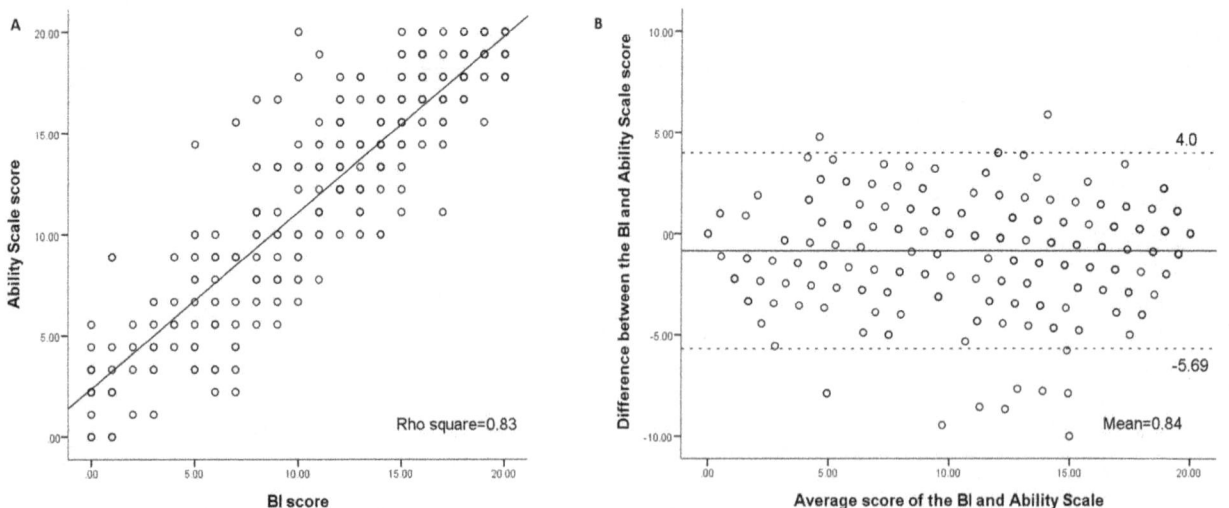

Figure 2. Correlation (A) and Bland-Altman plot (B) for the BI and Ability Scale. The Ability Scale scores were 0●20 transformed scores.

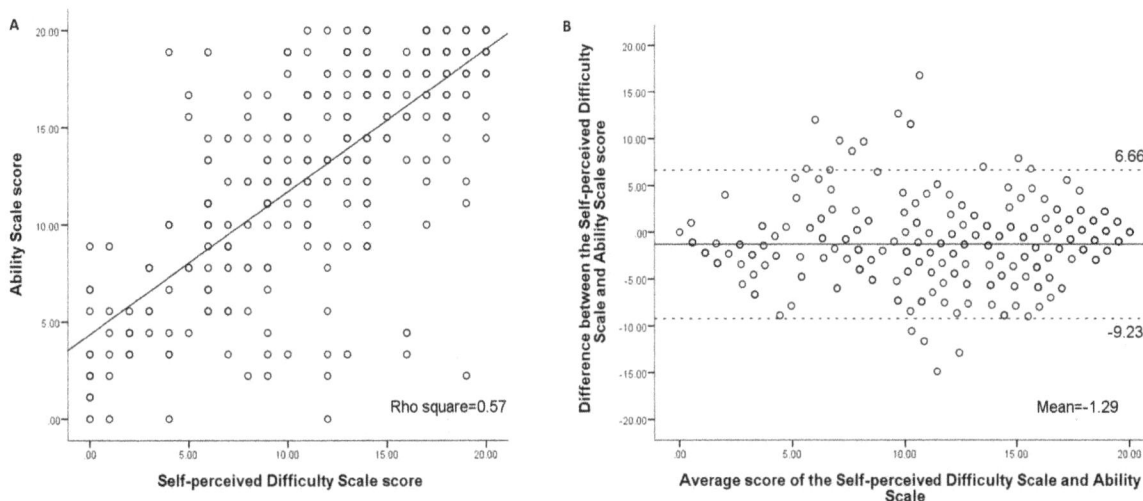

Figure 3. Correlation (A) and Bland-Altman plot (B) for the Self-perceived Difficulty Scale and Ability Scale. The Ability Scale scores were 0●20 transformed scores.

the patients who obtained extreme scores (either the highest score or the lowest score) on one scale did not obtain extreme scores on the other scale. Last, based on the aforementioned definitions, theoretically, each of the three ADL constructs has unique characteristics and has its own value and meaning, thus making each irreplaceable [8,10,13,18,35,36].Our results indicate that the three scales assess three unique constructs, which should be distinguished in clinical practice and research [13].

Mode of administration can have a substantial effect on the results of ADL assessments [5,37]. The BI assesses patients' actual performance in real life and is commonly assessed through face-to-face interview, which is easy and fast to administer [38]. However, self-reports by the patient and/or the patient's primary caregiver might overestimate or underestimate the patient's actual performance, and thus may affect the results of ADL assessment [5,39]. In such cases, it is important to measure patients' ADL function along with an objective measure (i.e., the Ability scale) to provide concrete information about what the patient can and cannot do on the tasks. Although the face-to-face interview has its own weakness, it is useful for assessing subjective feelings of difficulty (i.e., what the Self-perceived Difficulty Scale assesses) in performing ADL, as the level of difficulty is known only to the patient him/herself [10,40]. The effects of modes of administration may affect the results of the ADL assessments; thus, it is important to

use the most appropriate mode of administration to assess each construct of ADL [5].

The BI-SS is concise and quick to administer. The Self-perceived Difficulty Scale consisted of 10 items, and the Ability Scale contained only 8 items. The total time for completing both scales was appropriately 15 minutes. A short and quick-to-complete measure can lessen burdens on patients and clinicians, which is an especially important consideration for patients having severe disability. Therefore, the BI-SS appears useful in improving practice and enhancing the efficiency of administration.

It is strongly suggested that the BI-SS, which adopted the items from the original BI, be used in conjunction with the original BI to facilitate comparison and comprehensively obtain every aspect of patients' ADL functions. The Stroke Impact Scale-16 and the Physical Self-Maintenance Scale assess the constructs of self-perceived difficulty and ability, respectively [30,41,42]. However, it is ideal to use the same items to assess a patient's actual performance along with self-perceived difficulty and ability because this makes comparison of these three ADL functions of patients much more straightforward [8]. The resulting information could be useful for clinical reasoning and patient management, which may result in better treatment outcomes. In addition, using the BI-SS and the BI together can provide comprehensive (including different aspects of ADL functions) information that is useful for researchers in examining the impacts of stroke.

Table 3. The results of the agreement between the paired scales and the numbers of participants whose difference between 2 scales was beyond 1.85 points.

	Mean difference	Wilcoxon Z (p-value)	Number of participants with difference between 2 scales beyond 1.85 points (%)
BI score vs. Self-perceived Difficulty Scale score	0.44	−3.6 (<.001)	184 (60.1%)
BI score vs. Ability Scale score	−0.84	−5.3 (<.001)	128 (41.8%)
Self-perceived Difficulty Scale score vs. Ability Scale score	−1.29	−6.6 (<.001)	188 (61.4%)

The subjective feeling of difficulty in performing ADL might vary substantially between persons of different ethnicities. In addition, the tools/materials used for assessing the items of feeding, grooming, dressing, and bathing in the Ability Scale may be culture-specific. Particularly, chopsticks are the most common eating utensil in Taiwan and other Asian countries. However, chopsticks are less commonly used in North America and Europe. Thus, there is a need to cross-validate our results and use culture-specific items for different countries.

Three limitations of this study are addressed. First, we excluded patients with stroke who had cognitive impairment. It was determined that patients with cognitive impairment could not report their perceived difficulty on performing ADL and could not understand instructions to perform ADL. In addition, we also excluded patients with stroke who had co-morbidities such as dementia, Parkinsonism, limb amputation, or spinal cord injury. Thus, caution should be exercised in generalizing our findings to all stroke populations. Second, the reliability between raters has not yet been established, which may jeopardize our current validation of the BI-SS. Future studies are needed to examine the reliability of the BI-SS in patients with stroke. Third, the MID of the BI (i.e., 1.85 points) was used to act as a threshold to determine whether the patients' difference on the BI-SS had reached the MID. However, the cutoff value for the BI-SS may be different from that of the BI. The current results might be confounded by using the 1.85 cutoff as a marker for the difference in scores.

Future studies to estimate the MID of the BI-SS are needed to further validate our results.

Conclusion

The BI-SS was developed from the BI as supplementary scales in order to comprehensively assess ADL functions. The BI-SS had overall good construct validity in patients with stroke. The BI-SS could be a useful tool for assessing patients' ADL functions and identifying patients' difficulties in performing ADL tasks, planning intervention strategies, and assessing outcomes.

Supporting Information

File S1 Appendices. Appendix S1. Items and response categories of the Barthel Index (BI) and the BI-based Supplementary Scales (BI-SS). Appendix S2. A comparison of the ADL construct and characteristics of the Barthel Index, Self-perceived Difficulty Scale, and Ability Scale.

Author Contributions

Conceived and designed the experiments: IPH CLH. Performed the experiments: YCL SSC. Analyzed the data: YCL CLK KPY. Contributed reagents/materials/analysis tools: IPH CLH. Contributed to the writing of the manuscript: YCL CLK IPH CLH.

References

1. Williams LS, Weinberger M, Harris LE, Clark DO, Biller J (1999) Development of a stroke-specific quality of life scale. Stroke 30: 1362–1369.
2. Hsieh CL, Sheu CF, Hsueh IP, Wang CH (2002) Trunk control as an early predictor of comprehensive activities of daily living function in stroke patients. Stroke 33: 2626–2630.
3. Sijtsma K, Emons WH, Bouwmeester S, Nyklicek I, Roorda LD (2008) Nonparametric IRT analysis of Quality-of-Life Scales and its application to the World Health Organization Quality-of-Life Scale (WHOQOL-Bref). Qual Life Res 17: 275–290.
4. Kwakkel G, Wagenaar RC, Kollen BJ, Lankhorst GJ (1996) Predicting disability in stroke–a critical review of the literature. Age Ageing 25: 479–489.
5. Hsieh CL, Hoffmann T, Gustafsson L, Lee YC (2012) The diverse constructs use of activities of daily living measures in stroke randomized controlled trials in the years 2005–2009. J Rehabil Med 44: 720–726.
6. Wade DT, Collin C (1988) The Barthel ADL Index: a standard measure of physical disability. Int Disabil Stud 10: 64–67.
7. Jette AM (1994) Physical disablement concepts for physical therapy research and practice. Phys Ther 74: 380–386.
8. Holsbeeke L, Ketelaar M, Schoemaker MM, Gorter JW (2009) Capacity, capability, and performance: different constructs or three of a kind? Arch Phys Med Rehabil 90: 849–855.
9. Ostir GV, Volpato S, Kasper JD, Ferrucci L, Guralnik JM (2001) Summarizing amount of difficulty in ADLs: a refined characterization of disability. Results from the women's health and aging study. Aging (Milano) 13: 465–472.
10. Michielsen ME, de Niet M, Ribbers GM, Stam HJ, Bussmann JB (2009) Evidence of a logarithmic relationship between motor capacity and actual performance in daily life of the paretic arm following stroke. J Rehabil Med 41: 327–331.
11. Smith DS, Clark MS (1995) Competence and performance in activities of daily living of patients following rehabilitation from stroke. Disabil Rehabil 17: 15–23.
12. Barkat-Masih M, Saha C, Golomb MR (2011) ASKing the kids: how children view their abilities after perinatal stroke. J Child Neurol 26: 44–48.
13. Young NL, Williams JI, Yoshida KK, Bombardier C, Wright JG (1996) The context of measuring disability: does it matter whether capability or performance is measured? J Clin Epidemiol 49: 1097–1101.
14. WHO (2001) International classification of functioning, disability and health: ICF. Geneva: World Health Organization.
15. Wade DT (1992) Measurement in neurological rehabilitation. Oxford, UK: Oxford University Press.
16. Thoren-Jonsson AL, Grimby G (2001) Ability and perceived difficulty in daily activities in people with poliomyelitis sequelae. J Rehabil Med 33: 4–11.
17. Verbrugge LM, Jette AM (1994) The disablement process. Soc Sci Med 38: 1–14.
18. Grimby G, Andren E, Daving Y, Wright B (1998) Dependence and perceived difficulty in daily activities in community-living stroke survivors 2 years after stroke: a study of instrumental structures. Stroke 29: 1843–1849.

19. Hsueh IP, Lee MM, Hsieh CL (2001) Psychometric characteristics of the Barthel activities of daily living index in stroke patients. J Formos Med Assoc 100: 526–532.
20. Quinn TJ, Langhorne P, Stott DJ (2011) Barthel index for stroke trials: development, properties, and application. Stroke 42: 1146–1151.
21. Sangha H, Lipson D, Foley N, Salter K, Bhogal S, et al. (2005) A comparison of the Barthel Index and the Functional Independence Measure as outcome measures in stroke rehabilitation: patterns of disability scale usage in clinical trials. International Journal of Rehabilitation Research 28: 135–139.
22. Chen HC, Koh CL, Hsieh CL, Hsueh IP (2009) Test-re-test reliability of two sustained attention tests in persons with chronic stroke. Brain Inj 23: 715–722.
23. Collin C, Wade DT, Davies S, Horne V (1988) The Barthel ADL Index: a reliability study. Int Disabil Stud 10: 61–63.
24. van der Heijden PG, van Buuren S, Fekkes M, Radder J, Verrips E (2003) Unidimensionality and reliability under Mokken scaling of the Dutch language version of the SF-36. Qual Life Res 12: 189–198.
25. Koh CL, Hsueh IP, Wang WC, Sheu CF, Yu TY, et al. (2006) Validation of the action research arm test using item response theory in patients after stroke. J Rehabil Med 38: 375–380.
26. Yu WH, Chen KL, Chou YT, Hsueh IP, Hsieh CL (2013) Responsiveness and predictive validity of the hierarchical balance short forms in people with stroke. Phys Ther 93: 798–808.
27. van der Ark LA (2012) New developments in Mokken scale analysis in R. J Stat Softw 48: 1–27.
28. Stochl J, Jones PB, Croudace TJ (2012) Mokken scale analysis of mental health and well-being questionnaire item responses: a non-parametric IRT method in empirical research for applied health researchers. BMC Med Res Methodol 12: 74.
29. Salter K, Jutai JW, Teasell R, Foley NC, Bitensky J, et al. (2005) Issues for selection of outcome measures in stroke rehabilitation: ICF Participation. Disability & Rehabilitation 27: 507–528.
30. Lawton MP, Brody EM (1969) Assessment of older people: self-maintaining and instrumental activities of daily living. Gerontologist 9: 179–186.
31. Jaeschke R, Singer J, Guyatt GH (1989) Measurement of health status. Ascertaining the minimal clinically important difference. Control Clin Trials 10: 407–415.
32. Schunemann HJ, Guyatt GH (2005) Commentary–goodbye M(C)ID! Hello MID, where do you come from? Health Serv Res 40: 593–597.
33. Hsieh YW, Wang CH, Wu SC, Chen PC, Sheu CF, et al. (2007) Establishing the minimal clinically important difference of the Barthel Index in stroke patients. Neurorehabil Neural Repair 21: 233–238.
34. Bland JM, Altman DG (1986) Statistical methods for assessing agreement between two methods of clinical measurement. Lancet 1: 307–310.
35. Laditka SB, Jenkins CL (2001) Difficulty or dependency? Effects of measurement scales on disability prevalence among older Americans. J Health Soc Policy 13: 1–15.

36. Gill TM, Robison JT, Tinetti ME (1998) Difficulty and dependence: two components of the disability continuum among community-living older persons. Ann Intern Med 128: 96–101.

37. Sinoff G, Ore L (1997) The Barthel activities of daily living index: self-reporting versus actual performance in the old-old (> or = 75 years). J Am Geriatr Soc 45: 832–836.

38. Owens PL, Bradley EH, Horwitz SM, Viscoli CM, Kernan WN, et al. (2002) Clinical assessment of function among women with a recent cerebrovascular event: a self-reported versus performance-based measure. Ann Intern Med 136: 802–811.

39. Wilson R, Derrett S, Hansen P, Langley J (2012) Retrospective evaluation versus population norms for the measurement of baseline health status. Health Qual Life Outcomes 10: 68.

40. Lee YC, Chen YM, Hsueh IP, Wang YH, Hsieh CL (2010) The impact of stroke: insights from patients in Taiwan. Occup Ther Int 17: 152–158.

41. Flansbjer UB, Holmback AM, Downham D, Patten C, Lexell J (2005) Reliability of gait performance tests in men and women with hemiparesis after stroke. J Rehabil Med 37: 75–82.

42. Chang HY, Hsieh YW, Hsueh IP, Hsieh CL (2006) A forty-year retrospective of assessment of activities of daily living. Tw J Phys Med Rehabil 34: 63–71.

20

Rhinitis, Asthma and Respiratory Infections among Adults in Relation to the Home Environment in Multi-Family Buildings in Sweden

Juan Wang*, Karin Engvall, Greta Smedje, Dan Norbäck

Department of Medical Sciences, Uppsala University and University Hospital, Uppsala, Sweden

Abstract

Risk factors for rhinitis, asthma and respiratory infections in the home environment were studied by a questionnaire survey. Totally 5775 occupants ($\geq$18 years old) from a stratified random sample of multi-family buildings in Sweden participated (46%). 51.0% had rhinitis in the last 3 months (current rhinitis); 11.5% doctor diagnosed asthma; 46.4% respiratory infections in the last 3 months and 11.9% antibiotic medication for respiratory infections in the last 12 months. Associations between home environment and health were analyzed by multiple logistic regression, controlling for gender, age and smoking and mutual adjustment. Buildings constructed during 1960–1975 were risk factors for day time breathlessness (OR = 1.53, 95%CI 1.03–2.29). And those constructed during 1976–1985 had more current rhinitis (OR = 1.43, 95%CI 1.12–1.84) and respiratory infections (OR = 1.46, 95%CI 1.21–1.78). Cities with higher population density had more current rhinitis (p = 0.008) and respiratory infections (p<0.001). Rented apartments had more current rhinitis (OR = 1.23, 95%CI 1.07–1.40), wheeze (OR = 1.20, 95%CI 1.02–1.41), day time breathlessness (OR = 1.31, 95%CI 1.04–1.66) and respiratory infections (OR = 1.13, 95%CI 1.01–1.26). Living in colder parts of the country was a risk factor for wheeze (p = 0.03) and night time breathlessness (p = 0.002). Building dampness was a risk factor for wheeze (OR = 1.42, 95%CI 1.08–1.86) and day time breathlessness (OR = 1.57, 95%CI 1.09–2.27). Building dampness was a risk factor for health among those below 66 years old. Odor at home was a risk factor for doctor diagnosed asthma (OR = 1.49, 95%CI 1.08–2.06) and current asthma (OR = 1.52, 95%CI 1.03–2.24). Environmental tobacco smoke (ETS) was a risk factor for current asthma (OR = 1.53, 95%CI 1.09–2.16). Window pane condensation was a risk factor for antibiotic medication for respiratory infections (OR = 1.41, 95%CI 1.10–1.82). In conclusion, rhinitis, asthma and respiratory infections were related to a number of factors in the home environment. Certain building years (1961–1985), building dampness, window pane condensation and odor in the dwelling may be risk factors.

Editor: Oliver Schildgen, Kliniken der Stadt Köln gGmbH, Germany

Funding: The Swedish Research Council Formas supported the study through contract no. 244-2011-222. The funders had no role in study design, data collection and analysis, decision to publish, or preparation of the manuscript.

Competing Interests: The authors have declared that no competing interests exist.

* Email: juan.wang@medsci.uu.se

Introduction

Concern about possible health effects of indoor air pollution has been increasing especially with respects to allergies and asthma. The dwelling is an important indoor environment, since it is where we spend most time, usually 15–16 h per day [1].

Rhinitis can be divided into allergic rhinitis (AR) and non-allergic rhinitis (NAR). AR occurs when an allergen is the trigger for the nasal symptoms. NAR is when obstruction and rhinorrhea occurs in relation to non-allergic, noninfectious triggers, such as changes in the weather, cigarette smoke, etc [2]. Approximately 10%–25% of the world population is affected by AR [3]. The worldwide prevalence of allergic rhinitis among adults has been on the rise since at least 1990 [4–8]. In Sweden, the prevalence of AR increased from 22% to 31% from 1990 to 2008 in young adults [7]. However, less information is available on the prevalence or incidence of NAR. Generally, females [9,10], young adults [10–12], and those with allergic heredity [13,14] are at higher risk of having AR. Allergen sources in the home environment are

common, such as from pets [15], cockroaches [12,14], house dust mites, microbiologic agents [16,17], etc. Signs of dampness and indoor molds is another common exposure that has been widely studied in relation to both AR and NAR in home [17–19]. Other factors such as traffic-related air pollution, different lifestyle and socioeconomic conditions are quoted as adjuvant factors for AR [20].

Asthma is the most common chronic respiratory disease in the world. Approximately 300 million people in the world currently have asthma [21]. Epidemiological studies have suggested that the prevalence of asthma in adults is approximately 7–10% in different parts of the western world [22]. The current trend (since 1990's) in the prevalence of asthma among adults is unclear, some studies suggesting that asthma prevalence has stabilized or even decreased [5,7,22], while, others suggesting it is still increasing [4]. However, asthma prevalence among children in many parts of the world is still increasing [23]. Asthma frequently co-exist with rhinitis [3,24–26]. Adult asthma is more common among females [27–29], younger adults [27], and those with allergic heredity [27,29].

Smoking [30,31] and environmental tobacco smoke (ETS) [29,32–34] were found to be associated with asthma or asthma related symptoms. A common finding is the association between observed building dampness and molds and adults' asthma [35]. Exposures related to building dampness can be house dust mites, molds, bacteria, and even chemicals (from the degradation process of building materials). Studies has shown that adults' asthma or asthmatic symptoms were associated with higher levels of cockroach allergen [36], mouse allergen [36], house dust mites [37], fungal [38], airborne bacteria [37], formaldehyde [39,40] and total volatile organic compounds (VOC) [39,40] in dwellings, newly painted indoor surfaces [41], and combustion of wood, coal or biomass fuels [34].

Respiratory infections include infections of the lower and upper respiratory tract, and otitis media [42]. Preventive strategies include attempting to avoid contact with or spreading of infectious agents and covering sneezes and vaccination for influenza and pneumococcal pneumonia [42]. The presence of building dampness and molds are associated with increase in respiratory infections in adults [19,35,42,43]. Air movements in buildings and ventilation are essential for the transmission/spread of infectious diseases. There is some evidence of spread of infections by airborne transmission, such as measles, tuberculosis, chickenpox, influenza, smallpox and severe acute respiratory syndrome (SARS) [44]. There is however insufficient data to specify the minimum ventilation requirements to avoid the spread of infectious diseases via the airborne route [44,45].

The aging population is an important issue in many countries [46]. A better understanding of the health consequences of exposure to different risk factors among elderly, notably to environmental factors, is needed. There are only few studies investigating the influence of environment factors among respiratory health in the elderly [47,48]. Exposure to elevated levels of outdoor air pollution such as particle matter (PM), ozone (O_3), nitrogen dioxide (NO_2) and sulphur dioxide (SO_2) were associated with increased hospital admissions for asthma and chronic obstructive pulmonary disease (COPD) [47]. For indoor environment, the most consistent association was found between increased risk of COPD and exposure to ETS [48].

The first aim of this study was to investigate the prevalence of rhinitis, asthma and respiratory infections among occupants living in multi-family buildings in Sweden. The second of aim was to study occupants' health symptoms in relation to their home environment. The third aim was to study if there is any difference of these associations in relation to occupants' age (comparing those less than or equal to 65 years old with those more than 65 years old).

Material and Methods

Ethics Statement

The study and the consent procedure were approved by the Regional Ethical Committee in Uppsala, Sweden. All participants gave informed consent. An information letter sent together with the questionnaire stated that if the subjects answered and returned the questionnaire it meant they had given informed consent.

Selection of Buildings

The selection of multi-family buildings was performed by Statistics Sweden (SCB) [49]. The buildings were selected by a multi-stage sampling procedure with a first step to select 30 Swedish municipalities out of totally 290 municipalities across Sweden through a stratified random selection according to geographic and demographic characteristics (temperature zone and region), and degree of urbanization. The probability for a municipality to be selected was proportional to the size of the population of the municipality in December 31, 2006. The next step was selection of multi-family buildings from these 30 municipalities. Data on all multi-family buildings and their construction year were obtained from the central building register in Sweden. Stratified random sampling was used to sample buildings based on the construction year in 5 classes (before 1960, 1960–1975, 1976–1985, 1986–1995 and 1996–2005) aiming to get the same number of buildings in each age class. Since most buildings in Sweden are old, there was an over-sampling of new buildings in this study. Totally 690 multi-family buildings were sampled from the 30 municipalities.

Questionnaire and study population

The study population consisted of all adults (≥18 years old) living in the multi-family buildings included in the study. There were totally 8841 apartments and 12488 adults. The questionnaires were developed at Department of Medical Science, Uppsala University, based on previous studies [7,27,50–53]. The number of adults living in each apartment was identified by SCB from the Swedish civil registration register. Each adult (≥18 years) registered in the selected apartments received a personal questionnaire including medicine questions and personal factors. Moreover, one indoor environment questionnaire was sent to each apartment. The postal questionnaire was administered by SCB during the spring 2008. Two reminders were sent to those who did not reply the first time. Totally, 5775 adults participated in the study and returned the medical questionnaire (46%) and 4369 indoor environment questionnaires (49%) were returned.

Environmental questions

The home environment questionnaire included the following questions:

(1) Number of persons living at home;

(2) Ownership of the apartment (own/rented);

(3) Type of ventilation system (mechanical ventilation system/ only natural ventilation);

(4) Current pet-keeping status in the apartment: dog (no/yes); cat (no/yes);

(5) Whether anybody living in the apartment ride a horse or has in another way contact with horses (no/yes);

(6) Current environmental tobacco smoke at home (ETS) (no, if the answer is "never"/yes, if the answer is "daily", "weekly" or "monthly");

(7) Condensation on window panes in winter (no, if the answer is "never"/yes, if the answer is "less than 5 cm", "5–25 cm" or "more than 25 cm");

(8) New indoor painting in the last 12 months (no/yes);

(9) New floor materials in the last 12 months (no/yes);

(10) Any water leakage in the last 12 months (no/yes);

(11) Any floor dampness in the last 12 months (no/yes);

(12) Any visible molds in the last 12 months (no/yes);

(13) Any moldy odor in the last 12 months (no/yes);

(14) Any other odor in the last 12 months (no/yes);

(15) Any damp spot, visible mold or water leakage in the last 5 years (no/yes);

(16) Any technical building investigation of the apartment by a consulting company because of dampness, water damage or mold (no/yes);

One new variable "dampness in the last 12 months" was created based on four questions (which are question (10) – (13)) among all the 16 questions above, named as question (17). The options for this variable are: no, if the answers for the four questions are all "no"; yes, if the answer of any of the four question is "yes".

A dampness index was created based on question (15) and (17), which coded as: 0, both answers are "no"; 1, only one of the answers is "no"; 2, both answers are "yes".

A window-opening index was created based on two questions about window opening habit as follows: a) How often do you usually air the apartment by opening the windows during heating season (from September to April)? There are four options: daily, weekly, monthly and never, which were coded as 1, 2, 3 and 4; b) if you do, how long time? There are four options: the whole day/night, few hours, have cross-draught for a few minutes and never, which were coded as 1, 2, 3 and 4. The window-opening index was coded as: 0, if b) = 4; 1, if a) = 3 and b) = 3; 2, if a) = 2 and b) = 3, or a) = 3 and b = 2, or a) = 1 b) = 3; 3, if a) = 2 and b) = 2; or if a) = 3 and b) = 1, or a) = 2 and b) = 1; 4, if a) = 1 and b) = 2; 5, if a) = 1 and b) = 1. A higher window-opening index indicate more window opening.

Data about construction year of buildings were collected from the National Building Register, Real Property Register and were categorized into 5 groups (-1960/1961–1975/1976–1985/1986–1995/1996–2005). Data about population and area of each municipality were acquired from wikipedia website (http://sv.wikipedia.org/wiki/Lista_%C3%B6ver_Sveriges_kommuner). Population density (number of persons per km^2) were calculated based on population and area of each municipality. Data about temperature zone were collected from a Swedish government report [54], which has 4 catagories: 1, inner part of north Sweden (Norrland); 2, costal part of Norrland and some inner part of Svealand; 3, Svealand (main parts); 4, Göteland (main parts). A higher number indicate a warmer climate.

Personal questions

Medical questions in the personal questionnaire included the following:

(1) Gender (female/male);

(2) Age;

(3) Current rhinitis (Irritating, stuffy or runny nose in the last 3 months). There were three options: often (every week), sometimes, never;

(4) Any wheezing in the chest in the last 12 months (no/yes);

(5) Any daytime attack of time breathlessness at rest in the last 12 months (no/yes);

(6) Any daytime attack of time breathlessness after exercise in the last 12 months (no/yes);

(7) Woken by attack of time breathlessness at any time in the last 12 months (no/yes);

(8) Diagnosed with asthma by a doctor (no/yes);

(9) Asthma attack during the last 12 months (no/yes);

(10) Current asthma medication (no/yes);

(11) Number of respiratory infections (such as cold, throat infection or flu) in the last 3 months (no/yes)? The options were: never (no); 1 time and 2 or more times (yes);

(12) Antibiotic medication because of respiratory infections during the last 12 months (no/yes);

(13) Pollen allergy (no/yes);

(14) Furry pet allergy (no/yes).

The variable daytime breathlessness was created from question (5) and (6) coded as "no" if the answers to both questions is "no", and "yes" if any one of the answers is "yes".

Current asthma was created from question (9) and (10) coded as "no" if the answers to both questions is "no", and "yes" if any one of the answers is "yes".

The variable pollen or furry pet allergy was created from question (13) and (14) coded as "no" if the answers to both questions is "no", and "yes" if any one of the answers is "yes".

The rhinitis variable was further classified into 4 categories: no rhinitis, infection rhinitis, allergic rhinitis and non-allergic rhinitis. Infection rhinitis was defined as having both current rhinitis and any respiratory infections in the last 3 months. Allergic rhinitis was defined as having current rhinitis and pollen of furry pet allergy, but no respiratory infections. Non-allergic rhinitis was defined as having current rhinitis, but no pollen or furry pet allergy and no respiratory infections.

Statistical analysis

All statistical analyses were conducted with STATA 11.0 (STATA Corp, Texas, USA). The prevalence of symptoms and exposures were calculated for total subjects and age stratified groups. Ordinal regression models were used to study associations between current rhinitis, respiratory infections and home environment factors with adjustment for gender, age and current smoking. In the ordinal logistic regression OR is expressed for one step on the scale of the dependent variable. Mutual adjustment were then applied including all significant or nearly significant factors (p<0.1) with additional adjustment for gender, age and current smoking. As a next step, associations between different types of rhinitis symptoms and home environment factors were calculated by multi-nominal regression models with adjustment for gender, age and current smoking.

Multiple logistic regression was used to study associations between wheeze, day time breathlessness, night time breathlessness, doctor-diagnosed asthma, current asthma, respiratory infections and antibiotic medication for respiratory infections and home environment factors with adjustment for gender, age and smoking. Mutual adjustment were then applied including all significant or nearly significant factors (p<0.1) with additional adjustment for gender, age and current smoking.

In addition, sensitivity analyses were performed, by stratifying for age (≤65 years v.s >65 years old (elderly)).

Age interaction was studied in the mutual adjusted models (≤65 years old v.s elderly). Interaction was tested statistically if there were a marked numerical difference in OR when comparing the occupational active age group with elderly.

Associations were expressed as odds ratios (OR) with a 95% confidence interval (CI) for ordinal regression and logistic regression models. For multi-nominal regression models, associations were expressed as relative risk ratio (RRR) with a 95% confidence interval (CI). In all statistical analysis, two-tailed tests and a 5% level of significance were applied.

Results

Totally, 5775 personal (46%) and 4369 indoor environment questionnaires (49%) were returned. 73 subjects did not fill the question of their gender, and 49 subjects did not fill the question of their of age. Analysis of non-responders was performed by SCB Sweden. SCB Sweden analyzed differences between participants and non-participants based on background factors available from other population registers linked to the census [54]. For privacy reasons we did not have access to all these variables. The participation rate was higher among older persons, especially those older than 60 years. Married persons had a higher participation rate, as compared to those not being married. Moreover, the participation rate was related to degree of urbanization, with a slightly lower participation rate in larger cities and suburban municipalities. The participation rate was slightly lower in older buildings. There was no major difference in participation rate between different municipalities. The differences in participation rate between those being born in Sweden as compared to those foreign-born persons and between those having or not having Swedish citizenship were very small. All of the differences in participation rate were small, except for age and civil status.

The prevalence of smoking, allergy, rhinitis, asthma and respiratory infection symptoms in relation to gender and different age groups are shown in Table 1. In total 56.5% were female, 63.5% were 18 to 65 years old, and 36.5% were more than 65 years old; 12.0% were current smokers; 51.0% had current rhinitis; 17.7% wheeze; 11.7% day time breathlessness; 6.0% night time breathlessness; 11.5% doctor diagnosed asthma; 7.7% current asthma; 46.4% respiratory infections and 11.9% antibiotic medication for respiratory infections. The prevalence of current smoking, pollen allergy, furry pet allergy, current rhinitis, asthma attack, respiratory infections were lower among elderly. Wheeze, day time breathlessness, night time breathlessness were higher among elderly.

Descriptive data on home environment factors are shown in Table 2. Totally, 40.9% were living alone; 50.7% were living in rented apartments; 19.0% had window pane condensation; 14.7% had any dampness in the last 12 months and 19.3% in the last 5 years. Females were more living in rented apartments and more often in certain building years. Compared with subjects ≤65 years old, there were more elderly were living alone. The elderly had less cats, and less contact with horses, less exposure to ETS, less renovation (painting, new floors) and less dampness, visible molds and odors.

The associations between current rhinitis and home environment factors are shown in Table 3 (mutual adjustment). Current rhinitis was more common in those living in buildings constructed during 1976–1985, as compared to older buildings constructed before 1961 (reference category). Moreover, living in densely populated areas, living alone and living in rented apartments were associated with current rhinitis.

When dividing type of rhinitis into three groups (infection-allergic- and non-allergic rhinitis), infection rhinitis was more common among those living in buildings constructed during 1976–1985, as compared with older buildings constructed before 1961 and other buildings constructed after 1985. Moreover, it was more common in densely populated areas, among those living alone, those in rented apartments and in homes with window condensation in winter time. Living alone and window pane condensation were risk factors for allergic rhinitis. Non-allergic rhinitis was more reported among those living in rented apartments (Tables 4).

The associations between wheeze, day time breathlessness, night time breathlessness and home environment factors are shown in Table 5 (mutual adjustment). Wheeze was more common among those living in colder climate zones, in rented apartments and in homes with dampness problems (dampness index). Day time attacks of breathlessness was associated with living in buildings constructed during 1961–1975, in rented apartments, in homes with dampness problems, and in apartments with more window-opening (high window-opening index). The association between day time breathlessness and dampness close to significance for dampness index = 1 ($p = 0.05$). Night time breathlessness was more

reported in colder climate zones and in apartments with more window-opening time. The associations between doctor-diagnosed asthma, current asthma and home environment factors are shown in Table 6 (mutual adjustment). Doctor-diagnosed asthma was associated with living in homes with odor, other than moldy odor. Current asthma was more common in homes with ETS and in homes with odor, other than moldy odor.

The associations between respiratory infections, used antibiotic medication for respiratory infections and home environment factors are shown in Table 7 (mutual adjustment). Respiratory infections were associated with living in buildings constructed during 1976–1985, as compared with older buildings constructed before 1960, and in densely populated areas and in rented apartments. Antibiotic medication for respiratory infections was more common in homes with window pane condensation.

Among elderly, current rhinitis was less common among those in homes with dampness problems. Wheeze was more common in rented apartments. Day time attacks of breathlessness was associated with living in homes without mechanical ventilation and more common in homes with high window-opening index. Night time attacks of breathlessness was more reported among those living in colder climate zones. Doctor-diagnosed asthma was more common among those living in rented apartments. Respiratory infections was associated with living in buildings constructed during 1976–1985 and 1996–2005, as compared to older buildings constructed before 1961, and it was more commonly reported in less populated areas. Generally, for these associations OR were numerically higher among elderly as compared to subjects ≤65 years old.

Finally, statistical interaction was tested, comparing elderly with subjects ≤65 years old. There was an age interaction for the association between dampness index and the following health variables: current rhinitis (for interaction, p = 0.001), wheeze (for interaction, p = 0.001), day time attacks of breathlessness (for interaction, p = 0.002), night time attacks of breathlessness (for interaction, p = 0.004), doctor-diagnosed asthma (for interaction, p = 0.024), current asthma (for interaction, p = 0.021) and antibiotic medication for respiratory infections (for interaction, p = 0.015). There was a trend for age interaction between apartment ownership and doctor-diagnosed asthma (for interaction, p = 0.056). Moreover, there was an age interaction for the association between ownership and antibiotic medication for respiratory infections (for interaction, p = 0.015).

Discussions

Associations were demonstrated between home environmental factors in multi-family buildings and adults' rhinitis, asthma and respiratory symptoms. Densely populated areas (urbanization), colder climate zones, rented apartments, building dampness, certain construction years (1961–1975, 1976–1985), odor perception and ETS at home were risk factors for rhinitis, asthma symptoms and respiratory infections.

This study was made during the spring season, which is part of the pollen season in Sweden. Selection bias due to a low response rate can influence epidemiological studies. In this study, we included all subjects (≥18 years old) living in multi-family buildings, with no prior information on their health status. The sample size of this study was reasonably large, and is one of few covering a sample from a whole country. The response rate was not very high (46%). The participation rate was higher among elderly persons, married persons, and slightly lower in larger cities, suburban municipalities and in older buildings. However, we have found no major difference in participation rate between different

Table 1. Data on gender, smoking, allergy, rhinitis, asthma and respiratory infections.

Category	Subcategory	Male n=2483[b] (%)	Female n=3219[b] (%)	p value[d]	≤65 years old n=3637[c] (%)	>65 years old n=2089[c] (%)	p value[d]	Total n=5775 (%)
Female		-	-		54.2	60.4	<0.001	56.5
Current smoking		11.8	12.1	0.728	14.8	7.2	<0.001	12.0
Pollen allergy		23.9	23.7	0.891	28.3	15.7	<0.001	23.8
Furry pet allergy		12.2	11.6	0.505	15.5	5.4	<0.001	11.9
Pollen or furry pet allergy		27.4	27.1	0.847	32.7	17.6	<0.001	27.3
Rhinitis in the last 3 months	Never	49.4	48.7	<0.001	47.4	52.1	0.007	49.0
	Sometimes	41.3	37.2		40.3	36.7		39.1
	Weekly	9.3	14.1		12.3	11.2		11.9
Type of rhinitis	Never	49.6	49.0	0.308	47.6	52.4	<0.001	49.2
	Infection rhinitis	29.9	32.0		34.9	23.5		31.1
	Allergic rhinitis	8.2	7.3		8.3	6.5		7.7
	Non-allergic rhinitis	12.3	11.7		9.2	17.6		12.0
Wheeze in the last 12 months		17.3	17.8	0.642	16.4	19.9	0.001	17.7
Day time breathlessness in the last 12 months		10.8	12.3	0.078	10.3	14.0	<0.001	11.7
Night time breathlessness in the last 12 months		5.7	6.3	0.367	5.9	6.1	0.727	6.0
Doctor diagnosed asthma		9.9	12.6	0.002	12.0	10.3	0.056	11.5
Current asthma[a]		7.0	8.2	0.082	7.5	7.8	0.728	7.7
	Asthma attack	3.1	3.8	0.171	3.9	2.7	0.016	3.5
	Asthma medication	6.3	7.9	0.028	6.9	7.6	0.339	7.2
Respiratory infections in the last 3 months	No infection	53.1	53.9	0.191	48.0	63.1	<0.001	53.6
	One time	36.2	34.3		38.4	29.6		35.1
	Two or more times	10.6	11.8		13.6	7.3		11.3
Used antibiotic medication for respiratory infections in the last 12 months		9.7	13.5	<0.001	11.2	12.9	0.058	11.9

[a]Subjects who have had asthma attacks or have taken asthma medicine during the last 12 months.
[b]Subjects with missing data on gender (n=73) were excluded.
[c]Subjects with missing data on age (n=49) were excluded.
[d]p value by Chi-square test.

Table 2. Data on home building characteristics and indoor environment factors.

Home environment factors	Subcategory	Male n = 2483[e] (%)	Female n = 3219[e] (%)	p value[g]	≤65 years old n = 3637[f] (%)	>65 years old n = 2089[f] (%)	p value[g]	Total n = 5775 (%)
Temperature zone[a]	1	2.6	2.7	0.967	2.5	2.8	0.016	2.6
	2	11.0	11.1		10.1	12.6		11.0
	3	52.6	51.9		53.2	50.4		52.1
	4	33.9	34.4		34.2	34.1		34.3
Construction year	-1960	12.9	12.1	0.017	13.6	10.5	<0.001	12.5
	1961–1975	33.7	32.4		34.0	31.0		33.0
	1976–1985	16.8	18.6		17.0	19.1		17.9
	1986–1995	14.6	17.0		15.1	17.5		16.0
	1996–2005	21.9	19.8		20.2	21.9		20.7
Living alone		41.0	40.9	0.991	36.6	48.4	<0.001	40.9
Rented apartments		49.1	52.0	0.031	52.7	47.0	<0.001	50.7
Natural ventilation only		45.7	45.3	0.788	46.5	43.6	0.063	45.4
Have dog		7.5	7.7	0.726	8.1	6.9	0.112	7.7
Have cat		8.0	9.1	0.166	9.7	6.7	<0.001	8.7
Horse contact		3.2	3.6	0.376	4.4	1.8	<0.001	3.5
ETS		11.9	12.0	0.928	13.1	10.2	0.003	12.1
New indoor painting in the last 12 months		18.0	16.3	0.088	19.1	13.6	<0.001	17.1
New floor materials in the last 12 months		9.6	9.5	0.866	10.8	7.4	<0.001	9.5
Window pane condensation		19.4	18.7	0.535	21.3	15.2	<0.001	19.0
Water leakage in the last 12 months		7.1	6.4	0.306	7.4	5.4	0.004	6.7
Floor dampness in the last 12 months		6.3	7.0	0.287	7.6	5.1	<0.001	6.8
Visible molds in the last 12 months		4.0	3.5	0.355	4.5	2.4	<0.001	3.8
Moldy odor in the last 12 months		2.6	2.7	0.799	3.2	1.5	<0.001	2.7
Other odor in the last 12 months		8.2	8.7	0.611	9.2	7.2	0.026	8.5
Any dampness in the last 12 months[b]		15.0	14.4	0.536	16.4	11.4	<0.001	14.7
Any dampness in the last 5 years		20.1	18.5	0.156	21.3	15.3	<0.001	19.3
Consultant investigation for home dampness		15.4	13.9	0.177	15.8	12.4	0.003	14.5
Dampness index[c]	0	74.1	75.4	0.514	72.3	79.5	<0.001	74.7
	1	16.1	15.7		17.1	13.7		15.9
	2	9.7	9.0		10.6	6.9		9.3
Window-opening index[d]	0	2.0	1.8	0.912	2.2	1.4	<0.001	1.9
	1	2.9	2.6		3.1	2.0		2.7
	2	23.4	23.1		24.2	21.8		23.2
	3	11.2	10.8		11.9	9.3		11.0
	4	36.8	37.0		34.6	41.0		37.1

Table 2. Cont.

Home environment factors	Subcategory	Male n=2483[e] (%)	Female n=3219[e] (%)	p value[g]	≤65 years old n=3637[f] (%)	>65 years old n=2089[f] (%)	p value[g]	Total n=5775 (%)
	5	23.5	24.6		23.9	24.5		24.2

[a]Higher number stands for warmer climate.

[b]Subjects have reported one of the following dampness problems: water leakage, floor dampness, visible molds or moldy odor in the last 12 months.

[c]Dampness index, number of "yes" answers to "any dampness in the last 12 months" and "any dampness in the last 5 year": 0, answers were both "no"; 1, only one answer was "yes"; 2, answers were "yes" to both questions.

[d]Higher number stands for more window opening.

[e]Subjects with missing data on gender (n=73) were excluded.

[f]Subjects with missing data on age (n=49) were excluded.

[g]p value by Chi-square test.

municipalities, between those being born in Sweden as compared to those foreign-born persons, and between those having or not having Swedish citizenships. Furthermore, most of the differences in participation rate were small. The elderly in our study accounted for 36% in our study. It has been shown that elderly population (more than 65 years old) in Sweden are accounting for 23% of the adult population [55]. Elderly in our study were more prone to answer questionnaire, and retired people lives more in apartments other than in single-family buildings in Sweden. Recall bias can be a potential problem in questionnaire surveys. Subjects may overestimate or underestimate their personal symptoms or reports on indoor environment risk factors. However, some factors, such as building constructed year, population density were not collected by questionnaire. Moreover, we found some associations between specific home environmental risk factors and health status, not a similar association for all risk factors. Thus, we don't believe that our conclusions are seriously biased by selection or response errors.

Our study found that subjects living in colder climate zones reported more wheeze and night time breathlessness. This is in agreement with a previous study reported more asthma among Swedish conscripts in the colder parts of northern Sweden [56]. One possible explanation could be less ventilation to save energy.

Living in an area with a higher population density (persons/ km^2) was associated with current rhinitis, infection rhinitis and respiratory infections. One study in Swedish preschool children found that asthma prevalence increased by municipality population density measured the same way as in our study [57]. Population density is used as a proxy variable for degree of urbanization. Exposure to traffic air pollution is one factor associated with population density. Outdoor traffic related exposure was related to an increased risk of allergic rhinitis among adults in Italy [58] and in Sweden [59]. The risk for having infections would increase with the increase of population density because of increased probability of spending time in crowded environments.

Despite the low prevalence of ETS in the Swedish homes, we confirmed that ETS at home is still a risk factor for current asthma. ETS in homes is one of the most consistently factors associated with asthma and asthma-related symptoms among adults in homes [34].

Subjects renting their apartment had more current rhinitis, infection rhinitis, wheeze, day time breathlessness and respiratory infections. Renting apartment can be a proxy variable for lower socio-economic status (SES). One Swedish study on multi-family buildings in Stockholm found that dwellers renting their apartments reported more nasal symptoms than those owning their homes, and found a high correlation between different socio-economic factors (apartment ownership, income, education, and occupation) [60]. One study on SES (defined by parental education) and children's respiratory and allergic symptoms conducted in 13 diverse countries found that lower SES was related to decreased prevalence of allergy to aero-allergens [61]. The association between SES and asthma prevalence and incidence in adults is not well understood and is a matter of debate [62]. However, lower SES seems to be associated with more severe asthma or poorly controlled asthma [62]. Asthma prevalence was higher in lower SES groups among adults [63] and among children [61]. In Sweden, a large number of multi-family apartments of all construction periods are rental, owned by the community, with similar living standards and rental costs as private apartments [64]. However families with lower SES are overrepresented in buildings built from 1961–1975, mostly rented and today buildings prioritized for renovation. The influence of

Table 3. Associations between current rhinitis and building characteristics and indoor environment factors analyzed by ordinal regression models.

Factors	Subcategory	All subjects n = 5775 OR(95% CI)[c]	All subjects n = 5775 Mutual adj. OR(95% CI)[d]	≤65 years old, n = 3637[g], Mutual adj. OR(95% CI)[e]	>65 years old n = 2089[g], Mutual adj. OR(95% CI)[f]
Construction year	-1960	1.00	1.00	1.00	1.00
	1961–1975	1.23(1.03,1.46)*	1.12(0.90,1.41)	1.17(0.90,1.52)	1.12(0.73,1.72)
	1976–1985	1.34(1.10,1.63)**	1.43(1.12,1.84)**	1.45(1.07,1.96)*	1.54(0.97,2.46)
	1986–1995	1.18(0.96,1.44)	1.27(0.99,1.63)	1.30(0.96,1.74)	1.32(0.83,2.11)
	1996–2005	1.01(0.83,1.22)	1.15(0.91,1.46)	1.24(0.93,1.64)	1.12(0.71,1.76)
Population density/10000[a]		1.48(1.12,1.97)**	1.61(1.13,2.29)**	1.74(1.14,2.64)*	1.81(0.90,3.64)
Living alone		1.14(1.02,1.27)*	1.25(1.09,1.43)**	1.54(1.30,1.82)***	0.88(0.69,1.11)
Rented apartments		1.33(1.20,1.49)***	1.23(1.07,1.40)**	1.25(1.06,1.48)**	1.21(0.95,1.54)
Window pane condensation		1.23(1.07,1.42)**	1.16(0.98,1.38)	1.15(0.94,1.41)	1.22(0.88,1.68)
Odor, other than moldy odor in the last 12 months		1.21(0.98,1.50)	1.25(0.98,1.60)	1.30(0.97,1.73)	1.03(0.63,1.67)
Dampness index[b]	0	1.00	1.00	1.00	1.00
	1	1.10(0.94,1.28)	1.07(0.88,1.29)	1.32(1.05,1.67)*	0.67(0.46,0.98)*
	2	1.26(1.04,1.53)*	1.19(0.88,1.60)	1.46(1.03,2.06)*	0.64(0.34,1.21)

[a]The ORs were expressed per 10000 increase of the population density (number of persons per km²).
[b]Dampness index, number of "yes" answers to "any dampness in the last 12 months" and "any dampness in the last 5 year": 0, answers were both "no"; 1, only one answer was "yes"; 2, answers were "yes" to both questions.
[c]Adjusted for gender, age and smoking.
[d]Mutual adjustment models including gender, age and smoking for all subjects (inclusion criteria is $p<0.1$ in total sample).
[e]Mutual adjustment models including gender, age and smoking for younger and middle aged subjects (≤65 years old) (inclusion criteria is $p<0.1$ in total sample).
[f]Mutual adjustment models including gender, age and smoking for elderly (>65 years old) (inclusion criteria is $p<0.1$ in total sample).
[g]Subjects with missing data on age (n = 49) were excluded.
*** $p<0.001$,
** $p<0.01$,
* $p<0.05$.

Table 4. Associations between different types of rhinitis symptoms and building characteristics and indoor environment factors analyzed by multi-nominal logistic regression models.

Factors	Infection rhinitis n = 1568 RRR(95% CI)[a]	Allergic rhinitis n = 388 RRR(95% CI)[a]	Non-allergic rhinitis n = 605 RRR(95% CI)[a]
Construction year 1961–1975[b]	1.09(0.94,1.27)	1.16(0.91,1.48)	1.21(0.99,1.48)
Construction year 1976–1985[c]	1.32(1.11,1.57)**	0.93(0.68,1.28)	1.10(0.86,1.42)
Population density[d]	1.24(1.09,1.42)**	1.08(0.86,1.34)	1.00(0.84,1.20)
Living alone	1.16(1.02,1.33)*	1.37(1.10,1.69)**	1.03(0.85,1.23)
Rented apartments	1.28(1.12,1.46)***	1.16(0.93,1.45)	1.35(1.13,1.63)**
Window pane condensation	1.24(1.04,1.47)*	1.32(1.00,1.75)*	1.13(0.89,1.45)
Dampness index = 2[e]	1.21(0.96,1.53)	1.41(0.98,2.03)	0.98(0.69,1.40)

[a]Adjusted for gender, age and smoking.
[b]Buildings constructed during 1961–1975 compared with buildings constructed before 1960 and during 1986–2005 (excluding buildings constructed during 1976–1985).
[c]Buildings constructed during 1976–1985 compared with buildings constructed before 1960 and during 1986–2005 (excluding buildings constructed during 1961–1975).
[d]Population density (number of persons per km²) was used as a categorical variable in this analysis: population density >1000 persons/km² was compared with population density ≤1000 persons/km².
[e]Dampness index, number of "yes" answers to "any dampness in the last 12 months" and "any dampness in the last 5 year": 0, answers were both "no"; 1, only one answer was "yes"; 2, answers were "yes" to both questions. Dampness index = 2 was compared with dampness index = 0 in this analysis.
*** $p<0.001$,
** $p<0.01$,
* $p<0.05$.

Table 5. Associations between wheeze, day time breathlessness, night time breathlessness, building characteristics and indoor environment factors (by logistic regresson models).

Symptoms	Factors	Subcategory	All subjects n = 5775 OR(95% CI)[d]	All subjects n = 5775, mutual adj. OR(95% CI)[e]	≤65 years old n = 3637[h], mutual adj. OR(95% CI)[f]	>65 years old n = 2089[h], mutual adj. OR(95% CI)[g]
Wheeze in the last 12 months	Temperature zone[a]		0.91(0.83,1.01)	0.89(0.80,0.99)*	0.87(0.75,1.00)*	0.90(0.76,1.06)
	Rented apartments		1.35(1.16,1.56)***	1.20(1.02,1.41)*	1.10(0.89,1.35)	1.37(1.06,1.77)*
	Window pane condensation		1.20(0.99,1.43)	1.15(0.95,1.41)	1.13(0.89,1.44)	1.17(0.83,1.65)
	Dampness index[b]	0	1.00	1.00	1.00	1.00
		1	1.16(0.95,1.42)	1.06(0.85,1.33)	1.27(0.96,1.67)	0.77(0.52,1.15)
		2	1.53(1.20,1.94)**	1.42(1.08,1.86)*	1.90(1.38,2.62)***	0.69(0.38,1.22)
Day time breathlessness in the last 12 months	Construction year	-1960	1.00	1.00	1.00	1.00
		1961–1975	1.37(1.03,1.83)*	1.53(1.03,2.29)*	1.47(0.93,2.33)	2.13(0.91,4.99)
		1976–1985	1.25(0.91,1.72)	1.28(0.82,2.01)	1.11(0.65,1.91)	2.20(0.89,5.45)
		1986–1995	1.20(0.87,1.66)	1.39(0.89,2.18)	1.38(0.81,2.36)	1.94(0.78,4.81)
		1996–2005	0.76(0.54,1.05)	1.12(0.71,1.76)	0.95(0.55,1.63)	1.92(0.78,4.71)
	Rented apartments		1.60(1.34,1.90)***	1.31(1.04,1.66)*	1.25(0.93,1.69)	1.45(0.99,2.12)
	Natural ventilation only		1.35(1.12,1.63)**	1.13(0.90,1.42)	1.04(0.77,1.39)	1.47(1.01,2.14)*
	ETS		1.32(1.03,1.70)*	1.15(0.83,1.57)	1.03(0.70,1.54)	1.41(0.82,2.41)
	New indoor painting in the last 12 months		0.79(0.62,1.00)	0.71(0.50,1.01)	0.70(0.45,1.07)	0.76(0.39,1.47)
	New floor materials in the last 12 months		0.75(0.54,1.03)	0.62(0.38,1.00)	0.61(0.35,1.08)	0.62(0.24,1.55)
	Dampness index[b]	0	1.00	1.00	1.00	1.00
		1	1.35(1.07,1.70)*	1.35(1.00,1.81)*	1.44(1.00,2.07)	1.26(0.76,2.10)
		2	1.76(1.34,2.30)***	1.57(1.09,2.27)*	2.18(1.44,3.31)***	0.48(0.19,1.25)
	Window-opening index[c]		1.08(1.01,1.16)*	1.10(1.01,1.20)*	1.06(0.95,1.19)	1.20(1.02,1.40)*
Night time breathlessness in the last 12 months	Temperature zone[a]		0.85(0.74,0.99)*	0.74(0.61,0.90)**	0.76(0.59,0.97)*	0.69(0.50,0.97)*
	Construction year	-1960	1.00	1.00	1.00	1.00
		1961–1975	1.65(1.11,2.44)*	1.19(0.70,2.01)	1.39(0.76,2.57)	0.93(0.32,2.67)
		1976–1985	1.44(0.93,2.22)	1.23(0.69,2.18)	1.18(0.59,2.35)	1.54(0.51,4.64)
		1986–1995	1.42(0.91,2.22)	1.04(0.57,1.89)	0.95(0.45,1.99)	1.39(0.47,4.15)
		1996–2005	0.64(0.39,1.05)	0.55(0.29,1.05)	0.53(0.24,1.17)	0.63(0.19,2.06)
	Rented apartments		1.66(1.31,2.09)***	1.34(0.98,1.84)	1.27(0.85,1.89)	1.51(0.87,2.62)
	Natural ventilation only		1.25(0.97,1.62)	0.99(0.72,1.35)	1.02(0.69,1.50)	0.99(0.56,1.73)
	New indoor painting in the last 12 months		0.68(0.49,0.96)*	0.64(0.40,1.01)	0.53(0.31,0.92)*	0.95(0.42,2.19)
	Window pane condensation		1.35(1.02,1.80)*	1.10(0.76,1.59)	1.01(0.65,1.58)	1.28(0.64,2.55)
	Dampness index[b]	0	1.00	1.00	1.00	1.00
		1	1.41(1.04,1.90)*	1.10(0.72,1.68)	1.27(0.77,2.09)	0.87(0.39,1.92)
		2	1.46(1.01,2.13)*	1.60(0.96,2.64)	2.63(1.46,4.36)**	-
	Window-opening index[c]		1.12(1.02,1.24)*	1.18(1.04,1.34)*	1.13(0.97,1.32)	1.26(0.99,1.61)

[a]The ORs were expressed per 1 unit increase for temperature zone.
[b]Dampness index, number of "yes" answers to "any dampness in the last 12 months" and "any dampness in the last 5 year": 0, answers were both "no"; 1, only one answer was "yes"; 2, answers were "yes" to both questions.
[c]The ORs were expressed per 1 unit increase for window-opening index.
[d]Adjusted for gender, age and smoking.
[e]Mutual adjustment models including gender, age and smoking for all subjects (inclusion criteria is $p < 0.1$ in total sample).
[f]Mutual adjustment models including gender, age and smoking for subjects ≤65 years old (inclusion criteria is $p < 0.1$ in total sample).
[g]Mutual adjustment models including gender, age and smoking for subjects >65 years old (inclusion criteria is $p < 0.1$ in total sample).
[h]Subjects with missing data on age (n = 49) were excluded.
*** $p < 0.001$,
** $p < 0.01$,
* $p < 0.05$.

ownership on health in our study may also depend upon differences in building maintenance, e.g. a lack of control over the home environment because of renting rather than owning.

Our study found that reported building dampness (dampness index) was associated with wheeze and day time breathlessness. This finding is consistent with another Swedish study among adults living in multi-family buildings [65]. Building dampness problems in homes is associated with increased asthma prevalence, which has been shown in former studies [35,43,66,67]. A cohort study found that new onset of adult asthma was related to dampness/molds in dwellings in Europe, and concluded that the population-attributable risk was 3–14% for observed dampness/molds [68]. One meta-analysis showed that wheeze among adults were associated with damp homes, and concluded that building dampness and molds were associated with approximately 30–50% increases in a variety of respiratory and asthma-related health outcomes [43]. Building dampness is related to a complex mix of exposures, including house dust mite allergens [69], microbial

agents [70,71], bacteria [71–73], chemical emissions from degradation of building materials [74] as well as microbial volatile organic compounds (MVOC) [71].

Window pane condensation was associated with infection rhinitis, allergic rhinitis and antibiotic medication for respiratory infections. Window pane condensation is usually a marker of poor ventilation and a predictor of high relative air humidity (RH) indoors. A Japanese study found that window pane condensation in homes of female university students was related to wheeze symptoms [75]. Exhaled nitric oxide (NO) levels were associated with home window pane condensation among non-sensitized (skin prick tests for IgE sensitization) school children aged [76]. NO is a method introduced for non-invasive monitoring of airway inflammation.

We found that certain construction periods were associated with more respiratory illness. Buildings constructed from 1961–1975 were associated with more day time breathlessness. Buildings constructed from 1976–1985 were associated with more current

Table 6. Associations between doctor-diagnosed asthma, current asthma, building characteristics and indoor environment factors analyzed by logistic regression models.

Symptoms	Factors	Subcategory	All subjects n = 5775 OR(95% CI)[d]	All subjects n = 5775, mutual adj. OR(95% CI)[e]	≤65 years old n = 3637[h], mutual adj. OR(95% CI)[f]	>65 years old n = 2089[h], mutual adj. OR(95% CI)[g]
Doctor-diagnosed asthma	Temperature zone[b]		0.90(0.80,1.01)	0.95(0.83,1.08)	0.86(0.74,1.01)	1.16(0.90,1.50)
	Rented apartments		1.24(1.04,1.47)*	1.13(0.93,1.38)	0.97(0.76,1.23)	1.69(1.15,2.46)**
	Odor, other than moldy odor in the last 12 months		1.52(1.12,2.06)**	1.49(1.08,2.06)*	1.66(1.15,2.39)**	1.04(0.50,2.16)
	Dampness index[c]	0	1.00	1.00	1.00	1.00
		1	1.10(0.87,1.39)	1.14(0.87,1.49)	1.32(0.98,1.80)	0.67(0.36,1.25)
		2	1.34(1.01,1.78)*	1.20(0.79,1.81)	1.48(0.95,2.33)	0.50(0.15,1.66)
Current asthma[a]	Temperature zone[b]		0.89(0.78,1.02)	0.90(0.75,1.06)	0.78(0.64,0.95)*	1.25(0.90,1.74)
	Construction year	-1960	1.00	1.00	1.00	1.00
		1961–1975	1.17(0.84,1.62)	1.08(0.72,1.63)	0.99(0.62,1.58)	1.32(0.53,3.27)
		1976–1985	1.10(0.76,1.58)	1.02(0.64,1.62)	0.96(0.56,1.64)	1.26(0.47,3.35)
		1986–1995	1.09(0.75,1.59)	0.88(0.55,1.42)	0.73(0.42,1.28)	1.29(0.49,3.40)
		1996–2005	0.70(0.48,1.03)	0.70(0.43,1.13)	0.75(0.44,1.30)	0.60(2.12,1.72)
	Rented apartment		1.32(1.07,1.62)**	1.05(0.81,1.36)	0.95(0.69,1.29)	1.45(0.90,2.32)
	ETS		1.43(1.06,1.92)*	1.53(1.09,2.16)*	1.43(0.94,2.17)	1.79(0.97,3.34)
	New indoor painting in the last 12 months		0.73(0.54,0.98)*	0.69(0.47,0.99)*	0.69(0.45,1.04)	0.61(0.27,1.37)
	Odor, other than moldy odor in the last 12 months		1.64(1.15,2.33)**	1.52(1.03,2.24)*	1.71(1.10,2.65)*	1.05(0.43,2.52)
	Dampness index[c]	0	1.00	1.00	1.00	1.00
		1	1.14(0.86,1.52)	1.29(0.93,1.79)	1.57(1.07,2.29)*	0.76(0.37,1.58)
		2	1.50(1.08,2.08)*	1.14(0.68,1.92)	1.62(0.93,2.82)	0.22(0.03,1.63)

[a]subjects who have had asthma attacks or have taken asthma medicine during the last 12 months.
[b]The ORs were expressed per 1 unit increase for temperature zone.
[c]Dampness index, number of "yes" answers to "any dampness in the last 12 months" and "any dampness in the last 5 year": 0, answers were both "no"; 1, only one answer was "yes"; 2, answers were both "yes" to both questions.
[d]Adjusted for gender, age and smoking.
[e]Mutual adjustment models including gender, age and smoking for all subjects (inclusion criteria is $p<0.1$ in total sample).
[f]Mutual adjustment models including gender, age and smoking for subjects ≤65 years old (inclusion criteria is $p<0.1$ in total sample).
[g]Mutual adjustment models including gender, age and smoking for subjects >65 years old (inclusion criteria is $p<0.1$ in total sample).
[h]Subjects with missing data on age (n = 49) were excluded.
*** $p<0.001$,
** $p<0.01$,
* $p<0.05$.

Table 7. Associations between respiratory infections (by ordinal regression models), antibiotic medication for respiratory infections (by logistic regression models), building characteristics and indoor environment factors.

Symptoms	Factors	Subcategory	All subjects n = 5775 OR(95% CI)[d]	All subjects n = 5775, mutual adj. OR(95% CI)[e]	≤65 years old n = 3637[h], mutual adj. OR(95% CI)[f]	>65 years old n = 2089[h], mutual adj. OR(95% CI)[g]
Respiratory infections in the last 3 months	Construction year	-1960	1.00	1.00	1.00	1.00
		1961–1975	1.06(0.89,1.26)	1.07(0.90,1.28)	1.07(0.87,1.31)	1.11(0.79,1.56)
		1976–1985	1.41(1.17,1.71)***	1.46(1.21,1.78)***	1.33(1.06,1.68)*	1.87(1.30,2.69)**
		1986–1995	1.07(0.88,1.30)	1.08(0.88,1.31)	1.03(0.81,1.31)	1.25(0.86,1.80)
		1996–2005	1.09(0.91,1.31)	1.12(0.93,1.35)	0.97(0.78,1.21)	1.56(1.09,2.22)*
	Population density[a]		1.57(1.19,2.09)**	1.72(1.30,2.29)***	1.68(1.20,2.34)**	2.21(1.27,3.87)**
	Rented apartments		1.11(1.00,1.23)	1.13(1.01,1.26)*	1.13(0.99,1.29)	1.14(0.94,1.37)
Antibiotic medication for respiratory infections in the last 12 months	Population density[a]		1.67(1.08,2.58)*	1.63(0.94,2.85)	1.96(0.99,3.90)	1.53(0.58,4.09)
	Rented apartments		1.22(1.03,1.44)*	1.13(0.91,1.40)	1.46(1.10,1.92)**	0.84(0.59,1.20)
	Window pane condensation		1.33(1.08,1.64)**	1.41(1.10,1.82)**	1.49(1.09,2.03)*	1.23(0.78,1.94)
	Odor, other than moldy odor in the last 12 months		1.42(1.05,1.92)*	1.23(0.85,1.80)	1.20(0.75,1.91)	1.22(0.64,2.35)
	Dampness index[b]	0	1.00	1.00	1.00	1.00
		1	1.25(1.00,1.57)	1.08(0.80,1.47)	1.29(0.90,1.86)	0.77(0.42,1.39)
		2	1.43(1.08,1.89)*	1.40(0.92,2.12)	1.84(1.14,2.97)*	0.63(0.24,1.64)
	Window-opening index[c]		1.06(0.99,1.14)	1.09(1.00,1.18)	1.05(0.95,1.17)	1.13(0.97,1.31)

[a]The ORs were expressed per 10000 increase of the population density (number of persons per km²).
[b]Dampness index, number of "yes" answers to "any dampness in the last 12 months" and "any dampness in the last 5 year": 0, answers were both "no"; 1, only one answer was "yes"; 2, answers were "yes" to both questions.
[c]The ORs were expressed per 1 unit increase for window-opening index.
[d]Adjusted for gender, age and smoking.
[e]Mutual adjustment models including gender, age and smoking for all subjects (inclusion criteria is $p<0.1$ in total sample).
[f]Mutual adjustment models including gender, age and smoking for subjects ≤65 years old (inclusion criteria is $p<0.1$ in total sample).
[g]Mutual adjustment models including gender, age and smoking for subjects >65 years old (inclusion criteria is $p<0.1$ in total sample).
[h]Subjects with missing data on age (n = 49) were excluded.
*** $p<0.001$,
** $p<0.01$,
* $p<0.05$.

rhinitis, infection rhinitis and respiratory infections in the last 3 months. Our age classification of multi-family buildings were based on major changes in buildings technology in Sweden. Buildings from 1961–1975 were constructed during a building boom in suburbs of large cities rented by poorer people. They were mostly poor quality high-rise buildings with basements and only exhaust ventilation. These buildings have been reported to have the highest prevalence of dampness problems [77]. The next generation of multi-family buildings (constructed during 1976–1985) was influenced by energy saving demands, with many changes in construction techniques and new building materials [64]. The drastic increase of the oil price in 1974 initiated energy saving measures to reduce energy consumption in buildings during this period. Moreover, in 1977 self–level mortar containing the protein casein were introduced and used in Swedish buildings from 1977–1983. Due to severe indoor environmental problems this mortar was not used after 1983. Studies have shown that the problem was due to dampness causing chemical emissions such as ammonia and sulfhydryl compounds [78]. Later research identi-

fied another odorous compound, 2-acetophenone, emitted from the casein containing mortar. The compound is produced by degradation of the amino acid tryptophan [79]. It has a raw stuffy smell, and has been identified as a compound causing malodour in wine [80] and green tea [81]. The emission of ammonia from the mortar is known to cause blackening of parquet floors and degradation of acrylate polymers in water based glue and the plasticizer di-di-ethyl-hexyl-phthlate (DEHP) in polyvinylchloride (PVC) floor materials, causing emission of 2-etyl-1-hexanol to indoor air [82]. Epidemiological studies have shown that subjects staying in buildings with this type of mortar, and with emission of ammonia and 2-etyl-1-hexanol have a higher prevalence of mucosal inflammation and sick building syndrome [82] and asthma [74]. Thus, multifamily buildings constructed 1976-1984 had particular indoor exposures and were the first generation of buildings in Sweden with low ventilation due to increased energy saving demand and testing of new building materials on a large scale. This may have resulted in an impaired indoor environment leading to the elevated levels of health problems observed in this study.

More window-opening time (higher window-opening index) was associated increased risk of day time breathlessness and night time breathlessness. A review article concluded that higher ventilation rate was associated with less report of asthma or asthma-related symptoms [45]. The negative association between window-opening time and respiratory symptoms in our study is unclear. Polluted outdoor air entering the indoor environment when opening windows could be one explanation. However, this study included all multi-family buildings of the whole country, not only a small polluted area of Sweden. Another possible reason would be that those with asthma problems tried to improve ventilation situation by opening window more often (limitation of the cross sectional design).

We found associations between other odor perception (moldy odor was included in the dampness index) and doctor-diagnosed asthma and current asthma. Experimental studies have shown that odor thresholds are similar in asthmatic and non-asthmatic subjects [83]. Negative or positive attitudes to the odors may (cognitive bias) influence the occurrence of irritative symptoms on experimental exposure to odorous compounds [84]. As our results were based on mutual adjustment models, it is less likely that differences in personal factors or attitudes would have biased our results. Odor perception in our study may be an indicator of poor ventilation. Increased ventilation was found to be associated with less report of odor among university students in computer classrooms [85]. Reported odor was related to higher levels of total fungal DNA in Swedish daycare centers in Sweden [86]. Pungent odor, musty odor and stuffy odor in multi-family buildings in Sweden were associated with asthma symptoms among adults [65]. Self-report of odor perceptions in dwellings were also found to be associated with SBS among adults in China [87]. Thus, odor perception can be associated with different types of exposure and can be of importance for asthma.

New indoor painting in the last 12 months was negatively associated with current asthma, and there was a same trend for its association with night time breathlessness in our study. One former study found that self-reported domestic exposure to newly painted surfaces in the last 12 months in Swedish homes was positively associated with adults' nocturnal breathlessness [41]. The reason for the opposite finding in our study is not clear. Maybe some other activities that related to indoor painting improved the indoor environment but was not measured in our study. Paint used in indoor environment has becoming more and more environmental friendly with less and less chemical emissions, especially in developed countries like Sweden. One study compared new paint and conventional paint and found a significant increase in wheeze and breathlessness during use of conventional paint, but not with the new paint [88]. Painting is usually a part of a major renovation in buildings, which could benefit health by creating a better indoor environment with strategies of removing dust, house dust mites, molds etc.

The elderly in our study reported less pollen allergy, furry pet allergy, current rhinitis and respiratory infections in the last 3 months. The prevalence of environmental factors were also different. Two review articles have summarized articles on environment factors and respiratory health among the elderly [47,48]. The first review summarized 59 articles about the adverse respiratory effects of outdoor air pollution among individuals >65 years [47]. The second review included 33 relevant publications about exposure to major indoor air pollutants and respiratory diseases [48]. Few studies are available on adverse effects of building dampness and molds in relation to respiratory symptoms among subjects above 60 years [48]. Building dampness (dampness index) were associated with current rhinitis, wheeze, day time breathlessness, current asthma and used antibiotic medication for respiratory infections in the last 12 months among subjects less than or equal to 65 years old in our study (born during1943–2008), but no significant association were found among subjects more than 65 years old (born before 1943). The possible explanation for our finding could be that the effects of dampness problems and renting apartments were different between elderly and others in Sweden. The elderly in our study was born before 1943, and others were born during 1943 to 1990. The major increase in atopic diseases in Sweden started among those being born in the early 1960's and later [56,89]. The era with a lot of new chemical products started in the 1940s'. The elderly in our study was grown in a different environment (more exposed to a farming environment) compared with those younger (less than or equal to 65 years old), and which may make the elderly becoming less sensitive to building dampness and molds later in life. Sweden was a rural society in the old time and those born early were more often living on farms when they were young. Farming life experience in childhood was associated with a reduced risk of atopic sensitization [90] and less adult-onset of asthma [91].

Conclusions

Factors in multi-family dwellings, especially rented apartments, certain building years (especially 1961–1985), building dampness and molds, window pane condensation and odor perceptions at home can be risk factors for rhinitis, asthma and respiratory infections. Preventive measures could include avoiding building dampness and molds, repairing those buildings built during the 1961–1985 and increase ventilation flow in indoor environment.

Acknowledgments

Thanks to Boverket-The Swedish National Board of Housing, Building and Planning. Moreover, the authors would like thank all participants.

Author Contributions

Conceived and designed the experiments: KE. Performed the experiments: KE. Analyzed the data: JW. Contributed reagents/materials/analysis tools: KE GS DN. Contributed to the writing of the manuscript: JW KE GS DN.

References

1. Brasche S, Bischof W (2005) Daily time spent indoors in German homes—baseline data for the assessment of indoor exposure of German occupants. Int J Hyg Environ Health 208: 247–253.

2. Tran NP, Vickery J, Blaiss MS (2011) Management of rhinitis: allergic and non-allergic. Allergy Asthma Immunol Res 3: 148–156.

3. Bousquet J, Van Cauwenberge P, Khaltaev N (2001) Allergic rhinitis and its impact on asthma. J Allergy Clin Immunol 108: S147–334.

4. de Marco R, Cappa V, Accordini S, Rava M, Antonicelli L, et al. (2012) Trends in the prevalence of asthma and allergic rhinitis in Italy between 1991 and 2010. Eur Respir J 39: 883–892.

5. Verlato G, Corsico A, Villani S, Cerveri I, Migliore E, et al. (2003) Is the prevalence of adult asthma and allergic rhinitis still increasing? Results of an Italian study. J Allergy Clin Immunol 111: 1232–1238.

6. Braunstahl GJ (2009) United airways concept: what does it teach us about systemic inflammation in airways disease? Proc Am Thorac Soc 6: 652–654.

7. Bjerg A, Ekerljung L, Middelveld R, Dahlen SE, Forsberg B, et al. (2011) Increased prevalence of symptoms of rhinitis but not of asthma between 1990 and 2008 in Swedish adults: comparisons of the ECRHS and GA(2)LEN surveys. PLoS One 6: e16082.

8. Chinn S, Jarvis D, Burney P, Luczynska C, Ackermann-Liebrich U, et al. (2004) Increase in diagnosed asthma but not in symptoms in the European Community Respiratory Health Survey. Thorax 59: 646–651.

9. Eriksson J, Ekerljung L, Ronmark E, Dahlen B, Ahlstedt S, et al. (2012) Update of prevalence of self-reported allergic rhinitis and chronic nasal symptoms among adults in Sweden. Clin Respir J 6: 159–168.

10. Nihlen U, Greiff L, Montnemery P, Lofdahl CG, Johannisson A, et al. (2006) Incidence and remission of self-reported allergic rhinitis symptoms in adults. Allergy 61: 1299–1304.

11. Warm K, Backman H, Lindberg A, Lundback B, Ronmark E (2012) Low incidence and high remission of allergic sensitization among adults. J Allergy Clin Immunol 129: 136–142.

12. Ng TP, Tan WC (1994) Epidemiology of allergic rhinitis and its associated risk factors in Singapore. Int J Epidemiol 23: 553–558.

13. Radon K, Gerhardinger U, Schulze A, Zock JP, Norback D, et al. (2008) Occupation and adult onset of rhinitis in the general population. Occup Environ Med 65: 38–43.

14. Nyembue TD, Jorissen M, Hellings PW, Muyunga C, Kayembe JM (2012) Prevalence and determinants of allergic diseases in a Congolese population. Int Forum Allergy Rhinol 2: 285–293.

15. Bener A, Mobayed H, Sattar HA, Al-Mohammed AA, Ibrahimi AS, et al. (2004) Pet ownership: its effect on allergy and respiratory symptoms. Eur Ann Allergy Clin Immunol 36: 306–310.

16. Araki A, Kanazawa A, Kawai T, Eitaki Y, Morimoto K, et al. (2012) The relationship between exposure to microbial volatile organic compound and allergy prevalence in single-family homes. Sci Total Environ 423: 18–26.

17. Jaakkola MS, Quansah R, Hugg TT, Heikkinen SA, Jaakkola JJ (2013) Association of indoor dampness and molds with rhinitis risk: A systematic review and meta-analysis. J Allergy Clin Immunol 132: 1099–1110.e1018.

18. Kurt E, Metintas S, Basyigit I, Bulut I, Coskun E, et al. (2009) Prevalence and Risk Factors of Allergies in Turkey (PARFAIT): results of a multicentre cross-sectional study in adults. Eur Respir J 33: 724–733.

19. Kilpelainen M, Terho EO, Helenius H, Koskenvuo M (2001) Home dampness, current allergic diseases, and respiratory infections among young adults. Thorax 56: 462–467.

20. Wang DY (2005) Risk factors of allergic rhinitis: genetic or environmental? Ther Clin Risk Manag 1: 115–123.

21. Bahadori K, Doyle-Waters MM, Marra C, Lynd L, Alasaly K, et al. (2009) Economic burden of asthma: a systematic review. BMC Pulm Med 9: 24.

22. Lotvall J, Ekerljung L, Ronmark EP, Wennergren G, Linden A, et al. (2009) West Sweden Asthma Study: prevalence trends over the last 18 years argues no recent increase in asthma. Respir Res 10: 94.

23. Anandan C, Nurmatov U, van Schayck OC, Sheikh A (2010) Is the prevalence of asthma declining? Systematic review of epidemiological studies. Allergy 65: 152–167.

24. Yorgancioglu A, Ozdemir C, Kalayci O, Kalyoncu AF, Bachert C, et al. (2012) ARIA (Allergic Rhinitis and its Impact on Asthma) achievements in 10 years and future needs. Tuberk Toraks 60: 92–97.

25. Cruz AA, Popov T, Pawankar R, Annesi-Maesano I, Fokkens W, et al. (2007) Common characteristics of upper and lower airways in rhinitis and asthma: ARIA update, in collaboration with GA(2)LEN. Allergy 62 Suppl 84: 1–41.

26. Bousquet J, Annesi-Maesano I, Carat F, Leger D, Rugina M, et al. (2005) Characteristics of intermittent and persistent allergic rhinitis: DREAMS study group. Clin Exp Allergy 35: 728–732.

27. Janson C, Anto J, Burney P, Chinn S, de Marco R, et al. (2001) The European Community Respiratory Health Survey: what are the main results so far? European Community Respiratory Health Survey II. Eur Respir J 18: 598–611.

28. Leynaert B, Sunyer J, Garcia-Esteban R, Svanes C, Jarvis D, et al. (2012) Gender differences in prevalence, diagnosis and incidence of allergic and non-allergic asthma: a population-based cohort. Thorax 67: 625–631.

29. Lee YL, Hsiue TR, Lee CH, Su HJ, Guo YL (2006) Home exposures, parental atopy, and occurrence of asthma symptoms in adulthood in southern Taiwan. Chest 129: 300–308.

30. Backman H, Hedman L, Jansson SA, Lindberg A, Lundback B, et al. (2014) Prevalence trends in respiratory symptoms and asthma in relation to smoking - two cross-sectional studies ten years apart among adults in northern Sweden. World Allergy Organ J 7: 1.

31. Bjerg A, Ekerljung L, Eriksson J, Olafsdottir IS, Middelveld R, et al. (2013) Higher risk of wheeze in female than male smokers. Results from the Swedish GA 2 LEN study. PLoS One 8: e54137.

32. Meszaros D, Burgess J, Walters EH, Johns D, Markos J, et al. (2014) Domestic airborne pollutants and asthma and respiratory symptoms in middle age. Respirology.

33. Nadif R, Matran R, Maccario J, Bechet M, Le Moual N, et al. (2010) Passive and active smoking and exhaled nitric oxide levels according to asthma and atopy in adults. Ann Allergy Asthma Immunol 104: 385–393.

34. Jie Y, Ismail NH, Jie X, Isa ZM (2011) Do indoor environments influence asthma and asthma-related symptoms among adults in homes? a review of the literature. J Formos Med Assoc 110: 555–563.

35. WHO (2009). WHO Guidelines for Indoor Air Quality: Dampness and Mould. Geneva: World Health Organization.

36. Chew GL, Carlton EJ, Kass D, Hernandez M, Clarke B, et al. (2006) Determinants of cockroach and mouse exposure and associations with asthma in

37. families and elderly individuals living in New York City public housing. Ann Allergy Asthma Immunol 97: 502–513.

37. Bjornsson E, Norback D, Janson C, Widstrom J, Palmgren U, et al. (1995) Asthmatic symptoms and indoor levels of micro-organisms and house dust mites. Clin Exp Allergy 25: 423–431.

38. Hulin M, Moularat S, Kirchner S, Robine E, Mandin C, et al. (2013) Positive associations between respiratory outcomes and fungal index in rural inhabitants of a representative sample of French dwellings. Int J Hyg Environ Health 216: 155–162.

39. Norback D, Bjornsson E, Janson C, Widstrom J, Boman G (1995) Asthmatic symptoms and volatile organic compounds, formaldehyde, and carbon dioxide in dwellings. Occup Environ Med 52: 388–395.

40. Hulin M, Simoni M, Viegi G, Annesi-Maesano I (2012) Respiratory health and indoor air pollutants based on quantitative exposure assessments. Eur Respir J 40: 1033–1045.

41. Wieslander G, Norback D, Bjornsson E, Janson C, Boman G (1997) Asthma and the indoor environment: the significance of emission of formaldehyde and volatile organic compounds from newly painted indoor surfaces. Int Arch Occup Environ Health 69: 115–124.

42. Fisk WJ, Eliseeva EA, Mendell MJ (2010) Association of residential dampness and mold with respiratory tract infections and bronchitis: a meta-analysis. Environ Health 9: 72.

43. Fisk WJ, Lei-Gomez Q, Mendell MJ (2007) Meta-analyses of the associations of respiratory health effects with dampness and mold in homes. Indoor Air 17: 284–296.

44. Li Y, Leung GM, Tang JW, Yang X, Chao CY, et al. (2007) Role of ventilation in airborne transmission of infectious agents in the built environment - a multidisciplinary systematic review. Indoor Air 17: 2–18.

45. Sundell J, Levin H, Nazaroff WW, Cain WS, Fisk WJ, et al. (2011) Ventilation rates and health: multidisciplinary review of the scientific literature. Indoor Air 21: 191–204.

46. Christensen K, Doblhammer G, Rau R, Vaupel JW Ageing populations: the challenges ahead. (2009) The Lancet 374: 1196–1208.

47. Bentayeb M, Simoni M, Baiz N, Norback D, Baldacci S, et al. (2012) Adverse respiratory effects of outdoor air pollution in the elderly. Int J Tuberc Lung Dis 16: 1149–1161.

48. Bentayeb M, Simoni M, Norback D, Baldacci S, Maio S, et al. (2013) Indoor air pollution and respiratory health in the elderly. J Environ Sci Health A Tox Hazard Subst Environ Eng 48: 1783–1789.

49. The Swedish National Board of Housing Building and Planning (2009) Statistiska urval och metoder i Bovekets projekt BETSI. Sweden: The Swedish National Board of Housing, Building and Planning.

50. Norback D, Bjornsson E, Janson C, Palmgren U, Boman G (1999) Current asthma and biochemical signs of inflammation in relation to building dampness in dwellings. Int J Tuberc Lung Dis 3: 368–376.

51. Burney PG, Luczynska C, Chinn S, Jarvis D (1994) The European Community Respiratory Health Survey. Eur Respir J 7: 954–960.

52. Andersson K (1998) Epidemiological approach to indoor air problems. Indoor Air 8: 32–39.

53. Engvall K, Norrby C, Norback D (2003) Ocular, nasal, dermal and respiratory symptoms in relation to heating, ventilation, energy conservation, and reconstruction of older multi-family houses. Indoor Air 13: 206–211.

54. The Swedish National Board of Housing Building and Planning (2009) Enkätundersökning om boendes upplevda inomhusmiljö och ohälsa - resultat från projektet BETSI. Sweden: The Swedish National Board of Housing, Building and Planning.

55. Statistics Sweden (2009) The furture population of Sweden 2009–2060. Demographic reports.

56. Aberg N (1989) Asthma and allergic rhinitis in Swedish conscripts. Clin Exp Allergy 19: 59–63.

57. Broms K, Norback D, Eriksson M, Sundelin C, Svardsudd K (2009) Effect of degree of urbanisation on age and sex-specific asthma prevalence in Swedish preschool children. BMC Public Health 9: 303.

58. de Marco R, Poli A, Ferrari M, Accordini S, Giammanco G, et al. (2002) The impact of climate and traffic-related NO2 on the prevalence of asthma and allergic rhinitis in Italy. Clin Exp Allergy 32: 1405–1412.

59. Lindgren A, Stroh E, Nihlen U, Montnemery P, Axmon A, et al. (2009) Traffic exposure associated with allergic asthma and allergic rhinitis in adults. A cross-sectional study in southern Sweden. Int J Health Geogr 8: 25.

60. Engvall K, Hult M, Corner R, Lampa E, Norback D, et al. (2010) A new multiple regression model to identify multi-family houses with a high prevalence of sick building symptoms "SBS", within the healthy sustainable house study in Stockholm (3H). Int Arch Occup Environ Health 83: 85–94.

61. Gehring U, Pattenden S, Slachtova H, Antova T, Braun-Fahrlander C, et al. (2006) Parental education and children's respiratory and allergic symptoms in the Pollution and the Young (PATY) study. Eur Respir J 27: 95–107.

62. Le Moual N, Jacquemin B, Varraso R, Dumas O, Kauffmann F, et al. (2013) Environment and asthma in adults. Presse Med 42: e317–333.

63. Basagana X, Sunyer J, Kogevinas M, Zock JP, Duran-Tauleria E, et al. (2004) Socioeconomic status and asthma prevalence in young adults: the European Community Respiratory Health Survey. Am J Epidemiol 160: 178–188.

64. Engvall K, Norrby C, Bandel J, Hult M, Norback D (2000) Development of a multiple regression model to identify multi-family residential buildings with a high prevalence of sick building syndrome (SBS). Indoor Air 10: 101–110.

65. Engvall K, Norrby C, Norback D (2001) Asthma symptoms in relation to building dampness and odour in older multifamily houses in Stockholm. Int J Tuberc Lung Dis 5: 468–477.

66. Bornehag CG, Sundell J, Bonini S, Custovic A, Malmberg P, et al. (2004) Dampness in buildings as a risk factor for health effects, EUROEXPO: a multidisciplinary review of the literature (1998–2000) on dampness and mite exposure in buildings and health effects. Indoor Air 14: 243–257.

67. Wang J, Li B, Yu W, Yang Q, Wang H, et al. (2014) Rhinitis Symptoms and Asthma among Parents of Preschool Children in Relation to the Home Environment in Chongqing, China. PLoS One 9: e94731.

68. Norback D, Zock JP, Plana E, Heinrich J, Svanes C, et al. (2013) Mould and dampness in dwelling places, and onset of asthma: the population-based cohort ECRHS. Occup Environ Med 70: 325–331.

69. Zock JP, Jarvis D, Luczynska C, Sunyer J, Burney P (2002) Housing characteristics, reported mold exposure, and asthma in the European Community Respiratory Health Survey. J Allergy Clin Immunol 110: 285–292.

70. Bush RK, Portnoy JM, Saxon A, Terr AI, Wood RA (2006) The medical effects of mold exposure. J Allergy Clin Immunol 117: 326–333.

71. Sahlberg B, Gunnbjornsdottir M, Soon A, Jogi R, Gislason T, et al. (2013) Airborne molds and bacteria, microbial volatile organic compounds (MVOC), plasticizers and formaldehyde in dwellings in three North European cities in relation to sick building syndrome (SBS). Sci Total Environ 444: 433–440.

72. Nevalainen A, Seuri M (2005) Of microbes and men. Indoor Air 15 Suppl 9: 58–64.

73. Zhang X, Zhao Z, Nordquist T, Larsson L, Sebastian A, et al. (2011) A longitudinal study of sick building syndrome among pupils in relation to microbial components in dust in schools in China. Sci Total Environ 409: 5253–5259.

74. Norback D, Wieslander G, Nordstrom K, Walinder R (2000) Asthma symptoms in relation to measured building dampness in upper concrete floor construction, and 2-ethyl-1-hexanol in indoor air. Int J Tuberc Lung Dis 4: 1016–1025.

75. Takaoka M, Norback D (2011) The Home Environment of Japanese Female University Students - Association with Respiratory Health and Allergy. Indoor and Built Environment 20: 369–376.

76. Janson C, Kalm-Stephens P, Foucard T, Norback D, Alving K, et al. (2005) Exhaled nitric oxide levels in school children in relation to IgE sensitisation and window pane condensation. Respir Med 99: 1015–1021.

77. Engvall K, Norrby C, Norback D (2001) Sick building syndrome in relation to building dampness in multi-family residential buildings in Stockholm. Int Arch Occup Environ Health 74: 270–278.

78. Lundholm M, Lavrell G, Mathiasson L (1990) Self-leveling mortar as a possible cause of symptoms associated with "sick building syndrome". Arch Environ Health 45: 135–140.

79. Hoenicke K, Simat TJ, Steinhart H, Christoph N, Kohler HJ, et al. (1999) Determination of tryptophan and tryptophan metabolites in grape must and wine. Adv Exp Med Biol 467: 671–677.

80. Schmarr HG, Ganss S, Sang W, Potouridis T (2007) Analysis of 2-aminoacetophenone in wine using a stable isotope dilution assay and multidimensional gas chromatography-mass spectrometry. J Chromatogr A 1150: 78–84.

81. Kumazawa K, Masuda H (1999) Identification of potent odorants in Japanese green tea (Sen-cha). J Agric Food Chem 47: 5169–5172.

82. Wieslander G, Norback D, Nordstrom K, Walinder R, Venge P (1999) Nasal and ocular symptoms, tear film stability and biomarkers in nasal lavage, in relation to building-dampness and building design in hospitals. Int Arch Occup Environ Health 72: 451–461.

83. Caccappolo E, Kipen H, Kelly-McNeil K, Knasko S, Hamer RM, et al. (2000) Odor perception: multiple chemical sensitivities, chronic fatigue, and asthma. J Occup Environ Med 42: 629–638.

84. Andersson L, Claeson AS, Ledin L, Wisting F, Nordin S (2013) The influence of health-risk perception and distress on reactions to low-level chemical exposure. Front Psychol 4: 816.

85. Norback D, Nordstrom K (2008) An experimental study on effects of increased ventilation flow on students' perception of indoor environment in computer classrooms. Indoor Air 18: 293–300.

86. Cai GH, Broms K, Malarstig B, Zhao ZH, Kim JL, et al. (2009) Quantitative PCR analysis of fungal DNA in Swedish day care centers and comparison with building characteristics and allergen levels. Indoor Air 19: 392–400.

87. Wang J, Li B, Yang Q, Yu W, Wang H, et al. (2013) Odors and sensations of humidity and dryness in relation to sick building syndrome and home environment in Chongqing, China. PLoS One 8: e72385.

88. Beach JR, Raven J, Ingram C, Bailey M, Johns D, et al. (1997) The effects on asthmatics of exposure to a conventional water-based and a volatile organic compound-free paint. Eur Respir J 10: 563–566.

89. Aberg N, Hesselmar B, Aberg B, Eriksson B (1995) Increase of asthma, allergic rhinitis and eczema in Swedish schoolchildren between 1979 and 1991. Clin Exp Allergy 25: 815–819.

90. Leynaert B, Neukirch C, Jarvis D, Chinn S, Burney P, et al. (2001) Does living on a farm during childhood protect against asthma, allergic rhinitis, and atopy in adulthood? Am J Respir Crit Care Med 164: 1829–1834.

91. Varraso R, Oryszczyn MP, Mathieu N, Le Moual N, Boutron-Ruault MC, et al. (2012) Farming in childhood, diet in adulthood and asthma history. Eur Respir J 39: 67–75.

21

Effect of Transcranial Direct-Current Stimulation Combined with Treadmill Training on Balance and Functional Performance in Children with Cerebral Palsy: A Double-Blind Randomized Controlled Trial

Natália de Almeida Carvalho Duarte[1]*, Luanda André Collange Grecco[2], Manuela Galli[3], Felipe Fregni[4], Cláudia Santos Oliveira[5]

1 Master Program in Rehabilitation Sciences, Movement Analysis Lab, University Nove de Julho, São Paulo, São Paulo, Brazil, 2 Doctoral Program in Rehabilitation Sciences, Movement Analysis Lab, University Nove de Julho, São Paulo, São Paulo, Brazil, 3 Dept. of Electronic Information and Bioengineering, Politecnico di Milano and IRCCS San Raffaele Pisana, Rome, 4 Laboratory of Neuromodulation & Center of Clinical Research Learning, Department of Physical Medicine & Rehabilitation, Spaulding Rehabilitation Hospital and Massachusetts General Hospital, Harvard Medical School, Boston, MA, United States of America, 5 Professor, Master and Doctoral Programs in Rehabilitation Sciences, Movement Analysis Lab, University Nove de Julho, São Paulo, São Paulo, Brazil

Abstract

Background: Cerebral palsy refers to permanent, mutable motor development disorders stemming from a primary brain lesion, causing secondary musculoskeletal problems and limitations in activities of daily living. The aim of the present study was to determine the effects of gait training combined with transcranial direct-current stimulation over the primary motor cortex on balance and functional performance in children with cerebral palsy.

Methods: A double-blind randomized controlled study was carried out with 24 children aged five to 12 years with cerebral palsy randomly allocated to two intervention groups (blocks of six and stratified based on GMFCS level (levels I-II or level III).The experimental group (12 children) was submitted to treadmill training and anodal stimulation of the primary motor cortex. The control group (12 children) was submitted to treadmill training and placebo transcranial direct-current stimulation. Training was performed in five weekly sessions for 2 weeks. Evaluations consisted of stabilometric analysis as well as the administration of the Pediatric Balance Scale and Pediatric Evaluation of Disability Inventory one week before the intervention, one week after the completion of the intervention and one month after the completion of the intervention. All patients and two examiners were blinded to the allocation of the children to the different groups.

Results: The experimental group exhibited better results in comparison to the control group with regard to anteroposterior sway (eyes open and closed; p<0.05), mediolateral sway (eyes closed; p<0.05) and the Pediatric Balance Scale both one week and one month after the completion of the protocol.

Conclusion: Gait training on a treadmill combined with anodal stimulation of the primary motor cortex led to improvements in static balance and functional performance in children with cerebral palsy.

Trial Registration: Ensaiosclinicos.gov.br/RBR-9B5DH7

Editor: Barry J. Byrne, Earl and Christy Powell University, United States of America

Funding: The authors gratefully acknowledge financial support from the Brazilian fostering agencies Conselho Nacional de Desenvolvimento Científico e Tecnológico (CNPq), Coordenação de Aperfeiçoamento de Pessoal de Nível Superior (CAPES), and Fundação de Amparo á Pesquisa (FAPESP - 2012/24019-0). The funders had no role in study design, data collection and analysis, decision to publish, or preparation of the manuscript.

Competing Interests: The authors have declared that no competing interests exist.

* Email: natycarvalho_fisio@hotmail.com

Introduction

Cerebral palsy (CP) involves a set of neurophysiological impairments caused by a global reduction in subcortical activity that compromises the activity of corticospinal and somatosensory circuits [1], [2], [3], [4], [5], [6]. CP results in diminished activation of the central nervous system during the execution of movements [4]. A reduction in motor cortex excitability in children is associated with poor motor development [7]. Neurophysiological analyses have demonstrated global changes in cortex excitability in children with CP, even when the brain lesion is unilateral [8]. Such children have postural problems due to spasticity, muscle weakness and impaired muscle coordination. These postural problems can also affect motor development, leading to difficulties in performing basic functional actions, such as sitting, standing and walking [9], [10], [11], [12].

Adequate postural control involves a complex network of sensory and motor information. The integration of subcortical systems, such as the vestibular, sensorial and visual systems, is fundamental to the maintenance of balance. Moreover, posture is maintained through the combined efforts of the sensory motor cortex, supplementary motor area and pre-motor cortex [13].

While there is no cure for the brain lesion in CP, the manifestations of this condition can be minimized through neurorehabilitation [14]. Studies involving the administration of functional magnetic resonance on children with CP have demonstrated that rehabilitation resources are capable of promoting the activation of the primary motor cortex (M1) [14]. M1 is an important area of the brain that facilitates cerebral reorganization. Through a better understanding of the relationship between neuropathology and clinical function in CP, interventions can be individualized based on the neurological substrate available for recuperation, thereby maximizing the efficacy of the therapeutic process [15].

Recent studies have reported the benefits of gait training on a treadmill. Grecco *et al.* describe the positive effects of treadmill training in comparison to over-ground gait training on static and functional balance. The effects were found after 12 sessions of training at the aerobic threshold without body weight support. The benefits included an improvement in functional performance, suggesting that the motor effects can lead to greater independence in children with CP [10],[11].

Marchese *et al.* [16] suggest that repetitive sensory stimulation may favor the activation of important mechanisms that facilitate the motor learning process. Thus, like treadmill training, motor training may favor proprioceptive feedback, leading to adjustments for adequate postural balance and functional performance.

Transcranial direct-current stimulation (tDCS) is a safe, low-cost resource that can be used during motor therapy sessions and involves the administration of a weak electrical current to the scalp using sponge electrodes moistened with saline solution. The effects of stimulation are achieved by the movement of electrons due to electrical charges. The two poles are the anode (positive) and cathode (negative) electrodes. The electrical current flows from the positive pole to the negative pole, penetrating the skull and reaching the cortex, with different effects on biological tissues. Although most of the current is dissipated among the overlying tissues, a sufficient amount reaches the structures of the cortex and changes of membrane potential of the surrounding cells [17],[18]. tDCS is known to induce lasting changes in cortex excitability in both animals and humans. In rehabilitation processes, the aim of tDCS is to enhance local synaptic efficiency, thereby altering the maladaptive plasticity pattern that emerges following a cortex lesion. Stimulation is used to modulate the cortex activity by opening a pathway to increase and prolong functional gains achieved in physical therapy [19].

The authors believe that the combination of tDCS of the primary motor cortex and treadmill training can potentiate the effects on static balance. The hypothesis is that tDCS leads to the maintenance of the results following the interruption of the gait training protocol by inducing long-lasting changes in cortex excitability, thereby facilitating the learning process.

The aims of the present study were to determine the effects of tDCS applied over the primary motor cortex during ten sessions of treadmill gait training on balance and functional performance in children with PC and investigate whether the effects are maintained one month after the completion of the training sessions.

Materials and Methods

Ethics Statement

The protocol for this trial and supporting CONSORT checklist are available as supporting information; see Checklist S1 and Protocol S1. This study received approval from the Human Research Ethics Committee of the University Nove de Julho (Brazil) under process number 69803/2012 and was carried out in compliance with the ethical standards established by the Declaration of Helsinki. The study is registered with the Brazilian Registry of Clinical Trials under process number RBR-9B5DH7 (URL:http://www.ensaiosclinicos. gov.br/rg/RBR-9b5dh7/). There was a delay in releasing the record number for our study. To avoid delays in the conduct of the project or even loss of the sample, the recruitment of the sample was performed according to the previous schedule of the study. The authors confirm that all ongoing and related trials for this intervention are registered. All parents/guardians agreed to the participation of the children by signing a statement of informed consent.

Design

Full details about the trial protocol have previously been reported [20] and can be found in the supplementary appendix, available at http://www.biomedcentral.com. A phase II, prospective, analytical, double-blind, randomized, placebo-controlled clinical trial was carried out. Figure 1 presents the CONSORT [21] flow chart of the study.

Sample

The study took place at the Movement Analysis Lab, University Nove de Julho, Sao Paulo, Brazil, from November 2012 to September 2013. Twenty-nine children with CP were recruited from specialized outpatient clinics, from the physical therapy clinics of the University Nove de Julho and Center for Pediatric Neurosurgery, São Paulo, Brazil. The following were the inclusion criteria: diagnosis of spastic CP; classification on levels I, II or III of the Gross Motor Function Classification System (GMFCS); independent gait for at least 12 months; age between five and ten years; and degree of comprehension compatible with the execution of the procedures. The following were the exclusion criteria: history of surgery or neurolytic block in the previous 12 months; orthopedic deformities; epilepsy; metal implants in the skull or hearing aids.

All children who met the eligibility criteria (n = 24) were submitted to the initial evaluation and randomly allocated to an experimental group (treadmill training combined with active tDCS) and control group (treadmill training combined with placebo tDCS). Block randomization was used and stratified based on GMFCS level (levels I-II or level III). For each stratum, blocks of six were determined to minimize the risk of imbalance in the size of the separate samples. Numbered opaque envelopes were employed to ensure the concealment of the allocation. Each envelop contained a card stipulating to which group the child was allocated.

Evaluation

All evaluation procedures were carried out by two examiners who were blinded to the allocation of the children to the different groups. All patients were blinded for this study. Evaluations consisted of stabilometric analysis as well as the administration of the Pediatric Balance Scale (PBS) and Pediatric Evaluation of Disability Inventory (PEDI) one week before the intervention (Evaluation 1), one week after the completion of the intervention (Evaluation 2) and one month after the completion of the intervention (Evaluation 3). Each evaluation was held on a single

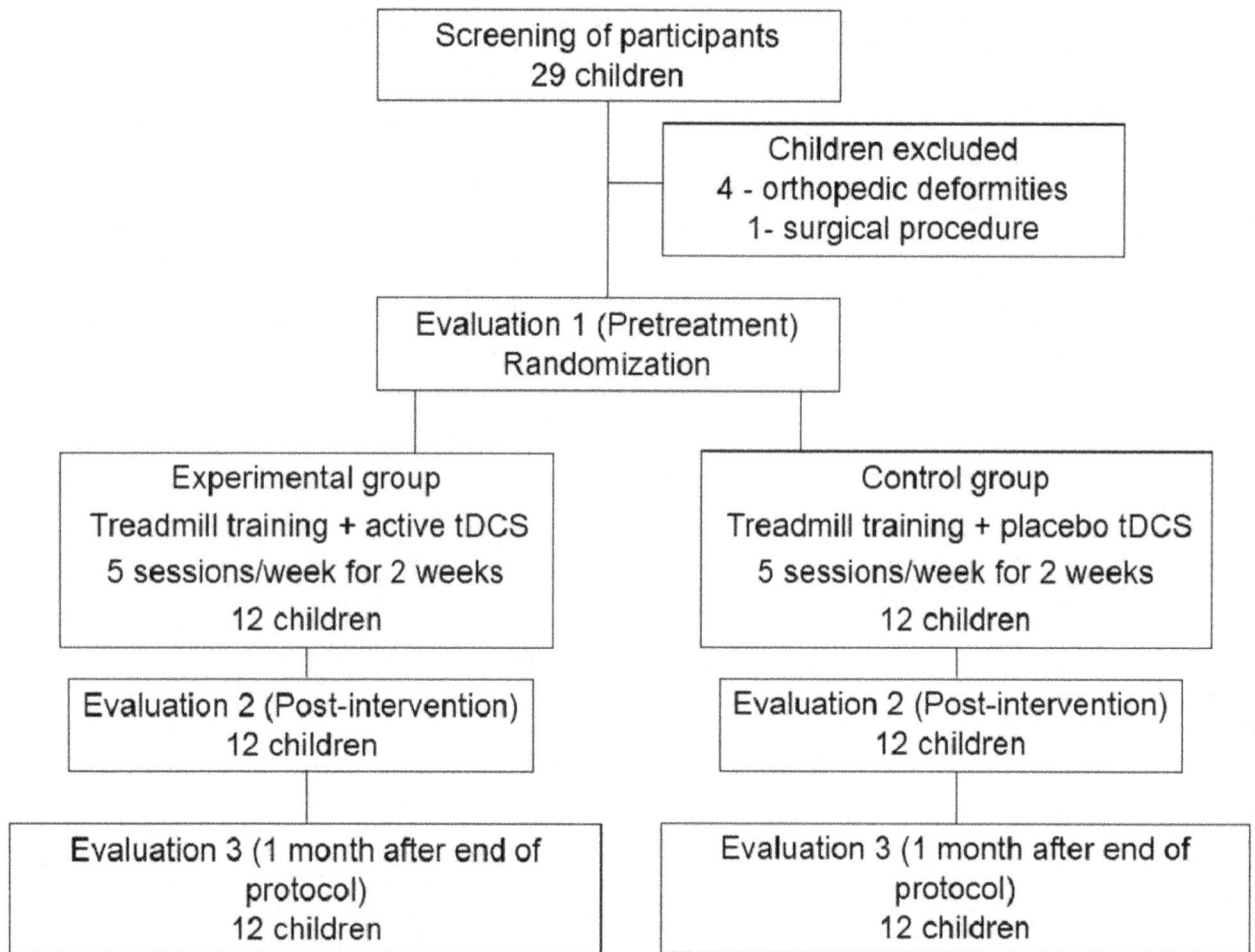

Figure 1. Flowchart of study based on Consolidated Standards of Reporting Trials.

day. The child first rested in a chair for 20 minutes. The stabilometric analysis was then performed, followed by the PBS and then by the PEDI.

Stabilometric analysis was performed for the evaluation of static balance. For such, a force plate (Kistler model 9286BA) was used, which allows the record of oscillations of the center of pressure (COP). The acquisition frequency was 50 Hz, captured by four piezoelectric sensors positioned at the extremities of the force plate, which measured 40×60 cm. The data were recorded and interpreted using the SWAY software program (BTS Engineering), integrated and synchronized to the SMART-D 140 system. The child was instructed to remain in a standing position on the force plate, barefoot, arms alongside the body, with an unrestricted foot base, heels aligned and gazed fixed on a point marked at a distance of one meter at the height of the glabellum (adjusted for each child). Children classified on level III of the GMFCS used their normal gait-assistance device, which was positioned off the force plate. Thirty-second readings were taken under two conditions: eyes open and eyes closed. Displacement of the COP was measured in the anteroposterior (x axis) and mediolateral (Y axis) directions under each visual condition.

The PBS consists of 14 tasks resembling activities of daily living. The items are scored on a five-point scale ranging from 0 (inability to perform the activity without assistance) to 4 (ability to perform the activity independently). The maximum score is 56. Scoring is based on the time in which a position is maintained, the distance to which the upper limb is able to reach out in front of the body and the time required to complete the task [19].

The PEDI allows a quantitative evaluation of functional performance. This questionnaire is administered in interview format to one of the caregivers, who offers information on the child's performance on routine activities and typical tasks of daily living. The test is composed of three parts. The first part addresses abilities in the child's repertoire, which are grouped into three functional domains: self-care (73 items), mobility (59 items) and social function (65 items). Each item on this part receives a score of either 0 (child is unable to perform the activity) or 1 (activity is part of the child's repertoire). The score of each domain is determined by the sum of the items [22], [23].

Intervention

One week after Evaluation 1, the children underwent the 10-session intervention protocol (5 weekly sessions for 2 weeks) involving treadmill training and tDCS (active or placebo). A specific test for children with CP was used to determine the treadmill training speed. This procedure was carried out based on the recommendations of Grecco *et al.* [9]. During the training sessions, the tDCS electrodes were positioned, the equipment was switched on and 20 minutes of gait training was performed simultaneously with anodal stimulation over the primary motor cortex (active or placebo). All children wore their normal braces during training, which were duly placed by the physiotherapist. Heart rate was monitored throughout the entire session to ensure an absence of overload on the cardiovascular system.

Gait training was performed on a treadmill (Inbramed, Millenium ATL, RS, Brazil). Two sessions were performed prior to the beginning of the protocol to familiarize the children with the treadmill. During these trial sessions, the children did not receive tDCS and treadmill speed was gradually increased based on the tolerance of each child. Training velocity was set at 80% of the maximum speed established during the exercise test [9].

Transcranial stimulation was applied with the tDCS Transcranial Stimulation device (Soterix Medical Inc., USA), using two sponge (non-metallic) electrodes (5×5 cm) moistened with saline solution. The anodal electrode was positioned over the primary motor cortex of the non-dominant hemisphere following the 10–20 International Electroencephalogram System [24] and the cathode was positioned in the supra-orbital region on the contralateral side.

To standardize the positioning of the electrodes of the diparetic patients, lower limb dominance was determined through self-reports; the children were asked: "Which leg is easier to move?" [25]. The anodal electrode was positioned over the hemisphere ipsilateral to the dominant lower limb. Thus, the patients were stimulated in the more compromised hemisphere. In cases of hemiparesis, stimulation was standardized over the lesioned hemisphere.

In the experimental group, a 1-mA current was applied over the primary motor cortex for 20 minutes as the children performed the treadmill training. The device has a button that allows the operator to control the intensity of the current. In the first ten seconds, stimulation was gradually increased until reaching 1 mA and gradually diminished in the last ten seconds of the session. In the control group, the electrodes were positioned at the same sites and the device was switched on for 30 seconds, giving the children the initial sensation of the 1 mA current, but no stimulation was administered during the rest of the time. This is a valid control procedure in studies involving tDCS.

The number of sessions attended, maximum speed during treadmill training, duration of treadmill training and distance travelled in each session were recorded on the follow-up chart. Any problems or injuries that occurred during training were also recorded. All participants were instructed to maintain their routine daily activities.

Statistical analysis

The sample size was calculated using the STATA 11 program and based on a study by Grecco et al. 2012 [9] [Effect of treadmill training without partial weight support on functionality in children with cerebral palsy: Randomized controlled clinical trial.] The PBS was selected as the primary outcome due to its proven validity and reliability in the literature for the evaluation of functional balance in children with CP and was therefore used in the sample size calculation. Based on a mean and standard deviation of 46.7 ± 7.6 in the experimental group and 34.9 ± 6.8 in the control group, 10 children in each group would be necessary for a bi-directional alpha of 0.05 and an 80% power. Twenty percent were added to each group to compensate for possible dropouts. Thus, the final sample was made up of 12 children in each group (total: 24 participants).

The Kolmogorov-Smirnov test was used to determine the adherence of the data to the Gaussian curve. The data proved to be parametric and were expressed as mean and standard deviation values. The effect size was calculated by the difference between

means of the pre-intervention and post-intervention evaluations and was expressed with respective 95% confidence intervals. Repeated-measures ANOVA was used for the intra-group analyses and one-way ANOVA was used for the inter-group analyses. A p-value <0.05 was considered statistically significant. The data were organized and tabulated using the Statistical Package for the Social Sciences v.19.0 (SPSS, Chicago, IL, USA).

Results

Twenty-nine children were screened and 24 were selected for participation in the present study, from November 2012 to September 2013. No losses occurred in either group. Table 1 displays the anthropometric characteristics and functional classification of the participants.

No statistically significant differences between groups were found regarding the anthropometric data, age or data referring to the primary or secondary outcomes at the baseline evaluation (p>0.05). Data as age, body mass, height and body mass index were analyzed by the independent t test. The GMFCS and topography was analyzed by the chi square test.

Table 2 displays the variables analyzed at baseline (Evaluation 1), after training (Evaluation 2) and at the follow up (Evaluation 3).

The PBS was chosen as the primary outcome due to the fact that this scale allows the evaluation of functional balance and has proven validity for use on children with CP. The experimental group exhibited the effect of training with tDCS, as demonstrated by the increase in the final score after training and at the follow up evaluation [F $(1.33) = 3.9$; p = 0.05] (Figure 2). In contrast, no significant effect on the PBS score was found in the control group after the intervention [F $(1.11) = 1.3$; p = 0.27].

The stabilometric evaluation revealed positive effects on the reduction in body sway in the anteroposterior direction with eyes open [F $(2.33) = 7.1$; p = 0.002], anteroposterior direction with eyes closed [F $(2.22) = 24.3$; p<0.0001], mediolateral direction with eyes open [F $(2.33) = 4.0$; p = 0.02] and mediolateral direction with eyes closed [F $(2.33) = 3.6$; p = 0.03] (Figure 3). The experimental group maintained these effects on anteroposterior and mediolateral sway with eyes open and closed after the intervention (p<0.05). In the control group, the effect was maintained at Evaluation 3 only with regard to mediolateral sway with eyes closed [F $(1.11) = 18.4$; p = 0.001].

Regarding the PEDI, an increase in the final score was found for the mobility [F $(2.22) = 19.2$; p<0.0001] and self-care [F $(2.22) = 9.90$; p = 0.0008] subscales. In the intra-group analysis, positive effects were found after treatment regarding self-care in both groups, but these effects were not maintained at Evaluation 3. Moreover, only the experimental group exhibited a positive effect regarding mobility after treatment (Evaluation 2). Figure 4 displays the PEDI results in both groups.

In the intra-group analysis, repeated-measures ANOVA revealed significant differences in both groups following motor training, with a reduction in oscillations of the COP one week after the end of the protocols. However, only the experimental group maintained this reduction one month after the protocol (Evaluation 3). The experimental group also exhibited improvements in regarding the balance scale. No significant intra-group differences were found with regard to self-care and functional mobility following treadmill training with tDCS.

In the inter-group analysis, one-way ANOVA revealed significant differences between groups. The experimental group exhibited significantly lower oscillations of the COP in the anteroposterior (experimental group with eyes open: 18.6 ± 3.9, 14.0 ± 2.7 and 14.2 ± 1.9 mm; experimental group with eyes

Table 1. Anthropometric characteristics and functional classification of children analyzed.

	Experimental group (n = 12)	Control group (n = 12)	
Age (years)*	7.8 (2.0)	8.1 (1.5)	p = 0.74
Body mass (Kg)*	27.9(2.5)	28.3(2.7)	p = 0.58
Height (cm)*	127.7(6.4)	128.2(7.4)	p = 0.73
Body mass index (Kg²/m)*	17.2(0.8)	17.8(1.5)	p = 0.39
GMFCS (I\II\III)**	(3\6\3)	(2\7\3)	p = 0.17
Topography (hemiparesis\diparesis)**	(3\9)	(2\10)	p = 0.77

Legend: GMFCS: Gross Motor Function Classification System.
*data expressed as mean (standard deviation); ** data representing frequency.

closed: 24.3±5.6, 17.1±4.3 and 17.7±4.6 mm; control group with eyes open: 20.3±4.5, 15.8±3.6 and 18.4±3.7 mm; control group with eyes closed: 24.2±4.8, 22.7±4.1 and 23.2±3.1 mm) and mediolateral (experimental group with eyes open: 20.3±4.5, 14.7±3.6 and 15.3±4.1 mm; experimental group with eyes closed: 25.4±18.9, 18.9±4.3 and 19.7±4.1 mm; control group with eyes open: 20.2±4.3, 18.6±3.2 and 18.8±3.1 mm; control group with eyes closed: 25.1±5.2, 22.9±4.2 and 22.8±3.6 mm) directions. These differences were found both one week and one month after the end of the interventions (Figure 2).

The experimental group also had better scores on the pediatric balance scale (experimental group: 40.5±9.4, 45.3±7.9 and 44.7±6.7; control group: 39.1±9.8, 39.7±8.9 and 39.5±9.3) (Figure 3).

However, no significant differences between groups were found regarding the self-care (experimental group: 46.1±10.8, 48.0±9.5 and 47.3±9.2; control group: 45.0±9.2, 45.5±9.3 and 45.6±8.9) or mobility (experimental group: 38.0±8.5, 41.7±7.4 and 40.9±7.7; control group: 39.3±7.4, 39.5±6.9 and 38.8±7.0) subscales of the PEDI (Figure 4).

Discussion

There has been increasing use of tDCS in the rehabilitation of patients with lasting neurological effects following a brain lesion, especially in cases of stroke. Studies have also demonstrated the benefits of this technique in patients with Parkinson's disease, pain

and depression. The method has proven to be promising and safe on adults [18].

Studies involving children also suggest that the method is safe, but requires lesser intensity of the electrical current. Through computations modeling, Minhas *et al.* (2012) [26] found that lesser intensity than that conventionally used on adults is capable of cortex stimulation in children. Based on the results achieved with stroke victims and studies that demonstrate an absence of adverse effects in children, the aim of the present investigation was to determine whether anodal stimulation of the primary motor cortex in the dominant hemisphere combined with treadmill training would lead to an increase in or the maintenance of the effect of treadmill training on static and functional balance in children with CP.

Previous studies have demonstrated that treadmill training without body support and at a speed determined by a prior exercise test leads to improvements in both static and functional balance and favors functional performance in children with CP [9]. In the present study, an established treadmill training protocol with effects demonstrated in the literature was used to determine whether tDCS is valid in children with CP classified on levels I, II and III of the GMFCS. The treadmill training had to be adapted to the tDCS procedures reported in the literature. The protocol described by Grecco *et al.* [9] was used as the basis for the present investigation. However, this protocol involves two weekly sessions of training over a seven-week period (total of 14 sessions). In the present study, five weekly sessions were held over a two-week

Table 2. Comparison of variables between experimental group and control group in three moments: Evaluation 1, Evaluation 2, and Evaluation 3.

	Experimental group			Control group		
	Evaluation 1	Evaluation 2	Evaluation 3	Evaluation 1	Evauation 2	Evaluation 3
PBS*	40.5(9.4)	45.3(7.9)	44.7(7.7)	39.1(9.8)	39.7(8.4)	39.5(9.3)
Oscillation AP EO*	18.6(3.9)	14.0(2.7)	14.2(2.6)	20.3(4.5)	15.8(3.6)	18.4(3.6)
Oscillation AP EC*	24.3(5.6)	17.1(4.3)	17.7(4.6)	24.2(4.8)	22.7(4.1)	23.2(4.1)
Oscillation ML EO*	20.3(4.5)	14.7(3.6)	15.3(4.1)	19.2(4.3)	18.6(3.2)	18.8(3.1)
Oscillation ML EC*	25.4(5.5)	18.9(4.3)	19.7(4.1)	25.1(5.2)	22.9(4.2)	22.8(3.6)
Self-care*	46.1(10.0)	48.0(9.5)	47.8(9.2)	45.0(9.2)	45.5(9.3)	45.6(9.4)
Mobility*	38.0(8.5)	41.7(7.4)	40.9(7.7)	38.3(7.4)	39.5(7.6)	38.8(7.0)

Legend: PBS (Pediatric Balance Scale), AP EO (Anteroposterior Eyes Open); AP EC (Anteroposterior Eyes Closed); ML EO (Mediolateral Eyes Open); ML EC (Mediolateral Eyes Closed).
*Data expressed as mean and standard deviation.

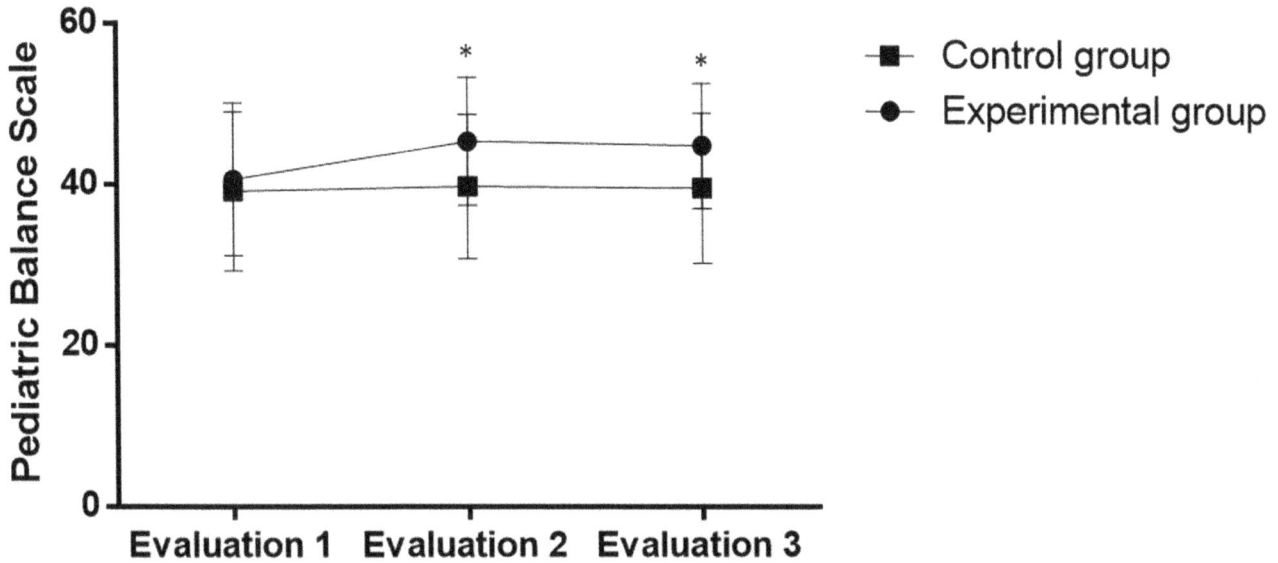

Figure 2. PBS scores in both groups before and after intervention. *statistically significant difference between groups (p<0.05).

period (total of 10 sessions). Thus, it was important to carry out a randomized controlled study involving a control group with placebo tDCS to determine the effects of treadmill training alone.

In a study involving patients with hemiparesis following a stroke, three sessions of anodal stimulation over the damaged motor cortex combined with specific training for the ankle of the paretic limb led to improvements in dorsiflexion and plantar flexion. This is in agreement with the present findings, as the strategies used by the ankle are fundamental to postural control and balance [27]. Another interesting study carried out by Kashi *et al.* (2013) [28] demonstrated that a single session of anodal stimulation in combination with balance and gait training resulted in improvements in balance, gait velocity and stride length in elderly individuals with leukoaraiosis (cerebral white matter lesion that

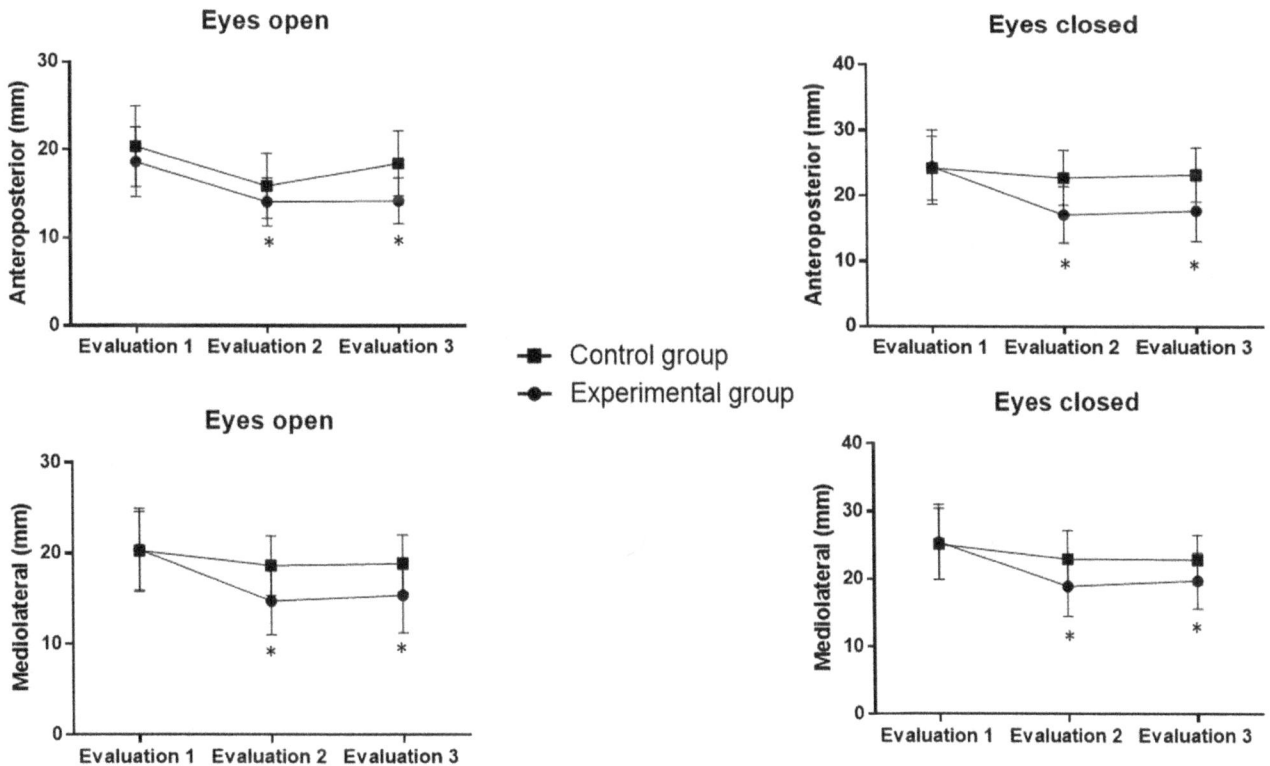

Figure 3. Oscillations of center of pressure. A) anteroposterior sway with eyes open; B) mediolateral sway with eyes open; C) anteroposterior sway with eyes closed; D) mediolateral sway with eyes closed. *Statistically significant difference between groups (p<0.05).

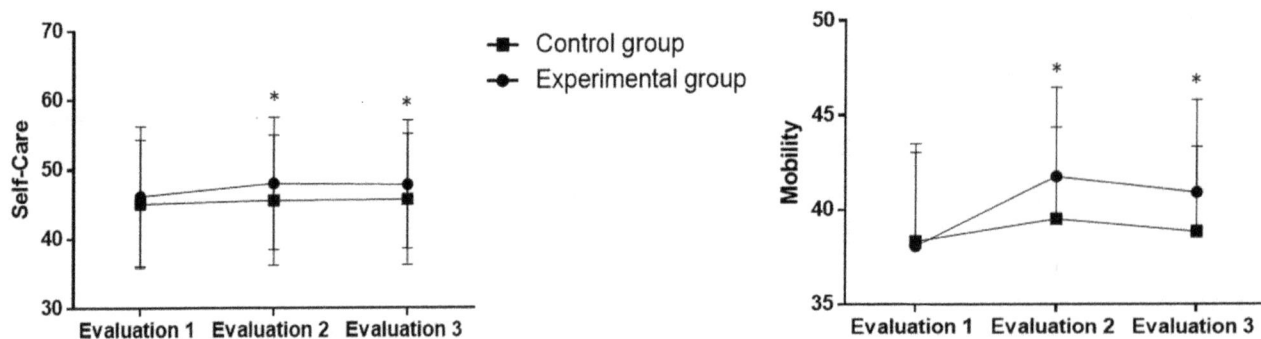

Figure 4. Self-care and mobility scores on PEDI in both groups before and after intervention.

affects gait and balance). In the present study, 10 consecutive sessions of tDCS were performed with the aim of potentiating the neuroplastic changes that occur from the combination of tDCS and motor training to determine whether the effects are persistent modifications of synaptic efficiency similar to long-term potentiation [29].

Kashi et al. (2012) [30] evaluated 30 healthy volunteers who received 15 minutes of anodal stimulation (2 mA; either active or placebo) of the prefrontal cortex while at rest prior to walking on a moving platform. The active group demonstrated improvements in postural control and gait velocity in comparison to the placebo group. These findings demonstrate that anodal tDCS is capable of causing changes in motor cortex excitability, thereby favoring motor control and lower limb movements.

In the present study, both groups demonstrated positive results following the different protocols. However, statistically significant differences between groups were found, with better results in the experimental group regarding anteroposterior sway, mediolateral sway and functional balance (PBS). These findings suggest that anodal stimulation of the primary motor cortex potentiated the results of treadmill training. The randomized, controlled study design allows the determination of the effect size, demonstrating the statistically significant effect of tDCS. One of the most important findings regards the fact that tDCS contributed to the maintenance of the effects of treadmill training. In clinical practice, the effects of physical therapy are often minimized or even completely lost following the interruption of the therapy sessions. In the present study, the gains achieved with the combination of treadmill training and tDCS remained one month after the completion of the protocol, suggesting the potential of tDCS to modify cortex excitability and favor neuroplasticity. The lack of an analysis of cortex excitability constitutes a limitation of this study. Although the aim was to analyze motor results, the measure of excitability could have allowed a more adequate explanation of the findings.

The possible adverse effects of tDCS should be addressed. However, the literature on tDCS in children is scarce and no previous papers involving motor training are found. In the present study, the children and their caregivers were asked about side effects at the end of each session and during the evaluations after the completion of the protocol. Three children in the experimental group experienced redness in the supra-orbital region (site of the cathode). No other adverse effects were reported, such as behavioral changes, headache or discomfort. During the sessions, 18 children (12 in the experimental group and 6 in the control group) reported a tingling sensation at the beginning of stimulation, but this sensation either ceased after a few seconds or was not considered bothersome. No children needed the intensity to be diminished or the stimulation to be stopped prior to the end of the 20-minute session. No children had difficulty performing treadmill training with tDCS and neither the wires nor the positioning of the electrodes hampered walking.

According to Kashi et al. (2012) [30], anodal tDCS induces changes in the excitability of the motor cortex referring to the lower limbs, with a consequent improvement in gait. Minhas et al. (2012) [26] carried out studies involving the administration of tDCS to children and found that the method is safe, but the current needs to be adjusted from 2 mA, which is used for adults, to 1 mA for children.

As a relatively new technique, few studies have employed tDCS on children with CP. Findings reported in the literature regard the use of transcranial magnetic stimulation as a method for analyzing the evoked potential [31] and cortex map [15]. This method has also been used to reduce spasticity in children with CP [32] in one or both hemispheres [15].

No studies were found addressing the effects of anodal tDCS over M1 on motor function or the combined use of tDCS and physical therapy, such as during gait training. Moreover, a limited number of studies discuss important clinical differences in CP, especially with regard to body sway and functional independence. For the present study, the findings described by Grecco et al. (2013) [20], who used the same treadmill training protocol, were considered clinically relevant.

The authors found no consensus in the literature or studies that specifically address a minimum difference that could be considered clinically important in the population with CP. However, as the present study involved a short intervention (2 weeks), the positive effect regarding the variables analyzed in the experimental group (gait training combined with anodal tDCS) at the follow up evaluation can be considered clinically important. The positive change in the PBS score in the experimental group allows one to infer that the quality of movement was optimized in these children. Indeed, the results demonstrate the effect size on functional balance in the experimental group vs. the control group at Evaluation 2 (5.6) and Evaluation 3 (5.2).

The findings of the present study demonstrate that the combination of treadmill training and anodal stimulation of the primary motor cortex in the dominant hemisphere was capable of potentiating improvements in static and functional balance in the children with cerebral palsy analyzed. Moreover, anodal stimulation favored the maintenance of the gains one month following the completion of the intervention. However, as this was a phase 2 study with a small sample size, further investigations with a larger number of participants and longer follow-up period are needed to confirm the results.

Author Contributions

Conceived and designed the experiments: ND LG MG FF CO. Performed the experiments: ND LG MG FF CO. Analyzed the data: ND LG MG FF CO. Contributed reagents/materials/analysis tools: ND LG MG FF CO. Wrote the paper: ND LG MG FF CO.

References

1. Burton H, Sachin D, Litkowski P, Wingert JR (2009) Functional connectivity for somatosensory and motor cortex in spastic diplegia. Somatosens Mot Res 26: 90–104.
2. Inder TE, Huppi PS, Warfield S, Kikinis R, Zientara GP, et al. (1999) Periventricular white injury in the premature infant is followed by reduced cerebral cortical gray matter volume at term. Ann Neurol 46:755–760.
3. Kurz MJ, Wilson TW (2011) Neuromagnetic activity in the somatosensory cortices if children with cerebral palsy. Neurosci Let 490:1-5.
4. Shin YK, Lee DR, Hwang HJ, You SJ (2012) A novel EEG-based brain mapping to determine cortical activation patterns in normal children and children with cerebral palsy during motor imagery tasks. NeuroRehabil 31: 349–55.
5. Rose S, Guzzetta A, Pannek K, Boyd R (2011) MRI structural connectivity, disruption of primary sensorimotor pathways, and hand function in cerebral palsy. Brain Connect 1: 309–16.
6. Chagas PSC, Mancini MC, Barbosa A, Silva PTG (2004) Análise das intervenções utilizadas para a promoção da marcha em crianças portadoras de paralisia cerebral: uma revisão sistemática da literatura. Rev Bras Fisioter 8: 155–63.
7. Pitcher JB, Schmeider LA, Burns NR, Drysdale JL, Higgins RD, et al. (2012) Reduced corticomotor excitability and motor skills development in children born preterm. J Physiol 590: 5827–44.
8. Nevalainen P, Pihko E, Maenpaa H, Valanne L, Nummenmaa L, et al. (2012) Bilateral alterations in somatosensory cortical processing in hemiplegic cerebral palsy. Dev Med Child Neurol 54:361–7.
9. Grecco LAC, Zanon N, Sampaio LMM, Oliveira CS (2013) A comparison of treadmill training and overground walking in ambulant children with cerebral palsy: randomized controlled clinical Trial. Clin Rehabil 27:674.
10. Rose J, Wolff DR, Jones VK, Bloch DA, Oehlert JW, et al. (2002) Postural balance in children with cerebral palsy. Dev Med Child Neurol 44:58–63.
11. Grecco LA, Tomita SM, Christovão TC, Pasini H, Sampaio LM, et al. (2013) Effect of treadmill gait training on static and functional balance in children with cerebral palsy: a randomized controlled trial. Rev Bras Fisioter 17:17–23.
12. Miranda PC, Lomarev M, Hallett M (2006) Modeling the current distribution during transcranial direct current stimulation. Clin Neurophysiol 117:1623–9.
13. Morris ME, Iansek R, Smithson F, Huxham F (2000) Postural instability in parkinson's disease: a comparison with and without a concurrent task. Gait and Posture 12: 205–216.
14. Dinomais M, Lignon G, Chinier E, Richard I, Ter MInassian A, et al. (2013) Effect of observation of simple hand movement on brain activations in patients with unilateral cerebral palsy: an fMRI study. Res Dev Disabil 34:1928–37.
15. Kesar TM, Sawaki L, Burdette JH, Cabrera MN, Kolaski K, et al. (2012) Motor cortical functional geometry in cerebral palsy and its relationship to disability. Clin Neurophysiol 123:1383–90.
16. Marchese R, Diverio M, Zucchi F, Lentino C, Abbruzzese G (2000) The role of sensory cues in the rehabilitation of parkisonian patients: a comparison of two physical therapy protocols. Movement Disorders 15: 879–883.
17. Wagner T, Fregni F, Fecteau S, Grodzinsky A, Zahn M, et al. (2007) Transcranial direct current stimulation: A computer-based human model study. Neuroimage 35:1113–24.
18. Mendonça ME, Fregni F (2012) Neuromodulação com estimulação cerebral não invasiva: aplicação no acidente vascular encefálico, doença de Parkinson e dor crônica. In:ASSIS, R.D. Manole. Condutas práticas em fisioterapia neurológica. São Paulo, p. 307–39.
19. Ries LGK, Michaelsen Soares PSA, Monteiro VC, Allegretti KMG (2012) Adaptação cultural e análise da confiabilidade da versão brasileira da Escala de Equilíbrio Pediátrica (EEP). Rev Bras Fisioter 16:205–215.
20. Grecco LAC, Duarte NAC, Mendonça ME, Pasini H, Lima VLCC, et al. (2013) Effect of transcranial direct current stimulation combined with gait and mobility training on functionality in children with cerebral palsy: study protocol for a double-blind randomized controlled clinical trial. BMC Pediatrics 13:168.
21. Moher D, Hopewell S, Schulz KF, Montori V, Gøtzsche PC, et al. (2010) CONSORT 2010 Explanation and Elaboration: updated guidelines for reporting parallel group randomised trial. J Clin Epi 63:e1–e37.
22. Feldman AB, Haley SM, Corvell J (1990) Concurrent and construct validity of the Pediatric Evaluation of Disability Inventory. Phys Ther 70:602–10.
23. Haley SM, Coster J, Faas RM (1991) A content validity study of the Pediatric Evaluation of Disability Inventory. Pediatr Phys Ther 3:177–84.
24. Homan RW, Herman J, Purdy P (1987) Cerebral location of international 10–20 system electrode placement. Electroencephalogr Clin Neurophysiol 66:376–82.
25. Sadeghi H, Allard P, Prince H, Labelle H (2000) Symmetry and limb dominance in able-bodied gait: a review. Gait & Posture 12:34–45.
26. Minhas P, Bikson M, Woods AJ, Rosen AR, Kessler SK (2012) Transcranial direct current stimulation in pediatric brain: A computational modeling study. Conf Proc IEEE Eng Med Biol Soc: 859–862
27. Stagg CJ, Bachtiar V, O'Shea J, Allman C, Bosnell RA, et al. (2012) Cortical activation changes underlying stimulation induced behavioral gains in chronic stroke. Brain 135: 276–84.
28. Kashi D, Dominguez RO, Allum JH, Bronstein AM (2013) Improving gait and balance in patients with leukoaraiosis using transcranial direct current stimulation and physical training: An exploratory study. Neurorehabil Neural Repair 27:864–71.
29. Liebetanz D, Nitsche MA, Tergau F, Paulus W (2002) Pharmacological approach to the mechanism of transcranial DC stimulation induced after effects of human motor cortex excitability. Brain 125:2238–47.
30. Kashi D, Quadir S, Patel M, Yousif N, Bronstein AM (2012) Enhanced locomotor adaptation after effect in the "broken escalator" phenomenon using anodal tDCS. J Neurophysiol 107:2493–2505.
31. Garvey MA, Mall V (2008) Transcranial magnetic stimulation in children. Clin. Neurophysiol 119:973–84.
32. Valle AC, Dionisio K, Pitskel NB, Pascual-Leone A, Orsati F, et al. (2007) Low and high frequency repetitive transcranial magnetic stimulation for the treatment of spasticity. Dev Med Child Neurol 49:534–8.

22

Clinical Effectiveness of Protein and Amino Acid Supplementation on Building Muscle Mass in Elderly People

Zhe-rong Xu[1], Zhong-ju Tan[1], Qin Zhang[1], Qi-feng Gui[1], Yun-mei Yang[2]*

1 Department of Geriatrics, First Affiliated Hospital, School of Medicine, Zhejiang University, Hangzhou, China, **2** State Key Laboratory for Diagnosis and Treatment of Infectious Diseases, Department of Geriatrics, First Affiliated Hospital, School of Medicine, Zhejiang University, Hangzhou, China

Abstract

Objective: A major reason for the loss of mobility in elderly people is the gradual loss of lean body mass known as sarcopenia. Sarcopenia is associated with a lower quality of life and higher healthcare costs. The benefit of strategies that include nutritional intervention, timing of intervention, and physical exercise to improve muscle loss unclear as finding from studies investigating this issue have been inconsistent. We have performed a systematic review and meta-analysis to assess the ability of protein or amino acid supplementation to augment lean body mass or strength of leg muscles in elderly patients.

Methods: Nine studies met the inclusion criteria of being a prospective comparative study or randomized controlled trial (RCT) that compared the efficacy of an amino acid or protein supplement intervention with that of a placebo in elderly people ($\geq$65 years) for the improvement of lean body mass (LBM), leg muscle strength or reduction associated with sarcopenia.

Results: The overall difference in mean change from baseline to the end of study in LBM between the treatment and placebo groups was 0.34 kg which was not significant (P = 0.386). The overall differences in mean change from baseline in double leg press and leg extension were 2.14 kg (P = 0.748) and 2.28 kg (P = 0.265), respectively, between the treatment group and the placebo group.

Conclusions: These results indicate that amino acid/protein supplements did not increase lean body mass gain and muscle strength significantly more than placebo in a diverse elderly population.

Editor: Conrad P. Earnest, Texas A&M University, United States of America

Funding: The authors have no support or funding to report.

Competing Interests: The authors have declared that no competing interests exist.

* Email: gbbf2000@sina.com

Introduction

Sarcopenia is an age related loss of muscle mass and strength, and is associated with a lower quality of life resulting from a reduced ability to perform daily living tasks [1]. Sarcopenia results in increased healthcare costs of approximately $900 per elderly adult which in the USA is approximately $18.5 billion per year [2]. Prevalence of sarcopenia differs by gender, living circumstances, and continent: 13.2% of Chinese men and 4.8% of Chinese women who are $\geq$70 years of age have sarcopenia, while 45–70% and 7–17.5% of American men and 2%–59% and 4–10% of American women have sarcopenia, respectively [3]. Age-related muscle loss is highly prevalent in nursing homes, with rates being as high as 68% in elderly men and 21% in elderly females [4], whereas community dwelling elderly have lower prevalence rates in males (10%) but higher rates in women (33%) [5].

Inadequate nutrition, oxidative stress, low physical activity levels, inflammation, and reduced hormone concentrations contribute to age related muscle loss [6]. Possible strategies that reliably increase muscle mass and strength in the elderly have been

actively investigated, but conclusions on the benefits of different nutritional interventions, timing of administration, and physical exercise from studies have been conflicting [7–20].

Several nutritional interventions such as creatine monohydrate, whey protein, caseinate, and essential amino acids appear to augment protein synthesis in muscles [1,21,22]. Numerous studies have found that these nutritional supplements enhance the magnitude of gain in lean body mass and muscle strength in older adults undergoing exercise training [1,6,15]. Essential amino acid and leucine supplementation have increased protein synthesis in muscles and are thought to be better strategies for offsetting muscle loss than intact protein [7,16,22–24], due in part to their higher absorption [22]. However, several studies that compared the effect of whey protein or amino acid supplementation on skeletal muscle mass, lean body mass, or strength in healthy elderly to that of placebos have not detected a significant difference between the two groups [8,17].

Many of the studies evaluating the impact of protein or amino acid supplementation on sarcopenia have been small and

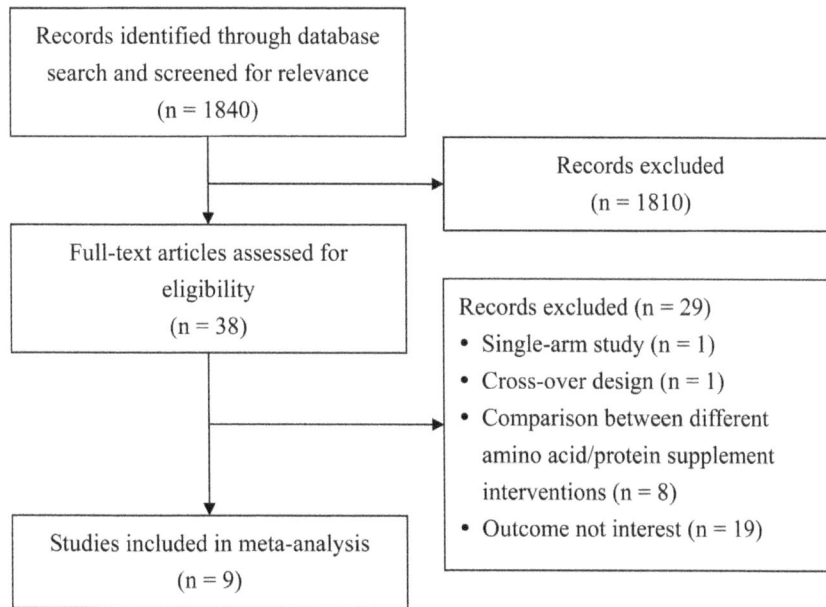

Figure 1. Flow diagram of study selection.

evaluated different supplements. In order to maximize the biostatical power of placebo controlled clinical trials, we have performed a meta-analysis to assess the ability of protein or amino acid supplementation to augment lean body mass or strength of leg muscles in elderly patients.

Experimental Methods

PubMed, Google Scholar, The Cochrane Library, EMBASE, and ClinicalTrials.gov were searched from inception to 13 Jun 2014 using combinations of the following terms: aging, elder, older, muscle loss or muscular atrophy, protein, amino acid. Inclusion criteria for the meta-analysis required that an article be published in a peer-reviewed reviewed journal that described a prospective study or randomized controlled trial (RCT) which compared the efficacy of an amino acid or protein supplement with placebo in improving lean body mass, leg muscle strength in elderly people ($\geq$65 years of age). Single group uncontrolled studies, cross sectional studies, or retrospective studies were excluded. Studies published as letters, comments, editorials, or case reports were also excluded, as well as studies that included people <65 years of age. We utilized the Delphi list to assess the quality of the included studies [25].

Data extraction

Full text articles for the relevant titles were assessed for eligibility which included studies that measured changes in lean body mass (LBM), and may have included evaluation of muscle strength of leg extension and double leg press. Two independent reviewers (coders) extracted the following information from each eligible study: cited reference, type of study, type and duration of interventions, participant number in the intervention and placebo groups, demographics of participants (age, sex, mean body mass index [BMI]), and mean values of the outcome measures (LBM, muscle strength in double leg press, muscle strength in leg extension) at baseline and post intervention. In case of a disagreement, a third reviewer resolved the issue.

To assess coder drift, agreement between coders was calculated by dividing the number of variables coded the same by the total number of variables. Mean agreement of $\geq$0.90 was considered to be acceptable.

Biostatistics

Treatment effectiveness was evaluated by comparison of LBM (primary outcome) and muscle strength of double leg press and leg extension (secondary outcomes) in elderly subjects at baseline and after nutritional intervention for 6 months (24 weeks). For treatment consistency, only studies providing protein supplementation were considered for meta-analysis. The means with standard deviations (SD) for the LBM, mean muscle strength (leg press and leg extension) were calculated for each group at baseline and post study completion. The difference in mean change (from baseline to end of study) with 95% confidence interval (95% CI) was calculated as the mean change of the protein intervention (treatment group) minus mean change of the placebo or non-nutritious supplements (control group) for each outcome.

Heterogeneity was determined by calculating Cochran Q and the I^2 statistic. The Q statistic indicated statistically significant heterogeneity at $P<0.10$. The I^2 statistic reflected the percentage of the observed between-study variability and provided a scale of heterogeneity: 0 to 24% = no heterogeneity; 25 to 49% = moderate heterogeneity; 50 to 74% = large heterogeneity; and 75 to 100% = extreme heterogeneity. If heterogeneity existed between studies (a Q statistic with $P<0.1$ or an I^2 statistic >50%), we performed the random-effects model (DerSimonian-Laird method). Otherwise, the fixed-effects model was recommended (Mantel-Haenszel method). Combined difference in mean change from baseline to end of study was calculated and a 2-sided P value <0.05 was considered to indicate statistical significance. Sensitivity analysis was performed using the leave-one-out approach. Publication bias was only assessed for lean body mass by constructing funnel plots and exacerbations rate by Egger's test. The absence of publication bias is indicated by the data points forming a symmetric funnel-shaped distribution and one-tailed significance level $P>0.05$ in Egger's test. All statistical analyses

Table 1. Quality assessment of the 9 studies included in the systematic review and meta-analysis as determined using the Delphi List.

Author (Year)	Was a method of randomization used?	Were the groups similar at baseline regarding the most important prognostic indicators?	Were the eligibility criteria specified?	Was the outcome assessor blinded?	Was the care provider blinded?	Was the patient blinded?	Were point estimate and measures of variability presented for the primary outcome measures?	Did the analysis include an intention-to-treat analysis?
Daly et al [27]	Yes	Yes	Yes	No	No	Yes	Yes	Yes
Vermeeren et al [28]	Yes	Yes	Yes	Yes	Yes	Yes	Yes	No
Chale et al [8]	Yes	Yes	Yes	Yes	Yes	Yes	Yes	Yes
Alemán-Mateo et al [29]	Yes	Yes	Yes	Yes	No	No	Yes	Yes
Tieland et al [20]	Yes	Yes	Yes	Yes	Yes	Yes	Yes	Yes
Tieland et al [26]	Yes	Yes	Yes	Yes	Yes	Yes	Yes	Yes
Leenders et al [19]	Yes	Yes	Yes	Yes	Yes	Yes	Yes	No
Ferrando et al [18]	Yes	Gender different, others similar	Yes	No	No	Yes	Yes	No
Verhoeven et al [17]	Yes	Yes	Yes	Yes	ND	Yes	Yes	No

ND, not described.

Study name	Comparison	Difference in means	Lower limit	Upper limit	Z-Value	P-Value
Daly et al (2014)	Protein vs. Control	0.50	-0.46	1.46	1.02	0.310
Vermeeren et al (2014)	Protein vs. Control	-0.10	-1.62	1.42	-0.13	0.897
Chale et al (2013)	Protein vs. Control	0.30	-3.55	4.15	0.15	0.879
Aleman-Mateo et al (2012)	Protein vs. Control	0.00	-3.97	3.97	0.00	1.000
Tieland et al (2012)a	Protein vs. Control	0.10	-4.63	4.83	0.04	0.967
Tieland et al (2012)b	Protein vs. Control	1.60	-3.46	6.66	0.62	0.535
		0.34	-0.42	1.10	0.87	0.386

Heterogeneity test: Q=0.71, df = 5, P = 0.982, I-square =0.00%

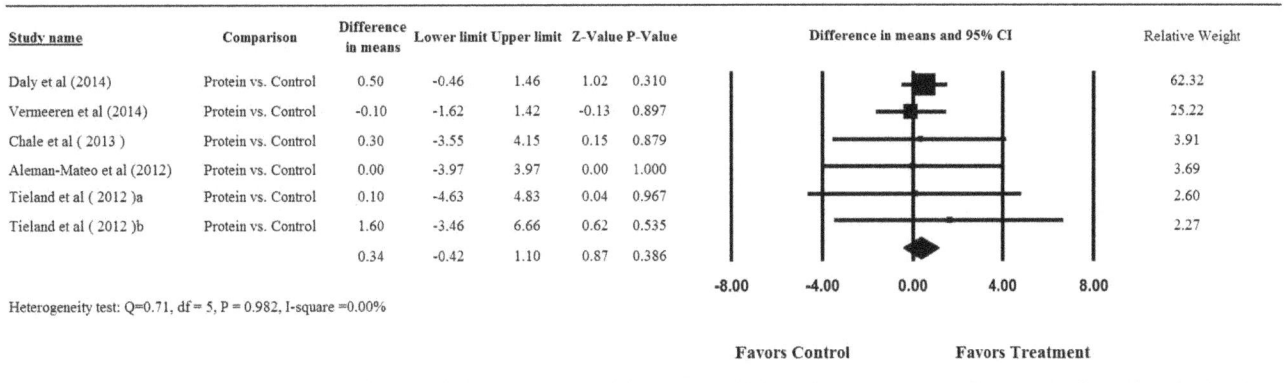

Figure 2. Forest plot showing results for the meta-analysis of difference in mean change from baseline in lean-body-mass after intervention: treatment vs. control. Abbreviation: CI, confidence interval.

were performed using the statistical software Comprehensive Meta-Analysis, version 2.0 (Biostat, Englewood, NJ, USA).

Results

Out of 1840 studies identified by the data base searches, 38 were screened for eligibility, and 29 were excluded for one of the following reasons: no comparison group (n = 1), no placebo (n = 8), cross over design (n = 1) or no value for mean muscle mass or leg muscle strength (n = 19) (Figure 1). Nine prospective studies met the inclusion criteria (Figure 1) [8,17–20,26–29].

All but one of the studies [18] were at least 75% compliant with the Delphi list (Table 1). Eight of the 9 studies were randomized, placebo-controlled clinical trials [8,17,19,20,26–29]. Five of the trials included an intention-to-treat analysis [8,20,26,27,29]. The 75%–100% compliance levels of 8 of the 9 studies to the Delphi criteria suggest that the studies provided high quality evidence. Coder drift was calculated to be 0.93, indicating satisfactory reliability between coders.

The number of total participants in all 9 studies who had taken the intervention was 267 (range, 10 to 53) and who had received placebo were 244 (range, 11 to 47). Six of the 9 studies provided a protein supplement (whey) to 203 elderly participants and placebo to 191 elderly subjects (controls) [8,20,26–29], 2 studies supplied leucine supplementation to 54 elderly participants and placebo to 42 controls [17,19], and one provided essential amino acids (EAA) to 10 elderly participants and 11 controls [18] (Table 2). The duration of intervention ranged from 10 days to 6 months (Table 2).

Lean Body Mass

Among the 6 studies with protein supplementation [8,20,26–29], three reported that nutritional supplementation significantly increased LBM in the elderly compared to placebo [8,26,27]. Two studies observed a significantly greater LBM in both the placebo and nutritional intervention groups [829]. Pooling of data from the 6 studies revealed no heterogeneity (Q = 0.71, df = 5, P = 0.982; $I^2 = 0.0\%$); therefore, a fixed-effects model was used to assess the difference in mean change in LBM from baseline to end of study between the placebo and protein supplementation groups. The difference in mean change of LBM from baseline to end of study between the placebo and protein supplementation groups ranged from −0.1 to 1.60 kg. The overall difference in mean change in LBM between treatment intervention and placebo was 0.34 kg

which was not significant (95% CI = −0.42 to 1.10 kg, P = 0.386, Figure 2).

We compared the health status of the participants in the 9 studies to determine whether the health status of the elderly correlated with the greater gain in LBM. No significant gains in LBM compared to the controls were observed in subjects with diabetes [19], chronic obstructive pulmonary disease [29], limited mobility, who were sedentary [8], moderately active [18], or healthy and independent [17] (Table 3).

Muscle strength: double leg press

Five of the 9 studies assessed the effect of nutritional intervention on muscle strength be double leg press [8,17,19,20,26]. Three of 5 studies reported that the strength of the leg press significantly increased in both placebo and intervention groups during the duration of the study and the mean change was similar in both groups [8]. Two studies reported no significant change in the strength of the leg press with respect to treatment time or group [17,20].

Three studies were included in the analysis of the influence of protein supplements on leg strength [8,20,26]. No heterogeneity was found among 3 studies (Q = 0.147, df = 2, P = 0.929; $I^2 = 0.0\%$); and the fixed-effects model revealed no significant difference in mean change in muscle strength by double leg press between the placebo and treatment groups. The difference in mean change from baseline to end of study ranged from −1.00 to 5 kg, with the overall difference in mean change being 2.14 kg (95% CI = −10.92 to 15.20 kg, P = 0.748, Figure 3A).

Muscle strength: leg extension

Six studies evaluated the effect of nutritional intervention on muscle strength by comparing leg extension muscle strength between the intervention and placebo groups [17,19,20,26–28]. Five of the 6 studies reported that the strength of the leg extension significantly increased in both groups during the duration of the study [8,19,26–28]. Two studies reported no significant change in the strength of the leg extension versus treatment time or group [17,20].

Among the 6 studies with protein supplementation, 2 did not provide the mean muscle strength of leg extension for both groups at baseline and at completion of study [8,17], hence the meta-analysis included 4 studies [20,26,28]. Since moderate heterogeneity was found among the studies (Q = 4.52, df = 3, P = 0.210; $I^2 = 33.66\%$), a fixed-effects model was used for the meta-analysis.

Table 2. Characteristics of studies included in the systematic review and meta-analysis.

Author (Year)	Study type	Comparison	Duration of Intervention	Number of cases	Mean Age (year)	Sex (Male %)	Mean BMI (kg/m²)	Lean body mass (kg)		Muscle strength (kg), double leg press		Muscle strength (kg), leg extension	
								Before	After	Before	After	Before	After
Daly et al [27]	RCT	Protein vs Control	4 months	53 vs 47	72 vs 74	0 v. 0	28 vs 28	0.6 (0.3, 0.8)* vs 0.1 (−0.4, 1.1)*	—	NA	NA	28 (18, 39)* vs 10 (−1, 21)*	NA
Vermeeren et al [28]	RCT	Protein vs Control	mean 9 days	23 vs 24	66 vs 65	61 vs 75	20 vs 21	Mean change from baseline: 0.5±2.6 vs −0.4±2.7		NA	NA	Mean change from baseline: 3±8 vs 2±9	
Chale et al [8]	RCT	Protein vs Control	6 months	42 vs 38	78 vs 77.3	40 vs 42	27 vs 26.9	46.7±8.6 vs 46.4±8.4	47.3±8.6 vs 46.7±8.4	125±39 vs 128±47	151±58 vs 149±54	NA	NA
Alemán-Mateo et al [29]	RCT	Protein vs Control	3 months	20 vs 20	75 vs 77	40 vs 45	27 vs 26	37.1±6.3 vs 36.8±6.4	37.9±6.5 vs 37.6±6.4	NA	NA	NA	NA
Tieland et al [20]	RCT	Protein vs Control	24 weeks	34 vs 31	78 vs 81	41.2 vs 48.9	27 vs 26.2	45.8±9.9 vs 46.7±9.5	45.8±9.9 vs 46.6±9.5	118±47 vs 124±50	136±47 vs 139±50	57±29 vs 57±28	68±29 vs 63±28
Tieland et al [26]	RCT	Protein vs Control	24 weeks	31 vs 31	78 vs 79	35 vs 32	28.7 vs 28.2	47.2±9.6 vs 45.7±8.9	48.5±9.4 vs 45.4±8.9	124±39 vs 116±36	169±39 vs 162±41	56±17 vs 58±17	77±18 vs 79±18
Leenders et al [19]	RCT	Leucine vs Control	24 weeks	39 vs 28	71 vs 71	100 vs 100	27.4 vs 27.2	61.9±6.9 vs 62.2±6.9	62.0±6.2 vs 62.2±6.9	202±44 vs 205±37	217±50 vs 218±42	80±12 vs 88±16	84±19 vs 94±21
Ferrando et al [18]	RCT	Amino acid vs Control	10 days	10 vs 11	71 vs 68	10 vs 50	NA	43.0±0.6 vs 46.8±1.0	42.1±0.6 vs 45.3±1.0	NA	NA	NA	NA
Verhoeven et al [17]	RCT	Leucine vs Control	12 weeks	15 vs 14	NA	100 vs 100	25.9 vs 26.3	54.6±5.8 vs 55.8±3.4	55.0±5.8 vs 56.2±4.1	170±8 vs 172±6	NA	85±3 vs 85±3	NA

NA, not available; RCT: randomized controlled trial.
*values are within-group mean absolutes of the change from baseline with 95% confidence intervals in parentheses.

Table 3. Summary of 9 trials included in the systematic review and meta-analysis.

Author (Year)	Condition of elderly	Supplement given	Significant increased LBM to baseline	Significant increased Leg press to baseline	Significant increased Leg extension to baseline	Significant increased Physical performance
Daly et al [27]	Healthy	Max.45 g protein/twice daily	Significant increased in protein group, different between groups	ND	Significant increased in protein group, different between groups	Significant increased in both group, similar between groups
Vermeeren et al [28]	COPD	125 ml/three times daily	Neither group	ND	Neither group	ND
Chale et al [8]	Mobility limited	20 g protein/day twice daily	Both groups improved, and also significant different between groups	Both groups to baseline	Both groups to baseline	Significant for whey group
Alemán-Mateo et al [29]	Healthy	15 g protein/day	Both groups improved, but no significant different between groups	ND	ND	ND
Tieland et al [20]	Pre-frail and frail	15 g protein twice daily	Neither group	Both groups to baseline	Both groups to baseline	Both groups
Tieland et al [26]	Pre-frail and frail	15 g protein twice daily	Significant increased in protein group, different between groups	Neither group	Trend toward significant improvement in protein group vs control.	Significant improvement in protein group vs control.
Leenders et al [19]	Type 2 diabetes	2.5 g leucine three times daily	None	Increased vs time in both groups, similar between groups	Increased vs time in both groups, similar between groups	ND
Ferrando et al [18]	Moderately active	15 g EAA three times daily	None	ND	ND	Increased vs time in both groups, similar between groups
Verhoeven et al [17]	Healthy	2.5 g leucine three times daily	None vs time or groups	None vs time or groups	None vs time or groups	ND

COPD, chronic obstructive pulmonary disease; EAA, essential amino acids; LBM, lean body mass; ND, not described.

The difference in mean change from baseline to end of study in the 4 studies ranged from 0 to 18 kg with the overall difference in mean change from baseline to end of study being 2.28 kg (95% CI = −1.73 to 6.29 kg, P = 0.265, Figure 3B). The combined difference in mean change of muscle strength by leg extension from baseline to end of study revealed no significant difference between the control and treatment groups.

Sensitivity analysis

To assess the effect of a single study on the results of the meta-analysis, we removed each study in turn for LBM (Figure 4A), muscle strength by double leg press (Figure 4B), and muscle strength by leg extension (Figure 4C). The removal of any study did not alter the magnitude and direction; taken together, these results indicated that the meta-analysis showed good reliability.

Publication Bias

Publication bias (Figure 5) was assessed using the LBM results only as more than 5 studies reported results for this outcome (note: more than five studies are required to detect funnel plot asymmetry [30]). Egger's test results showed that there was no publication bias in LBM results among studies (Figure 5, t = 0.046, one-tailed P = 0.483).

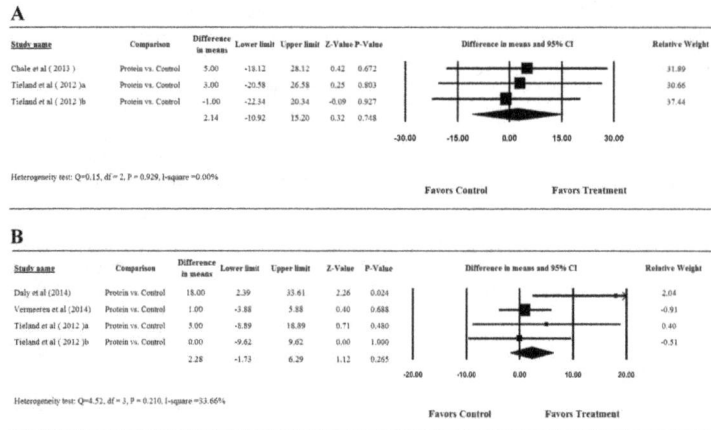

Figure 3. Forest plot showing results for the meta-analysis of difference in mean change from baseline in (A) muscle strength of double leg press and (B) muscle strength of leg extension after intervention: treatment vs. control. Abbreviation: CI, confidence interval.

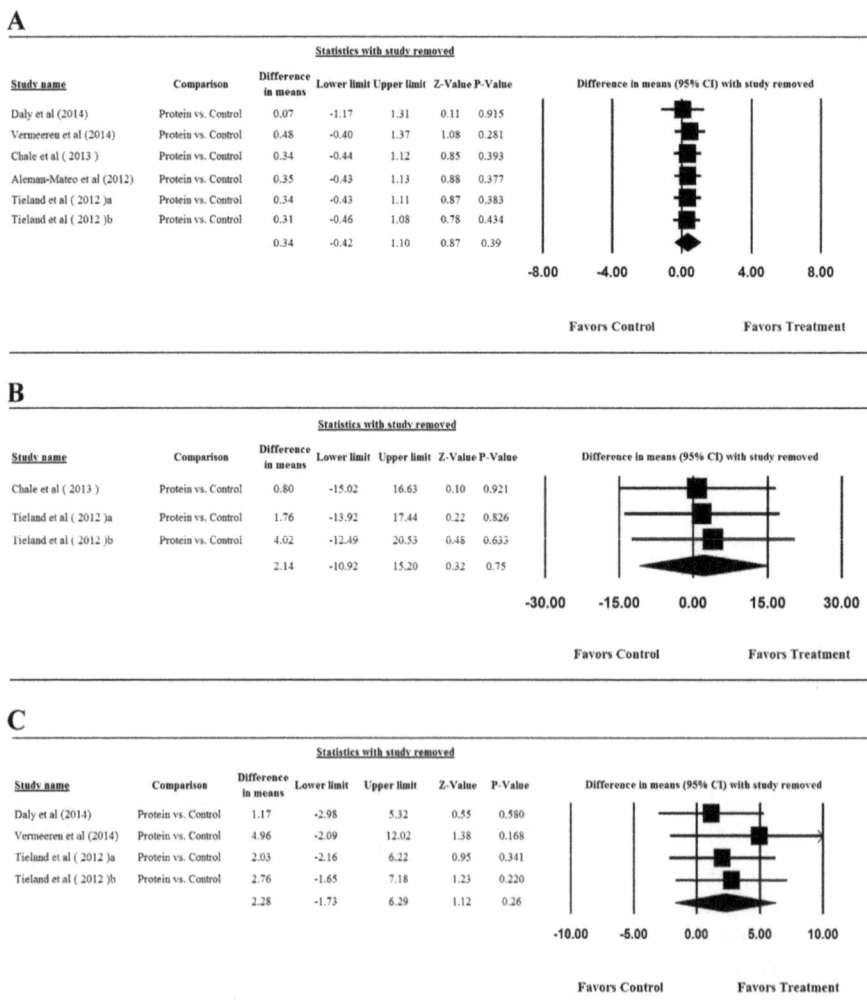

Figure 4. Results of sensitivity analysis to examine the influence of individual studies on pooled estimates as determined using the leave-one-out approach: (A) lean-body-mass; (B) muscle strength of double leg press. Abbreviation: CI, confidence interval.

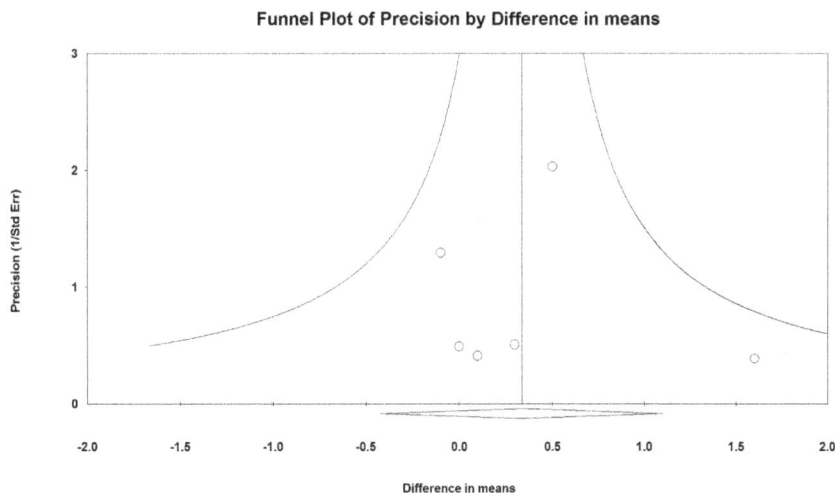

Figure 5. Funnel plot for the assessment of publication bias for studies included in the meta-analysis of the assessment of the mean change from baseline in lean body mass after intervention.

Discussion

This meta-analysis of 9 placebo-controlled studies assessed protein and amino acid supplementation on improving LBM in elderly subjects. Our analysis detected no significant differences between placebo and treatment groups in mean change from baseline to the end of the studies of LBM or muscle strength as measured by double leg press or leg extension in a mixed elderly population.

Multiple studies, several of which were included in our meta-analysis, found no significant benefit of protein supplementation compared to placebo in improving LBM [8,20,26–29,31]. However, protein supplementation has increased LBM and strength in some studies [32]. This inconsistency raises questions of whether it may be due to differences in study design, difference in efficacy of the supplements tested, or differences among the populations analyzed. Identification of the variables that influence the outcome of high protein intake towards a significant increase in LBM or leg strength would provide important guidance for physicians and for cost effective usage of protein supplementation.

The health and physical status of the patient may influence outcomes. Physical condition may affect response to protein or amino acid supplementation. One study showed that whey supplementation augmented LBM significantly more than placebo in pre-frail and frail elderly subjects receiving resistance training [20] but not in another study of elderly subjects with limited mobility that also received protein supplements and resistance training [8]. These findings suggest that the physical condition of the elderly is not solely responsible for the divergent results. Undernourishment may be another condition that significantly affects the outcome [33]. An earlier meta-analysis showed that protein supplementation induced significant weight gain in undernourished elderly subjects and may reduce mortality [33]. In addition, some elderly subjects may have reduced sensitivity to the amino acid induced anabolic signals and thus have a higher propensity to muscle wasting [21]. Addition of leucine appeared to normalize these anabolic signals [14,32]. The health status or stage of the skeletal muscle (whether the person does or does not have sarcopenia) may also affect their ability to respond to protein or amino acid supplementation.

The provided supplement or its dosage also may impact treatment outcomes since supplementation with essential amino acid was not as efficacious in increasing LBM in elderly subjects as whey protein in a direct comparison [32]. Both whey and caseinate supplementation induced a similar increase in protein synthesis after heavy resistance training in healthy elderly participants [12]. Interestingly, a fortified, hydrolyzed collagen protein supplement added to a relatively low-protein diet maintained LBM to a greater extent than whey protein [34]. In some studies [7,11,13], supplementation with essential amino acids improved LBM or muscle protein synthesis rate in elderly subjects; however, another study did not find any benefit of supplementing with amino acids [14].

Loss of muscle tissue or development of sarcopenia is accelerated by bed rest and lack of physical activity [23]. The elderly in the Tieland et al study [26] performed resistance-type exercise 2 times per week for 24 weeks and had a significant increase in LBM in the supplement group, whereas 5 of the included studies involved participants on bed rest [18], no exercise program [17,20,29], or patients who were hospitalized [28]. All participants in the study reported by Daly et al [27] performed resistance training. Consistent with the findings of Tieland et al [26], Daly et al [27] found that participants in supplement group had a significant increase in LBM compared with participants in the control group. The participants of the Chale et al study [8] also performed resistance training and both treatment and placebo groups had similar increases in LBM and leg muscle strength; although, the whey group showed a significant improvement in physical performance [8]. Similarly, in the study by Leenders et al [19] both treatment and control groups reported a mean of 1.55 h physical exercise daily and both groups had similar but significant increases in mean leg strength (both leg press and extension). The resistance training regimen in the study by Tieland et al [26] included several more types of exercises than that of Chale et al [8], while the training regimen in the study of Daly et al [27] involved progressive resistance training. Hence, the beneficial interaction between resistance training and whey protein supplementation on muscle mass and strength gain may depend to some extent on the type of resistance training regimen used. In support for the benefits of concurrent resistance training, a meta-analysis of six studies of older participants reported that protein supplementation augmented loss of fat free mass [35].

There are several limitations to this analysis that should be considered when interpreting the findings. There are a number of outcomes that this analysis did not assess primarily due to limitations of the included studies. These outcomes included (but are not limited to) gender, physical performance and activity, and muscle stage. We also included only RCT. Some non-RCT trials have been done that indicate protein or amino acid supplementation may improve LMB [36]. The relatively small number of included studies, the small subject populations, diverse supplements administered, different outcomes measured and study designs used in the 9 included studies further confounds the analysis. In particular, several studies incorporated exercise (for both intervention and control participants) as part of the study [8,26,27], while the others did not. Although our meta-analysis suggests that exercise had little effect on the change in LBM in the individual studies, this possibility clearly warrants examination in appropriately designed studies. In addition, it is not clear whether our findings will be applicable to elderly subjects who receive other types of supplements, had different exercise regimens, or health status than those used in the 9 included studies. The small number of RCTs that address the question of the use of protein or amino acid supplements to reduce muscle loss in elderly subjects highlights the need for more controlled studies to address this medically important question.

In conclusion, these results indicate that amino acid or protein supplements did not increase lean body mass gain and muscle strength significantly more than placebo in a diverse elderly population. The ability of protein or amino acid supplementation to augment muscle mass and strength may depend on the nutritional physical status of the participants, or their ability to digest protein and absorb the amino acids, the sensitivity of the anabolic pathways in muscles, and the resistance training regimen itself.

Author Contributions

Conceived and designed the experiments: ZRX YMY. Performed the experiments: QZ. Analyzed the data: QZ. Wrote the paper: QFG. Definition of intellectual content, literature research, data acquisition: ZJT. Manuscript preparation, literature research, guarantor of integrity of the entire study: ZRX.

References

1. Forbes SC, Little JP, Candow DG (2012) Exercise and nutritional interventions for improving aging muscle health. Endocrine 42: 29–38.
2. Janssen I, Shepard DS, Katzmarzyk PT, Roubenoff R (2004) The healthcare costs of sarcopenia in the United States. J Am Geriatr Soc 52: 80–85.
3. Cheng Q, Zhu X, Zhang X, Li H, Du Y, et al. (2014) A cross-sectional study of loss of muscle mass corresponding to sarcopenia in healthy Chinese men and women: reference values, prevalence, and association with bone mass. J Bone Miner Metab 32: 78–88.
4. Landi F, Liperoti R, Fusco D, Mastropaolo S, Quattrociocchi D, et al. (2012) Prevalence and risk factors of sarcopenia among nursing home older residents. J Gerontol A Biol Sci Med Sci 67: 48–55.
5. Masanes F, Culla A, Navarro-Gonzalez M, Navarro-Lopez M, Sacanella E, et al. (2012) Prevalence of sarcopenia in healthy community-dwelling elderly in an urban area of Barcelona (Spain). J Nutr Health Aging 16: 184–187.
6. Candow DG, Forbes SC, Little JP, Cornish SM, Pinkoski C, et al. (2012) Effect of nutritional interventions and resistance exercise on aging muscle mass and strength. Biogerontology 13: 345–358.
7. Dillon EL, Sheffield-Moore M, Paddon-Jones D, Gilkison C, Sanford AP, et al. (2009) Amino acid supplementation increases lean body mass, basal muscle protein synthesis, and insulin-like growth factor-I expression in older women. J Clin Endocrinol Metab 94: 1630–1637.
8. Chale A, Cloutier GJ, Hau C, Phillips EM, Dallal GE, et al. (2013) Efficacy of whey protein supplementation on resistance exercise-induced changes in lean mass, muscle strength, and physical function in mobility-limited older adults. J Gerontol A Biol Sci Med Sci 68: 682–690.
9. Fiatarone MA, O'Neill EF, Ryan ND, Clements KM, Solares GR, et al. (1994) Exercise training and nutritional supplementation for physical frailty in very elderly people. N Engl J Med 330: 1769–1775.
10. Groen BB, Res PT, Pennings B, Hertle E, Senden JM, et al. (2012) Intragastric protein administration stimulates overnight muscle protein synthesis in elderly men. Am J Physiol Endocrinol Metab 302: E52–60.
11. Baier S, Johannsen D, Abumrad N, Rathmacher JA, Nissen S, et al. (2009) Year-long changes in protein metabolism in elderly men and women supplemented with a nutrition cocktail of beta-hydroxy-beta-methylbutyrate (HMB), L-arginine, and L-lysine. JPEN J Parenter Enteral Nutr 33: 71–82.
12. Dideriksen KJ, Reitelseder S, Petersen SG, Hjort M, Helmark IC, et al. (2011) Stimulation of muscle protein synthesis by whey and caseinate ingestion after resistance exercise in elderly individuals. Scand J Med Sci Sports 21: e372–383.
13. Koopman R, Verdijk LB, Beelen M, Gorselink M, Kruseman AN, et al. (2008) Co-ingestion of leucine with protein does not further augment post-exercise muscle protein synthesis rates in elderly men. Br J Nutr 99: 571–580.
14. Koopman R, Verdijk L, Manders RJ, Gijsen AP, Gorselink M, et al. (2006) Co-ingestion of protein and leucine stimulates muscle protein synthesis rates to the same extent in young and elderly lean men. Am J Clin Nutr 84: 623–632.
15. Kim HK, Suzuki T, Saito K, Yoshida H, Kobayashi H, et al. (2012) Effects of exercise and amino acid supplementation on body composition and physical function in community-dwelling elderly Japanese sarcopenic women: a randomized controlled trial. J Am Geriatr Soc 60: 16–23.

16. Solerte SB, Gazzaruso C, Bonacasa R, Rondanelli M, Zamboni M, et al. (2008) Nutritional supplements with oral amino acid mixtures increases whole-body lean mass and insulin sensitivity in elderly subjects with sarcopenia. Am J Cardiol 101: 69E–77E.
17. Verhoeven S, Vanschoonbeek K, Verdijk LB, Koopman R, Wodzig WK, et al. (2009) Long-term leucine supplementation does not increase muscle mass or strength in healthy elderly men. Am J Clin Nutr 89: 1468–1475.
18. Ferrando AA, Paddon-Jones D, Hays NP, Kortebein P, Ronsen O, et al. (2010) EAA supplementation to increase nitrogen intake improves muscle function during bed rest in the elderly. Clin Nutr 29: 18–23.
19. Leenders M, Verdijk LB, van der Hoeven L, van Kranenburg J, Hartgens F, et al. (2011) Prolonged leucine supplementation does not augment muscle mass or affect glycemic control in elderly type 2 diabetic men. J Nutr 141: 1070–1076.
20. Tieland M, van de Rest O, Dirks ML, van der Zwaluw N, Mensink M, et al. (2012) Protein supplementation improves physical performance in frail elderly people: a randomized, double-blind, placebo-controlled trial. J Am Med Dir Assoc 13: 720–726.
21. Cuthbertson D, Smith K, Babraj J, Leese G, Waddell T, et al. (2005) Anabolic signaling deficits underlie amino acid resistance of wasting, aging muscle. FASEB J 19: 422–424.
22. Paddon-Jones D, Sheffield-Moore M, Katsanos CS, Zhang XJ, Wolfe RR (2006) Differential stimulation of muscle protein synthesis in elderly humans following isocaloric ingestion of amino acids or whey protein. Exp Gerontol 41: 215–219.
23. Phillips SM (2012) Nutrient-rich meat proteins in offsetting age-related muscle loss. Meat Sci 92: 174–178.
24. Leenders M, van Loon LJ (2011) Leucine as a pharmaconutrient to prevent and treat sarcopenia and type 2 diabetes. Nutr Rev 69: 675–689.
25. Verhagen AP, de Vet HC, de Bie RA, Kessels AG, Boers M, et al. (1998) The Delphi list: a criteria list for quality assessment of randomized clinical trials for conducting systematic reviews developed by Delphi consensus. J Clin Epidemiol 51: 1235–1241.
26. Tieland M, Dirks ML, van der Zwaluw N, Verdijk LB, van de Rest O, et al. (2012) Protein supplementation increases muscle mass gain during prolonged resistance-type exercise training in frail elderly people: a randomized, double-blind, placebo-controlled trial. J Am Med Dir Assoc 13: 713–719.
27. Daly RM, O'Connell SL, Mundell NL, Grimes CA, Dunstan DW, et al. (2014) Protein-enriched diet, with the use of lean red meat, combined with progressive resistance training enhances lean tissue mass and muscle strength and reduces circulating IL-6 concentrations in elderly women: a cluster randomized controlled trial. Am J Clin Nutr 99: 899–910.
28. Vermeeren MA, Wouters EF, Geraerts-Keeris AJ, Schols AM (2004) Nutritional support in patients with chronic obstructive pulmonary disease during hospitalization for an acute exacerbation; a randomized controlled feasibility trial. Clin Nutr 23: 1184–1192.
29. Aleman-Mateo H, Macias L, Esparza-Romero J, Astiazaran-Garcia H, Blancas AL (2012) Physiological effects beyond the significant gain in muscle mass in sarcopenic elderly men: evidence from a randomized clinical trial using a protein-rich food. Clin Interv Aging 7: 225–234.

30. Sutton AJ, Duval SJ, Tweedie RL, Abrams KR, Jones DR (2000) Empirical assessment of effect of publication bias on meta-analyses. BMJ 320: 1574–1577.

31. Nissen SL, Sharp RL (2003) Effect of dietary supplements on lean mass and strength gains with resistance exercise: a meta-analysis. J Appl Physiol (1985) 94: 651–659.

32. Katsanos CS, Chinkes DL, Paddon-Jones D, Zhang XJ, Aarsland A, et al. (2008) Whey protein ingestion in elderly persons results in greater muscle protein accrual than ingestion of its constituent essential amino acid content. Nutr Res 28: 651–658.

33. Milne AC, Potter J, Avenell A (2005) Protein and energy supplementation in elderly people at risk from malnutrition. Cochrane Database Syst Rev: CD003288.

34. Hays NP, Kim H, Wells AM, Kajkenova O, Evans WJ (2009) Effects of whey and fortified collagen hydrolysate protein supplements on nitrogen balance and body composition in older women. J Am Diet Assoc 109: 1082–1087.

35. Cermak NM, Res PT, de Groot LC, Saris WH, van Loon LJ (2012) Protein supplementation augments the adaptive response of skeletal muscle to resistance-type exercise training: a meta-analysis. Am J Clin Nutr 96: 1454–1464.

36. Borsheim E, Bui QU, Tissier S, Kobayashi H, Ferrando AA, et al. (2008) Effect of amino acid supplementation on muscle mass, strength and physical function in elderly. Clin Nutr 27: 189–195.

23

Outcomes in Cochrane Systematic Reviews Addressing Four Common Eye Conditions: An Evaluation of Completeness and Comparability

Ian J. Saldanha*, Kay Dickersin, Xue Wang, Tianjing Li

Department of Epidemiology, Johns Hopkins Bloomberg School of Public Health, Baltimore, Maryland, United States of America

Abstract

Introduction: Choice of outcomes is critical for clinical trialists and systematic reviewers. It is currently unclear how systematic reviewers choose and pre-specify outcomes for systematic reviews. Our objective was to assess the completeness of pre-specification and comparability of outcomes in all Cochrane reviews addressing four common eye conditions.

Methods: We examined protocols for all Cochrane reviews as of June 2013 that addressed glaucoma, cataract, age-related macular degeneration (AMD), and diabetic retinopathy (DR). We assessed completeness and comparability for each outcome that was named in ≥25% of protocols on those topics. We defined a completely-specified outcome as including information about five elements: *domain, specific measurement, specific metric, method of aggregation,* and *time-points.* For each domain, we assessed comparability in how individual elements were specified across protocols.

Results: We identified 57 protocols addressing glaucoma (22), cataract (16), AMD (15), and DR (4). We assessed completeness and comparability for five outcome domains: quality-of-life, visual acuity, intraocular pressure, disease progression, and contrast sensitivity. Overall, these five outcome domains appeared 145 times (instances). Only 15/145 instances (10.3%) were completely specified (all five elements) (median = three elements per outcome). Primary outcomes were more completely specified than non-primary (median = four versus two elements). Quality-of-life was least completely specified (median = one element). Due to largely incomplete outcome pre-specification, conclusive assessment of comparability in outcome usage across the various protocols per condition was not possible.

Discussion: Outcome pre-specification was largely incomplete; we encourage systematic reviewers to consider all five elements. This will indicate the importance of complete specification to clinical trialists, on whose work systematic reviewers depend, and will indirectly encourage comparable outcome choice to reviewers undertaking related research questions. Complete pre-specification could improve efficiency and reduce bias in data abstraction and analysis during a systematic review. Ultimately, more completely specified and comparable outcomes could make systematic reviews more useful to decision-makers.

Editor: Kypros Kypri, University of Newcastle, Australia, Australia

Funding: This project was funded by the National Eye Institute, grant number 1U01EY020522 (http://www.nei.nih.gov/). The funder had no role in study design, data collection and analysis, decision to publish, or preparation of the manuscript.

Competing Interests: All authors are affiliated with the US Satellite of the Cochrane Eyes and Vision Group (the group responsible for producing the Cochrane Reviews evaluated as part of this work): Drs. Kay Dickersin and Tianjing Li are Faculty members; Dr. Xue Wang is a Methodologist; and Dr. Ian Saldanha is a Research Assistant. Drs. Kay Dickersin, Tianjing Li, and Xue Wang have authored several Cochrane systematic reviews that are assessed as part of this study.

* Email: isaldan1@jhmi.edu

Introduction

In clinical trials, an outcome is an event or measure in study participants that is used to assess the effectiveness and/or safety of the intervention being studied [1]. Choosing relevant outcomes is a critical early step in the design of clinical trials and systematic reviews for a number of reasons [2]. In clinical trials, expected effect sizes on critical outcomes are used to determine sample size [3]. In addition, there is general agreement that by pre-specifying the primary and secondary outcomes and limiting the number of statistical analyses, clinical trialists reduce the likelihood of Type I error (i.e., finding a statistically significant treatment effect just by chance, in the absence of a true treatment effect) and outcome reporting bias (i.e., selectively reporting outcomes based on the strength and/or direction of the findings). Although satisfactory solutions have not yet been developed, there is growing recognition that these issues also apply to systematic reviews [4]–[5]. Indeed, the Cochrane Collaboration recommends that systematic reviewers limit the number of and pre-specify all outcomes for their systematic review [6]–[7].

The process of conducting a systematic review of intervention effectiveness begins with formulating a research question, and then, finding and synthesizing the evidence from studies that address the question. In formulating the question, the systematic reviewer defines the population, intervention, comparison, and outcomes (PICO) to be examined. Studies that address the review question, typically clinical trials, should be broadly similar on the population, intervention and comparison groups, but frequently report different outcomes from those chosen by the systematic reviewer. Clinical trialists typically measure numerous outcomes, sometimes in the hundreds [8]. It is likely that these outcomes are different from those chosen by the systematic reviewer; overlap of the chosen outcomes can vary from none to complete (Figure 1). In many cases, the primary outcome of interest to the systematic reviewers may not have been an outcome of interest to the clinical trialists [9], or may not be reported clearly or consistently in the clinical trial reports or associated documents [10]. Systematic reviewers thus face an important decision: should they choose outcomes to be examined based on what they believe to be important outcomes ("systematic review author judgment") or based on what they know is reported in the relevant clinical trials ("clinical trialist judgment")?

How systematic reviewers choose outcomes and pre-specify them in systematic review protocols is currently unclear. One view is that, unlike clinical trialists, systematic reviewers should not base outcome choice on sample size/power calculations and Type I error rates. Instead, the objective of medical research should be to draw conclusions based on all sources of available evidence [11]. Systematic reviews, which are often used to inform clinical practice guidelines and policy, could and even should include all the outcomes that patients, clinicians, and policy-makers need to know about. Systematic reviews also allow elucidation of existing research gaps in a given field [12], for example, when outcomes are not examined in trials and should be.

In our view, regardless of who chooses the outcomes to be assessed in a systematic review and how those outcomes are chosen, all outcomes need to be specified completely and clearly if they are to be of use to decision-makers.

The objective of our study was to assess the completeness of pre-specification and comparability of outcomes in all Cochrane reviews addressing four common eye conditions. Our purpose is not to hold systematic review protocols to a standard that may not

have been described at the time they were published, rather it is to initiate a discussion on important questions for systematic reviewers: how should systematic reviewers choose outcomes to address in the review; how should these outcomes be reported (i.e., which elements are necessary for complete reporting) by systematic reviewers; and if outcomes are pre-specified in systematic review protocols, should these protocols be formally updated with amendments to reflect changing outcome specification?

Methods

Review protocols examined

The Cochrane Collaboration publishes and archives all its systematic review protocols, completed reviews, and updates in *The Cochrane Database of Systematic Reviews*. Protocols for systematic reviews, hereafter referred to as 'protocols', were eligible for our study if they were published by the Cochrane Eyes and Vision Group (CEVG) in *The Cochrane Database of Systematic Reviews* in or before June 2013 (Issue 6), and if they addressed any of the following four eye conditions: glaucoma, age-related macular degeneration (AMD), cataract, and diabetic retinopathy (DR). We selected these four conditions because of their high disease burden across populations and the range of interventions addressing them [13]. For each eligible review, we identified the oldest available protocol and, when no protocol could be found for a review, we contacted CEVG editors and review authors via email to ask whether they had a copy. When these efforts were not successful, we used the most recent version of the completed review in place of the protocol.

Five elements of a completely specified outcome

We used an outcome definition that includes five elements: (1) the *domain* or outcome title (e.g., visual acuity); (2) the *specific measurement* or technique/instrument used to make the measurement (e.g., Snellen chart); (3) the *specific metric* or format of the outcome data from each participant that will be used for analysis (e.g., value at a time-point, change from baseline); (4) the *method of aggregation* or how data from each group will be summarized (e.g., mean, percent/proportion); and (5) the *time-points* that will be used for analysis (e.g., 3 months) (Figure 2). Whereas Zarin et al. specify these same elements [8], they define the first four elements and consider time-points related to each of those four.

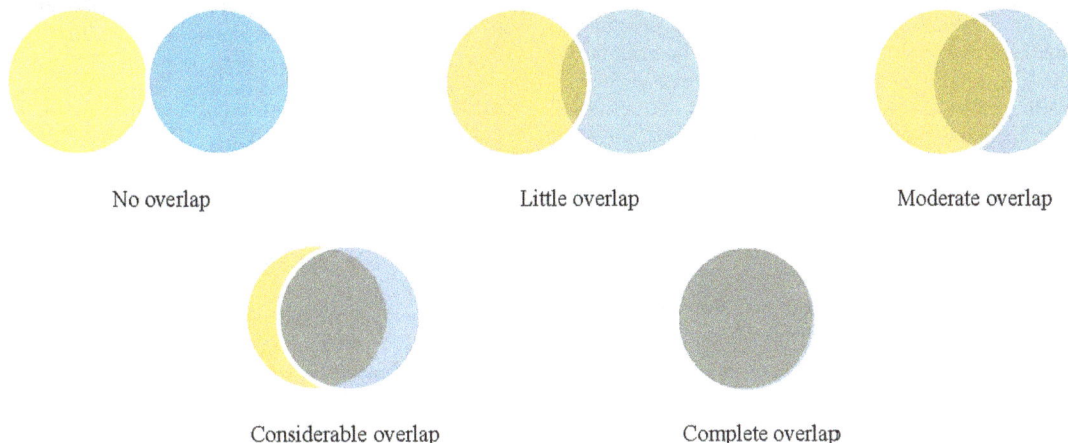

Figure 1. Examples of extent of overlap of possible outcome domains chosen by clinical trialists and systematic reviewers. Yellow - Outcomes chosen by clinical trialists. Blue - Outcomes chosen by systematic reviewers. Grey - Outcomes chosen by BOTH clinical trialists and systematic reviewers.

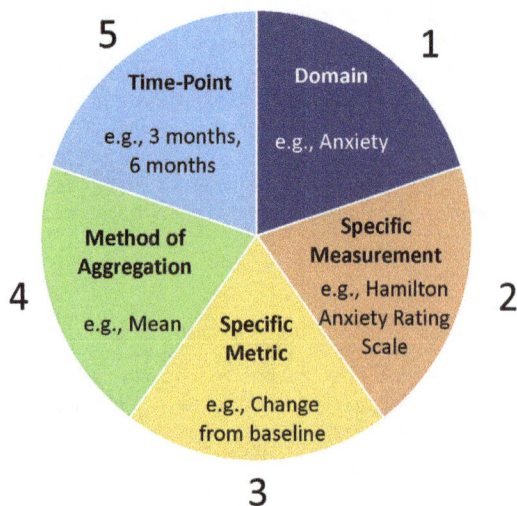

Figure 2. Five elements of a completely specified outcome, with anxiety as an example.

Selecting outcome domains for data extraction

Before beginning data extraction, one investigator (IS) identified all outcome domains in the Methods sections of included protocols. We then selected for data extraction those outcome domains appearing in at least 25% of eligible protocols. Then, for those eligible protocols with published completed reviews, we compared the Methods section of the protocol with the Methods section of the most recent version of the corresponding completed review, noting any differences in the specified outcome domains. We did this step to evaluate whether focusing on the protocols, some of which were published a while ago, would mean that we were assessing a different set of outcome domains than those currently being evaluated by the review authors.

Data extraction

We designed, tested, and finalized a data extraction form using Google Forms©. Two investigators (IS and XW) extracted data independently and resolved discrepancies through consensus or discussion with a third author (TL). We extracted data about the eye condition and year of publication of each protocol. We extracted from the Methods section the following data pertaining to each eligible outcome: type of outcome (primary, non-primary, or unclear [if not specified]) and each of the five outcome elements described earlier. For element 2, we extracted all specific measurements that were specified, or classified the specific measurement as unclear (if not specified). We classified element 3 (specific metric) into one or more of the following categories: (i) value at a time-point, (ii) time-to-event, (iii) change from baseline, and (iv) unclear (if not specified). We classified element 4 (method of aggregation) into one or more of the following categories: (i) mean, (ii) median, (iii) percent/proportion, (iv) absolute number, and (v) unclear (if not specified). For element 5, we extracted all time-points that were specified, or classified the time-points as unclear (if not specified).

Data analysis

We assessed the extent of completeness using the number of elements specified out of five possible, and considered an outcome specified in the Methods section as "complete" if all five elements were specified. For each outcome, we calculated median,

interquartile range (IQR), and proportion of outcome elements specified. We performed Kruskal-Wallis tests for nonparametric comparisons of medians and distributions of extent of completeness by condition addressed, year of protocol publication, type of outcome, and outcome domain.

We assessed the frequency and comparability of outcome elements (i.e., similarity of categories for each element) for elements 3 and 4 across protocols addressing each of the four eye conditions. Protocols could specify more than one category for a given element. Comparability was therefore assessed as the distribution of those categories across protocols. As an example, if one protocol specified visual acuity at a time-point as well as change in visual acuity from baseline, we counted both categories for specific metric (element 3). In another example, protocols addressing cataract and assessing the outcome of visual acuity were considered to be comparable in method of aggregation (element 4) if they all specified mean or all specified median or both. However, they would not be comparable in element 4 if some specified mean and others specified median.

Statistical significance was defined at the 5% level. All data were analyzed using STATA© version 12 (College Station, TX).

Results

Characteristics of protocols examined

Our search identified 57 eligible systematic reviews (Table 1). We were able to find protocols for 54 reviews (94.7%), and used the Methods section of completed reviews for the remaining three (5.3%). An updated protocol was published for one of the 54 protocols. Glaucoma was the most frequently addressed condition (22 protocols), followed by cataract (16 protocols), AMD (15 protocols), and DR (4 protocols). Approximately half of the protocols (29/57; 50.9%) were published between 2006 and 2010. Thirty-four protocols were associated with a completed review, the most recent version of which was published a median of five (IQR 4–8, range 0–15) years after publication of the protocol.

Outcome domains used in protocols

We examined five outcome domains named in at least 25% of the eligible protocols (Table 2): quality-of-life (47/57 protocols; 82.5%), visual acuity (47/57; 82.5%), intraocular pressure (21/57; 36.8%), disease progression (15/57; 26.3%), and contrast sensitivity (15/57; 26.3%). One protocol did not name any of these five outcome domains. For most completed systematic reviews (30/34; 88.2%), these five outcome domains were similar to what was named in their corresponding protocols. Compared to their protocols, two completed systematic reviews dropped quality-of-life while one completed review added it. One completed systematic review dropped contrast sensitivity.

Completeness of outcome pre-specification

Across the 57 protocols, the five most frequent outcome domains appeared 145 times ('instances'); however, only 15/145 instances (10.3%) involved complete pre-specification (i.e., where all five elements of the outcome were specified). Overall, a median of three (IQR 2–4) elements were specified per outcome (Table 3). Extent of completeness was not statistically significantly different by condition. Completeness of outcome specification may be better in protocols published later compared to earlier, (median of three [IQR 2–4] elements specified in 2006–2010 versus one [IQR 1–3] in 2000 or earlier), although the difference was not statistically significant (p = 0.1635).

Fifty-four of 57 protocols (94.7%) specified at least one primary outcome. Among the five outcome domains evaluated in our

Table 1. Number of protocols and outcome domains by condition, year published, and whether specified as primary outcome.

Characteristic	Number (%) of protocols	Number (%) of outcomes
All	57[1] (100)	145[2] (100)
Condition addressed		
Glaucoma	22 (38.6)	51 (35.2)
Cataract	16 (28.1)	35 (24.1)
Age-related macular degeneration (AMD)	15 (26.3)	47 (32.4)
Diabetic retinopathy (DR)	4 (7.0)	12 (8.3)
Year of protocol publication		
2000 or earlier	6 (10.5)	13 (9.0)
2001 to 2005	15 (26.3)	37 (25.5)
2006 to 2010	29 (50.9)	76 (52.4)
2011 or later	7 (12.3)	19 (13.1)
Type of outcomes domain specified	Not applicable	
Outcomes specified as primary		48 (33.1)
Outcomes specified as non-primary		88 (60.7)
Type of outcome unclear		9 (6.2)

[1] 54 protocols and 3 completed reviews; One protocol did not include any of the outcome domains selected for detailed data extraction.
[2] 139/145 of the outcomes were described in the 54 protocols.

study, at least one was a primary outcome in 48/57 (84.2%) protocols. Extent of completeness appeared to differ by outcome type, with primary outcomes being most completely specified and outcomes with type unclear being least completely specified (median four versus one respectively, p = 0.0001). Intraocular pressure was the most completely specified outcome in our sample, with a median of four (IQR 3–4) elements specified (Table 2). Quality-of-life was least completely specified, with a median of one (IQR 1–2) element specified. The patterns of completeness of individual elements were similar across outcomes (Figure 3). Method of aggregation was specified least often, while domain and time-points were specified more often than other elements. The completeness of individual elements for the quality-of-life outcome was less than for other outcomes, overall. Although intraocular pressure was the most completely specified outcome, only 24% of protocols assessing it specified the specific measurement. Patterns of completeness of individual outcome elements also appeared to be similar across conditions, except for outcomes in DR protocols, where there were only four protocols and so the percentages are unlikely to be reliable (Figure 4).

Table 4 provides some examples of incomplete specification of outcomes in our sample of systematic reviews.

Comparability of outcome elements

Table 5 shows the distribution of specific metrics (element 3) and methods of aggregation (element 4) across instances of usage of outcome domain, by condition. The specific metric was unclear for large proportions of individual instances (often as high as 100% for the 16 instances of usage of quality-of-life in protocols addressing glaucoma and for the four instances of usage of contrast sensitivity in protocols addressing cataract). For instances where the specific metric was specified, the most frequent specific metrics were 'value at a time-point' and 'change from baseline'.

The method of aggregation was unclear for large proportions of individual instances (often as high as 100% for the 16 instances of usage of quality-of-life in protocols addressing glaucoma and for the four instances of usage of visual acuity in protocols addressing DR). For instances where the method of aggregation was specified, the most frequent methods of aggregation were 'mean' and 'percent/proportion'.

Table 2. Completeness (number of completely-specified elements out of five possible) by outcome domain.

Characteristic	Number (%) of protocols	Median (IQR) number of completely-specified elements per outcome	p-value
All	57[1] (100)	3.0 (2.0–4.0)	-
Outcome domain			
Quality-of-life	47 (82.5)	1.0 (1.0–2.0)	0.0001
Visual acuity	47 (82.5)	3.0 (2.0–4.0)	
Intraocular pressure	21 (36.8)	4.0 (3.0–4.0)	
Disease progression	15 (26.3)	3.0 (2.0–4.0)	
Contrast sensitivity	15 (26.3)	2.0 (1.0–3.0)	

[1] One protocol did not include any of the outcome domains selected for detailed data extraction.

Table 3. Completeness (number of completely-specified elements out of five possible) by type of protocol/outcome.

Characteristic	Median (IQR) number of completely specified elements per outcome	p-value
All[1]	3.0 (2.0–4.0)	NA
Condition addressed		
Glaucoma	3.0 (2.0–4.0)	0.1218
Cataract	3.0 (2.0–4.0)	
Age-related macular degeneration (AMD)	2.0 (1.0–3.0)	
Diabetic retinopathy (DR)	3.0 (1.5–4.0)	
Year of protocol publication		
2000 or earlier	1.0 (1.0–3.0)	0.1635
2001 to 2005	2.0 (2.0–4.0)	
2006 to 2010	3.0 (2.0–4.0)	
2011 or later	2.0 (2.0–3.0)	
Type of outcome domain specified		
Outcomes specified as primary	4.0 (3.0–4.0)	0.0001
Outcomes specified as non-primary	2.0 (1.0–3.0)	
Type of outcome not specified	1.0 (1.0–2.0)	

[1] 54 protocols and 3 completed reviews; Median 3.0 (2.0–4.0) for outcomes in the 54 protocols and 1.5 (1.0–2.0) for outcomes in the 3 reviews (p = 0.0627); One protocol did not include any of the outcome domains selected for detailed data extraction.

Discussion

Summary of main findings

We have shown that, if outcome pre-specification in systematic review protocols is judged using recommended standards for clinical trials, then it is largely incomplete. Although completeness appears to have improved somewhat over time, on average, only three of five standard elements of an outcome were pre-specified. Due to largely incomplete outcome pre-specification, a conclusive assessment of comparability in outcome elements across the various protocols per condition was not possible. However, we observed variation in specific metrics and methods of aggregation.

Completeness of outcome pre-specification

There are some reasons that might explain why outcomes were not completely specified in our study of systematic review protocols. First, although we believe complete specification of all five elements is necessary for a number of reasons, the idea is new to the systematic review community. This is demonstrated by the fact that the Cochrane Handbook states only that the name of the

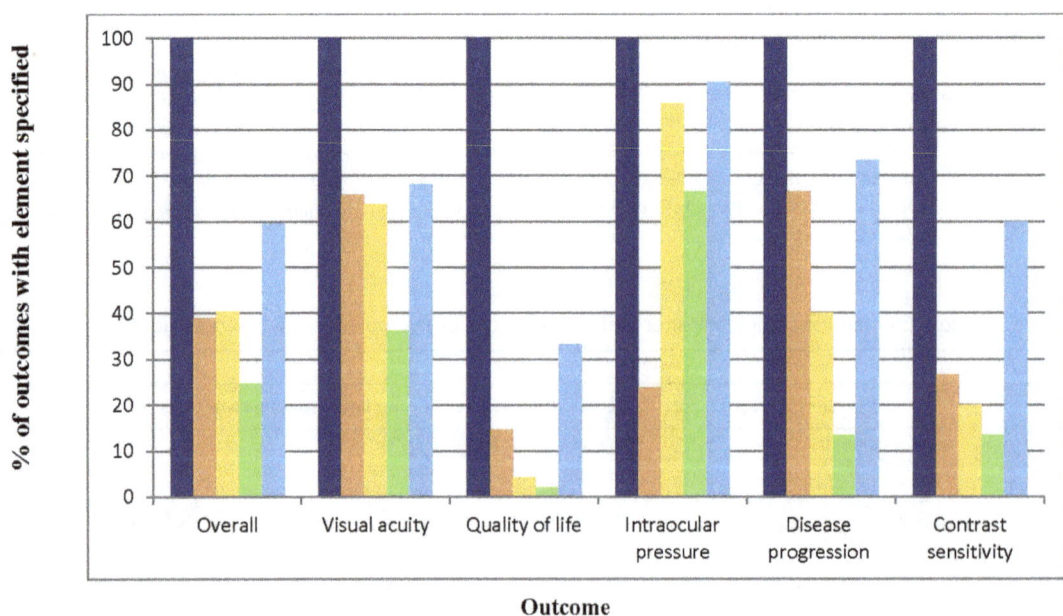

Figure 3. Completeness of specification of outcome elements, by outcome. Navy blue - Domain. Orange – Specific measurement. Yellow – Specific metric. Green – Method of aggregation. Blue – Time-point(s).

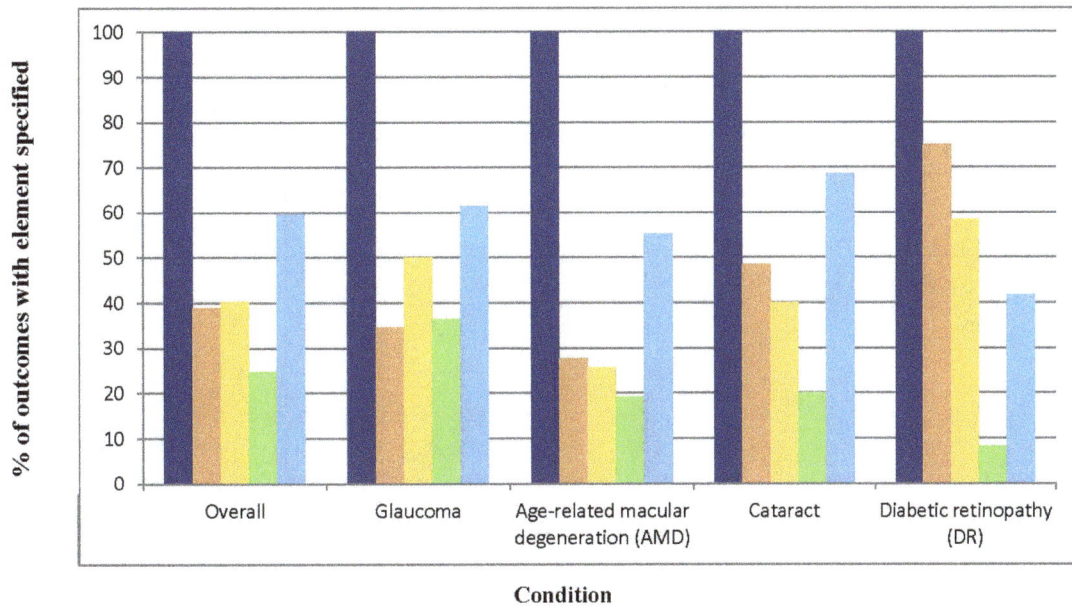

Figure 4. Completeness of specification of outcome elements, by condition. Navy blue - Domain. Orange – Specific measurement. Yellow – Specific metric. Green – Method of aggregation. Sky blue – Time-point(s).

outcome (equivalent to *domain* [element 1]), type of scale (equivalent to *specific measurement* [element 2]), and timing of measurement (equivalent to *time-points* [element 5]) must be pre-specified[6]; and there is no explicit mention of pre-specification of *specific metric* (element 3) or *method of aggregation* (element 4). Indeed, elements 1 and 5 were the most often-specified elements in our sample of protocols, though element 2 was frequently not specified (70% of the time) (Figure 3).

Another possible explanation for incomplete pre-specification of outcomes is that choice of outcomes could be influenced by the findings of (and outcomes examined in) the clinical trials that would be included in the review. We did not assess the outcomes examined at the level of the clinical trials to determine the likelihood that this occurred, but suggest that doing so may contribute to a better understanding of how review outcomes are chosen. Are they chosen because systematic reviewers consider them the most important outcomes to examine, because they are the outcomes that have been examined in clinical trials, or both? If the review outcomes were chosen purely because they were the outcomes that have been reported in clinical trials, this is troubling because of the possibility of "meta-bias". We know, for example,

that outcomes reported in clinical trials could have been selectively reported because of desirable or undesirable findings [14]–[15]. By pre-specifying in the protocol the outcomes to be examined in the review, systematic reviewers minimize the potential for bias [5], [16], and reassure readers that the choice of outcomes was not influenced by the results of individual clinical trials. That said, systematic reviewers are usually familiar with their field and *a priori* aware of potentially eligible clinical trials and/or how the outcome in question is frequently measured. Complete pre-specification also could improve efficiency in data abstraction and analysis during a systematic review.

Systematic reviewers may also anticipate potential variation in outcomes across included clinical trials, and may allow for this by pre-specifying the elements of the outcome domain of interest in broad rather than specific terms (e.g., "visual acuity" versus "change in visual acuity from baseline to 1 year, as measured using a Snellen chart"). If such variation is suspected, systematic reviewers could explicitly state that all variations of a given element(s) will be included. This could minimize the occurrence of what Page et al. refer to as "selective inclusion" in systematic reviews [5].

Table 4. Examples of incomplete outcome pre-specification.

Exact text from methods section of protocol	Number of completely-specified elements (out of five possible)
"The primary outcome for the review will be visual acuity."	1
"When available quality of life data will be described for those with operated and unoperated cataract."	1
"Postoperative visual acuity"	1
"Quality of life"	1
"Contrast sensitivity"	1
"Vision-related quality of life at one year"	2
"Mean IOP"	2

Table 5. Frequency of categories of specific metric (element 3) and method of aggregation (element 4) across instances of usage of outcome domains by condition.

Condition/Outcome domain (Number of protocols/Number of instances)	Categories of specific metric (element 3) (% of instances)				Categories of method of aggregation (element 4) (% of instances)			
	Value at a time-point	Time-to-event	Change from baseline	Unclear	Mean	Percent/proportion	Absolute number	Unclear
Glaucoma (22 protocols)								
Quality-of-life (16 instances)	-	-	-	100	-	-	-	100
Visual acuity (13 instances)	31	-	31	46	8	39	-	54
Intraocular pressure (20 instances)	55	10	25	15	50	10	-	40
Disease progression (2 instances)	-	50	50	-	-	-	-	100
Cataract (16 protocols)								
Quality-of-life (12 instances)	17	-	-	83	-	8	-	92
Visual acuity (15 instances)	53	-	20	33	-	33	-	67
Intraocular pressure (1 instance)	100	-	-	-	100	100	-	-
Disease progression (3 instances)	-	-	33	67	-	-	-	100
Contrast sensitivity (4 instances)	-	-	-	100	-	-	-	100
Age-related macular degeneration (15 protocols)								
Quality-of-life (15 instances)	-	-	-	100	-	-	-	100
Visual acuity (15 instances)	47	-	33	40	20	13	13	60
Disease progression (6 instances)	-	-	-	100	-	-	17	83
Contrast sensitivity (11 instances)	18	-	9	73	18	18	-	82
Diabetic retinopathy (4 protocols)								
Quality-of-life (4 protocols)	-	-	-	100	-	-	-	100
Visual acuity (4 instances)	100	-	25	-	-	-	-	100
Disease progression (4 instances)	50	25	-	25	25	-	-	75

Notes:
- If there was no instance of usage of a certain outcome domain across all reviews addressing a given condition, the above table does not include a row for that outcome domain for that condition.
- Percentages are row percentages (adding up individual categories within an element). Percentages sometimes total more than 100% for an element because some protocols used more than one category for that element.
- No reviews used "median" as a method of aggregation (element 4).

We assume that primary outcomes for both clinical trials and systematic reviews are chosen based on perceived clinical importance and/or importance to patients; and that they are usually measured and reported more thoroughly than non-primary outcomes [17]. Not surprisingly, in our study, primary outcomes were more completely specified than other outcome types. Our estimate of 94.7% protocols pre-specifying a primary outcome is somewhat higher than the 88% that has been reported as pre-specified in clinical trial protocols [18], and this could be related to the fact that we were examining protocols entered into software that requests the domain names of the pre-specified outcomes.

In our study, the most incompletely pre-specified outcome was quality-of-life, a key patient-important outcome. This finding is concordant with other studies that have found that outcome reporting in clinical trials is a bigger problem for patient-important outcomes than other types of outcomes [19]–[20]. Further, when patient-important outcomes are not primary outcomes in clinical trials, the likelihood that reporting is complete is further reduced [20]. Our study aimed to evaluate the completeness and comparability of all outcomes, both patient-important and not.

Our recommendation is that systematic reviewers should engage in discussion about and strongly consider pre-specifying all five elements of each outcome they wish to examine. When explicit pre-specification of all five elements of a given outcome is not possible, for example when all possible options for a given outcome element are not known or are too numerous, the systematic reviewers should enumerate all known acceptable options for each element and explicitly state that all options for that element would be accepted, or provide rationale for why it is impossible to completely pre-specify an element.

The Preferred Reporting Items for Systematic Reviews and Meta-analyses Protocols (PRISMA-P) is currently under development [21]. We hope that the availability of reporting guidelines (including details about outcome specification) will improve the completeness of specification of outcomes. Assuming that the Cochrane Collaboration recognizes the importance of completeness of pre-specification, there are some possible ways to ensure that review authors are aware of the five elements of a completely specified outcome. First, editorial teams at Cochrane Review Groups (CRGs) should make all review authors aware of the five outcome elements early in the process (no later than the protocol development stage). Second, peer reviewers should be directed to consider whether the outcomes are completely pre-specified and not likely to have been chosen based on the strength and direction of the findings for those outcomes. Third, the Cochrane Handbook and other systematic review guidance materials, in addition to training workshops and other educational avenues, should incorporate explicit descriptions of all five outcome elements. Other organizations producing guidance on systematic review methodology (e.g., Agency for Healthcare Research and Quality [AHRQ], the Centre for Reviews and Dissemination [CRD]) should also incorporate descriptions of the five outcome elements in their guidance materials.

Organizations such as the Cochrane Collaboration suggest limiting the number of outcomes examined in a systematic review [6]. However, in order to evaluate whether the effect of an intervention persists over time, an otherwise identical outcome (i.e., identical in the other four elements) is often measured at a number of time-points. For the purpose of counting the number of outcomes measured, we recommend that these repeated measurements be counted as one outcome regardless of the number of time-points at which the outcome is assessed.

Comparability of outcome elements

In the era of evidence-based medicine, decision-makers in healthcare (e.g., patients, clinicians, and policy-makers) increasingly rely on systematic reviews. It is important that decision-makers have access to high quality and up-to-date individual systematic reviews as well as are able to compare results across systematic reviews. Cochrane "overviews" (Cochrane reviews which compile evidence from related reviews of interventions into a single accessible and usable document) [6], and network meta-analyses (analyses of three or more interventions for a given condition in one meta-analysis) [22]–[23] are examples of formal comparisons across systematic reviews. To better feed into these formal comparisons and clinical practice guidelines, the elements of outcomes used in the various systematic reviews addressing a given condition should be comparable. In our study, the largely incomplete pre-specification of outcomes in protocols restricted our ability to assess comparability in outcome elements across protocols. In cases where the various elements were specified, however, we observed variation in specific metrics and methods of aggregation. An example of such variation is: one protocol pre-specified that the outcome domain of visual acuity would be measured as mean change in visual acuity (number of letters) from baseline to one year, while another protocol pre-specified that visual acuity would be measured as percent of participants with improvement in visual acuity of at least three letters at one year. While both protocols specified the same outcome domain at the same time-point, differences in the specific metric (mean change versus value at a time-point) and method of aggregation (mean versus percent) would preclude a direct comparison of the visual acuity results.

Efforts to promote comparability of outcomes across related clinical trials have led to the creation of core outcome measures within research fields [24]–[26]. One such effort is the Core Outcome Measures in Effectiveness Trials (COMET) Initiative [27], whose investigators have produced guidance on methods for identifying core outcome sets [28]. Because the issue of comparability of outcomes across systematic reviews is complex, we recommend that researchers within a field (e.g., systematic reviewers, Cochrane review group editors, clinical trialists) and patients consider developing comparable outcomes across systematic reviews, adding to a core list over time as appropriate.

There are pros and cons of establishing comparability in outcomes across reviews, however. Increased comparability will likely facilitate formal comparisons across systematic reviews and development of clinical practice guidelines. In addition, decision-makers would be better able to compare more directly the effectiveness of treatment options. For example, hundreds of measurement scales (*specific measurements*) have been used to assess mental status in schizophrenia [29] and quality-of-life [30], making comparability across clinical trials very challenging. Finally, use of comparable outcomes could discourage authors from 'cherry-picking' outcomes to be used in their studies [31].

On the other hand, comparability across reviews is not always possible or desirable. Limiting outcomes to those used by previous researchers risks excluding an outcome that is in fact important, or authors may be compelled to include an outcome that they do not consider important. Additionally, it might not be possible to identify *a priori* all relevant outcomes and outcome elements for a rapidly evolving field or for a field with a large number of relevant outcomes.

Availability of protocols and amendments to protocols

We were unable to obtain 3/57 (5.3%) protocols associated with our sample of Cochrane reviews. This poses a concern for investigators conducting methodological research in systematic reviews, and for users of systematic reviews generally. Although we do not believe that relying on the Methods sections of three completed Cochrane reviews in the cases where we could not find the protocols is likely to have influenced our findings, we believe that all protocols and previous versions of completed systematic reviews should be made available to researchers. Furthermore, an updated protocol was published for only one of the protocols we examined. The Cochrane Collaboration should consider keeping all protocols up-to-date by publishing updated versions of protocols or publishing protocol amendments for all its reviews. In this way, Cochrane review protocols would be formally amended in the same way that clinical trial protocols are amended and made available, providing an accessible audit trail. This practice will facilitate Cochrane's contribution of its protocols and updates to PROSPERO [32]–[33], an international database of prospectively registered systematic reviews.

Our focus on Cochrane reviews is both a strength and a limitation. Assuming that Cochrane reviews are among the most rigorously conducted and reported systematic reviews [34]–[35], it is likely that completeness and comparability of outcomes are higher in our sample of reviews than in other reviews. It would be useful to know how others producing systematic reviews (e.g., AHRQ, CRD, independent authors) choose and describe outcomes in their systematic reviews.

As discussed, we did not examine the individual clinical trials examined by each Cochrane review in our sample to learn more about the source of non-comparability in outcome elements. Nor did we test for empirical evidence of outcome reporting bias on the part of the systematic reviewers. Because our assessments of completeness and comparability were based on what was reported in the protocols (and some completed reviews), it is possible that our findings were a consequence of unsatisfactory reporting and that the rationale for the outcomes chosen could not be determined without asking the systematic review authors directly.

Our study should be replicated in other disease areas and on a larger scale to assess the applicability of our findings to other fields.

Although we have compared the outcomes pre-specified in the protocol with what is in the corresponding completed review's Methods section, a next step would be to compare the outcomes in the Methods with those in the Results section. This would allow a confirmation of the potential bias by systematic reviewers that has been demonstrated by Kirkham et al. using a cohort of Cochrane reviews [36] and by various investigators studying this issue in clinical trials [14], [17], [37]–[38].

Conclusions

We recommend that systematic review authors strongly consider pre-specifying all outcomes of interest using the five elements of a completely specified outcome (domain, specific measurement, specific metric, method of aggregation, and time-points), amending the protocol formally, as needed. We further suggest that researchers and other stakeholders, such as patients, carefully consider the pros and cons of establishing comparability in outcomes across systematic reviews addressing a given condition.

Acknowledgments

We acknowledge the contributions of Deborah Zarin, MD; Karen Robinson, MA, PhD; Swaroop Vedula, MD, MPH, PhD; and Evan Mayo-Wilson, MSc, MPA, DPhil for their comments on previous versions of this manuscript. We also acknowledge the contributions of Michael Marrone, MPH, Kristina Lindsley, MS, and James Heyward, BA for their help with data abstraction and locating systematic review protocols for this study.

Author Contributions

Conceived and designed the experiments: IJS KD XW TL. Performed the experiments: IJS KD XW TL. Analyzed the data: IJS KD XW TL. Contributed reagents/materials/analysis tools: IJS KD XW TL. Wrote the paper: IJS KD XW TL.

References

1. Meinert CL (2012) Clinical trials dictionary: Terminology and usage recommendations. 2nd edition. Wiley. Hoboken, NJ.

2. Institute of Medicine (2011) Finding what works in health care: standards for systematic reviews. Available: http://www.iom.edu/Reports/2011/Finding-What-Works-in-Health-Care-Standards-for-Systematic-Reviews.aspx. Accessed 2014 September 12.

3. Campbell MJ, Julious SA, Altman DG (1995) Estimating sample sizes for binary, ordered categorical, and continuous outcomes in two group comparisons. BMJ 311(7013): 1145–1148.

4. Bender R, Bunce C, Clarke M, Gates S, Lange S, et al. (2008) Attention should be given to multiplicity issues in systematic reviews. J Clin Epidemiol 61(9): 857–865.

5. Page MJ, McKenzie JE, Forbes A (2013) Many scenarios exist for selective inclusion and reporting of results in randomized trials and systematic reviews. J Clin Epidemiol 66(5): 524–537.

6. Higgins JPTGreen S, (editors) (2011) Cochrane Handbook for Systematic Reviews of Interventions Version 5.1.0 [updated March 2011]. The Cochrane Collaboration. Available: www.cochrane-handbook.org. Accessed 2014 September 12.

7. Chandler J, Churchill R, Higgins J, Tovey D (2012) Methodological standards for the conduct of new Cochrane Intervention Reviews. Version 2.2. 17, December 2012. Available: http://www.editorial-unit.cochrane.org/sites/editorial-unit.cochrane.org/files/uploads/MECIR_conduct_standards%202.2%2017122012.pdf. Accessed 2014 September 12.

8. Zarin DA, Tse T, Williams RJ, Califf RM, Ide NC (2011) The ClinicalTrials.gov results database–update and key issues. N Engl J Med 364(9): 852–860.

9. Singh S, Loke YK, Enright PL, Furberg CD (2011) Mortality associated with tiotropium mist inhaler in patients with chronic obstructive pulmonary disease: systematic review and meta-analysis of randomised controlled trials. BMJ 14; 342:d3215. doi: 10.1136/bmj.d3215

10. Jefferson T, Jones MA, Doshi P, Del Mar CB, Heneghan CJ, et al. (2012) Neuraminidase inhibitors for preventing and treating influenza in healthy adults and children. Cochrane Database Syst Rev (1):CD008965.

11. Goodman SN (1989) Meta-analysis and evidence. http://www.ncbi.nlm.nih.gov/pubmed/2666026Control Clin Trials 10(2): 188–204.

12. Robinson KA, Saldanha IJ, Mckoy NA (2011) Development of a framework to identify research gaps from systematic reviews. J Clin Epidemiol 64(12): 1325–1330.

13. National Eye Institute (2010) Statistics and Data Available: http://www.nei.nih.gov/eyedata. Accessed 2014 September 12.

14. Vedula SS, Bero L, Scherer RW, Dickersin K (2009) Outcome reporting in industry-sponsored trials of gabapentin for off-label use. N Engl J Med 361(20): 1963–1971.

15. Dwan K, Altman DG, Cresswell L, Blundell M, Gamble CL, et al. (2011) Comparison of protocols and registry entries to published reports for randomised controlled trials. Cochrane Database Syst Rev Issue 1. Art. No.: MR000031. doi: 10.1002/14651858.MR000031.pub2

16. Stewart L, Moher D, Shekelle P (2012) Why prospective registration of systematic reviews makes sense. Syst Rev 1: 7. doi:10.1186/2046-4053-1-7

17. Kirkham JJ, Dwan KM, Altman DG, Gamble C, Dodd S, et al. (2010) The impact of outcome reporting bias in randomised controlled trials on a cohort of systematic reviews. BMJ 340: c365. doi: 10.1136/bmj.c365

18. Mathieu S, Boutron I, Moher D, Altman DG, Ravaud P (2009) Comparison of registered and published primary outcomes in randomized controlled trials. JAMA 302(9): 977–984.

19. Wieseler B, Kerekes MF, Vervolgyi V, Kohlepp P, McGauran N, et al. (2012) Impact of document type on reporting quality of clinical drug trials: a comparison registry reports, clinical study reports, and journal publications. BMJ 344 d8141 doi: 10.1136/bmj.d8141

20. Wieseler B, Wolfram N, McGauran N, Kerekes MF, Vervolgyi V, et al. (2013) Completeness of reporting of patient-relevant clinical trial outcomes: comparison

of unpublished clinical study reports with publicly available data. PLOS Med 10 (10) e1001526. doi: 10.1371/journal.pmed.1001526

21. EQUATOR Network (2014) Reporting Guidelines under development. Available: http://www.equator-network.org/library/reporting-guidelines-under-development/#99. Accessed 2014 September 12.

22. Caldwell DM, Ades AE, Higgins JP (2005) Simultaneous comparison of multiple treatments: combining direct and indirect evidence. BMJ 331(7521): 897–900.

23. Li T, Puhan M, Vedula SS, Singh S, Dickersin K for the Ad Hoc Network Meta-analysis Methods Meeting Working Group (2011) Network meta-analysis – highly attractive and more methodological research is needed. BMC Medicine 9(1): 79. doi:10.1186/1741-7015-9-79

24. Miller AB, Hoogstraten B, Staquet M, Winkler A (1981) Reporting results of cancer treatment. Cancer 47(1): 207–214.

25. Tugwell P, Boers M, Brooks P, Simon LS, Strand V (2007) OMERACT: An international initiative to improve outcome measures in rheumatology. Trials 8: 38.

26. Dworkin RH, Turk DC, Farrar JT, Haythornthwaite JA, Jensen MP, et al. (2005) Core outcome measures for chronic pain trials: IMMPACT recommendations. Pain 113(1–2): 9–19.

27. COMET Initiative (2014) Overview. Available: http://www.comet-initiative.org/about/overview. Accessed 2014 September 12.

28. Williamson PR, Altman DG, Blazeby JM, Clarke M, Devane D, et al. (2012) Developing core outcome sets for clinical trials: issues to consider. Trials 13(132). doi: 10.1186/1745-6215-13-132

29. Thornley B, Adams C (1998) Content and quality of 2000 controlled trials in schizophrenia over 50 years. BMJ 317(7167): 1181–1184.

30. Salek S (1999) Compendium of Quality of Life Instruments. Wiley. ISBN: 0-471-98145-1.

31. Clarke M (2007) Standardising outcomes for clinical trials and systematic reviews. Trials 8: 39.

32. Booth A, Clarke M, Dooley G, Ghersi D, Moher D, et al. (2012) The nuts and bolts of PROSPERO: an international prospective register of systematic reviews. Sys Rev 1: 2. doi: 10.1186/2046-4053-1-2

33. Booth A, Clarke M, Dooley G, Ghersi D, Moher D, et al. (2013) PROSPERO at one year: an evaluation of its utility. Sys Rev 2: 4. doi: 10.1186/2046-4053-2-4

34. Jadad AR, Cook DJ, Jones A, Klassen TP, Tugwell P, et al. (1998) Methodology and reports of systematic reviews and meta-analyses: A comparison of Cochrane reviews with articles published in paper-based journals. JAMA 280(3): 278–280.

35. Moher D, Tetzlaff J, Tricco AC, Sampson M, Altman DG (2007) Epidemiology and reporting characteristics of systematic reviews. PLoS Med 4(3): e78.

36. Kirkham JJ, Altman DG, Williamson PR (2010) Bias due to changes in prespecified outcomes during the systematic review process. PLoS One 5(3): e9810. doi: 10.1371/journal.pone.0009810

37. Chan AW, Altman D (2005) Identifying outcome reporting bias in randomized trials on PubMed: review of publications and survey of authors. BMJ 330(7494): 753.

38. Chan AW, Hrobjartsson A, Haahr MT, Gøtzsche PC, Altman DG (2004) Empirical evidence for selective reporting of outcomes in randomized trials: comparison of protocols to published articles. JAMA 291(20): 2457–2465.

Immune Biomarkers Predictive of Respiratory Viral Infection in Elderly Nursing Home Residents

Jennie Johnstone[1]*, Robin Parsons[2], Fernando Botelho[2], Jamie Millar[2], Shelly McNeil[3], Tamas Fulop[4], Janet McElhaney[5], Melissa K. Andrew[6], Stephen D. Walter[1], P. J. Devereaux[1,7], Mehrnoush Malekesmaeili[8], Ryan R. Brinkman[8,9], James Mahony[10,11], Jonathan Bramson[2,10,11]¶, Mark Loeb[1,7,10,11]*¶

1 Department of Clinical Epidemiology and Biostatistics, McMaster University, Hamilton, Ontario, Canada, 2 McMaster Immunology Research Centre, McMaster University, Hamilton, Ontario, Canada, 3 Canadian Center for Vaccinology, IWK Health Centre and Capital Health, Dalhousie University, Halifax, Nova Scotia, Canada, 4 Department of Medicine, Geriatrics Division, Research Center on Aging, University of Sherbrooke, Sherbrooke, Quebec, Canada, 5 Department of Medicine, Northern Ontario School of Medicine, Sudbury, Ontario, Canada, 6 Department of Medicine, Dalhousie University, Halifax, Nova Scotia, Canada, 7 Department of Medicine, McMaster University, Hamilton, Ontario, Canada, 8 Terry Fox Laboratory, British Columbia Cancer Agency, Vancouver, British Columbia, Canada, 9 Department of Medical Genetics, University of British Columbia, Vancouver, British Columbia, Canada, 10 Department of Pathology and Molecular Medicine, McMaster University, Hamilton, Ontario, Canada, 11 Institute for Infectious Disease Research, McMaster University, Hamilton, Ontario, Canada

Abstract

Objective: To determine if immune phenotypes associated with immunosenescence predict risk of respiratory viral infection in elderly nursing home residents.

Methods: Residents ≥65 years from 32 nursing homes in 4 Canadian cities were enrolled in Fall 2009, 2010 and 2011, and followed for one influenza season. Following influenza vaccination, peripheral blood mononuclear cells (PBMCs) were obtained and analysed by flow cytometry for T-regs, CD4+ and CD8+ T-cell subsets (CCR7+CD45RA+, CCR7-CD45RA+ and CD28-CD57+) and CMV-reactive CD4+ and CD8+ T-cells. Nasopharyngeal swabs were obtained and tested for viruses in symptomatic residents. A Cox proportional hazards model adjusted for age, sex and frailty, determined the relationship between immune phenotypes and time to viral infection.

Results: 1072 residents were enrolled; median age 86 years and 72% female. 269 swabs were obtained, 87 were positive for virus: influenza (24%), RSV (14%), coronavirus (32%), rhinovirus (17%), human metapneumovirus (9%) and parainfluenza (5%). In multivariable analysis, high T-reg% (HR 0.41, 95% CI 0.20–0.81) and high CMV-reactive CD4+ T-cell% (HR 1.69, 95% CI 1.03–2.78) were predictive of respiratory viral infection.

Conclusions: In elderly nursing home residents, high CMV-reactive CD4+ T-cells were associated with an increased risk and high T-regs were associated with a reduced risk of respiratory viral infection.

Editor: Christine Bourgeois, INSERM, France

Funding: This work was supported by Canadian Institutes of Health Research (CIHR), Public Health Agency of Canada (PHAC)/CIHR Influenza Research Network (PCIRN), National Institues of Health (R01 EB008400/EB/NIBIB), Natural Sciences and Engineering Research Council of Canada. The funders had no role in study design, data collection and analysis, decision to publish, or preparation of the manuscript.

Competing Interests: The authors have declared that no competing interests exist.

* Email: johnsj48@mcmaster.ca (JJ); loebm@mcmaster.ca (ML)

¶ JB and ML are co-senior authors on this work.

Introduction

The burden of respiratory viral infection in elderly nursing home residents is high [1]. With active surveillance the incidence of respiratory viral infection is estimated to range from 1.4–2.8 per 1000 resident days [2]. Influenza and respiratory syncytial virus (RSV) are the viruses commonly responsible for morbidity and mortality associated with infection, but other respiratory viruses including parainfluenza, human metapneumovirus, coronavirus and rhinovirus can also cause severe disease in this population [1,3–7]. It is a widely held belief that immunosenescence, the waning of immune function associated with old age, is responsible for this increased risk and severity of infection [8]; however, only sparse data exist to substantiate this position [9].

As a first step towards the identification of immune biomarkers predictive of respiratory viral infection in elderly nursing home residents, we characterized immune phenotypes in elderly nursing home residents [10]. Whole blood analysis of circulating CD4+ and CD8+ T-cell subsets was performed in a cross-sectional study involving 262 nursing home elderly participants and immune phenotypes were compared to immune phenotypes from healthy adults. In addition, we explored how individual immune phenotypes were influenced by age, sex, frailty and nutritional status in the nursing home elderly [10]. We observed lower naïve CD8+ T-cells (CD8+CD45RA+CCR7+) and higher terminally differentiated memory T-cells (CD8+CD45RA+CCR7-) and senescent T-cells (CD8+CD28−) when compared to healthy adults [10], consistent with prior findings in elderly people [11–14]. It is hypothesized that the reduced numbers of naïve CD8+ T-cells observed in the elderly due to thymic involution, coupled with an accumulation of poorly functioning terminally differentiated memory T-cells and senescent cells possibly arising from chronic antigenic stimulation by cytomegalovirus (CMV) [15,16], predisposes elderly people to infection [17].

Supporting this hypothesis, senescent CD8+ T-cells and high titres of CMV antibody have been found to be associated with influenza vaccine failure in older people [18–20]. Whether these same CD4+ T-cell subsets are associated with infection is less clear. The accumulation of a separate class of T-cell, the regulatory CD4+ T-cell (T-regs) in elderly people has also been observed in elderly nursing home residents [10] and community dwelling elderly people [21]. While T-regs are known to be responsible for controlling the magnitude of CD4+ and CD8+ T-cell responses to viral infections [22], whether the accumulated T-regs in the elderly lead to impairment of host control of infection is not known.

To our knowledge, the relationship between immune phenotypes associated with immunosenescence and risk of respiratory viral infection has not been studied. If a relationship is established, this could help identify elderly nursing home residents at highest risk of become ill and could provide more focused care through targeted prevention. To this end, we sought to identify immune biomarkers predictive of respiratory viral infection during the ensuing respiratory viral season, in an elderly nursing home cohort.

Methods

Subjects and Setting

In this prospective cohort study, elderly participants were recruited from 32 nursing homes in 4 Canadian cities (Halifax, Nova Scotia, Sherbrooke, Quebec, Hamilton, Ontario and Vancouver, British Columbia) in September and October 2009, 2010 and 2011. Residents recruited for a separate study [10] were also eligible for inclusion in this study. Residents ≥65 years of age were eligible for the study. Exclusion criteria included individuals: not planning to be vaccinated against influenza, receiving immunosuppressive medications (including cancer chemotherapy, oral corticosteroid use >21 days, methotrexate, post-transplant medications and/or anti-cytokine or B-lymphocyte depletion therapies), or expected to die within 30 days, as determined by the supervising physician. Written informed consent was obtained from all participants or their legally appointed guardian in the event they were not competent to provide consent themselves. The study protocol was approved by the Research Ethics Board at each participating institution and nursing home.

Trained research personnel abstracted baseline demographics from the participants based on an interview, examination and chart review. Frailty was rated according to the Clinical Frailty Scale, an 8-point scale ranging from 1–8 as follows: (1) very fit, (2) well, (3) well with treated comorbid illness, (4) apparently vulnerable, (5) mildly frail defined as dependence in instrumental activities of daily living (ADL), (6) moderately frail defined as required assistance with basic ADL, (7) severely frail defined as completely dependent on others for ADL and (8) very severely frail

[23]. The Clinical Frailty Scale has been validated in the nursing home population [23]. Participants received the seasonal influenza vaccine, typically in October or November, by public health nurses in accordance with guideline recommendations for the given year [24–26]. Peripheral blood mononuclear cells (PBMCs) were drawn from participants 21 days post vaccination.

Residents were actively followed by research staff for the influenza season immediately following the PBMC draw. The influenza season was defined as spanning from the first week ≥5% of specimens submitted to the local public health laboratory for viral testing were positive for influenza and ending when <5% were positive for influenza for 2 consecutive weeks. The influenza season was chosen as the period of follow-up as the rate of respiratory viral infection is highest during the winter months [2]. Trained research personnel reviewed each participant for the presence of symptoms or signs of respiratory illness twice weekly or more often if notified of symptoms by nursing home staff. Nasopharyngeal swabs (Copan ESwab, Copan Diagnostics Inc., Murrieta, California) were obtained by the research staff when a resident had one or more of the following new symptoms or signs: fever (≥38°Celsius), worsening cough, nasal congestion, sore throat, headache, sinus problems, muscle aches, fatigue, ear ache or infection, chills, not otherwise explained by an alternative diagnosis.

Peripheral Blood Mononuclear Cell Analysis and Flow Cytometry

Blood was obtained from participants between 0700 and 1000 hours and hand delivered to the research laboratory for immediate processing. PBMCs were isolated and frozen using a validated common standard operating procedure [27].

T-cell immune phenotypes were determined by thawing patient PBMCs as previously described [28]. Viability of the PBMCs was found to range between 87% and 98% and the average viability was 94.6%. An aliquot (0.5–16×10^6 cells/stain) was placed in round-bottom 96-well plates with anti-CD3-Qdot605, anti-CD8-Alexa Flour 700, anti-CD4-Pacific Blue, anti-CD45RA-PE Texas Red, anti-CD28-PE, anti-CD57-FITC, anti-CCR7-PE Cy7. T-regs were identified using anti-CD3-FITC, anti-CD4-Pacific Blue, anti-CD127-PerCP-Cy5.5, anti-CD25-PE, and anti-FoxP3-Alexa-Fluor700. The following antibodies were purchased from BD Bioscience: anti-CD4-Pacific Blue, anti-CD28-PE, anti-CCR7-PE-Cy7 and anti-CD25-PE. The following antibodies were purchased from eBioscience: anti-CD3-FITC, anti-CD127-PerCP-Cy5.5, anti-FoxP3-AlexaFluor700. The anti-CD3-Qdot605 was purchased from Invitrogen. The anti-CD57-FITC and anti-CD45RA-PE-TexasRed antibodies were purchased from Beckman Coulter. We defined the T-cell subsets as follows: naïve (CD45RA+CCR7+), terminally differentiated (CD45RA+CCR7-) and senescent (CD28-CD57+). T-regs were defined as CD4+CD25^hiC-D127^lo Foxp3+. CD4+ and CD8+ immune phenotypes and T-regs were expressed as a percentage of CD3+. Antibody staining was performed using a Beckman Coulter Biomek NX^P Laboratory Automation Workstation (Beckman Coulter, Ontario) as previously described [29], followed by analysis using an LSR II flow cytometer with a high-throughput sampler (BD Biosciences, NJ, USA). T-regs were analyzed using FlowJo 9.6 (Treestar Inc, Ashland, OR). T-cell subset analysis employed an automated gating pipeline using the flowDensity algorithm [30]. This approach uses customized threshold calculations for the different cell subsets to mimic a manual gating scheme based on expert knowledge of hierarchical gating order and 1D density information. Population identification is individually tuned to each cell population in a data driven manner. T-cell subpopulations were identified using characteristics of their density distribution such as the number of peaks, height and width of each peak, change of the slope in the distribution curve, standard deviation, and median density (Figure S1). CD45RA thresholds were estimated based on control samples, which where then applied automatically to stimulated samples. CCR7 thresholds were estimated based on CD57+ populations given the explicit instruction that CD57+ cells are CCR7- (Figure S1). A total of 17 populations identified by this approach using high performance computing resources at the Michael Smith Genome Sciences Centre in order to reduce computational time.

CMV-reactive T-cells were identified by stimulating PBMCs with a pool of overlapping peptides spanning the immunodominant pp65 protein of CMV (PepTivator pp65, Miltenyi Biotec) according to our published protocols [28]. Briefly, thawed PBMCs were cultured overnight at 37°C and stimulated with CMV peptides (2 ug/ml) for 1 hr at 37°C. A matched set of PBMCs were stimulated with DMSO as a negative control. Brefeldin A (BD Biosciences) was then added according to the manufacturer's instructions and the cells were incubated for an additional 4 hours. The cells were stained with anti-CD4-PacificBlue and anti-CD8-AlexaFluor700, permeabilized and finally stained with anti-IFN-γ-APC, anti-TNF-α-FITC and anti-CD3-QDot605. CMV-reactive T-cells were identified as CD3+ (CD4+ or CD8+) IFN-γ+ TNF-α+.

Respiratory Virus Detection

Using 200 ul of nasopharyngeal swab material, nucleic acid was extracted by the bioMerieux easyMAG automated extractor. Specimens were tested using the xTAG Respiratory Virus Panel (RVP) assay for influenza A (subtype H1 and H3), influenza B, RSV (subtype A and B), parainfluenza (1–4), coronavirus (NL63, OC43, HKU1 and 229E), human metapneumovirus, enterorhinovirus, and adenovirus as per the manufacturer's protocol (Luminex Molecular Diagnostics, Inc., Toronto, Ontario).

Statistical analysis

The immune phenotype distributions as well as the age distribution were skewed, and so the distributions of these continuous variables were summarized as medians and interquartile ranges (IQR). The age and sex for those who had PBMCs obtained and those who did not were compared using Mann-Whitney U and chi-square test as appropriate. Complete case analysis of immune phenotypes was planned if there was <10% missing data for each parameter [31].

Unadjusted hazard ratios (HR) and 95% confidence intervals (CIs) using Cox proportional hazards model were first constructed to explore the relationship between immune phenotypes and time to symptomatic respiratory viral infection. In the event a resident had multiple respiratory viral infections, only the first infection was included as an outcome. If a participant died prior to a respiratory viral infection, their time was censored on the date of death. We hypothesized that the following immune phenotypes associated with immunosenescence would be associated with increased risk of infection [12–17,21]: low CD4+ and CD8+ naïve T-cells and high CD4+ and CD8+ terminally differentiated and senescent T-cells as well as high CMV-reactive CD4+ and CD8+ T-cells and high T-regs. Low was defined as immune phenotypes in the first quartile of the distribution and high was defined as immune phenotypes in the fourth quartile of the distribution. A priori, it was decided that age, sex and frailty would be included in the final model, given their potential for confounding with the effects of primary interest in this population [32]. Immune phenotypes with a p-value <0.20 in univariable analysis were included in the final multivariable model. The final model was determined using backwards elimination. A sandwich variance estimator was used to account

for the clustering effect at the level of the nursing homes [33]. The proportional hazards assumption for continuous variables was explored graphically by plotting partial residuals against time to event and tested by regressing the partial residuals against time. The proportional hazards assumption for categorical variables was examined by a log-minus-log graph to ensure the plotted lines remained parallel. The presence of multicollinearity was examined using the variance inflation factor (VIF); presence of multicollinearity was defined as VIF >5.

P-values and 95% CIs were constructed using 2-tailed tests. P-values <0.05 were considered statistically significant. Statistical analyses were performed using R, version 3.0.2 [34].

Results

Nursing Home Cohort

In total, 1165 residents were enrolled in the study and of these, and PBMC were obtained from 1087 (93%). Reasons for not obtaining PBMCs were either refusal of influenza vaccine or refusal of blood draw. There was no statistically significant difference in age (median, 86 (IQR 80–90) versus 85 (IQR 79–89) without PBMCs, p = 0.42) or sex (%female, 72% versus 64% without PBMCs, p = 0.12) between those that did and did not have PBMCs obtained. Fifteen participants (1%) withdrew before the end of the study, leaving 1072 as our final sample size. Seventy-three participants died before a respiratory viral infection could be identified.

Baseline Characteristics

Baseline characteristics of the final cohort are summarized in Table 1. The median age was 86 years (IQR 80–90 years) and the ages ranged from 65–102 years. Eight persons were ≥100 years. Most (93%) had at least one co-morbidity, and almost half (44%) scored either 7 or 8 on the Clinical Frailty Scale, which is defined as severely and very severely frail respectively. Figures 1, 2 and 3 describe the gating strategies used to define the immune phenotypes. The medians and corresponding IQRs for each immune cell type tested in this study can be found in Table 1.

Respiratory Virus Infection

In total, 269 swabs were obtained from 233 symptomatic people. Nasopharyngeal swabs were positive for viruses in 87 symptomatic residents (Table 2). Coronavirus (32%), influenza (24%), rhinovirus (17%) and RSV (14%) were the most common viruses found. One nasopharyngeal swab positive for influenza A also had rhinovirus present.

Predictors of Respiratory Virus Infection

We subsequently investigated whether a relationship existed between specific immune cell populations and respiratory virus infection. The proportional hazards assumption was satisfied for all covariates included in the model and there was no concerning evidence of multicollinearity (all VIFs were <3). In univariable analyses, low naïve CD8+ T-cell% (HR 0.69, 95% CI 0.51–0.95) and high T-reg% (HR 0.47, 95% CI 0.26–0.85) were associated with a reduced risk of respiratory viral infection and high terminally differentiated CD8+ T-cell% (HR 1.57, 95% CI 1.10–2.24), high senescent CD8+ T-cell% (HR 1.55, 95% CI 1.11–2.17) and high CMV-reactive CD4+ T-cell% (HR 1.82, 95% CI 1.13–2.94), were associated with an increased risk of respiratory viral infection (Table 3). In multivariable analysis adjusted for age, sex and frailty, only high T-reg% (HR 0.41, 95% CI 0.20–0.81) and high CMV-reactive CD4+ T-cell% (HR 1.69, 95% CI 1.03–

Table 1. Baseline characteristics of the nursing home elderly.

	Total n = 1072
Demographics [n(%)]	
Age (years)	
65–74	131 (12)
75–84	337 (31)
85–94	508 (47)
≥95	96 (9)
Sex (F)	776 (72)
Prior co-morbidity	
COPD	186 (17)
Coronary artery disease	346 (32)
Diabetes	290 (27)
Heart failure	148 (14)
Stroke	273 (25)
Dementia	511 (48)
≥5 medications	966 (90)
Frailty	
4	76 (7)
5	174 (16)
6	354 (33)
7	460 (43)
8	8 (1)
Immune Phenotypes [median (IQR)]	
CD8+ T-cell	
Naïve CD8+ T-cell%	1.10 (0.60–1.82)
Terminally differentiated CD8+ T-cell%	8.95 (4.72–14.80)
Senescent CD8+ T-cell%	5.87 (2.40–11.58)
CD8+ CMV T-cell%	0.32 (.03–1.53)
CD4+ T-cell	
Naïve CD4+ T-cell%	13.2 (6.90–22.85)
Terminally differentiated CD4+ T-cell%	8.46 (4.93–14.04)
Senescent CD4+ T-cell%	1.66 (0.28–4.54)
CD4+ CMV T-cell%	0.06 (0.006–0.40)
T-reg	
T-reg%	2.73 (2.12–3.45)

2.78) remained predictive of respiratory viral infection in the final model (Table 3 and Figure 4).

Discussion

In this prospective cohort study of elderly nursing home residents, CD4+ T cells, in particular T-regs and CMV-reactive CD4+ T-cells were predictive of respiratory viral infection during the ensuing respiratory viral season in multivariable analysis. In contrast, CD8+ T-cells were not found to be predictive in multivariable analysis. To our knowledge, this is the first study to identify immune biomarkers predictive of respiratory viral infection in elderly people.

T-regs are responsible for creating the balance between the immune response to pathogens and the harmful sequelae of inflammation that arises with this response [35]. High T-regs have

been consistently observed in elderly people when compared to healthy adults [10,21], and it has been hypothesized that this shift may be associated with increased risk of infection seen in the elderly [21,36]. It is intriguing that in our study higher levels of circulating T-regs were associated with reduced risk of symptomatic respiratory virus infection. We did not systematically test all residents in our study for respiratory virus throughout the study, so we cannot determine whether the association between high T-regs and reduced risk of infection was due to absence of infection or whether there was a higher incidence of asymptomatic infections in the high T-reg group. Little is known about the role of T-regs in preventing acute respiratory viral infection in humans [35]. In mice, a robust T-reg response has been observed during influenza [37] and RSV infection [38] and depletion of T-regs delays RSV viral clearance from lungs [38] suggesting that T-regs play an important role in controlling the immune response to respiratory

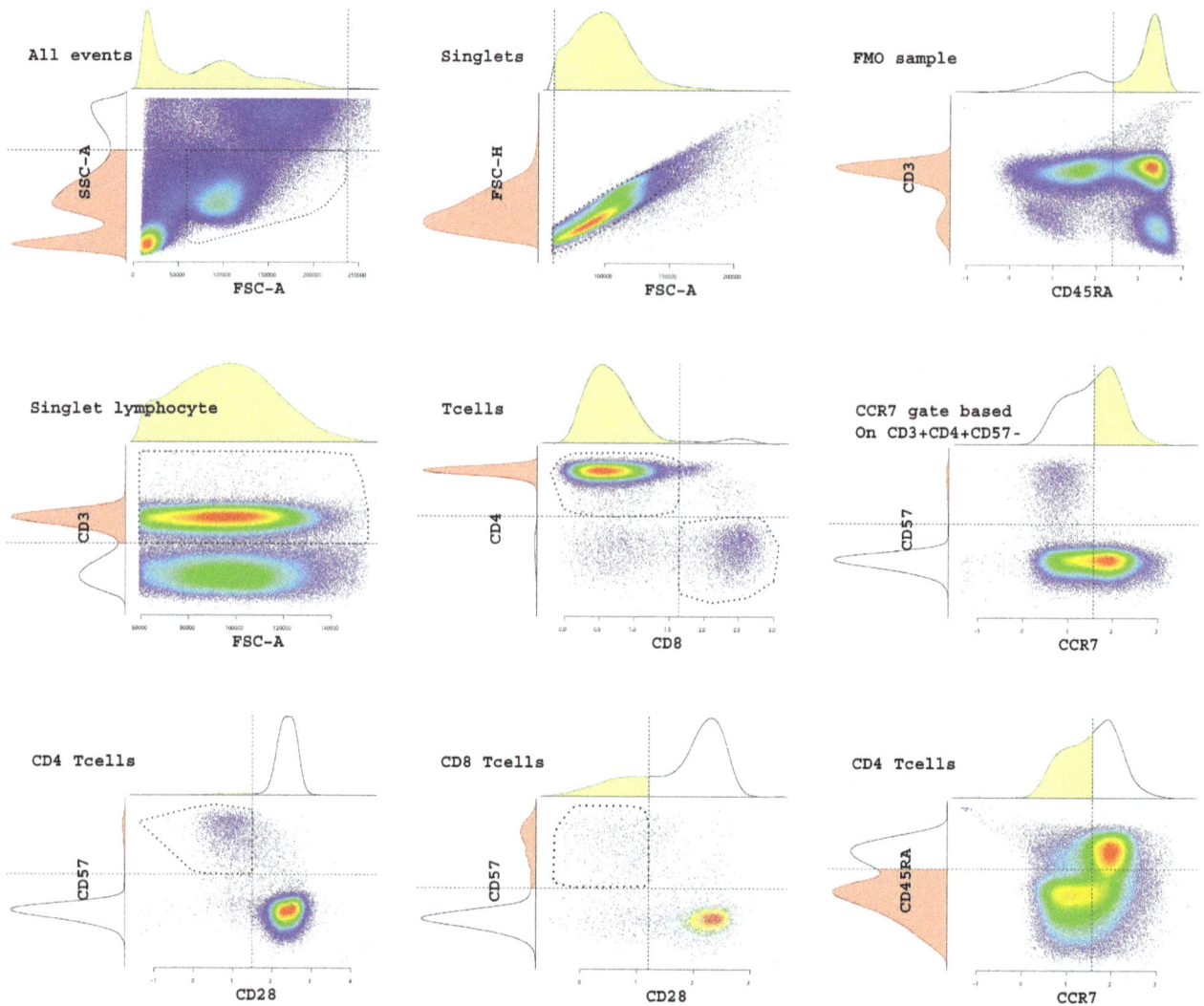

Figure 1. Gating strategy for T-cell phenotypes. T cell phenotypes were defined using the flowDensity software package. Lymphocytes were first gated from non-margin events, and then singlets were gated. CD45RA thresholds were calculated based on singlet lymphocytes FMO. CD3+ cells were gated and then separated into CD4+CD8- and CD4-CD8+. Expression of CD57, CD28, CD45RA and CCR7 was analyzed on either CD4+CD8- or CD8-CD4+.

viral infection. In aged mice, higher percentages of T-regs are observed at baseline and during acute influenza infection when compared to younger mice, and their presence is thought to contribute to a decrease and delay of CD8+ T-cell response during acute influenza infection [39]. In consideration of the murine data, we speculate that elevated levels of T-regs may suppress immune pathology associated with anti-viral immunity.

CMV has been proposed as the chronic antigenic stimulus responsible for accelerated immunosenescence, including the accumulation of senescent CD8+ T-cells [40,41]. There have been at least three studies looking at the association between CMV infection and influenza vaccine response in the elderly [20,42,43]. In one, CMV was associated with influenza vaccine non-response [20], however two other studies found no association [42,43]. In contrast to the reports on seropositivity, we focused on the T-cell response to CMV and observed that elevated frequencies of CMV-reactive CD4+ T-cells, but not CMV-reactive CD8+ T-cells, were associated with an increased risk of respiratory viral infection. We are unaware of any other study linking CMV-

reactive CD4+ T-cells to increased risk of respiratory viral infection. It is difficult to speculate on the possible biological relationship between the CMV-reactive CD4+ T cells and susceptibility to infection. Given the observation that CD4+ T-regs also correlate with susceptibility, we interpret these collective data as an indication that the distribution of functional cells (i.e. effector, suppressor, Th1, Th2, etc...) within the CD4+ T cell compartment has a strong influence on host resistance in the elderly. Most research to date has focused on CD8+ T-cells in the elderly and these observation strongly support a new line of research in the elderly to understand how and why skewing of the CD4+ T-cell compartment contributes significantly to the outcome of respiratory infection.

Low naïve CD8+ T-cells, high terminally differentiated CD8+ T-cells and senescent CD8+ T-cells have been described in elderly populations [10–14] and have been hypothesized to predict risk of infection [9,17]. Although there were associations between these immune phenotypes and risk of respiratory viral infection in univariable analyses, after adjustment for known confounders such

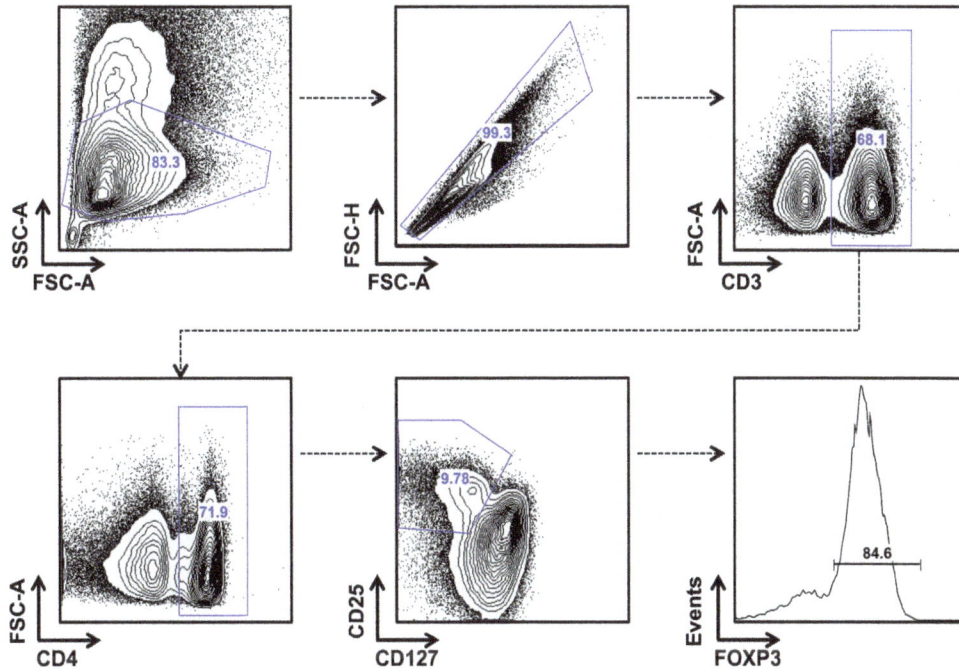

Figure 2. Gating strategy of T-reg. Lymphocytes and singlets were selected. Gates were then set up for CD3+ cells and CD4+. To identify the T-regs, a gate was set up to select CD25+CD127 $^{lo/-}$ and T-regs were defined as CD25+CD127 $^{lo/-}$ FOXP3+.

as age, sex and frailty, CD8+ T cells were not predictive of respiratory viral infection once all immune phenotypes with suspected association with respiratory viral infection were included in the model. This illustrates the need for a robust statistical

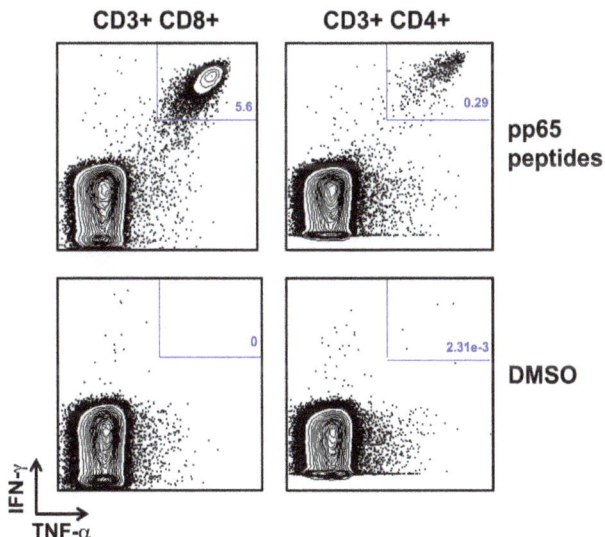

Figure 3. Gating strategy for CMV-reactive T cells. PBMC were stimulated with pp65 peptides to identify CMV-reactive T-cells. As a negative control, PBMC were stimulated with DMSO. Subsequently, the T-cells were stained for surface markers and intracellular cytokines. To define the CMV-reactive T-cells, the flow data was gated on singlet lymphocytes (as shown in Figures 1 and 2) and subsequently gated on CD3+CD8+ cells and CD3+CD4+. The plots show intracellular cytokine staining results for a single patient. CMV-reactive T-cells were defined as IFN-γ+ TNF-α+.

approach, including adequate sample size allowing for adjustment for known confounders and other immune phenotypes when exploring associations between immune biomarkers and outcomes.

Frailty is a "state variable" which aims to capture a person's vulnerability to adverse health outcomes. The Clinical Frailty Scale used here has been previously validated in nursing home residents and has been shown to robustly predict outcomes including mortality, disability and cognitive decline [23]. Frailty influences health outcomes through a number of mechanisms, including overall burden of disease/comorbidity and reduced reserve to tolerate further insults. Frailty has also been associated with immunosenescence [44]. Because of its importance as a measure of overall health and its relevance to immune function, it was a relevant measure to include in this study.

Our analysis was greatly facilitated by an automated analysis approach which eliminated what would have otherwise been an extremely time-consuming process of manual gating over 1,000 FCS files using an approach that was unbiased relative to manual gating with variability as low or even lower than manual gating. This approach should help facilitate the efficiency of future large studies of immune biomarkers.

This study provides insights into the role of immunosenescence and the risk of respiratory viral infection in elderly nursing home residents. Although our study was designed to identify associations and not causation, our findings suggest the possibility that strategies to boost circulating T-regs [45] or vaccines to prevent infection with CMV [46] or prophylactic anti-viral therapy to prevent re-activation of CMV may reduce respiratory viral infections in this high-risk population. In addition, those identified at increased risk of respiratory viral infection could be offered alternative prevention strategies such as heightened surveillance during the highest risk periods, which could help prevent nursing home outbreaks and transmission to healthcare workers and their families.

Table 2. Respiratory viruses present in symptomatic elderly nursing home residents.

	Nasopharyngeal swabs positive for respiratory virus* n = 87 n(%)
Influenza	21 (24)
Influenza A	16 (18)
Influenza B	5 (6)
RSV	12 (14)
RSV A	10 (11)
RSV B	2 (2)
Coronavirus	28 (32)
Coronavirus OC43	15 (17)
Coronavirus NL63/229E	9 (10)
Coronavirus HKU1	4 (5)
Rhinovirus	15 (17)
Human metapneumovirus	8 (9)
Parainfluenza	4 (5)
Parainfluenza 1	3 (3)
Parainfluenza 2	1 (1)

*One patient had mixed influenza A and rhinovirus.

Limitations of this study include lower than expected influenza viral infection. Although influenza is not necessarily the most common virus isolated in nursing homes, [1], we expected to see more than 21 cases in 1072 residents during the influenza season based on prior respiratory viral infection surveillance studies conducted in nursing homes [1,2]. We do not believe that cases were missed. Indeed, we performed prospective active surveillance for symptomatic respiratory viral infection, and approximately one third of the nasopharyngeal swabs were positive for virus, comparable to another study, which performed active surveillance

Table 3. Immune phenotype predictors of respiratory viral infection in univariable and multivariable analysis.

	HR (95% CI) Unadjusted	P-value	HR (95% CI) Final Model*	P-value
Age	0.99 (0.97–1.01)	0.35	0.99 (0.98–1.01)	0.30
Sex				
Male	Reference		Reference	
Female	1.13 (0.65–1.98)	0.66	1.03 (0.58–1.84)	0.92
Clinical Frailty Scale				
4	Reference		Reference	
5	1.44 (0.34–6.17)	0.62	2.68 (0.58–12.47)	0.21
6	1.99 (0.59–6.70)	0.27	3.67 (1.06–12.67)	0.04
7 or 8	1.41 (0.39–5.07)	0.60	2.45 (0.55–10.86)	0.24
CD8+ T-cell				
Low naïve CD8+ T-cell%	0.69 (0.51–0.95)	0.02		
High terminally differentiated CD8+ T-cell%	1.57 (1.10–2.24)	0.01		
High senescent CD8+ T-cell%	1.55 (1.11–2.17)	0.01		
High CMV-reactive CD8+ T-cell%	1.15 (0.65–2.03)	0.64		
CD4+ T-cell				
Low naïve CD4+ T-cell%	0.85 (0.61–1.18)	0.33		
High terminally differentiated CD4+ T-cell%	0.96 (0.60–1.55)	0.88		
High senescent CD4+ T-cell%	1.08 (0.71–1.64)	0.73		
High CMV-reactive CD4+ T-cell%	1.82 (1.13–2.94)	0.01	1.69 (1.03–2.78)	0.04
T-reg				
High T-reg%	0.47 (0.26–0.85)	0.01	0.41 (0.20–0.81)	0.01

*Final model adjusted for age, sex, frailty, high T-reg% and high CMV-reactive CD4+ T-cell%.

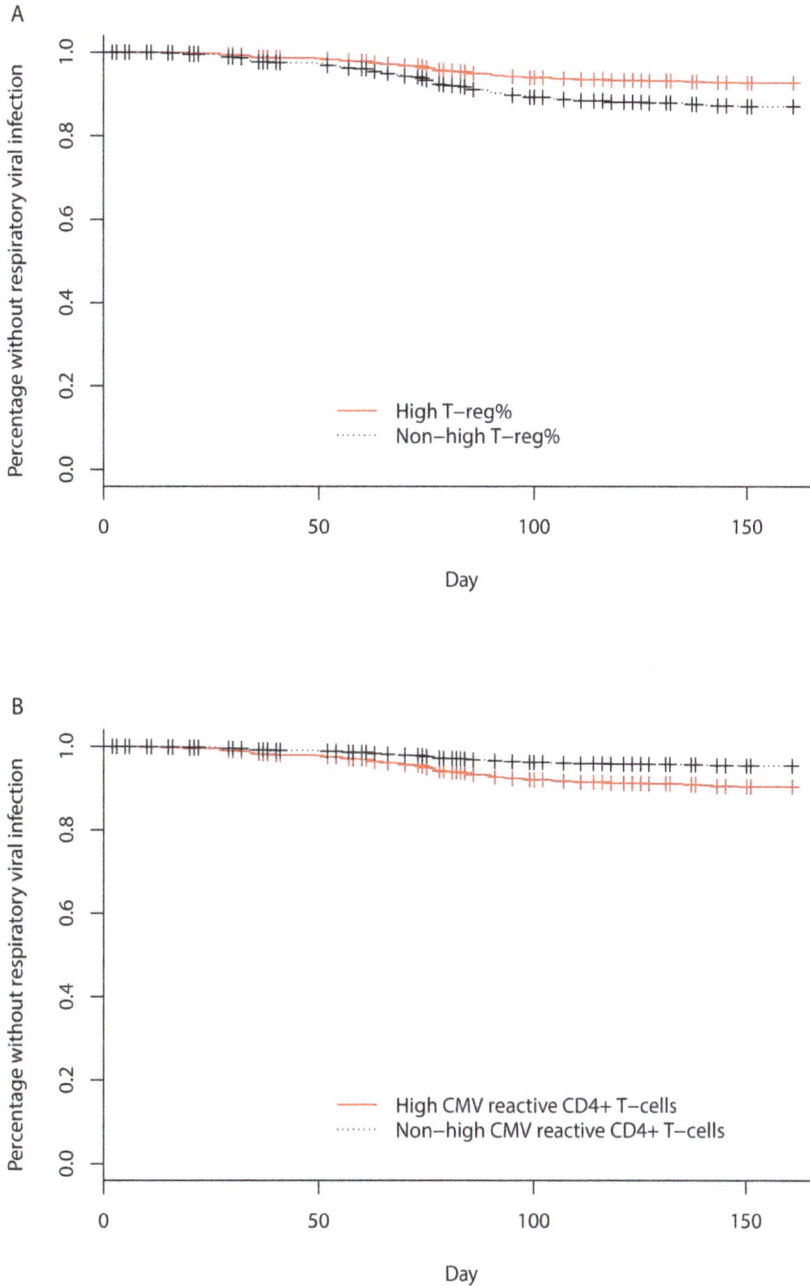

Figure 4. Time to respiratory viral infection stratified by a) T-reg%, adjusted for age, sex, frailty and CMV-reactive CD4+ T-cell%) and b) CMV-reactive CD4+ T-cell%, adjusted for age, sex, frailty and T-reg%.

for respiratory infections in nursing homes in Canada [2]. Instead, we believe the lower numbers were due to circulation of pandemic H1N1, an influenza strain that had less impact on older people during the 2009–2010 influenza season than pre-pandemic years and the relatively low incidence of influenza during 2010-2011 influenza season [47]. In addition, the lower numbers could have been due to the fact that we only included residents who had been vaccinated against influenza. We felt that influenza vaccination status was too important a confounder to manage statistically, both because of its potential ability to prevent influenza infection and because of its association with the healthy user bias [48,49]. It remains possible that there are different immune predictors for

each of the different respiratory viruses in this vaccinated cohort and combining the respiratory viruses together in one combined endpoint limited its generalizability; however we chose *a priori* to combine the respiratory viruses together in a combined endpoint based on the fact they result in similar outcomes in this population [1,3–7]. The low number of participants with influenza precluded our ability to perform a sensitivity analysis, looking at immune phenotypes predictive of influenza infection.

An additional limitation was that we were unable to include immune phenotypes as continuous variables in the analysis. In general, maintaining data as continuous is preferred over categorizing data [50]; however an analysis including immune phenotype data as continuous was not feasible as it led to estimates with wide confidence intervals. Thus, the analysis was performed using categorized variables, similar to other aging studies [51–55]. Although seventy-three participants died prior to developing a respiratory viral infection, we do not believe this competing risk introduced significant bias. Competing risks are unlikely to bias the result when the follow-up is short, or the proportion of participants experiencing a competing risk is less than the proportion of participants experiencing the outcome [56]. In this study, the follow-up was short (only one influenza season) and the proportion of participants who died was less than those who developed a respiratory viral infection. Last, these results were obtained in a frail elderly population and may not be generalizable to community dwelling elderly.

In conclusion, in elderly nursing home residents, high CMV-reactive CD4+ T-cells were predictive of increased risk of respiratory viral infection and high T-regs were predictive of reduced risk during the ensuing respiratory viral season. These findings provide insights into immunosenescence and risk of infection and may help guide future prevention strategies.

Supporting Information

Figure S1 Comparison of automated versus manual gating for T-cell phenotypes. The same gating hierarchy was used for manual (top row) and automated (bottom row) approaches for the T-cell panel as described in the text. Similar results were obtained for both methods.

Acknowledgments

We wish to acknowledge the hard work and dedication of the clinical research staff on this project including Chenai Muzamhindo, Diane Dakers, Ashley Chin, Louise Rochon, Eliette Théberge, Sarah DeCoutere and Gale Tedder as well as the Canada's Michael Smith Genome Sciences Centre, Vancouver, Canada for high performance computing support. Dr. Jennie Johnstone receives salary support from CIHR. Mark Loeb holds the Michael G. DeGroote Chair in Infectious Diseases at McMaster University. Jonathan Bramson holds a Canadian Research Chair in Translational Cancer Immunology and the John Bienenstock Chair in Molecular Medicine.

Author Contributions

Conceived and designed the experiments: JJ SM TF J. McElhaney MA JB ML. Performed the experiments: RP FB J. Millar MM RB JM JB. Analyzed the data: JJ SW PD JB ML. Contributed reagents/materials/analysis tools: RB J. Mahony JB. Wrote the paper: JJ RP FB J. Millar SM TF J. McElhaney MA SW PD MM RB J. Mahoney JB ML.

References

1. Falsey A, Dallal G, Formica M, Andolina G, Hamer D, et al. (2008) Long-term care facilities: a cornucopia of viral pathogens. J Am Geriatr Soc 56: 1281–1285.
2. Loeb M, McGeer A, McArthur M, Peeling RW, Petric M, et al. (2000) Surveillance for outbreaks of respiratory tract infections in nursing homes. CMAJ 162: 1133–1137.
3. Drinka P, Gravenstein S, Langer E, Krause P, Shult P (1999) Mortality following isolation of various respiratory viruses in nursing home residents. Infect Control Hosp Epidemiol 20: 812–815.
4. Louie J, Yagi S, Nelson F, Kiang D, Glaser C, et al. (2005) Rhinovirus outbreak in a long-term care facility for elderly persons associated with unusually high mortality. Clin Infect Dis 41: 262–265.
5. Hicks L, Shepard C, Britz P, Erdman D, Fischer M, et al. (2006) Two outbreaks of severe respiratory disease in nursing homes associated with rhinovirus. J Am Geriatr Soc 54: 284–289.
6. Falsey A, McCann R, Hall W, Criddle M, Formica M, et al. (1997) The "common cold" in frail older person: impact of rhinovirus and coronavirus in a senior daycare center. J Am Geriatr Soc 45: 706–711.
7. Boivin G, De Serres G, Hamelin M, Côté S, Argouin M, et al. (2007) An outbreak of severe respiratory tract infection due to human metapneumovirus in a long-term care facility. Clin Infect Dis 44: 1152–1158.
8. Smith P, Bennett G, Bradley S, Drinka P, Lautenbach E, et al. (2008) SHEA/APIC Guideline: Infection prevention and control in the long-term care facility; Society for Healthcare Epidemiology of America (SHEA); Association for Professionals in Infection Control and Epidemiology (APIC). Am J Infect Control 36: 504–535.
9. Fulop T, Pawelec G, Castle S, Loeb M (2009) Immunosenescence and vaccination in nursing home residents. Clin Infect Dis 48: 443–448.
10. Johnstone J, Millar J, Lelic A, Verschoor C, Walter S, et al. (2014) Immunosenescence in the nursing home elderly. BMC Geriatrics 14: 50.
11. Saule P, Trauet J, Dutriez V, Lekeux V, Dessaint J, et al. (2006) Accumulation of memory T cells from childhood to old age: central and effector memory cells in CD4+ versus effector memory and terminally differentiated memory cells in CD8+ compartment. Mech Ageing Dev 127: 274–281.
12. Fahey J, Schnelle J, Boscardin J, Thomas J, Gorre M, et al. (2000) Distinct categories of immunologic changes in frail elderly. Mech Ageing Dev 115: 1–20.
13. Effros R, Boucher N, Porter V, Zhu X, Spaulding C, et al. (1994) Decline in CD28+ T cells in centenarians and in long-term T cell cultures: a possible cause for both in vivo and in vitro immunosenescence. Exp Gerontol 29: 601–609.
14. Boucher N, Dufeu-Duchesne T, Vicaut E, Farge D, Effros R, et al. (1998) CD28 expression in T cell aging and human longevity. Exp Gerontol 33: 267–282.
15. Wikby A, Johansson B, Olsson J, Löfgren S, Nilsson B, et al. (2002) Expansion of peripheral blood CD8 T-lymphocyte subpopulations and an association with cytomegalovirus seropositivity in the elderly: the Swedish NONA immune study. Exp Gerontol 37: 445–453.
16. Looney R, Falsey A, Campbell D, Torres A, Kolassa J, et al. (1999) Role of cytomegalovirus in the T-cell changes seen in elderly individuals. Clin Immunol 90: 213–219.

17. Fulop T, Larbi A, Wikby A, Mocchegiani E, Hirokawa K, et al. (2005) Dysregulation of T-cell function in the elderly: scientific basis and clinical implications. Drugs Aging 22: 589–603.
18. Goronzy J, Fulbright J, Crowson C, Poland G, O'Fallon W, et al. (2001) Value of immunological markers in predicting responsiveness to influenza vaccination in elderly individuals. J Virol 75: 12182–12187.
19. Saurwein-Teissl M, Lung T, Marx F, Gschösser C, Asch E, et al. (2002) Lack of antibody production following immunization in old age: association with CD8+ CD28- T cell clonal expansions and an imbalance in the production of Th1 and Th2 cytokines. J Immunol 168: 5893–5899.
20. Trzonkowski P, Mysliwska J, Szmit E, Wieckiewicz J, Lukaszuk K, et al. (2003) Association between cytomegalovirus infection, enhanced proinflammatory response and low level of anti-hemagglutinins during the anti-influenza vaccination – an impact of immunosenescence. Vaccine 21: 3826–3836.
21. Wang L, Xie Y, Zhu L, Chang T, Mao Y, et al. (2010) An association between immunosenescence and CD4+CD25+ regulatory T-cells: a systematic review. Biomed Environ Sci 23: 327–332.
22. Rowe J, Ertelt J, Way S (2012) Foxp3+ regulatory T-cells, immune stimulation and host defence against infection. Immunology 136: 1–10.
23. Rockwood K, Abeysundera M, Mitnitski A (2007) How should we grade frailty in nursing home patients? J Am Med Dir Assoc 8: 595–603.
24. Langley J, Warshawsky B, Ismail S, Crowcroft N, Hanrahan A, et al. (2009) Statement on seasonal trivalent inactivated influenza vaccine for 2009–2010. CCDR 35: ACS-6.
25. Langley J, Warshawsky B, Ismail S, Crowcroft N, Hanrahan A, et al. (2010) Statement on seasonal trivalent inactivated influenza vaccine for 2010–2011. CCDR 36: ACS-6.
26. Langley J, Warshawsky B, Cooper C, Crowcroft N, Hanrahan A, et al. (2011) Statement on seasonal trivalent inactivated influenza vaccine for 2011–2012. CCDR 37: ACS-5.
27. Disis M, dela Rosa C, Goodell V, Kuan L, Chang J, et al. (2006) Maximizing the retention of antigen specific lymphocyte function after cryopreservation. J Immunol 308: 13–18.
28. Lelic A, Verschoor C, Ventresca M, Parsons R, Evelegh C, et al. (2012) The polyfunctionality of human memory CD8+ T cells elicited by acute and chronic virus infections is not influenced by age. PLoS Pathog 8: e1003076.
29. Verschoor C, Johnstone J, Millar J, Dorrington M, Habibagahi M, et al. (2013) Blood CD33(+)HLA-DR(-) myeloid-derived suppressor cells are increased with age and a history of cancer. J Leukoc Biol 93: 633–637.
30. Submitted as an R package in Bioconductor: An open source, open development software project to provide tools for the analysis and comprehension of high-throughput genomic data.
31. Marshall A, Altman D, Holder R (2010) Comparison of imputation methods for handling missing covariate data when fitting a Cox proportional hazards model: a resampling study. BMC Med Res Methodol 31: 112.
32. Fulop T, Larbi A, Witkowski J, McElhaney J, Loeb M, et al. (2010) Aging, frailty and age-related disease. Biogerontology 11: 547–563.

33. Wei L, Lin D, Weissfeld L (1989) Regression-analysis of multivariate incomplete failure time data by modeling marginal distributions. J Am Stat Assoc 84: 1065–1073.

34. R Core Team (2013) R: A language and environment for statistical computing. R Foundation for Statistical Computing, Vienna, Austria. ISBN 3-900051-07-0. Available: http://www.R-project.org/.

35. Keynan Y, Card C, McLaren P, Dawood M, Kasper K, et al. (2008) The role of regulatory T-cells in chronic and acute viral infections. Clin Infect Dis 46: 1046–1052.

36. Lages C, Suffia I, Velilla P, Huang B, Warshaw G, et al. (2008) Functional regulatory T cells accumulate in aged hosts and promote chronic infectious disease reactivation. J Immunol 181: 1835–1848.

37. Betts R, Prabhu N, Ho A, Lew F, Hutchinson P, et al. (2012) Influenza A virus infection results in a robust, antigen-responsive, and widely disseminated Fox3+ regulatory T cell response. J Virol 86: 2817–2825.

38. Fulton R, Meyerholz D, Varga S (2010) Foxp3+ CD4 regulatory T cells limit pulmonary immunopathology by modulating the CD8 T cell response during respiratory syncytial virus infection. J Immunol 185: 2382–2392.

39. Williams-Bey Y, Jiang J, Murasko D (2011) Expansion of regulatory T cells in aged mice following influenza infection. Mech Ageing Dev 132: 163–170.

40. Koch S, Larbi A, Ozcelik D, Solana R, Gouttefangeas C, et al. (2007) Cytomegalovirus: A driving force in human T-cell immunosenescence. Ann NY Acad Sci 1114: 23–25.

41. Pawelec G, Derhovanessian E, Larbi A, Strindhall J, Wikby A, et al. (2009) Cytomegalovirus and human immunosenescence. Rev Med Virol 19: 47–56.

42. den Elzen W, Vossen A, Cools H, Westendorp R, Kroes A, et al. (2011) Cytomegalovirus infection and responsiveness to influenza vaccination in elderly residents of long-term care facilities. Vaccine 29: 4869–4874.

43. Derhovanessian E, Theeten H, Hahnel K, Van Damme P, Cools N, et al. (2013) Cytomegalovirus-associated accumulation of late-differentiated CD4 T-cells correlates with poor humoral response to influenza vaccination. Vaccine 31: 685–690.

44. McElhaney J, Zhou X, Talbot H, Soethout E, Bleackley R, et al. (2012) The unmet need in the elderly: How immunosenescence, CMV infection, co-morbidities and frailty are a challenge for the development of more effective influenza vaccines. Vaccine 30: 2060–2067.

45. Sehrawat S, Rouse B (2011) Tregs and infections: on the potential value of modifying their function. J Leukoc Biol 90: 1079–1087.

46. Krause P, Bialek S, Boppana S, Griffiths PD, Laughlin C, et al. (2013) Priorities for CMV vaccine development. Vaccine 32: 4–10.

47. Mitchell R, Taylor G, McGeer A, Frenette C, Suh K, et al. (2013) Understanding the burden of influenza infection among adults in Canadian hospitals: a comparison of the 2009–2010 pandemic season with the prepandemic and postpandemic seasons. Am J Infect Control 41: 1032–1037.

48. Jackson L, Jackson M, Nelson J, Neuzil K, Weiss N (2006) Evidence of bias in estimates of influenza vaccine effectiveness in seniors. Int J Epidemiol 35: 337–344.

49. Jackson L, Nelson J, Benson P, Neuzil K, Reid R, et al. (2006) Functional status is a confounder of the association of influenza vaccine and risk of all cause mortality in seniors. Int J Epidemiol 35: 345–352.

50. Bennette C, Vickers A (2012) Against quantiles: categorization of continuous variables in epidemiologic research, and its discontents. BMC Med Res Methodol 12: 21.

51. Izaks G, Remarque E, Becker S, Westendorp R (2003) Lymphocyte count and mortality risk in older persons. The Leiden 85-plus study. J Am Geriatr Soc 51: 1461–1465.

52. Leng S, Xue Q, Tian J, Huang Y, Yeh S, et al. (2009) Associations of neutrophil and monocyte counts with frailty in community-dwelling disabled older women: results from the Women's Health and Aging Studies I. Experimental Gerontol 44: 511–516.

53. Collerton J, Martin-Ruiz C, Davies K, Hilkens C, Isaacs J, et al. (2012) Frailty and the role of inflammation, immunosenescence and cellular ageing in the very old: cross-sectional findings from the Newcastle 85+ study. Mech Ageing Dev 133: 456–466.

54. Wang G, Kao W, Murakami P, Xue Q, Chiou R, et al. (2010) Cytomegalovirus infection and the risk of mortality and frailty in older women: a prospective observational cohort study. Am J Epidemiol 171: 1144–1152.

55. Mathei C, Vaes B, Wallemacq P, Degryse J (2011) Associations between cytomegalovirus infection and functional impairment and frailty in the BEFRAIL cohort. J Am Geriatr Soc 59: 2201–2208.

56. Berry S, Ngo L, Samelson E, Kiel D (2010) Competing risk of death: an important consideration in studies of older adults. J Am Geriatr Soc 58: 783–787.

Permissions

The contributors of this book come from diverse backgrounds, making this book a truly international effort. This book will bring forth new frontiers with its revolutionizing research information and detailed analysis of the nascent developments around the world.

We would like to thank all the contributing authors for lending their expertise to make the book truly unique. They have played a crucial role in the development of this book. Without their invaluable contributions this book wouldn't have been possible. They have made vital efforts to compile up to date information on the varied aspects of this subject to make this book a valuable addition to the collection of many professionals and students.

This book was conceptualized with the vision of imparting up-to-date information and advanced data in this field. To ensure the same, a matchless editorial board was set up. Every individual on the board went through rigorous rounds of assessment to prove their worth. After which they invested a large part of their time researching and compiling the most relevant data for our readers.

The editorial board has been involved in producing this book since its inception. They have spent rigorous hours researching and exploring the diverse topics which have resulted in the successful publishing of this book. They have passed on their knowledge of decades through this book. To expedite this challenging task, the publisher supported the team at every step. A small team of assistant editors was also appointed to further simplify the editing procedure and attain best results for the readers.

Apart from the editorial board, the designing team has also invested a significant amount of their time in understanding the subject and creating the most relevant covers. They scrutinized every image to scout for the most suitable representation of the subject and create an appropriate cover for the book.

The publishing team has been an ardent support to the editorial, designing and production team. Their endless efforts to recruit the best for this project, has resulted in the accomplishment of this book. They are a veteran in the field of academics and their pool of knowledge is as vast as their experience in printing. Their expertise and guidance has proved useful at every step. Their uncompromising quality standards have made this book an exceptional effort. Their encouragement from time to time has been an inspiration for everyone.

The publisher and the editorial board hope that this book will prove to be a valuable piece of knowledge for researchers, students, practitioners and scholars across the globe.

List of Contributors

Martin Griebe, Michael G. Hennerici, Achim Gass and Kristina Szabo
Department of Neurology, MR Research Neurology, Universitäts Medizin Mannheim, University of Heidelberg, Mannheim, Germany

Michael Amann
Department of Neurology, University Hospital Basel, Basel, Switzerland
Division of Diagnostic and Interventional Neuroradiology, Department of Radiology, Basel, Switzerland

Jochen G. Hirsch
Fraunhofer MEVIS, Institute for Medical Image Computing, Bremen, Germany

Lutz Achtnichts
Department of Neurology, University Hospital Basel, Basel, Switzerland

Felix Grassmann, Peter G. A. Schoenberger and Bernhard H. F. Weber
Institute of Human Genetics, University of Regensburg, Regensburg, Germany

Caroline Brandl
Institute of Human Genetics, University of Regensburg, Regensburg, Germany
Department of Ophthalmology, University Hospital Regensburg, Regensburg, Germany

Tina Schick and Sascha Fauser
Department of Ophthalmology, University Hospital of Cologne, Cologne, Germany

Daniele Hasler and Gunter Meister
Biochemistry Center Regensburg (BZR), Laboratory for RNA Biology, University of Regensburg, Regensburg, Germany

Monika Fleckenstein and Moritz Lindner
Department of Ophthalmology, University of Bonn, Bonn, Germany

Horst Helbig
Department of Ophthalmology, University Hospital Regensburg, Regensburg, Germany

Wai H. Lim
University of Western Australia School of Medicine and Pharmacology, Sir Charles Gairdner Hospital Unit, Perth, Australia
Department of Renal Medicine, Sir Charles Gairdner Hospital, Perth, Australia

Joshua R. Lewis and Richard L. Prince
University of Western Australia School of Medicine and Pharmacology, Sir Charles Gairdner Hospital Unit, Perth, Australia
Department of Endocrinology and Diabetes, Sir Charles Gairdner Hospital, Perth, Australia

Germaine Wong
entre for Kidney Research, Children's Hospital at Westmead, Sydney, Australia
School of Public Health, Sydney Medical School, The University of Sydney, Sydney, Australia

Robin M. Turner
School of Public Health, The University of New South Wales, Sydney, Australia

Ee M. Lim
Department of Renal Medicine, Sir Charles Gairdner Hospital, Perth, Australia
PathWest, Sir Charles Gairdner Hospital, Perth, Australia

Peter L. Thompson
Department of Cardiovascular Medicine, Sir Charles Gairdner Hospital, Perth, Australia

Peng-Ching Hsiao
Graduate Institute of Medical Sciences, National Defense Medical Center, Department of Nursing, Tri Service General Hospital, Taipei, Taiwan

Chi-Ming Chu
Section of Health Informatics, Institute of Public Health, National Defense Medical Center and University, Taipei, Taiwan

Pei-Yi Sung
Department of Nursing, Taoyuan Branch, Taipei Veterans General Hospital, Taoyuan, Taiwan

Wann-Cherng Perng
Division of Pulmonary and Critical Care Medicine, Department of Internal Medicine, Tri-Service General Hospital, National Defense Medical Center, Taipei, Taiwan

Kwua-Yun Wang
Graduate Institute of Medical Sciences, National Defense Medical Center, Department of Nursing, Taipei Veterans General Hospital, Taipei, Taiwan

Nicolas Carvalho and Gilles Chopard
Department of Clinical Psychiatry, University Hospital, Besanc,on, France
E.A. 481, Laboratory of Neurosciences, University of Franche-Comté, Besanc,on, France

Nicolas Noiret
Department of Clinical Psychiatry, University Hospital, Besanc,on, France
E.A. 3188, Laboratory of Psychology, University of Franche-Comté, Besanc,on, France

Pierre Vandel and Julie Monnin
Department of Clinical Psychiatry, University Hospital, Besanc,on, France
E.A. 481, Laboratory of Neurosciences, University of Franche-Comté, Besanc,on, France
CICIT 808 Inserm, Besanc,on University Hospital, Besanc,on, France

Eric Laurent
E.A. 3188, Laboratory of Psychology, University of Franche-Comté, Besanc,on, France
UMSR 3124/FED 4209 MSHE Ledoux, CNRS and University of Franche-Comté, Besanc,on, France

John Gounarides, Jennifer S. Cobb, Jing Zhou, Frank Cook, Xuemei Yang, Hong Yin and Erik Chang Rao
Analytical Sciences, Novartis Institutes for Biomedical Research, Cambridge, MA, United States of America

Meredith and Muneto Mogi
Global Discovery Chemistry, Novartis Institutes for Biomedical Research, Cambridge, MA, United States of America

Qian Huang and YongYao Xu
Developmental and Metabolic Pathways, Novartis Institutes for Biomedical Research, Cambridge, MA, United States of America

Karen Anderson, Andrea De Erkenez, Sha-Mei Liao, Maura Crowley, Natasha Buchanan, Stephen Poor, Yubin Qiu, Elizabeth Fassbender, Siyuan Shen, Amber Woolfenden, Amy Jensen, Rosemarie Cepeda, Bijan Etemad-Gilbertson, Shelby Giza, Bruce Jaffee and Sassan Azarian
Ophthalmology, Novartis Institutes for Biomedical Research, Cambridge, MA, United States of America

Masashige Saito
Department of Social Welfare, Nihon Fukushi University, Aichi, Japan

Katsunori Kondo
Center for Preventive Medical Science, Chiba University, Chiba, Japan

Naoki Kondo
Department of Health Economics and Epidemiology Research, The University of Tokyo, Tokyo, Japan

Aya Abe
Department of Empirical Social Security Research, National Institute of Population and Social Security Research, Tokyo, Japan

Toshiyuki Ojima
Department of Community Health and Preventive Medicine, Hamamatsu University School of Medicine, Shizuoka, Japan

Kayo Suzuki
Department of Social Studies, Aichi Gakuin University, Aichi, Japan

Xue Chen
Department of Ophthalmology, The First Affiliated Hospital of Nanjing Medical University and State Key Laboratory of Reproductive Medicine, Nanjing Medical University, Nanjing, China
Department of Ophthalmology & Visual Sciences, The Chinese University of Hong Kong, Hong Kong, China

Shi Song Rong, Li Jia Chen, Mårten E. Brelén, Chi Pui Pang, Pancy O. S. Tam and Fang Yao Tang
Department of Ophthalmology & Visual Sciences, The Chinese University of Hong Kong, Hong Kong, China

Qihua Xu
Department of Ophthalmology, The First Affiliated Hospital of Nanjing Medical University and State Key Laboratory of Reproductive Medicine, Nanjing Medical University, Nanjing, China
Department of Ophthalmology, The Affiliated Jiangyin Hospital of Southeast University Medical College, Jiangyin, China

Yuan Liu and Chen Zhao
Department of Ophthalmology, The First Affiliated Hospital of Nanjing Medical University and State Key Laboratory of Reproductive Medicine, Nanjing Medical University, Nanjing, China

Hong Gu
Department of Ophthalmology & Visual Sciences, The Chinese University of Hong Kong, Hong Kong, China
Department of Ophthalmology, Ningbo Medical Treatment Center Lihuili Hospital, Ningbo, China

Chen-Ying Hung
Cardiovascular Center, Taichung Veterans General Hospital, Taichung, Taiwan
Department of Internal Medicine, Taipei Veterans General Hospital, Hsinchu Branch, Hsinchu County, Taiwan

Kuo-Yang Wang
Cardiovascular Center, Taichung Veterans General Hospital, Taichung, Taiwan
Department of Internal Medicine, Taipei Veterans General Hospital, Hsinchu Branch, Hsinchu County, Taiwan
School of Medicine, Chung Shan Medical University, Taichung, Taiwan

Tsu-Juey Wu and Jin-Long Huang
Cardiovascular Center, Taichung Veterans General Hospital, Taichung, Taiwan
Department of Internal Medicine, Taipei Veterans General Hospital, Hsinchu Branch, Hsinchu County, Taiwan

School of Medicine, Chung Shan Medical University, Taichung, Taiwan
Department of Internal Medicine, Faculty of Medicine, Institute of Clinical Medicine, Cardiovascular Research Center, National Yang-Ming University School of Medicine, Taipei, Taiwan

Yu-Cheng Hsieh
Cardiovascular Center, Taichung Veterans General Hospital, Taichung, Taiwan
Department of Internal Medicine, Faculty of Medicine, Institute of Clinical Medicine, Cardiovascular Research Center, National Yang-Ming University School of Medicine, Taipei, Taiwan

El-Wui Loh
Kaohsiung Municipal Kai-Syuan Psychiatric Hospital, Kaohsiung, Taiwan

Ching-Heng Lin
Department of Medical Research, Taichung Veterans General Hospital, Taichung, Taiwan

Lei Feng
Department of health service management, School of Health Service Administration, Anhui medical university, Hefei, Anhui, China
Medical Department, The people's hospital of Xinjiang Uighur autonomous region, Urumqi, Xinjiang, China

Ping Li, Xihua Wang, Yanli Ben, Xiaolin Cao, Min Ling, Anshuan Gou, Yanmei Wang, Jiangqin Xiao, Ming Hou, Xiuli Wang, Bo Lin and Faxing Wang
Medical Department, The people's hospital of Xinjiang Uighur autonomous region, Urumqi, Xinjiang, China

Zhi Hu and Ying Ma
Department of health service management, School of Health Service Administration, Anhui medical university, Hefei, Anhui, China

Weiming Tang
Project-China, University of North Carolina, Guangzhou, China, Department of STI Control Guangdong Center for Skin Diseases and STI Control, Guangzhou, China

Tanmay Mahapatra and Sanchita Mahapatra
Department of Epidemiology, Fielding School of
Public Health, University of California Los
Angeles, Los Angeles, California, United States of
America

**Chris P. Verschoor, Jamie Millar, Robin Parsons,
Alina Lelic**
Department of Pathology and Molecular Medicine,
McMaster University, Hamilton, Ontario, Canada,

Jennie Johnstone
Department of Clinical Epidemiology and
Biostatistics, McMaster
University, Hamilton, Ontario, Canada,

Mark Loeb
Department of Pathology and Molecular Medicine,
McMaster University, Hamilton, Ontario, Canada,
Department of Clinical Epidemiology and
Biostatistics, McMaster
University, Hamilton, Ontario, Canada,
Department of Medicine, McMaster University,
Hamilton, Ontario, Canada,
Institute for Infectious Diseases Research, McMaster
University, Hamilton, Ontario, Canada

Jonathan L. Bramson and Dawn M. E. Bowdish
Department of Pathology and Molecular Medicine,
McMaster University, Hamilton, Ontario, Canada,
Institute for Infectious Diseases Research, McMaster
University, Hamilton, Ontario, Canada

Index

Index

www.ingramcontent.com/pod-product-compliance
Lightning Source LLC
Chambersburg PA
CBHW061253190326
41458CB00011B/3658